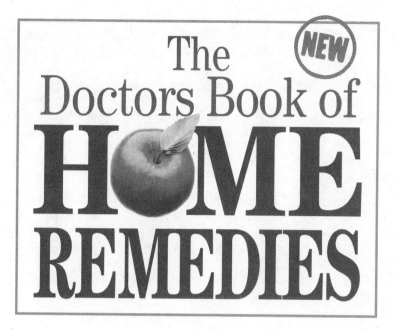

The
Doctors Book of
NEW
H⬤ME
REMEDIES

# The Doctors Book of HOME REMEDIES

NEW

Simple, Doctor-Approved

Self-Care Solutions for

146 Common Health Conditions

By the Editors of **PREVENTION**
Health Books

RODALE

Printed in the United States of America
Rodale Inc. makes every effort to use acid-free ∞, recycled paper ♻.

Interior and cover design by Christina Gaugler

**Library of Congress Cataloging-in-Publication Data**

The doctors book of home remedies : simple, doctor-approved self-care
    solutions for 146 common health conditions / by the editors of
    Prevention Health Books.
        p.      cm.
    Includes index.
    ISBN 1–57954–611–0 hardcover
    1. Medicine, Popular.    2. Self-care, Health.
RC81 .D648   2002
610–dc21                                            2002009240

**Distributed to the book trade by St. Martin's Press**

2   4   6   8   10   9   7   5   3        hardcover

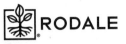

**RODALE**

WE **INSPIRE** AND **ENABLE** PEOPLE TO IMPROVE
THEIR LIVES AND THE WORLD AROUND THEM

FOR PRODUCTS & INFORMATION

**WWW.RODALESTORE**.COM
**WWW.PREVENTION**.COM

(800) 848-4735

## About *Prevention* Health Books

The editors of *Prevention* Health Books are dedicated to providing you with authoritative, trustworthy, and innovative advice for a healthy, active lifestyle. In all of our books, our goal is to keep you thoroughly informed about the latest breakthroughs in natural healing, medical research, alternative health, herbs, nutrition, fitness, and weight loss. We cut through the confusion of today's conflicting health reports to deliver clear, concise, and definitive health information that you can trust. And we explain in practical terms what each new breakthrough means to you, so you can take immediate, practical steps to improve your health and well-being.

Every recommendation in *Prevention* Health Books is based upon reliable sources, including interviews with qualified health authorities. In addition, we retain top-level health practitioners who serve on our board of advisors. *Prevention* Health Books are thoroughly fact-checked for accuracy, and we make every effort to verify recommendations, dosages, and cautions.

The advice in this book will help keep you well-informed about your personal choices in health care—to help you lead a happier, healthier, and longer life.

## Notice

# CONTENTS

# C

# D

# H

# I

# J

# K

# L

# M

# N

# O

# P

# R

# S

# INTRODUCTION

When we decided to write the original *Doctors Book of Home Remedies* back in 1990, we knew we were tapping into a broad interest. Lots of people wrote to *Prevention* magazine's "Mailbag" editor with their own home remedies for everything from dandruff to ingrown toenails. Most of the remedies made good sense, but some were, well, wacky. We needed a home remedies authority, someone who could say, "Yes, it's okay to put Krazy Glue on a paper cut," or "No, you don't want to apply kerosene to an itch—or anything else!"

And that's when we thought about doctors. They get poison ivy, heartburn, leg cramps, and hemorrhoids, just like the rest of us. And they probably hate going to the doctor just as much. What do they do?

Lucky for us, doctors are as enthusiastic as their patients when it comes to home remedies. Specialists in their fields are likely to have seen and heard everything—and to know what really works and why. We interviewed more than 500 doctors and other health care professionals and gathered more than 2,000 safe, effective self-care tips to create *The Doctors Book of Home Remedies*.

The original *Doctors Book* become an immediate success, going on to sell more than 16 million copies in the United States and around the world. It's been published in 22 languages and 31 countries. From what we've heard, there are dog-eared copies of the book sitting on bookshelves around the globe, a familiar reference whether you speak Chinese, Swedish, or Croatian.

It was those worn-out copies that got us wishing that people could have a fresh, new *Doctors Book*—one without tattered corners. So that's what we did.

Our new revision is better than ever. It offers 500 new home remedies, updated to reflect some of the latest applications in alternative, herbal, and nutritional medicine. It helps people make the best use of new over-the-counter products. And it offers the same kind of practical advice on diet, lifestyle changes, and stress reduction that you might get from a good doctor who actually has the time to address these issues during an office visit.

The new *Doctors Book* contains 40 new chapters, some covering completely new topics reflective of our times. In 1990, we weren't all that concerned with topics like burnout, hostility, or seasonal affective disorder. And we'd never even heard of road rage. But these topics do concern many people now, and we're happy to report that there really are things you can do about them without going to the doctor. Feeling angry? Try screaming in your car—windows rolled up, of course—for as long as you need to release pent-up hostility. Feeling burned out at work? Take an extra-long lunch break, and let the boss worry about things. Hey, it's what the doctor recommends!

We've added an herb/drug interaction chart that you can check for any possible safety issues that you need to know before trying a remedy. That's especially important given that herbal remedies can have just as powerful an effect as conventional medications.

And we've added three new special features: "When to Call a Doctor" offers critical advice about when it's not safe to self-treat. "Do Just 1 Thing" saves you time and energy by pointing out the remedies most likely to give you an immediate benefit. And "Cures from the Kitchen" highlights remedies using foods that you may have on hand, such as drinking a cup of well-steeped sage tea to stop menopause-related night sweats.

As much as things change, some have stayed the same. Today, more than ever, people want to handle their own health problems when it makes sense to do so. That's in part because of the realities of today's world. If you call your doctor about something minor, you'll be lucky to get a call back the same day. This book saves you the phone call. It's on call, 24 hours a day, right in your own home. Trusted, valued, and essential, the new, revised *Doctors Book of Home Remedies* is as useful today as it was in 1990.

—The Editors of *Prevention* Health Books

# The Doctors Book of HOME REMEDIES

NEW

# ACNE

## 14 Remedies for Smoother Skin

Acne is so common among teenagers—about 80 percent of young men and women develop pimples, half of them severe enough to require physician treatment—it is considered a natural rite of passage. Adolescents get acne because hormones called androgens, which increase the amount of oil the skin produces, circulate at higher levels in their blood.

Yet teenagers aren't the only ones plagued by nasty skin eruptions. Acne can also bedevil women in the midst of hormone changes triggered by menstruation, birth control pills, pregnancy, even early menopause.

"Women can have flare-ups at 25 or 35 years old and even older," says James E. Fulton Jr., M.D., Ph.D. "In fact, my mother was still breaking out when she was 62."

Acne is really a catchall term for a variety of symptoms, including pimples, whiteheads, blackheads, and skin cysts, says Peter E. Pochi, M.D. "It's a condition where the pores of the skin become clogged and you get inflamed and non-inflamed lesions."

Contrary to popular misconceptions, chocolate and dirty hair or skin do not cause acne outbreaks. Usually, it's hereditary, says Dr. Fulton.

If both of your parents had acne, three out of four of your brothers and sisters will also get it. But if your sister is pimple-free while your face is a war zone, it's because other factors can aggravate an acne outbreak, says Dr. Fulton, including stress, sun exposure, seasonal changes, and climate. Certain types of makeup, as well as oral contraceptives, can also cause breakouts.

"Working women are especially vulnerable," adds Dr. Fulton. "They're prone to lots of stress, plus they tend to wear a lot of makeup."

So here's some blemish-free advice.

**Change your makeup.** "Oil-based makeup is the problem," says Dr. Fulton. "The pigments in foundation, rouges, cleansing creams, or night moisturizers aren't the problem, and neither is the water in the products. It's just the oil. The oil is usually a derivative of fatty acids that are more potent than your own fatty acids. Use a non-oil-based makeup if you are prone to acne."

## WHEN TO CALL A DOCTOR

No doubt that a huge pimple on the end of your nose can make you feel like Rudolph. But acne can get much more serious than a simple blemish.

Acne is classified in four grades, the first being a mild bout, with a few whiteheads and blackheads. At the other end of the spectrum, grade four cases are often accompanied by severe inflammation that becomes red or purple. Consider it a flashing light to see a dermatologist.

Severe acne can result in permanent scarring if it isn't treated properly, says Peter E. Pochi, M.D. A dermatologist can offer prescription medications that will take care of severe acne very well, including topical creams, gels, or lotions with vitamin A or benzoyl peroxide to help unblock the pores and reduce bacteria.

**Read the labels.** Avoid cosmetic products that contain lanolins, isopropyl myristate, sodium lauryl sulfate, laureth-4, and D & C red dyes. Like oil, these ingredients are too rich for the skin.

**Rinse off that rouge.** "Wash your makeup off thoroughly every night," says Dr. Fulton. "Use a mild soap twice a day and make sure you rinse the soap entirely off your face. Rinsing six or seven times with fresh water should do it."

**Go for the natural look.** "Whatever makeup you use, the less you use of it, the better," says Dr. Fulton.

**Blame it on the Pill.** Dr. Fulton's research suggests that certain birth control pills, such as Ovral (norgestrel and ethinyl estradiol), Loestrin (norethindrone acetate and ethinyl estradiol), and Norinyl (norethindrone and ethinyl estradiol) can aggravate acne. If you're on the Pill and have an acne problem, discuss it with your doctor. She may be able to switch you to another pill or prescribe a different birth control method.

The makers of Ortho Tri-Cyclen (norgestimate and ethinyl estradiol) claim that theirs is the only birth control pill clinically proven to help reduce moderate acne and maintain clearer skin. These pills are sometimes used to treat acne.

Birth control pills can improve acne or make it worse—and the acne often flares up 10 days after pills are stopped.

**Leave well enough alone.** "You shouldn't squeeze pimples or whiteheads," says Dr. Pochi. "A pimple is an inflammation, and you could add to the inflammation by squeezing it. You may cause an infection." Squeezing a whitehead could break open the wall of the skin pore, allowing contents to leak out onto the skin and cause a pimple. The one exception is a pimple with a little central yellow pus head in it. "Gentle squeezing usually pops these open very nicely. Once the pus is out, the pimple will heal more quickly," he adds.

Otherwise, there isn't much you can do to a pimple to make it go away faster. "Normally a pimple will last from 1 to 4 weeks, but it will always go away," says Dr. Pochi.

**Attack blackheads.** You can also get rid of a blackhead by squeezing the skin that surrounds it. "A blackhead is a very blocked pore. The material inside the blocked pore is solid, and the surface of the pore is widened," explains Dr. Pochi. The black part of a blackhead is not dirt. In fact, dermatologists aren't really sure what it is, but whatever it is, squeezing won't result in a pimple.

**Use OTCs to knock out acne.** You can fight back an acne attack with over-the-counter products. "Use OTCs with benzoyl peroxide in them," says Dr. Fulton. "The benzoyl part pulls the peroxide into the pore and releases oxygen, which kills the bacteria that aggravates acne. It's like two drugs in one. The benzoyl also suppresses the fatty acid cells that irritate the pores." OTC acne products come in various forms, such as gels, liquids, lotions, or creams. He suggests a water-based gel, which is least likely to irritate the skin. Put it on for an hour or so in the evening, washing it off very thoroughly at bedtime, especially in the areas around the eyes and neck.

They also come in concentrations ranging from 5 to 10 percent. The percentage, however, has little to do with the product's effectiveness. "In most tests that have been conducted, the lower-strength products were as effective as the upper-strength ones," says Thomas Gossel, Ph.D., R.Ph.

"Make sure you clean your skin thoroughly before applying any over-the-counter acne medication," he adds.

**Stop the spread of acne.** Apply acne medication about ½ inch around the affected area, says Dr. Fulton, to help keep the acne from spreading. "The medication really doesn't fight the pimple you already have," he explains. "It acts more like a pimple preventive." Acne moves across the face from the nose out to the ear. You need to treat beyond the red inflammatory area.

**Give dry skin extra care.** Dry skin can be sensitive to benzoyl peroxide, so Dr. Gossel recommends that you start with a lower-strength product first, then increase the concentration slowly. "You're going to get reddening of the skin when you put it on, but that is a normal reaction," he says.

# How Hollywood Hides Blemishes

While pimples are bad enough, they're positively horrendous if you're a movie star. That teeny bump on the side of your nose? Put it on the big screen, and watch it grow to garbage can size. Even Julia Roberts' smile couldn't hide that puppy.

Ah, but when's the last time you saw Julia or Tom Hanks or any other movie star with a zit? Don't celebrities ever break out? "You bet they do," says Hollywood makeup artist Maurice Stein. "The difference is, they can't let their pimples or any other blemish show."

Stein has been a makeup artist for more than 30 years, touching up famous faces in such movies as *M*A*S*H, Funny Girl,* and the original *Planet of the Apes* films.

Guerrilla warfare is the only way to fight the pimple that always sprouts at the wrong time. So here are a few combat tips from the trenches in Hollywood. Stein says that he has used these on "some of the most expensive faces in the world."

**Go undercover.** You can totally block out the discoloration, whether it's pink, red, or purple, if you find a foundation makeup with a high pigment level, says Stein. The normal range for most foundations is 12 to 15 percent. While you can't really tell the pigment level by looking at a product, you can tell by sampling it. "Take a drop of it and rub it on your skin," suggests Stein. "If it's so solid in color that you can't see your own skin underneath it, then you know it has a high pigment level and will do well in covering your blemish."

**Try it the stars' way.** "When I cover a pimple on an entertainer's face, I use two thin layers of foundation with a layer of loose translucent powder between each layer," Stein says. This helps set each layer.

**Stay out of the sun.** Acne medications may cause adverse reactions to the sun. "Minimize exposure to sunlight, infrared heat lamps, and sunscreens until you know how you will react," cautions Dr. Gossel. For those with especially sensitive skin, a dermatologist can arrange for a skin (patch) test to check on susceptibility to topical toxicity from ultraviolet light.

**Use one treatment at a time.** Be careful not to mix treatments. If you use an OTC acne product, stop using it if you get prescription medication for your acne. "Benzoyl peroxide is a close cousin to Retin-A and other products containing vitamin A derivatives," says Dr. Gossel. Don't use both at the same time.

## PANEL OF ADVISORS

**James E. Fulton Jr., M.D., Ph.D.,** is a dermatologist and founder of the Acne Research Institute in Newport Beach, California. He is also coauthor of *Dr. Fulton's Step-by-Step Program for Clearing Acne* and codiscoverer of Retin-A (synthetic vitamin A), a prescription drug used to treat a variety of skin problems.

**Thomas Gossel, Ph.D., R.Ph.,** is a professor of pharmacology and toxicology at Ohio Northern University in Ada. He is an expert on over-the-counter products.

**Peter E. Pochi, M.D.,** is a former professor of dermatology at Boston University School of Medicine.

**Maurice Stein** is a cosmetologist and Hollywood makeup artist. He is the owner of Cinema Secrets, a full-service beauty supplier for the public and a theatrical beauty supplier for the entertainment industry in Burbank, California.

# ADDICTION
## 11 Steps to Recovery

Imagine a man who knocks back a few stiff drinks after work. Is he a "pleasure" drinker or an alcoholic? What about the woman who raids the refrigerator when she's tired or depressed, or the millions of Americans who spend hours sitting in front of the television or cruising the Internet?

Harmless diversions—or addictions?

Most people have some kind of addiction. They find something they like that makes them feel good, and they may use it again and again as a kind of coping mechanism, says Tom Horvath, Ph.D.

We tend to think of addictions in their most severe forms: the drug abuser who craves the next fix, for example, or the compulsive gambler who empties the family bank account into the slot machines. But millions of Americans have milder addictions. They crave substances or experiences that make them feel good temporarily but that often have harmful long-term consequences.

If you suspect that you have an addiction—to cigarettes, gambling, food, the Internet, or anything else—ask yourself this question: Has the behavior caused enough problems for you to consider stopping or cutting back? If the answer is yes, it's time to make a few changes to break the addiction's grip.

## WHEN TO CALL A DOCTOR

Denial is one of the hallmarks of addiction. People with drug, alcohol, or other addictions often insist that their behavior is normal, even when the destruction is all around them.

Are friends, family members, or coworkers gently suggesting that you may have a problem? Listen to them. Look at your recent behavior. Ask yourself if they're seeing something that you don't.

"Try to solve the problems on your own," advises Tom Horvath, Ph.D. "Try cutting back or quitting entirely—and get the support of the people around you. If you've made one or several attempts that don't seem to be going far or fast enough, then it's time to get professional help."

**Start by listing pros and cons.** It's difficult for most people to recognize that they have an addiction. One way to find out is to list the pros and cons of the behavior that's worrying you.

First, write down all the things that you like about the substance or activity. If you drink, for example, the list might include things such as "It helps me unwind" or "I like the feeling of euphoria."

Second, write down the benefits of quitting: "I'd be more productive if I didn't drink" or "I'd have fewer Friday night fights with my spouse."

Now, compare the lists. Does it appear that the costs of your behavior outweigh the benefits? Congratulations. You've just recognized that you have some problems—the first step toward making the necessary changes, says Dr. Horvath.

And you've done it alone. You need to decide for yourself when you're ready to make the necessary—and often difficult—changes to free yourself from addictions, he adds.

**Taper off—or stop completely.** Some people wean themselves from addictions by initially smoking 10 fewer cigarettes each day, for example, or gambling once a week instead of every night. Others find it easier to go cold turkey.

Both approaches can be effective. "With weaning, people are generally less scared, so they're more motivated," says Dr. Horvath. Going cold turkey is harder initially, but it makes the whole process go more quickly. "You pay more up front, but it's easier to maintain because there is a shorter transition period," he explains.

**Distance yourself from cravings.** Anyone who curtails addictive substances or behaviors will go through a withdrawal period. The cravings—for one more cigarette, one more drink, one more day at the track—can be almost unbearably intense.

"I advise people to keep their cravings at a distance," says Dr. Horvath. In other words, acknowledge how you're feeling. Admit to yourself how uncomfortable you are. But don't give in. Distract yourself. Call a friend. Walk around the block. Wash the dishes. Do whatever it takes to take your mind off the craving.

"Just because you have an itch doesn't mean you have to scratch," he adds. Be strong. Individual cravings will disappear in minutes or even seconds, and the entire experience of cravings will often evaporate in a month or two.

**Stay busy.** "A lot of people who make the commitment to quit doing something find themselves sitting at home all the time," says Peter A. DeMaria Jr., M.D. If you don't keep busy—with exercise, hobbies, or other activities that keep your mind and body active—you'll find yourself focusing more and more on the cravings.

"Exercise can be especially helpful because it's a way of reconnecting to things that are healthy," Dr. DeMaria adds.

**Get your mind racing.** One way to distract yourself from cravings is to think about something—anything—at high speed. Count ceiling tiles as quickly as you can. Try reading book titles backward. Do repetitious math problems in your head—such as subtracting 7 from 1,000, 7 from 993, and so on.

"When you do these sorts of things quickly, they take up your entire mind, which will help you get past the craving," says Dr. Horvath.

**Avoid behavior triggers.** If you've just quit smoking, the last thing you need is an evening at a smoke-filled party. If you've been obsessed with the Internet, online Christmas shopping is probably not a good idea.

Alcoholics Anonymous (AA) and other self-help programs teach members to avoid people, places, or things that are associated with their addictions. "Some people will alter their walking or driving routes in order to avoid parts of the city where they used to buy drugs or to avoid people they used to hang out with," says Dr. DeMaria. "With smoking, talking on the phone may be a trigger. You have to recognize what your triggers are and figure out how to respond when you're confronted."

As time goes by, you'll find that addiction triggers will lose most or all of their pull. "Even AA members can go to a bar once in a while when they've achieved stable sobriety," Dr. Horvath explains.

**Substitute good behaviors for bad ones.** Avoidance is helpful in the early stages of fighting addictions, but no one can avoid all sources of temptation indefinitely. You can, however, develop substitute habits. When you feel an urge for a cigarette, for example, chew gum. When the television beckons, read a magazine. After a while, your new habits will take the place of the old ones.

**Make it harder to indulge.** Addictions are grounded in habits, which means people sometimes indulge without really thinking about what they're doing.

Smokers, for example, may find themselves three puffs into a cigarette that they don't remember lighting. People with eating problems may raid the refrigerator without being consciously aware that they left the living room.

One way to break unconscious habits is to make them harder to practice. A smoker, for example, might put a pack of cigarettes inside a box and wrap the whole thing with rubber bands. You still may decide to smoke, but at least you won't be doing it automatically.

The same approach works with other addictions. Turn off the computer when you sign off the Internet—and maybe crawl under the desk to pull the plug. Clear the house of alcohol, pornography, or other "forbidden" things. Putting obstacles between you and your addiction will force you to think about what you're doing, which in turn will make the addiction easier to overcome, says Dr. Horvath.

### Find new sources of satisfaction.

It's not enough merely to give up unhealthy behaviors. If you're going to be successful, you need to replace addictions with something positive.

"In order to develop new habits, you need to gradually change the sources of satisfaction in your life," says Dr. Horvath. This could be as simple as creating healthier lifestyle habits. Instead of spending the night in front of the television, for example, go to bed early and get more rest. You might focus more of your energy on eating healthful foods, exercising regularly, or even donating several hours a week to a charity.

### Do just 1 thing

Join a group. There are thousands of self-help groups for overcoming every sort of addiction—to alcohol, drugs, sex, overeating, and the Internet, to name just a few.

Self-help groups are free, they don't require insurance, and they can be very effective, either by themselves or in combination with therapy, says Peter A. DeMaria Jr., M.D.

At self-help groups, you spend time with people in various stages of recovery, says Dr. DeMaria. "They've been through it all before, and they can act as role models and mentors."

Every support group has a different mix of messages and personalities. If you find yourself in a gathering that doesn't feel right, don't give up on the idea. "I usually advise people to go to at least six different meetings in order to find one they like," he says.

**Learn from setbacks.** Nearly everyone who struggles with addictions slips on occasion. Expect it, says Dr. Horvath. Don't get discouraged, and don't give up.

"When slips happen, ask yourself why they happened. Turn them into a learning situation," says Dr. Horvath. "Persistence is the most important virtue.

Everyone who keeps going is going to be successful. Eventually, you run out of ways to make mistakes."

## PANEL OF ADVISORS

**Peter A. DeMaria Jr., M.D.,** is an associate professor of psychiatry and human behavior in the division of substance abuse programs at Jefferson Medical College of Thomas Jefferson University in Philadelphia.

**Tom Horvath, Ph.D.,** is president of Practical Recovery Services, an addiction treatment center in La Jolla, California, and president of SMART Recovery, an abstinence-oriented support group for those with addictive behaviors.

# AGE SPOTS
## 9 Ways to Out the Spots

It sounds like something Jerry, George, and Elaine might quibble about in the diner on *Seinfeld*: Are age spots really a by-product of old age? And if they aren't, shouldn't they have their name changed?

Actually, the term *age spots* is a misnomer. These flat, rounded, brown areas that commonly appear on the backs of hands as well as on necks, faces, and shoulders are actually large, sun-induced freckles with no relation to age, says Audrey Kunin, M.D.

"The reason they're called age spots is that they usually occur because of sun exposure over time—which means that for a lot of people they won't show up on their skin until they get a little older," she says.

While age spots are common in older people, someone who's had significant sun exposure can get them as early as their late twenties or thirties. Sunlight contains ultraviolet (UV) rays that cause suntans and sunburns. As time goes by, this sun damage causes more pigment than normal to be deposited in the skin. This eventually leads to these flat, brown skin freckles known as age spots, liver spots, or sun spots.

No matter what they're called, they're unsightly. And, if they change in size, they may actually be skin cancers, which is why it's always a good idea to have a dermatologist examine your skin at least once a year.

But, assuming they are indeed age spots, here are some tips on concealing or fading them (as well as preventing more).

## WHEN TO CALL A DOCTOR

If your age spots have a mind of their own and don't respond to home remedies or if you have an age spot that bleeds, itches, tingles, or changes in size or color, it's time to see your doctor. Some skin cancers, such as melanoma, can look like age spots.

If your age spots are simply stubborn, then many doctors recommend a prescription-strength fade cream with 4 percent hydroquinone called Lustra as the first line of action. "Rub it on twice per day for 21 to 28 days, and you should see marked improvement," says C. Ralph Daniel III, M.D.

For a stronger, quicker bleaching effect, some doctors prescribe vitamin A creams such as Retin-A and Renova along with prescription-strength hydroquinone, Dr. Kunin says.

And if creams fail to do the trick, your doctor has several treatment options at his disposal to make age spots disappear, says Dr. Daniel. For instance, your doctor can freeze them with liquid nitrogen. After 4 to 6 days, the spots peel off. "This is a highly effective procedure," he says.

A second treatment procedure is a chemical peel—done with trichloroacetic acid (TCA) or glycolic acid. These treatments can be quite effective for all body areas but may cause scarring and whitening of the skin if not done properly, says Mitchel Goldman, M.D. The upper layer of affected skin takes 2 to 3 days to peel from your face or 5 to 7 days from your arms and chest.

A third and much more expensive procedure (average cost ranges between $2,000 and $6,000, depending on how large an area is treated) is laser resurfacing. During this procedure, the doctor uses pulses of laser light to fade the spots. The laser resurfacing procedure can take a half-hour to an hour to perform and 2 to 6 weeks to heal, says Dr. Goldman.

**Lighten up.** If your age spots aren't too big or too dark, over-the-counter bleaching agents could help fade them, Dr. Kunin says. Look for over-the-counter products like Porcelana or Palmer's Skin Success Cream, which contain 2 percent hydroquinone, the best-known active ingredient used in many types of bleaching agents. Hydroquinone lightens age spots until they become less noticeable or even disappear. It works best with a glycolic acid moisturizer, like Neutrogena Pore Refining Cream or Alpha Hydrox Enhanced Crème, which smooths out the skin.

Apply the bleaching agent twice a day to your sun spots, carefully following the manufacturer's directions. Dab the cream directly onto the age spots with a cotton swab so that you don't bleach the pigment in unaffected areas.

"Be patient," says Dr. Kunin. "You won't see results overnight. These lightening agents often take 6 to 12 months to do the job." Stop the treatment when the age spots disappear, or the affected area may become lighter than your normal skin tone.

**Keep the rays away.** Because these brown blotches are caused by the sun's UV rays, limiting your exposure to the sun is the first important step in the battle against age spots. That means you should use a quality sunscreen each and every time you go outdoors for an extended period of time, says C. Ralph Daniel III, M.D.

Even if you already have age spots, sunscreen keeps existing ones from darkening and helps prevent more from popping up, says Dr. Kunin.

Buy a broad-spectrum sunblock (which protects you from both the UVA and UVB rays of the sun) with a sun protection factor (SPF) of at least 15. Apply it to exposed skin 10 to 15 minutes before you go outside, says Dr. Daniel. Tests show that SPF 15 sunblock protects the skin against about 93 percent of the sun's UV rays while it is on the patient, he adds.

If you plan to spend the better part of the day on the golf course, tennis court, or ski slope, use a broad-spectrum sunscreen with an SPF of 30, says Dr. Kunin. Ditto if you spend a lot of time on a boat or at the beach, because the sun reflects off the water. And since perspiration and water can wash off your sunscreen, reapply it periodically.

**Use your head.** Whether you're heading to the beach or spending extended time in the midday sun, wear a hat with a 4-inch-wide brim to keep the sun off your face and neck, says Dr. Kunin.

Baseball caps, assuming they're worn with the bill in front, don't protect your ears, the back of your neck, or even most of your face from full-bore sun, says Dr. Kunin. Straw hats don't usually offer much protection either. If the hats are unlined and loosely woven, the sun shines directly through them.

"Choose a hat with an extra-long bill and sun-protective cloth inside," says Dr. Kunin. "It will give you the extra protection that helps limit your chances of developing age spots."

**Protect your lips.** The lips are an area that most people don't think about guarding from the sun. But age spots can pop up on your lips, too. Many women think that their lipstick

## Cures from the Kitchen

Cut a few lemon slices and place them directly on your age spots for 10 to 15 minutes once a day, suggests Audrey Kunin, M.D. "The acid in the fresh lemon juice helps lighten the age spots in some cases." It won't happen overnight, though. Dr. Kunin says that you'll notice a difference in 6 to 12 weeks. Watch carefully. Overuse may cause the upper layer of skin to peel away.

**What the Doctor Does ...** There is a wart-remover product called Wart Stick that contains 40 percent salicylic acid, which is also the beta hydroxy acid that doctors use to treat wrinkles. "Because the stick allows you to concentrate on one specific spot or area to treat, I got the idea to use the Wart Stick for people who have brown spots, dark circles, and roughened areas of the skin," explains Nelson Lee Novick, M.D. "It's convenient, it doesn't run, and it works." He recommends applying it at bedtime. It may take 8 to 12 months to see results. Wart Stick is available at some drugstores, at mass merchandisers, and online.

will protect them. The sun, however, can penetrate many lighter shades, and lipstick typically wears off throughout the day, leaving the lips naked and unprotected.

Apply either a lip balm or lipstick with an SPF of 15 to 30 before you head outside. Dr. Kunin recommends English Ideas brand lip balm, available online and at Dillard's or Sephora stores. If you still want to wear your favorite non-SPF lipstick, apply the lipstick over a layer of the protective balm.

**Shun the sun.** "Avoid the sun as much as possible during peak hours (10:00 A.M. to 4:00 P.M. during spring, summer, and fall or 10:00 A.M. to 2:00 P.M. during winter), when the ultraviolet radiation is the strongest," says Dr. Kunin. If you have outdoor chores like gardening to do, perform them early in the morning or in the evening. And remember that sunblock is needed even during winter and on cloudy days.

**Act somewhat shady.** Since excessive sun exposure causes age spots, periodically retreat to a shady spot on sunny days. At the beach or a backyard barbecue, park yourself under a big umbrella. Also, whenever you're in the sun, wear tightly woven, light-colored clothing if it's not too hot out. It helps keep UV rays from penetrating your skin. "It sounds simple, but protecting yourself with sunblock or staying out of the sun are the two best ways to keep new age spots from cropping up on your skin," says Dr. Kunin.

**Launch a cover-up.** If the other at-home remedies don't do the trick and you don't want to spend the money on a dermatologist-administered chemical peel or a laser resurfacing treatment, you can always reach into your cosmetics bag. "Brown age spots can be concealed by applying a cream-based or water-based concealer," says Dr. Kunin. Pick a lighter version of your skin tone to best hide age spots.

# ALLERGIES
## 16 Ways to Alleviate the Symptoms

Allergies are the result of an immune system run amok. They develop when your immune system overreacts to a normally harmless substance, such as pollen, cat dander, or dust. About one in five Americans are plagued by sneezing, coughing, wheezing, chest tightness, difficulty breathing, itchy eyes, hives, and rashes, which are all hallmarks of allergy symptoms.

Allergies come in almost infinite variety. But most triggers, called allergens, stimulate the immune system through four basic routes: ingestion (eating peanuts or shrimp, for example), injection (such as getting a penicillin shot), absorption through the skin (touching poison ivy), and inhalation (breathing in cat dander).

For food and drug allergies, avoidance is the only option. To prevent or treat contact allergies caused by poison plants, see Poison Plant Rashes on page 468. But when you want relief from inhalant allergies, the answer is probably right under your own nose, since house dust, pollen, pet dander, and mold are the most common triggers.

"You find a bit of everything in house dust," says Thomas Platts-Mills, M.D. "Different people are allergic to different things—pieces of cockroach are pretty potent, actually—but the single biggest cause of problems is the dust mite."

The dust mite is an almost microscopic relative of ticks and spiders. But living mites are not the problem. People react, instead, to the fecal material that mites expel on carpets, bedding, and upholstered furniture. The bodies of dead mites also trigger allergies.

When scientists visited 831 residents across the United States in the late 1990s to conduct the first national allergy survey, they discovered that almost one in four houses harbor dust mites. Only the western United States was relatively spared. Cockroach allergens were found in homes throughout America, especially in homes where scientists also found food debris.

The other common airborne allergens are equally hard to escape. Pollen fills the air in almost every region with seasonal regularity. Mold grows wherever it's dark and humid, under carpets, in dank basements, and in leaky garages and storage sheds. And with 68 million dogs and 73 million cats in America, it's not easy to escape pet dander. If you're sensitive to any of these allergens—most likely because you've inherited the tendency—contact with them will trigger a sneezing, wheezing, itchy reaction.

Fortunately, there's much you can do to minimize the misery. The following doctor-tested and recommended tips will plant you firmly on the path to easy breathing and dry eyes.

**Treat your symptoms.** A certain amount of exposure to whatever bothers you is unavoidable. Allergy shots, available from your doctor, are a great way to make sure that your forays into the outside world are pleasant instead of painful. But you don't have to rely on them. Over-the-counter antihistamines, available from your local druggist, work wonders on drippy noses and red, itchy eyes.

"For the most part, they do a good job," says Richard Podell, M.D. "But if you have an allergy that persists for more than 5 to 7 days, you should probably see your doctor."

**Air-condition your car.** If walking outside makes you start wheezing and sneezing, imagine what tearing through all those pollen clouds at 55 miles per

## Do just 1 thing

Air-condition your house. This is probably the single most important thing that you can do to alleviate pollen problems, and it can help with two other chief inhalants: mold and dust mites.

"The basic idea is to create an oasis of sorts," says Richard Podell, M.D. "You want your home to be a place of sanctuary, a place you can count on to provide escape."

Air-conditioning units help in two ways. They keep humidity low, which discourages mites and mold, and they can filter the air in the course of cooling it—if you also install an air cleaner. But it's the sealing of the house that provides the real benefit, Dr. Podell says. If you have the windows open, the inside of the house is essentially the same environment as the outside of the house—full of pollen.

## WHEN TO CALL A DOCTOR

If you have a known allergy, notice any of the following symptoms, and have never experienced them before during an allergy attack, you should see your doctor.

- Welts that spring up in response to exposure to an allergen, also known as hives. They may indicate the onset of anaphylactic shock, an allergic reaction severe enough to kill. Anaphylactic shock is most commonly associated with bee or fire ant stings, but it can occur in response to other allergens, too. Seek medical attention promptly.
- Wheezing—a whistling sound when you breathe.
- Asthma—congestion of the chest severe enough to make breathing difficult, often accompanied by wheezing.
- An allergy attack that doesn't respond to over-the-counter medications within a week.

hour is going to do. Be sensible and remember to use the air conditioner in your car. Of course, it's not the same as letting the wind rip through your hair, but, remember, you're doing it for your health.

**Install an air filter.** Keeping the air clean in your home can bring relief from pollen, mold, and pet dander. HEPA (high-energy particulate-arresting) filters are most efficient. When you use an air filter in your room, remember to keep the door closed so that the machine won't get overburdened with too much air to clean.

Air filters aren't much use against dust mites, however. The mites are so heavy that they hang in the air only for a few minutes and aren't floating around for the filter to draw them in.

**Buy a dehumidifier.** Keeping the air in your home dry will help put a stop to dust mite problems.

Dust mites don't do very well in humidity below about 45 percent, Dr. Platts-Mills says. "Generally, the drier, the better."

Remember to empty the unit's water often and clean it regularly, according to the manufacturer's instructions, so that it doesn't become a haven for mold. If your dehumidifier creates a problem for a child or someone else sensitive to dry air, try putting a small room humidifier close to his bed.

**Keep it clean.** People with allergies fare better when dust and grime are kept to a minimum. Try not to use aerosol sprays or products containing harsh chemicals or odors that may irritate your airways. But your home will need

## How the Home Became a Dust Mite Haven

In the 1940s, American home-owners welcomed the vacuum cleaner with enthusiasm. Before long, no homemaker could live without one.

But the same technology that makes our lives easier today has indirectly contributed heavily to one common medical problem: allergies to dust mites.

"The vacuum cleaner made carpeting more attractive than throw rugs," says David Lang, M.D. With central heating, homes tended to stay warm year-round. Add very tight, well-insulated homes and cold-water washes to the package (courtesy of the energy crisis), and you end up with a perfect environment for dust mites.

more than a dusting with a dry cloth, which just propels allergens into the air. Instead, wipe down hard surfaces and floors with a slightly damp cloth. In humid areas, use a bleach solution.

Bleach kills mold, and, unlike some other exotic (and potentially dangerous) chemicals, you can get it at the grocery store. Wipe down surfaces in your bathroom as needed. The label on Clorox bleach suggests that you clean floors, vinyl, tile, and your kitchen sink with a solution of ¾ cup of Clorox bleach per gallon of water. Let it stand for 5 minutes and then rinse. Use a regular fungicide for tough locations, like the basement. Of course, don't use it on fabrics, or they'll get bleached.

If you're allergic to house dust, pet dander, or another common household allergen, get someone else to take care of cleaning that carpet, such as a teenager or a professional cleaning service. The cost of hiring a helper is a small price to pay to avoid an allergic reaction.

**Isolate your pets.** The furry friends that occupy America's homes cause a staggering number of allergy exacerbations every year. Cat dander usually causes the most problems, but dogs, birds, rabbits, horses, and other pets with hair or fur also cause allergies in those who are susceptible. If you can't bear to part with your pet, make your bedroom a haven, sealed off from the rest of the house and absolutely forbidden territory for critters.

"One walk a week through a room is all it takes for a pet to keep a dander allergy going," Dr. Podell says.

**Wear a face mask.** Use one when doing anything that's likely to expose you to an allergen that you know will cause you problems. A simple chore like vacuuming can throw huge quantities of dust and whatever else is in your home into the air, where it will hang for several minutes, says David Lang, M.D. Similarly, gardening can expose you to huge volumes of pollen. A small mask that covers your nose and mouth, known professionally as a dust and mist respirator, can keep the allergen from reaching your lungs. The 3M Company makes an inexpensive version that comes highly recommended and can be found in most hardware stores.

**Enforce a no-smoking policy.** Tobacco smoke is a significant irritant for the smoker and anyone else breathing nearby. Smoke can make allergies worse. You'll breathe easier if you keep your home, office, and car smoke-free zones.

**Make your bed a mite-free zone.** Encase your pillows, mattress, and box spring in allergen-proof covers. These covers, sold by allergy-supply companies such as American Allergy Supply, National Allergy Supply, Allergy Control Products, and Stopallergy.com, provide a barrier between you and any allergens that may be housed inside them. Look for a fabric weave tight enough to keep out dust mite allergens (10 microns wide).

**Choose the hot cycle on laundry day.** Linens should be washed in water that is at least 130°F to rid them of dust mites and their wastes. To test your water temperature, stop the washer once it's filled and dip a meat thermometer into the water. If you're worried about scalding people by setting your water heater that high, consider taking your bedding to a professional laundry service where you're assured that the bedding will be washed at a sufficiently high temperature.

**Throw out your carpets.** Carpets may look nice, but they make an almost perfect home for dust mites and mold. Plus, tightly woven carpets very effectively attract and hold pollen and pet dander. Even steam cleaning may not help.
"It's not hot enough to kill the mites," says Dr. Platts-Mills. All steam cleaning really does is make it warmer and wetter underneath—an ideal climate for both mites and mold.

**Buy throw rugs.** Replace your carpets with throw rugs, and you'll achieve two major benefits. First, you'll eliminate your home's biggest collector of dust, pollen, pet dander, and mold. Second, you'll make keeping your home allergen-free much easier. Rugs *can* be washed at temperatures hot enough to kill dust mites. Also, the floors underneath—courtesy of a rug's loose weave—stay cooler and drier, conditions distinctly hostile to mold and mites.
"Mites can't survive on a dry, polished floor," Dr. Platts-Mills says. "That kind of floor dries in seconds versus days for a steam-cleaned carpet."

**Buy synthetic pillows.** Dust mites like synthetic (Hollofil or Dacron) pillows just as much as those made from down and foam, but synthetic pillows have one major advantage: You can wash them in hot water.

**Minimize clutter.** Dried flowers, books, stuffed animals, and other homey touches collect dust and allergens. Try to keep knickknacks in closets or drawers or rid your home of them entirely.

**Make at least one room a sanctuary.** If you can't afford central air and don't want to rip the wall-to-wall carpeting out of every room in your house, there's still hope. Make just *one* room a sanctuary.

"Most people spend the largest part of their time at home in the bedroom," Dr. Platts-Mills says. Making just that one room an allergen-free area can do a great deal to alleviate the allergy.

Do it by air-conditioning the room in summer, sealing it from the rest of the house (by keeping the door closed), replacing carpets with throw rugs, encasing linens in allergen-proof cases, and keeping it dust-free.

## PANEL OF ADVISORS

**David Lang, M.D.,** is the section chief of allergy and immunology at Thomas Jefferson University in Philadelphia.

**Thomas Platts-Mills, M.D.,** is a professor of medicine and head of the division of allergy and immunology at the University of Virginia Medical Center in Charlottesville.

**Richard Podell, M.D.,** is an associate clinical professor in the department of family medicine at the University of Medicine and Dentistry of New Jersey–Robert Wood Johnson Medical School in Piscataway.

# ANAL FISSURES AND ITCHING
## 14 Soothing Solutions

Even though the symptoms are comparable—pain, bleeding, and itching—the similarities between anal fissures and hemorrhoids are largely superficial. Hemorrhoids are generally swollen veins. In contrast, fissures are ulcers, or breaks in the skin, which just happen to occur in the same general area.

Fissures are very much like those painful tears that sometimes develop in the corners of your mouth, says J. Byron Gathright Jr., M.D. Both the oral and anal variety occur where skin meets delicate mucous membrane. In the anus, a common cause of such tears is the passing of a large, hard stool, he says.

New research points to anatomical problems that can contribute to chronic anal fissures, as opposed to isolated problems with the painful lesions. Increased pressure in the internal anal sphincter muscle and reduced bloodflow to the area where fissures occur may make you more prone to chronic problems.

If you have fissures, you know these little sores can make your life—at least your sitting life—miserable. Take comfort in the fact that about 60 percent of anal fissures heal within a few weeks. In severe, chronic cases, surgery may be required, but it carries considerable risks, including the possibility of fecal incontinence if the anal sphincter is injured. Fortunately, a number of nonsurgical remedies exist to alleviate the pain and to prevent fissures from recurring. Here's what our experts suggest.

**Ban hard stools with fiber and fluid.** The anal opening was never meant to accommodate large, hard stools. Generally a by-product of a Western diet lacking in fiber, rock-hard stools tug and tear at the anal canal, which can result in anal fissures as well as hemorrhoids.

The solution? Adapt yourself to a diet high in fiber and fluids that produce soft bowel movements. Eating more fruit, vegetables, and whole grains and drinking six to eight glasses of water a day are the best remedies and preventive measures you can use for anal fissures, says Dr. Gathright. Once your stool is soft and pliable, your anal fissures should begin to heal on their own.

## WHEN TO CALL A DOCTOR

Fissures generally don't require special medical attention, unless they persist.

"The real caution with fissures is not to put them off forever—an ulcer that doesn't heal may be a cancer," says Lewis R. Townsend, M.D.

"If you have fissures that don't heal within 4 to 8 weeks, get them evaluated," says Dr. Townsend. "A sore that will not heal is one of the seven classic warning signs of cancer."

In addition, if you notice a mucous discharge from your anus, have it checked out by a doctor. "Abscesses can be very serious in that area," says John O. Lawder, M.D.

**Try the petroleum solution.** Eating more fiber will soften your stool, but you can also protect your anal canal by lubricating it before each bowel movement. A dab of petroleum jelly inserted about ½ inch into the rectum may help the stool pass without causing any further damage, says Edmund Leff, M.D.

**Buff yourself with talcum.** Following each shower or bowel movement, brush yourself with baby powder. This helps keep the area dry, which can help to reduce friction throughout the day, says Marvin Schuster, M.D.

**Avoid diarrhea.** It may seem odd, but not only can hard, constipated stools worsen anal fissures—so can diarrhea. Watery stools can soften the tissues around them, and they also contain acid that can burn the raw anal area and give you a form of "diaper rash" to add additional misery to your condition, says Dr. Schuster.

**Don't scratch.** Anal fissures may be itchy as well as painful, but using sharp fingernails on your tender anus can tear at the already sore tissue, says John O. Lawder, M.D.

**Shed those excess pounds.** The more weight you carry, the more likely you are to sweat. Perspiration in your anal area only slows your fissures' healing, says Dr. Lawder.

**Minimize swelling with hydrocortisone.** Nonprescription topical creams containing hydrocortisone can help reduce the inflammation that often comes with anal fissures, says Dr. Gathright.

**Try a vitamin solution.** Nonprescription ointments containing vitamins A and D may be particularly helpful for soothing pain and helping fissures heal, says Dr. Schuster.

**Soak in a hot tub.** Whether you fill your bathtub with hot water or slip into an outdoor hot tub, warm water helps relax the muscles of the anal sphincter and reduce much of the discomfort of fissures, says Dr. Leff.

**Steer clear of certain foods.** While no food causes fissures, some foods may provide excess irritation and discomfort to the anal canal as they pass through the bowels. Beware of spicy and pickled foods, says Dr. Schuster.

**Buy yourself a special pillow.** Alleviate the pain associated with sitting on a fissure by picking up a doughnut-shaped or liquid-filled pillow at a drugstore or medical supply store, says Dr. Lawder.

**Wipe gently.** Rough toilet paper and overzealous wiping slows healing of your fissures. Use only white, unscented, top-quality toilet paper. Perfumes and colorings can provide irritation to the already irritated area, says Dr. Lawder. You can soften toilet paper by moistening it under the faucet before wiping.

**Substitute facial tissue.** The very best toilet paper isn't a toilet paper at all. Facial tissues coated with moisturizing lotion offer the least amount of friction to your fissure-plagued bottom, says Dr. Lawder.

**Try liquid toilet tissue.** A company in Seaford, New York, has developed an alternative to irritating toilet tissue.

ClenZone, from Hepp Industries, diverts water from your bathroom faucet to underneath your toilet seat in a kind of portable bidet. A narrow stream of water, aimed right where you need it most, does all your "wiping" for you. There's no need for toilet paper, except for one or two sheets to pat yourself dry.

"This is a neat little appliance that offers a real nice way to get clean after a bowel movement," says John A. Flatley, M.D., who says he uses a ClenZone in his own home. He says that this product, intended for both fissures and hemorrhoids, is not a cure, but it does offer a gentle, soothing way of cleaning. "I'd suggest it for anybody," he says.

The ClenZone costs from $25 to $70 and is available through Hepp Industries, Inc., 687 Kildare Crescent, Seaford, NY 11783.

## PANEL OF ADVISORS

**John A. Flatley, M.D.,** is a colon-rectal surgeon in Kansas City, Missouri, where he also served as a clinical instructor of surgery at the University of Missouri–Kansas City School of Medicine.

**J. Byron Gathright Jr., M.D.,** is chairman emeritus of the department of colon and rectal surgery at the Ochsner Clinic Foundation and clinical professor of surgery at Tulane University, both in New Orleans. He is also past president of the American Society of Colon and Rectal Surgeons, and Secretary General of the International Society of University Colon and Rectal Surgeons.

**John O. Lawder, M.D.,** is a family practitioner specializing in nutrition and preventive medicine in Torrance, California.

**Edmund Leff, M.D.,** is a colon and rectal surgeon in Phoenix and Scottsdale, Arizona.

**Marvin Schuster, M.D.,** is director emeritus of the Marvin M. Schuster Center for Digestive and Motility Disorders at the Hopkins Bayview Medical Center, and professor emeritus of medicine and psychiatry at Johns Hopkins University School of Medicine, both in Baltimore.

**Lewis R. Townsend, M.D.,** is a clinical instructor of obstetrics and gynecology at Georgetown University Hospital and former director of the physicians' group at Columbia Hospital for Women Medical Center, both in Washington, D.C.

# ANGINA
## 12 Long-Life Strategies to Protect the Heart

More than a few people have confused the symptoms of angina with those of a heart attack. Angina isn't quite that serious, but it's close. Think of it as a heart *warning*.

Angina (the full name is angina pectoris) occurs when the heart gets insufficient blood and oxygen, which may result in temporary nausea, dizziness, or a burning or squeezing pain in the chest. Angina itself isn't a disease. It's a symptom of underlying problems, usually coronary artery disease.

"When you have chronic angina, you're at a much higher risk of having a sudden 'cardiac event,' such as a heart attack or sudden cardiac arrest," says David M. Capuzzi, M.D., Ph.D. "Unfortunately, most people who experience acute cardiac events do not have prior angina to warn them."

Anything that increases the heart's demand for oxygen, such as exercise or emotional stress, can trigger bouts of angina. The attacks normally last less than 5 minutes and are unlikely to cause permanent damage to the heart. The underlying problems, however, can be life-threatening.

The discomfort of angina can be relieved with nitroglycerine, beta-blockers, or other medications that dilate arteries or reduce the heart's demand for oxygen. In addition, it's essential to make some lifestyle changes to reduce attacks and prevent the problem from getting worse.

**Keep cholesterol under control.** Along with other fatty substances in the blood, cholesterol slowly accumulates on the linings of arteries and restricts

## WHEN TO CALL A DOCTOR

Most people with angina have a form called chronic stable angina. This means that it occurs in predictable ways when they're active—during exercise, for example, or at times of emotional stress—with the pain lasting 5 minutes or less. Most chronic stable angina can easily be managed with medications in combination with lifestyle changes.

Unstable angina, on the other hand, is much more serious. The discomfort can occur out of the blue, even when you're resting, and the pain may last 20 minutes or more.

"If there's any change in your usual pattern of angina—if symptoms such as pain or shortness of breath get more intense or insistent—get to an emergency room right away," says David M. Capuzzi, M.D., Ph.D.

"Before your trip to the ER, chew one or two aspirin tablets. Aspirin thins the blood and can help dissolve blood clots that may be blocking circulation to the heart. It's important for people with angina or other evidence of coronary disease to have chewable aspirin always available," says Dr. Capuzzi.

bloodflow to the heart. If you're having episodes of angina, it probably means fatty buildups have reached dangerous levels, says Howard Weitz, M.D.

Keep your total cholesterol below 200. In addition, levels of low-density lipoproteins (LDL, the "bad" cholesterol) should ideally be below 100. Apart from the use of medications, reducing the amount of saturated fat in your diet is one of the most effective ways to control cholesterol.

Saturated fat is mainly found in meats, rich desserts, and snack foods. If you have high cholesterol, limit red meat to no more than twice a week and avoid snack foods made with butter or other fats, says Kristine Napier, R.D.

**Increase the fiber in your diet.** Found in whole grains, legumes, fruits, and other plant foods, fiber helps prevent cholesterol from passing through the intestinal wall into the bloodstream. High-fiber foods are also filling, which means you'll naturally eat smaller amounts of other, fattier foods, Napier says.

**Eat vegetarian.** A meat-free diet isn't for everyone, but it's an ideal way for those with angina to partially control the underlying coronary artery disease. Not only is a vegetarian diet low in fat, it provides a bounty of antioxidants—chemical compounds that help prevent cholesterol from sticking to artery walls.

"Diet alone can lower cholesterol up to 20 percent," says Dr. Weitz. "At the same time, it decreases your risk of heart attack as much as 25 percent if you can lower LDL levels to 100 or less, which makes arterial plaques more stable and less likely to rupture and form clots. Patients frequently require cholesterol-lowering medication to achieve this goal, however."

**Exercise often.** "Exercise is a major lifestyle component to prevent coronary disease, although we usually make sure people also take the appropriate medication," says Dr. Weitz. Strive to exercise 20 to 30 minutes for 6 to 7 days a week.

Obviously, talk to your doctor before starting an exercise plan if you experience angina. You'll be advised to gradually build up your fitness—by starting with short walks or swims, for example, and increasing the exertion over a period of weeks or months.

"We worry about the weekend warrior who tries to get all of his exercise at once," Dr. Weitz notes.

**Exercise later in the day.** Morning can be a risky time for people with angina because fight-or-flight hormones, such as cortisol and norepinephrine, rise overnight and peak in the morning, says Dr. Capuzzi. The levels stay elevated until about noon, and intensive morning exercise is probably not a good idea for most patients with angina.

"Don't sprint in the morning or do any heavy lifting or other stressful exercises," Dr. Capuzzi advises. "Ease into the morning and follow your doctor's advice."

**Eat lightly.** Large meals are a common angina trigger because blood diverted to the intestine during digestion is then not available to the heart, Dr. Weitz explains. Many people can avoid discomfort by eating smaller meals five or six times a day, rather than two or three large meals.

**Stay at a healthful weight.** Those extra pounds that tend to accumulate over the years put an incredible load on the heart. For one, the heart has to work harder to supply blood to all that extra body tissue. Additionally, being overweight can result in elevated levels of cholesterol, which makes it harder for blood to circulate.

**Stay away from smoke.** Whether you smoke yourself or are exposed to secondhand smoke on a regular basis, now's the time to clear the air. Smoking even one cigarette temporarily reduces your heart's supply of oxygen, which can result in painful angina.

**Take aspirin.** If your stomach can handle it, experts generally agree that taking one 325-milligram aspirin daily is good protection. It won't stop the pain of angina, but it does reduce the risk of blood clots that can lead to heart attacks. In fact, taking an aspirin each day can reduce the risk of coronary heart disease by 28 percent.

**Supplement with vitamin E.** An antioxidant nutrient, vitamin E helps prevent a process called oxidation, in which unstable oxygen molecules in the blood damage cholesterol, making it more likely to stick to arteries and reduce bloodflow to the heart. "Vitamin E is particularly helpful for smokers or those with diabetes, who have high oxidative stress," says Dr. Capuzzi. He recommends taking 400 IU of vitamin E daily.

**Get extra vitamin C.** Like vitamin E, vitamin C is an antioxidant that helps prevent cholesterol from accumulating in the arteries. Take 500 milligrams daily, Dr. Capuzzi advises. "However, there is some evidence that high doses of vitamins E or C can actually increase oxidative stress and may do more harm than good," he adds.

**Get some calm in your life.** Emotional stress is an inevitable part of daily life, but when tension and anxiety soar, the body's demand for blood and oxygen increases, which can result in angina. Regular exercise is an excellent way to reduce stress. Some people meditate. Others practice yoga or deep breathing. Experiment a bit and find what works best for you.

## PANEL OF ADVISORS

**David M. Capuzzi, M.D., Ph.D.,** is a professor of medicine, biochemistry, and molecular pharmacology and director of the Cardiovascular Disease Prevention Center at Thomas Jefferson University Hospital in Philadelphia.

**Kristine Napier, R.D.,** is nutrition director of Nutrio.com, author of *Eat to Heal,* and coauthor of *Eat Away Diabetes.*

**Howard Weitz, M.D.,** is codirector of the Jefferson Heart Institute of Thomas Jefferson University Hospital and deputy chairman of the department of medicine at Jefferson Medical College, both in Philadelphia.

# ANXIETY

## 21 Ways to Control Excessive Worrying

Anxiety, or hand-wrenching, tummy-turning worry, is a natural reaction to some of life's most challenging situations.

A little bit of anxiety can be good. It helps motivate you to meet a deadline, pass a test, or deliver a well-crafted presentation at work. It also keeps you from walking head-on into danger. As part of the fight-or-flight response, anxiety causes your heart rate to increase and your muscles to tense should you need to act.

At its extreme, however, worry runs amok. Once it begins to interfere with everyday life, worry is considered an anxiety disorder. About 25 million Americans experience these disorders, which include panic attacks, generalized anxiety disorder, phobias, post-traumatic stress syndrome, and obsessive-compulsive disorder. Anxiety disorders require medical attention and sometimes medication.

Millions of people fall somewhere in between these two extremes, however. They worry too much but don't have an actual disorder. Chronic worriers are able to function from day to day, but the anxiety eats away at their emotional and physical health. Edward M. Hallowell, M.D., calls this "persistent toxic worry."

"We virtually train ourselves to worry, which only reinforces the habit," Dr. Hallowell says. "Worriers often feel vulnerable if they're not worrying."

Worriers have good reason to stop. Excessive worry, or anxiety, is associated with increased risk for depression, heart disease, and other medical conditions.

Here are some tips for getting a handle on excessive worry.

**Breathe.** "Regulating the breath is the most effective antianxiety measure I know," says Andrew Weil, M.D., who recommends the yogic relaxing breath. Simply inhale though your nose for 4 seconds, hold your breath for 7 seconds, and exhale through your mouth for 8 seconds. Practice this technique regularly throughout the day for about a minute at a time.

**Make contact.** The more isolated you feel, the more likely you are to worry, says Dr. Hallowell, who recommends daily doses of human contact. Go to a

## WHEN TO CALL A DOCTOR

The line between normal worrying and an anxiety disorder can be hard to discern. "If your life is restricted by anxiety, get medical attention," advises Bernard Vittone, M.D. Also see a doctor if you:

- Experience more than one panic attack a month or fear having a second attack

- Are nervous or anxious most of the time, particularly if your worry is attached to situations that would not make other people anxious

- Frequently experience insomnia, shakiness, poor concentration, tight muscles, or heart palpitations

- Feel nervous in or avoid facing particular situations, such as crossing bridges or tunnels

- Take refuge from fear or worry by using drugs, including alcohol, or overeating

- Can't stop obsessing or ruminating about the past

- Are in an emotional crisis, and the support of caring friends, family, or clergy doesn't seem to help

- Fear you might harm yourself or others

restaurant, a supermarket, or a library and start a conversation with someone. Call a friend or relative. Feeling connected reduces anxiety, Dr. Hallowell says.

**Meditate.** Do some sort of meditative activity for at least 15 minutes, up to three or four times each day. Research shows that meditation can significantly lower anxiety. Find a quiet environment, clear your mind, and actively relax, says Bernard Vittone, M.D. "Focus on a mantra or make your mind a blank slate, whatever works for you."

**Stay in the present.** Focus on what's happening *now*, not on the past or the future. Take 1 day, 1 hour, or even 1 minute at a time, says Dr. Vittone.

**Pass up passivity.** Don't be a passive victim, says Dr. Hallowell. If you're worried about your job, health, or finances, for instance, create a plan to solve potential problems. Start a savings account or schedule a work evaluation with your boss. Taking action reduces anxiety.

**Get real.** Or, at least, get the facts, says Dr. Hallowell. Exaggerated worry often stems from a lack of information. If your CEO snubs you in the hall, you may worry that you're not doing a good job. But the CEO may have been pondering a personal matter, not even aware that you were there.

**Stop the stimulus.** People who are too anxious need to decrease stimulation, says Dr. Vittone. Eliminate some of the racket vying for your attention. Turn off the car radio, don't answer the telephone at home, take a lunch break away from your office—and away from your cell phone.

**Take a "news fast."** Turn off the television. Leave the morning paper on the porch. "Taking a break from the news for a few days may decrease feelings of anxiety and lessen personal worries," says Dr. Weil.

**Envision the worst.** Ask yourself, "What's the worst that could happen?" "How bad would it be?" "What's the likelihood of it happening?"

The worst thing that can happen usually isn't that bad, Dr. Vittone says. What's more, it seldom happens. Later, you may even wonder why you worried at all.

**Write it down.** Journaling, or putting your anxious thoughts on paper, can help to defuse them and restore calm, says Dr. Weil.

**Prepare to sleep.** At night, that is. "Give yourself time to unwind and relax," says Dr. Vittone. Take 30 to 50 minutes to do something quiet and nonstressful before bed. Read a light novel or watch a television comedy. Avoid active tasks such as housework.

**Laugh at yourself.** Take another view of your worries. Ask yourself: "What's funny about this situation?" "When I think about this 2 years from now, will I laugh?"

If we can find humor in a situation, we immediately defuse the danger, Dr. Vittone says.

**Share your worry.** Never worry alone. "When we talk about our worries, the toxicity dissipates," says Dr. Hallowell. Talking it through helps us find solutions and realize that our concerns aren't so overwhelming.

**Let it go.** Chronic worriers have a tough time letting go. You may hold on to worry as though it will fix the

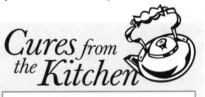

### Cures from the Kitchen

To calm yourself before bedtime, reach for a glass of warm milk. "The old wives' tale of having warm milk really does help," says Bernard Vittone, M.D. Milk contains the amino acid tryptophan, which can cause a certain amount of relaxation.

problem, Dr. Hallowell says. It won't. So practice, practice, practice. Train yourself to let go. He suggests meditation or visualization, but you can develop your own technique. One patient "sees" worries in the palm of her hand and blows them away. Another takes a shower and "watches" worries go down the drain. "Don't feel like a failure if you can't do it at first," he says. Keep practicing.

**Handle with less care.** Stop treating yourself as fragile. If you believe that you're fragile, it becomes a self-fulfilling prophecy. Instead, learn to make anx-

---

# How to Choose a Therapist

Edward M. Hallowell, M.D., offers these tips for choosing a mental-health professional, such as a licensed clinical social worker, psychologist, or psychiatrist. To start, consult two or three licensed professionals with good reputations in your community. Keep these questions in mind as you talk with each of them.

- Does she have a pleasant disposition and a sense of humor?

- Do you feel safe and at ease with her?

- Is she sincere about trying to understand and help you?

- Does she treat you with dignity and respect?

- Is she honest, nondefensive, and kind?

- Is she willing to explain her approach, including strategies, goals, and length of treatment?

- Does she make you feel accepted?

- Can she understand your background and cultural heritage, if relevant?

- Does she treat you like an equal— or as though you are flawed or defective?

- Do you leave the sessions feeling more hopeful and empowered most of the time?

- Do you feel that she understands your pain?

- Do you feel safe disclosing your innermost feelings and that they are held in confidence?

- Does she give you homework assignments between sessions?

As you talk with potential therapists, keep in mind that research shows that the therapist's personal style, such as empathy, is more important in determining therapeutic success than is a therapist's theoretical persuasion or choice of techniques, Dr. Hallowell says.

These tips also apply if you're seeking help for depression, the symptoms of which are often intertwined with those of anxiety, or other serious mental disorders. (For more information on depression, see page 159.)

iety a stimulus and not a handicap. If you're about to give a speech, for instance, imagine it as a thrill instead of a threat.

**Find your challenge.** Anxiety often arises when people have too many things going on at once. Instead of viewing your busyness as negative, think of life as action-filled, rich, or challenging. If you're raising a family, for example, consider how one day you will miss your children's presence at home. The way you interpret things makes all the difference in the world, Dr. Vittone says.

**Avoid alcohol.** Beer, wine, and other alcoholic beverages can exacerbate anxiety. "Alcohol reduces the anxiety when you first take it in," says Dr. Vittone. "But when it wears off, it has the opposite effect." People are often more anxious the day after a night of heavy drinking, he says. Avoid alcohol, or limit consumption to one or two drinks a day.

**Consider kava.** This over-the-counter herbal supplement is a natural relaxant, says Dr. Weil. What's more, it's a nonaddictive alternative to anxiety-busting prescriptive medications. Look for tablets containing 40 to 70 milligrams of kavalactones, the active ingredients. Take no more than two tablets each day. "You may notice your level of anxiety diminishing within a week after you begin to take kava," he says. "But the maximum benefit usually doesn't appear for 4 to 8 weeks." Don't take kava if you have a history of liver problems or drink alcohol regularly.

---

## Put a Cap on Caffeine

Nothing is worse for anxiety than caffeine, says Bernard Vittone, M.D.

Found in foods like chocolate; beverages such as coffee, tea, and colas; and medications like Excedrin, caffeine affects neurotransmitters in the brain, which causes anxiety. Research shows that people who are predisposed to anxiety and those with panic disorders are especially sensitive to caffeine's effects.

Caffeine is deceptive, says Dr. Vittone. When you drink a cup of coffee, for example, you're likely to feel more vivacious for up to an hour. Two to 12 hours after that, caffeine's anxiety-producing effects kick in. Because of this delayed reaction, people rarely connect anxiety to their morning java.

If you consume a lot of caffeine, try this test: Abstain from coffee and other caffeine-containing foods for 2 weeks. Then, drink three cups in one sitting and see how you feel. You're likely to notice a tightening of muscles, worry, nervousness, or apprehension several hours later.

"I really advocate trying to cut out caffeine completely," Dr. Vittone says. If that's asking too much, then limit coffee, tea, or colas to one cup a day.

Bernard Vittone, M.D., who considers himself "more anxious than the average individual," banishes worry by jogging 30 to 40 minutes every day after work.

If you experience anxiety, he suggests exercising for at least ½ hour each day. Try running, cycling, walking, yoga, or stretching. The more vigorous the exercise, the more anxiety you'll work out of your system.

## PANEL OF ADVISORS

**Edward M. Hallowell, M.D.,** is a psychiatrist and founder of the Hallowell Center for Cognitive and Emotional Health in Sudbury, Massachusetts. He is the author of *Worry: Hope and Help for a Common Condition* and *Connect: 12 Vital Ties That Open Your Heart, Lengthen Your Life, and Deepen Your Soul.*

**Bernard Vittone, M.D.,** is a psychiatrist and founder of the National Center for the Treatment of Phobias, Anxiety, and Depression in Washington, D.C.

**Andrew Weil, M.D.,** is a clinical professor of medicine and director of the program in integrative medicine at the University of Arizona in Tucson. He is the author of several books, including *8 Weeks to Optimum Health.*

# ASTHMA
## 28 Steps to Better Breathing

You may think of asthma as a childhood illness, not one that's much of a problem for adults. Yet approximately 5 percent of American adults and 5 to 10 percent of children have asthma. It accounts for some 500,000 hospital admissions every year.

Asthma isn't always serious enough to require hospitalization, of course. It may cause only occasional and short-lived symptoms, such as breathlessness, coughing, or wheezing. But unless your asthma is well-controlled, it subtly interferes with normal activity and may get out of hand quickly.

Asthma occurs when the main air passages in the lungs, called bronchioles, become inflamed and overly sensitive to "triggers." During attacks, the lungs produce extra mucus and the bronchiole walls narrow, making breathing difficult.

No cure exists yet, but nearly everyone can dramatically reduce—and maybe even eliminate—symptoms. Even if you currently use medications to treat your asthma, you may be able to reduce the dose or frequency more than 50 percent by practicing good lifestyle control, says Thomas F. Plaut, M.D.

Here are some doctor-recommended approaches.

**Look into allergies.** More than 80 percent of adults with asthma have allergies that trigger or worsen symptoms. "Everyone who takes medications daily for asthma needs to find out if they have allergies," says Dr. Plaut. Think about when your symptoms occur and what you are doing at the time. Any patterns may help indicate what you're allergic to. You might want to keep an asthma journal.

**Keep a food diary.** Food allergies are quite rare, but they're worth considering if you have asthma. For one thing, people with asthma tend to have more serious reactions to the allergens in foods. In addition, about 8 percent of those with severe asthma also have a food allergy, says Dr. Plaut.

Almost any food can cause reactions in those with asthma. The main culprits are preservatives and additives, such as the sulfites added to some wines, beers, dried fruits, and frozen foods. If you write down everything you eat for a month or two and jot down the dates of asthma episodes and the severity of symptoms, you'll get a good sense if anything in your diet is contributing to the problem, says Dr. Plaut.

## Do just 1 thing

If you take medications for asthma control, get in the habit of using a peak-flow meter. Available in drugstores, it's a device that measures the speed at which air leaves the lungs. It's an invaluable way to detect the airway narrowing that occurs prior to asthma attacks. Treating asthma at the earliest possible time can help prevent emergencies.

A reading between 80 to 100 percent indicates that your breathing is healthy, says Thomas F. Plaut, M.D. Lower scores may indicate that you need higher doses of medication or your asthma isn't adequately controlled.

It's also important to keep a daily diary that lists the following: peak-flow levels, the frequency and severity of symptoms, how frequently you're using medicines, and possible triggers you've been exposed to.

By consulting the diary regularly, you'll be able to detect factors that cause your asthma to get worse—and those that cause it to improve, Dr. Plaut explains.

**Avoid plant pollen.** It's a main asthma trigger. Plants pollinate at specific times of the year, so once you know which pollens are your triggers, take steps to

## WHEN TO CALL A DOCTOR

The symptoms of asthma are often subtle at first, but they can get much worse in a hurry. Any changes in your usual breathing patterns need to be checked by a doctor.

If you're already being treated for asthma, see your doctor if you're needing the asthma medication more frequently. In addition, if your wheeze, cough, or shortness of breath gets worse even after the medicine has been given time to work, you need to call your doctor. *Anytime you have an attack, it means the asthma isn't as well-controlled as it should be.*

avoid them. Stay indoors between 5:00 and 10:00 A.M. and on dry, hot, windy days, for example, when pollen counts tend to be highest. During the warm months, keep your windows closed and cool your house with an air conditioner.

Of Americans who are allergic to pollen, 75 percent are allergic to ragweed. Ragweed season runs from August to November, usually peaking in mid-September. Check out your local television or newspaper weather reports for daily pollen counts so that you'll know when it's a good idea to stay inside.

**Switch on the bathroom fan.** Mold is a common asthma trigger, and it thrives in bathrooms and other high-moisture areas. Good ventilation is essential. Use the bathroom fan every time you bathe or shower to help remove the moisture that mold needs to thrive.

Also try using a squeegee on the bathroom tiles. It takes about 30 seconds, wipes off extra moisture, and is a terrific strategy for preventing mold, says Dr. Plaut.

**Wash your pets weekly.** Dogs and cats are loaded with dander—a combination of skin cells and allergy-causing proteins that can provoke asthma attacks. Some people with asthma who are allergic to pets will need to find new homes for them. At the very least, wash your pets weekly—with or without shampoo—to remove the dander.

**Open windows when you cook.** Strong food odors—from a smoky frying pan, for example, or the pungent oils in raw onions and garlic—often irritate airways and trigger asthma attacks. Open the windows or use an exhaust fan when you cook to help vent the odors outside.

**Keep dust under control.** It's impossible to eliminate all dust, but the more you get rid of, the less likely you are to have asthma attacks, says Dr. Plaut.

A few times a week, run a dust-busting cloth over picture frames, windowsills, and other areas where dust accumulates. Mop linoleum and hardwood floors, and use a vacuum equipped with a HEPA (high-energy particulate-arresting) filter, which traps dust particles and keeps them out of harm's way.

**Change furnace filters.** During the cold months, central heating systems unleash veritable clouds of dust, Dr. Plaut says. One of the best things that you can do is replace the standard furnace filters with electronic air cleaners. Available from heating contractors, the devices act almost like dust magnets.

**Get rid of dust mites.** Despite the name, these microscopic creatures thrive on dead skin cells, not dust. They're an asthma trigger—and because people shed millions of skin cells every day, dust mites cannot be totally eliminated. They can be reduced, however.

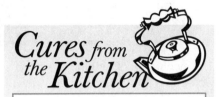

## Cures from the Kitchen

If you or anyone in your family has asthma, put fish on the menu at least twice a week.

Fatty fish such as tuna, salmon, and mackerel contain beneficial fats called omega-3 fatty acids. Asthma is an inflammatory disease, and the omega-3s help to damp down many of the body's processes that create inflammation.

Vacuuming the house—not just the floors but also upholstery—goes a long way toward reducing mite populations. It's also important to wash sheets, pillowcases, and bathroom towels at least once a week. Use water that's at least 130°F to kill adult mites as well as the eggs, says Dr. Plaut.

"It's also important to encase pillows, mattresses, and box springs with covers made specifically to act as a barrier against dust mites. These covers are available at allergy supply stores," he adds.

**Keep your house pest-free.** Studies have shown that roaches—which thrive in the same areas as humans—can trigger asthma.

These pests can be extremely difficult to get rid of, even if your house is always squeaky-clean. One of the safest ways to control roaches is to sprinkle boric acid in areas where they congregate—around drainpipes, for example, or along kitchen and bathroom baseboards.

"Don't have an exterminator spray the house if you can help it," says Dr. Plaut. The fumes can irritate the airways for days, making asthma symptoms much worse.

**Make your house a smoke-free zone.** Cigarette smoke is extremely irritating. It not only triggers asthma attacks but also can increase the risk of asthma in children. If you smoke, take advantage of nicotine patches, prescription medications, or smoking-cessation programs. Let others know that smoking in the house is *verboten*.

**Load your diet with flavonoids.** To fight the inflammation that accompanies asthma, consume foods loaded with flavonoids—tiny crystals in foods like onions, apples, blueberries, and prickly pears that give them their blue, yellow, or reddish hues. Flavonoids not only strengthen the capillary walls, they are antioxidants, and so they help protect the membranes in the airways from being damaged by pollution. Eat a couple of servings of flavonoid-rich foods every day.

**Take magnesium.** Extra magnesium may help to decrease muscle tension and airway spasms, explains Kendall Gerdes, M.D. Take 100 to 500 milligrams one to three times a day. Because high doses of magnesium (350 milligrams or more) can cause cramps, gas, or diarrhea for some people, Dr. Gerdes suggests starting with the lowest dosage and increasing it gradually until you experience these side effects. Then cut back the dosage until problems subside.

*Note:* If you have heart or kidney problems, talk to your doctor before taking supplemental magnesium.

**Supplement with quercetin.** Quercetin is a flavonoid extracted from certain fruits and vegetables, such as apples and onions, that helps inhibit the allergic reaction that can lead to asthma. Take 250 milligrams per day, advises Elson Haas, M.D. Because asthma is a serious, highly individualized condition, it's a good idea to talk with your doctor before making any changes to your treatment plan, he adds.

**Stay active.** An active lifestyle can help control asthma much better than a sedentary one. Physical activity helps improve lung capacity and may enable people to use lower doses of medications or to use them less often. All asthma patients should discuss a fitness program with their physicians.

**Exercise in warm weather.** Breathing cold air while skiing or skating, for example, can irritate the airways and trigger asthma attacks. Make sure you wear a mask to create a reservoir of warm air, advises Dr. Plaut. If you notice that you're having more asthma episodes during the cold months, consider shifting to warm-weather activities. Swimming is especially good because the moist air soothes the airways and reduces the risk of attacks.

**Change your breathing style.** Most people breathe using their chest muscles only. This makes it difficult to fully empty air from the lungs. For those with asthma, it's important to use the diaphragm as well. This large muscle between the chest and abdomen adds power to your breathing and helps remove "used" air from the lungs, which can reduce feelings of breathlessness, explains Dr. Plaut.

It takes practice to get in the habit of diaphragmatic breathing (also called abdominal breathing). Several times a day, lie on your back with one hand on your belly and the other on your chest. As you breathe in, the hand on your belly should rise slightly, while the hand on your chest should barely move.

**Take up a wind instrument.** Playing such an instrument, like the oboe, saxophone, or trumpet, requires diaphragmatic breathing, Dr. Plaut says. Even if you aren't especially musical, it's great practice for breathing muscles.

**Practice stress control.** Yoga, self-hypnosis, deep breathing, and other techniques for reducing stress are helpful for asthma because they help the airways open more fully, says Dr. Plaut.

**Wash your hands often.** Asthma episodes tend to surge in the autumn and winter, when people tend to get more colds. Even a mild case of the sniffles can make asthma harder to control. A viral infection is a common trigger of an asthma attack.

Cold viruses can survive for hours on doorknobs, handrails, and even money. Washing your hands often—at least every few hours—will flush away the viruses before they have a chance to take hold.

**Think twice about aspirin.** About 5 percent of those with asthma are sensitive to aspirin, ibuprofen, and related pain relievers, known as nonsteroidal anti-inflammatory drugs (NSAIDs), says Dr. Plaut. For those who are sensitive, an asthma attack or other respiratory problems can begin within 2 hours of taking the drugs.

If you need long-term pain relief—because of arthritis, for example—your doctor may advise you to switch to acetaminophen or other analgesics that are less likely to trigger asthma attacks.

**Don't put up with heartburn.** The upward surge of stomach acids that cause the telltale pain of heartburn can also trigger asthma attacks. One of the best ways to prevent heartburn is to eat four or more small meals daily, instead of two or three large meals, Dr. Plaut advises. Also, don't eat just before bedtime. To help prevent stomach acid from going "upstream," raise the head of your bed 4 to 6 inches by putting blocks under the legs of the bed.

You can also quell heartburn with over-the-counter antacids or with acid-suppressing drugs such as cimetidine (Tagamet).

**Flush your sinuses.** Millions of Americans get sinus infections every year, and the inflammation and mucous drainage can make asthma worse. Sinusitis often requires treatment with antibiotics, but you may be able to prevent infections by flushing your sinuses at home, says Dr. Plaut.

Mix ½ teaspoon of salt in 1 cup of warm water. Pour the solution into your cupped palm and inhale it with one nostril while holding the other nostril closed. Then repeat with the other nostril. People who get frequent sinus infections should repeat the treatment once daily. If you get infections less often, it's fine to flush the sinuses only when you have a cold or when your allergies are worse than usual.

**Act quickly if asthma strikes.** Don't ignore early signs of asthma attacks, even if the symptoms—wheezing, coughing, or faster breathing—seem mild at first. Use your rescue medication promptly. It will help reverse airway narrowing before the attack gets more serious, says Dr. Plaut.

**Keep track of inhaler "puffs."** If you use medication to control asthma, the worst thing is to discover that your inhaler is empty right when you need it. To prevent that, put a piece of masking tape on the inhaler and make a mark on the tape every time you use it.

**Or use the Doser.** Available at allergy supply stores and catalogs, the Doser attaches to metered inhalers and automatically keeps track of how many doses you have left.

## PANEL OF ADVISORS

**Kendall Gerdes, M.D.,** is director of Environmental Medicine Associates in Denver.

**Elson Haas, M.D.,** is the director of the Preventive Medical Center of Marin, an integrated health-care facility in San Rafael, California, and author of seven books on health and nutrition, including *The False Fat Diet* and *Staying Healthy with Nutrition.*

**Thomas F. Plaut, M.D.,** is medical consultant to *Asthma Update* newsletter and the author of *Dr. Tom Plaut's Asthma Guide for People of All Ages* and *One-Minute Asthma.*

# ATHLETE'S FOOT
## 16 Ways to Get Rid of It

You don't have to be an athlete to catch athlete's foot. The fungal infection, which is caused by an organism that lives on the skin and breeds best under warm, moist conditions, can be caught simply by letting your bare feet touch moist areas in locker rooms, pools, and bathrooms. And even though these balmy climates encourage the growth of the fungus, sweaty footwear is more often the culprit.

Athlete's foot is the most common form of tinea, a fungal infection of the nails, skin, hair, or body. The fungus triggers redness, swelling, cracking, burning, scaling, and intense itching between your toes, and your skin may also appear puckered.

Once you have the fungus, it will take at least 4 weeks to make headway against a savage case. Worse, it will return unless you stamp out the conditions that caused it in the first place. So here are some tips on dealing with an active infection and some ways to guard against an encore.

**Baby your foot.** Athlete's foot can come on suddenly and be accompanied by oozing blisters and an intermittent burning sensation, says Frederick Hass, M.D. When you're going through this acute stage, baby your foot. Keep it uncovered and at constant rest. Although the inflammation itself is not dangerous, it can get worse, leading to a bacterial infection if you're not careful.

**Soothe the sores.** Use soothing compresses to cool the inflammation, ease the pain, lessen the itching, and dry the sores, says Dr. Hass. Dissolve one packet of Domeboro powder or 2 tablespoons of Burow's solution (both available without a prescription in drugstores) in 1 pint of cold water. Soak an untreated white cotton cloth in the liquid and apply three or four times daily for 15 to 20 minutes.

**Look for a (salty) solution.** Soak your foot in a mixture of 2 teaspoons of salt per pint of warm water, says Glenn Copeland, D.P.M. Do this for 5 to 10

## WHEN TO CALL A DOCTOR

How do you know if that red, itching splotch between your toes is a true case of athlete's foot? And when should tinea between your toes send you scrambling to see a doctor?

According to Thomas Goodman Jr., M.D., that rash probably isn't athlete's foot if:

- It's on a child's foot. (It's very rare for a child below the age of puberty to have a fungus infection of the foot.)

- It's on top of the toes. (Eruptions on the tops of toes and the top of the foot are probably some form of contact dermatitis caused by shoes.)

- The foot is red, swollen, sore, blistered, and oozing. Call a doctor because you may have an acute form of dermatitis.

If you have a true case of athlete's foot, be wary of infection. You cannot assume that athlete's foot will go away of its own accord, says Suzanne M. Levine, D.P.M. An unchecked fungal infection can lead to cracks in the skin and invite a nasty bacterial infection.

Frederick Hass, M.D., recommends that you consult your physician if:

- The inflammation proves incapacitating.

- Swelling occurs in the foot or the leg at any time during the attack, and you develop a fever.

- Pus appears in the blisters or the cracked skin.

minutes at a time, and repeat until the problem clears up. The saline solution provides an unappealing atmosphere for the fungus and lessens excess perspiration. What's more, it softens the affected skin so that antifungal medications can penetrate deeper and act more effectively.

**Medicate your foot.** Now's the time to apply an over-the-counter antifungal medication, which may contain either miconazole nitrate (found in Micatin products, for example), tolnaftate (Aftate or Tinactin), or fatty acids (Desenex). According to dermatologist Thomas Goodman Jr., M.D., lightly apply the medication to the area involved and rub in gently. Continue two or three times a day for 4 weeks (or for 2 weeks after the problem seems to have cleared up).

**Treat your little piggies.** For athlete's foot between your toes, says Dr. Goodman, apply an aluminum chloride solution. This clear liquid not only kills fungus but also helps dry the area, discouraging regrowth. Ask your pharmacist to make a solution of 25 percent aluminum chloride in water. Use a cotton swab to apply the liquid between your toes two or three times a day. Continue for 2 weeks after the infection clears up.

A word of warning from Dr. Goodman: Don't use aluminum chloride on skin that is cracked or raw—it will sting like crazy. Heal the cracks first with an antifungal agent.

**Rub in baking soda.** For fungus on your feet, especially between the toes, apply a baking soda paste, suggests Suzanne M. Levine, D.P.M. Add a little lukewarm water to 1 tablespoon of baking soda. Rub the paste on the fungus, then rinse and dry thoroughly. Finish the treatment by dusting on cornstarch or powder.

**Scrub away dead skin.** When the acute phase of the attack has settled down, says Dr. Hass, remove any dead skin. "It houses living fungi that can reinfect you. At bath time, work the entire foot lightly but vigorously with a bristle scrub brush. Pay extra attention to spaces between toes—use a small bottle brush or test-tube brush there." If you scrub your feet in the bathtub, shower afterward to wash away any bits of skin that could attach themselves to other parts of the body and start another infection.

**Pay attention to toenails.** Toenails are favorite breeding spots for the fungus, says Dr. Hass. Scrape the undersides of your nails clean at least every second or third day. Be sure to use an orange stick, toothpick, or wooden match rather than a metal nail file, which could scratch the nails and provide niches for the fungus to collect in.

**Keep applying cream.** Once your infection has cleared, help guard against its return by continuing to use (less often) the antifungal cream or lotion that cured your problem, says Dr. Goodman. This is especially prudent during warm weather. Use your own judgment as to how often to use it; from once a day to once a week is fine.

**Choose proper shoes.** Avoid plastic shoes and footwear that has been treated to keep water out, says Dr. Copeland. They trap perspiration and create a warm, moist spot for the fungus to grow. Natural materials such as cotton and leather provide the best environment for feet, while rubber and even wool may induce sweating and hold moisture.

**Change them often.** Don't wear the same shoes 2 days in a row, says podiatrist Dean S. Stern, D.P.M. It takes at least 24 hours for shoes to dry out thoroughly. If your feet perspire heavily, change shoes twice a day.

**Keep them dry—and clean.** Dust the insides of your shoes frequently with antifungal powder or spray. Another good idea, says Neal Kramer, D.P.M., is to spray some disinfectant (such as Lysol) on a rag and use it to wipe out the insides of your shoes every time you take them off. That kills any fungus spores.

**Air them.** Dr. Hass recommends giving your shoes a little time in the sun to air out. Remove the laces and prop each shoe open. You should even leave sandals outdoors to dry between wearings. And wipe the undersides of their straps clean after every wearing to remove any fungi-carrying dead skin. The idea is to reduce even the slightest possibility of reinfection.

**Sock the infection.** If your feet perspire heavily, says Dr. Hass, change your socks three or four times a day. And wear only clean cotton socks, not those made with synthetic yarns. Be sure to rinse them thoroughly during laundering, because detergent residue can aggravate your skin problem. And to help kill fungus spores, says Dr. Kramer, wash your socks twice in extra-hot water.

**Powder your toes.** To further keep your feet dry, allow them to air-dry for 5 to 10 minutes after a shower before putting your shoes and socks on, says Diana Bihova, M.D. To speed complete drying, hold a hair dryer about 6 inches from your foot, wiggle your toes, and dry between them. Then apply powder. To avoid the mess of loose powder, place it in a plastic or paper bag, then put your foot into the bag and shake it well.

**Cover up in public places.** You can decrease your exposure to the fungus, says Dr. Goodman, by wearing slippers or shower shoes in areas where other people go barefoot. That includes gyms, spas, health clubs, locker rooms, and even around swimming pools. If you're prone to fungal infections, you can pick them up almost any place that is damp—so be prudent.

## PANEL OF ADVISORS

**Diana Bihova, M.D.,** is a dermatologist affiliated with the dermatology department at the Columbia University College of Physicians and Surgeons in New York City.

**Glenn Copeland, D.P.M.,** is a podiatrist at the Women's College Hospital in Toronto. He is also consulting podiatrist for the Canadian Back Institute and a podiatrist for the Toronto Blue Jays baseball team.

**Thomas Goodman Jr., M.D.,** is a dermatologist and former assistant professor of dermatology at the University of Tennessee Health Science Center in Memphis. He is the author of *Smart Face*.

**Frederick Hass, M.D.,** is a general practitioner in San Rafael, California. He is on the staff of Marin General Hospital in Greenbrae.

**Neal Kramer, D.P.M.,** is a podiatrist in Bethlehem, Pennsylvania.

**Suzanne M. Levine, D.P.M., P.C.,** is a podiatrist and a podiatric attending physician at New York–Presbyterian Hospital. She is the author of *Your Feet Don't Have to Hurt.*

**Dean S. Stern, D.P.M.,** is a podiatrist at Rush–Presbyterian–St. Luke's Medical Center in Chicago.

# BACKACHE
## 24 Pain-Free Ideas

Back pain may be one of the most pervasive ailments in America. Two-thirds of American adults will experience back pain at some time in their lives. As a result, back pain is the leading cause of disability in Americans under age 45.

Back pain comes in two varieties: acute and chronic.

## Acute Back Pain

Acute pain comes on suddenly and intensely. It's the kind you usually experience from doing something that you shouldn't be doing or from doing it the wrong way. The pain can come from sprains, strains, or pulls of muscles in your back. It may hurt like crazy for several days, but doctors say that you can be pain-free without any lasting effects by following these self-help tips.

**Stay active.** Forget the old adage to get plenty of bed rest. In a study at the Texas Tech University Health Sciences Center School of Nursing in Lubbock, researchers found that patients who exercised returned to work more quickly than those who didn't.

**If you must go to bed, keep it short.** "Most people think that a week of bed rest will take away the pain," says back expert David Lehrman, M.D. "But that's not so. For every week of bed rest, it takes 2 weeks to rehabilitate."

Research at the University of Texas Health Sciences Center bears this out. Researchers there studied 203 patients who came into a walk-in clinic complaining of acute back pain. Some were told to rest for 2 days, others for 7

## WHEN TO CALL A DOCTOR

When does your back need medical backup? When you experience any of the following:

- Back pain that comes on suddenly for no apparent reason
- Back pain that is accompanied by other symptoms, such as fever, stomach cramps, chest pain, or difficulty breathing
- An acute attack that lasts for more than 2 or 3 days without any pain relief
- Chronic pain that lasts more than 2 weeks without relief
- Back pain that radiates down your leg to your knee or foot

You shouldn't always assume that back pain is a sign that something is wrong with just your back, notes Milton Fried, M.D. It could be a sign of some other disorder.

days. There was no difference in the length of time it took the pain to diminish in either group, reports Richard A. Deyo, M.D., who was one of the researchers. But those who got out of bed after only 2 days returned to work sooner.

**Put your pain on ice.** The best way to cool down an acute flare-up is with ice, says pain researcher Ronald Melzack, Ph.D. It helps reduce swelling and the strain on your back muscles. For best results, he says, try ice massage. "Put an ice pack on the site of the pain and massage the spot for 7 to 8 minutes." Do this every few hours for a day or two.

**Try some heat relief.** After the first day or two of ice, physicians recommend that you switch to heat, says Milton Fried, M.D. Take a soft towel and put it in a basin of very warm water. Wring it well and flatten it so that there are no creases in it. Lie on your stomach, with pillows under your hips and ankles, and fold the towel across the painful part of your back. Put some plastic wrap over that, then put a heating pad set on medium on top of the plastic. If possible, place something on top that will create pressure, like a telephone book. "This creates moist heat and will help reduce muscle spasms," he explains. You may need another person's help with this.

**Use heat *and* cold.** For those of you who can't make up your mind which feels better, it's okay to use both methods, says Edward Abraham, M.D. It may even have an added bonus. "An intermittent regimen of heat and ice will actually make you feel better," he says. "Do 30 minutes of ice, then 30 minutes of heat, and keep repeating the cycle."

**Stretch to smooth a spasm.** Stretching a sore back will actually enhance the healing process, says Dr. Lehrman, by helping the muscle "calm down" sooner than by just waiting for it to calm down on its own. He recommends the following stretch for lower back pain: Gently bring your knees up from the bed and to your chest. Once there, put a little pressure on your knees. Stretch, then relax. Repeat.

**Roll out of bed.** Each morning, when you get out of bed, doctors advise that you roll out—carefully and slowly.

"You can minimize the pain of getting out of bed by sliding to the edge of the bed," says Dr. Lehrman. "Once there, keep your back rigid and then let your legs come off the bed first. That motion will act like a springboard, lifting your upper body straight up off the bed."

## Chronic Back Pain

For some people, back pain is chronic, a part of everyday life. For whatever reason, the pain lingers on and on for what can seem like an eternity. Other people experience recurring pain; any little movement can set it in motion. The following tips are particularly helpful for those with chronic pain, although people with acute pain can benefit from them as well.

**Lumber up.** Lumber under the mattress will help the lumbar on top. "The object is to have a bed that doesn't sag in the middle when you sleep on it," says Dr. Fried. "A piece of plywood between the mattress and the box spring will end the sagging problem."

**Drown pain with a waterbed.** An adjustable waterbed that doesn't make a lot of waves is excellent for most types of back trouble, says Dr. Fried.

Dr. Abraham agrees. "In waterbeds, you get an equalized change in the pressure on various segments of your body," he says. "You can lie in one position for the entire night because of this."

**Become a "lazy S" sleeper.** A bad back can't stomach lying facedown. "The best position for someone resting in bed is what we call the lazy S position," says Dr. Abraham. "Put a pillow under your head and upper neck, keep your back relatively flat on the bed, then put a pillow under your knees."

When you straighten your legs, your hamstring muscles pull and put pressure on your lower back, he explains. Keeping your knees bent puts slack into the hamstrings and takes the pressure off your back.

# Exercise Your Pain Away

Exercise may be the last thing you want to think about when your back aches, but specialists say that exercise is the best thing going for chronic back pain.

"For people who suffer daily from back pain, especially if the pain varies throughout the day, exercise can be beneficial," says Roger Minkow, M.D.

If you're under a doctor's care for back pain, be sure to get the okay before you begin. Here are some doctor-recommended exercises.

**Play press-up.** Press-ups are something like half of a pushup. "Lie on the floor on your stomach. Keep your pelvis flat on the floor and push up with your hands, arching your back as you lift your shoulders off the floor," says Dr. Minkow.

This helps strengthen your lower back. Dr. Minkow recommends doing it once in the morning and once in the afternoon.

**Move into a crunch.** While you're on the floor, turn over onto your back and do what's called a crunch situp. Lie flat with both feet on the floor and your knees bent. Cross your arms and rest your hands on your shoulders. Raise your head and shoulders off the floor as high as you can while keeping your lower back on the floor. Hold for 1 second, then repeat.

**Swim on dry land.** You don't need a deep-pile rug to swim on your floor. Lie on your stomach and raise your left arm and your right leg. Hold for 1 second, then alternate with your left leg and right arm as if you were swimming.

This will extend and strengthen your lower back, says Dr. Minkow.

**Get into the pool.** "Swimming is great exercise for the back," reports Milton Fried, M.D. "A good exercise for acute lower-back pain is to get into a warm pool and swim."

**Put your mettle to the pedal.** "Ride a stationary bike with a mirror set up so that you can see yourself," says Dr. Minkow. "Be sure to sit up straight without slouching. If you have to, raise the handlebars so that you're not bent over forward."

**Remember: "No pain, no gain" equals no brain.** Be careful and know your limit with these and any other exercises, Dr. Minkow advises. "If the exercise you're doing hurts or aggravates your condition, don't do the exercise anymore," he says. "You're not going to improve anything by gritting your teeth and doing one more repetition. If you feel fine the day after or 2 days after you exercise, then it's safe to continue exercising."

**Develop fetal attraction.** You'll sleep like a baby if you sleep on your side in the fetal position. "It's a good idea to stick a pillow between your knees when you sleep on your side," says Dr. Fried. "The pillow stops your leg from sliding forward and rotating your hips, which puts added pressure on your back."

**Take an aspirin a day.** It can keep back pain away, claim the experts. Back pain is often accompanied by inflammation around the site of the pain, says Dr. Fried, and simple over-the-counter anti-inflammatory drugs, such as aspirin and ibuprofen, can help take it away. "It can even help for a fairly severe amount of inflammation," he adds.

Acetaminophen is not as effective, because it is not an anti-inflammatory drug.

**Bark up the right tree.** If you're looking for a natural anti-inflammatory, try some white willow bark, which can be found in capsule form in health food stores. "It is a natural salicylate, the active ingredient that gives aspirin its anti-inflammatory power," says Dr. Fried. "Taken after meals, it shouldn't hurt your stomach, and it works very well on mild to moderate back pain. Those who have ulcers or heartburn, however, should not use it."

**Visualize yourself pain-free.** The middle of the night can be the worst time for pain. Pain wakes you up, and it keeps you up. "Using visualization is a particularly good thing to do at times like this," says Dennis Turk, Ph.D.

"Close your eyes and imagine a lemon on a white china plate. See a knife next to it. See yourself pick up the knife and slice the lemon. Hear the sound it makes cutting through. Smell the aroma. Bring the lemon up to your face and imagine its taste."

The idea is to bring as much detail to the image as possible. The more involved the image is, the more you are engaged with it and the quicker you will become distracted from the pain, says Dr. Turk.

**Turn your pain upside down.** "Gravity inversion works wonders on back pain," says Dr. Fried. "Your spine is constantly compressed when you're standing. Gravity separates it all and provides relief." With this therapy, you strap yourself to a special device that tilts back and allows you to hang upside down. "Gradually doing inversion traction with a proper, safe inversion apparatus for 30 minutes a day will really work to rid you of lower back pain," he says. You can find an apparatus in most health catalogs and online. Make sure that you purchase a sturdy inversion unit with inversion boots, he adds. You should, however, have your doctor's okay to use this kind of therapy, especially if you have disk problems. And those who have glaucoma or are at risk for developing it should not use it.

**Try tai chi to untie muscle knots.** Tai chi is an ancient Chinese discipline of slow, fluid movements. "It's a great relaxation method that helps the muscles in your back," says Dr. Abraham, who uses the method himself. "There are a lot of breathing exercises and stretching activities that foster a harmony within the body."

Tai chi takes time and self-discipline to learn, but Dr. Abraham says that it's worth it.

# Car Seat Comfort

Does your back drive you crazy every time you buckle up? It could be that what you're sitting on is the seat of your problem. While there are many causes for back pain, most people have what is called mechanical back pain, or pain related to sitting, standing, lifting, or bending, says Roger Minkow, M.D., who designs seats for airplane and automobile manufacturers. "Riding in the car can be a real source of pain for people in this category."

**Take a new car for a "test-sit."** Next time you're in the market for a car, Dr. Minkow suggests testing for cushion comfort as well as cruise-ability. Adjust the seat so that your legs are slightly bent when you push on the pedals. The back of the seat should push against your lower back around your waist. A smart thing to do is rent the same make and model for a weekend and take a long drive to see how comfortable the seat is.

**Inflate a pillow.** If you are not in the market for a new car, a blow-up cushion is a cheap fix for mechanical back pain, says Dr. Minkow. "There are several on the market, but I am familiar with the Back Support Air Pillow by MedicAir. Be careful to put only two or three puffs of air into this cushion, so that it's floppy and not fully inflated. This cushion fills in the space in the curve of the lower back, putting the spine into 'neutral' and preventing slouching." Blow-up cushions are available in health catalogs and online.

## PANEL OF ADVISORS

**Edward Abraham, M.D.,** is an assistant clinical professor of orthopedics at the University of California, Irvine, College of Medicine, and has a practice in Santa Ana. He originated the concept for outpatient back therapy in the United States.

**Richard A. Deyo, M.D.,** is a professor of medicine and health services and director of the Center for Cost and Outcomes Research at the University of Washington in Seattle.

**Milton Fried, M.D.,** is the founder and director of the Milton Fried Medical Clinic in Atlanta. He also holds degrees in chiropractic and physical therapy.

**David Lehrman, M.D.,** is an orthopedic surgeon affiliated with Mount Sinai Hospital and the Miami Heart Institute in Miami Beach, Florida.

**Ronald Melzack, Ph.D.,** is a professor emeritus of psychology at McGill University in Montreal.

**Roger Minkow, M.D.,** is a back specialist and founder and director of Backworks, a rehabilitation facility for people with back injuries, located in Petaluma, California.

**Dennis Turk, Ph.D.,** is the John and Emma Bonica professor of anesthesiology and pain research at the University of Washington in Seattle.

# BAD BREATH
## 16 Ways to Overcome It

In Roman times, people used sticks for toothbrushes and tooth powder so abrasive that it ground away the surface of the teeth, exposing the pulp. When their teeth hurt, they applied olive oil in which earthworms had been boiled. After all of that, it's safe to say, they had bad breath.

Today, dental hygiene is big business, and the space allocated to it in the average grocery store rivals that of the produce section. But still, people worry about their breath. The good news is that for the most part—with proper dental care—bad breath, also called halitosis, can be avoided for good. Here's how.

**Don't dine with the garlic family.** Highly spiced foods like to linger long after the party's over. Certain tastes and smells recirculate through the essential oils that they leave in your mouth. Depending on how much you eat, the odor can remain up to 24 hours, no matter how often you brush your teeth. Some foods to avoid include onions, hot peppers, and garlic.

**Meat at the deli later.** Spicy deli meats such as pastrami, salami, and pepperoni also leave oils behind long after you have swallowed them. You breathe. They breathe. If an occasion calls for sweet-smelling breath, avoid these meats for 24 hours beforehand to keep them from talking for you.

## WHEN TO CALL A DOCTOR

If your halitosis hangs on for more than 24 hours without an obvious cause, call your dentist or doctor, says Roger P. Levin, D.D.S. It can be a sign of gum disease, gastrointestinal problems, or even more serious diseases, such as cancer and tuberculosis. Bad breath can also be a sign of dehydration or zinc deficiency, or it can be caused by some drugs, including penicillamine and lithium.

**Say, "Please, no cheese."** Camembert, Roquefort, and blue cheese are called strong for good reason—they get a hold on your breath and don't let go. Other dairy products may have the same effect.

**Don't fish for compliments.** Some fish, like the anchovies on your pizza or even the tuna you tuck into your brown-bag lunch, can leave a lasting impression.

**Stick with water.** Coffee, beer, wine, and whiskey are at the top of the list of liquid offenders. Each leaves a residue that can attach to the plaque in your mouth and infiltrate your digestive system. Each breath you take spews traces back into the air.

**Carry a toothbrush.** Some odors can be eliminated—permanently or temporarily—if you brush immediately after a meal. The main culprit in bad breath is a soft, sticky film of living and dead bacteria that clings to your teeth and gums, says Eric Shapira, D.D.S. That film is called plaque. At any time, there are 50 trillion of these microscopic organisms loitering in your mouth. They sit in every dark corner, eating each morsel of food that passes your lips, collecting little smells, and producing little odors of their own. As you exhale, the bacteria exhale. So brush away the plaque after each meal and get rid of some of the breath problem.

**Rinse out your mouth.** Even when you can't brush, you can rinse. Take a sip of water after meals, swish it around, and wash the smell of food from your mouth, says Jerry F. Taintor, D.D.S.

**Gargle a minty mouthwash.** If you need 20 minutes of freedom from bad breath, gargling with a mouthwash is a great idea. But like Cinderella's

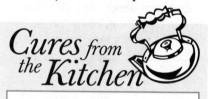

## Cures from the Kitchen

**Eat your parsley.** Parsley adds more than green to your lunch plate; it's also a breath-saver, because it contains chlorophyll, a known breath deodorizer. So pick up that sprig garnishing your plate and chew it thoroughly. Or toss a few handfuls (even add some watercress to the mix) in a juicer. Sip the juice anytime you need to refresh your breath.

**Think "spice is nice."** Other herbs and spices in your kitchen are natural breath enhancers. Carry a tiny plastic bag of cloves, fennel, or anise seeds to chew after odorous meals.

**Try a gargle special.** Mix extracts of sage, calendula, and myrrh gum (all available at health food stores) in equal proportions and gargle with the mixture four times a day. Keep the mouthwash in a tightly sealed jar at room temperature.

## How to Test Your Breath

How horrible is your halitosis? If you don't have a friend to tell you the truth, there are a couple of ways you can test your breath, says Eric Shapira, D.D.S.

**Cup your hands.** Breathe into them with a great, deep "ha-a-a-a." Sniff. If it smells rank to you, then it's deadly to those you come in contact with, says Dr. Shapira.

**Floss.** Not to clean your teeth, although that's a great idea, but to find out just how bad your breath might be, pull the floss gently between your teeth and then sniff some of the gunk you unearth. If it smells bad, you smell bad.

coach-turned-pumpkin, when your time is up, the magic will be gone, and you'll be back to talking from behind your hand again.

**Choose your mouthwash by color and flavor.** Amber and medicine-flavored mouthwashes contain essential oils such as thyme, eucalyptus, peppermint, and wintergreen, as well as sodium benzoate or benzoic acid. Red and spicy mouthwashes may contain zinc compounds. Both types neutralize the odor-producing waste products of your mouth bacteria.

**Chew a mint or some gum.** Like mouthwash, a breath mint or minty gum is just a cover-up, good for a short interview, a short ride in a compact car, or a very short date.

**Brush your tongue.** "Most people overlook their tongues," says Dr. Shapira. "Your tongue is covered with little hairlike projections, which under a microscope look like a forest of mushrooms. Under the caps of the 'mushrooms,' there's room to harbor plaque and some of the things we eat. That causes bad breath."

His advice? While brushing, gently sweep the top of your tongue, too, so that you don't leave food and bacteria behind to breed bad breath.

### PANEL OF ADVISORS

**Roger P. Levin, D.D.S.,** is the chief executive officer of the Levin Group, a dental practice in Baltimore.

**Eric Shapira, D.D.S.,** is an assistant clinical professor and lecturer at the University of the Pacific School of Dentistry in San Francisco and a dentist in Half Moon Bay, California.

**Jerry F. Taintor, D.D.S.,** is chairman of endodontics at the University of Tennessee College of Dentistry in Memphis. He is the author of *The Complete Guide to Better Dental Care.*

# BED-WETTING
## 5 Options for Sleep-Through Nights

Bed-wetting, also called enuresis, is such a common childhood challenge that as many as 7 million boys and girls over the age of 5 wake up to sopping sheets and pajamas. And boys are twice as likely to experience this condition than girls.

The causes are varied: an overproduction of urine at night, slow physical development, and an inability to recognize that the bladder is full during sleep. After the age of 4, anxiety may also play a role. Finally, genetics may be to blame; in 1995, Danish scientists found a site on human chromosome 13 that is at least partly responsible for bed-wetting.

The good news? Almost all kids eventually outgrow bed-wetting. In the meantime, try these remedies.

**Be realistic.** "Don't praise and don't punish," says child-care expert Anne Price. "Just change the bed and don't say a word. It'll go away by itself. Kids don't do it on purpose, so don't praise them when they are dry or punish them when they are wet."

**Change for the better.** To help minimize psychological stress, Price recommends arranging the bedroom so that the child can change the sheets himself. "And set out a felt-covered rubber pad so when he has an accident he can lay it over the wet part of the bed. Also, put out a pair of dry pajamas he can change into. That way, at least he won't feel babyish."

**Don't be alarmed.** "Bed-wetting alarms can work," says Bryan Shumaker, M.D. "But you'd better have patience. The alarm is loud, and chances are good it'll wake up everybody in the house when it goes off."

Bed-wetting alarms emit a buzzing or ringing sound when the child is wet. The theory is that the sound will condition him to awaken when he needs to urinate. Eventually, wetting will ease, and a full bladder will signal the child to awaken.

Most children respond to this type of conditioning strategy within 60 days, says Dr. Shumaker. Bed-wetting is considered cured when the child remains dry for 21 consecutive nights.

The newer alarms are much smaller and more sensitive to wetness than the bulky, complicated mats and pads of yesterday. Today's alarms run on hearing-aid batteries and boast moisture sensors that attach directly to the underwear. Best of all, those who use modern alarms have relapse rates of only 10 to 20 percent, compared to the 50 percent relapse rate of older models. Even kids who relapse often find lasting success with a second round of alarm use.

**Boost bladder muscles.** "If the child's daytime pattern is one in which he goes to the bathroom fairly often, then bladder-stretching exercises may work," says pediatric nurse practitioner Linda Jonides. Her recommendation: Have the child drink lots of liquids during the daytime, then practice bladder control by holding off urination for as long as possible.

**Practice patience and love.** "Understand that all kids outgrow bed-wetting at a rate of 15 percent a year," says Dr. Shumaker. "Which means by the time they go through puberty, less than 1 or 2 percent will still wet the bed. So be patient and supportive. No kid wants to wet on himself. It's unpleasant, uncomfortable, and cold, and besides 'only babies do that'—and no kid wants to be a baby. Patience and support is the bottom line."

## PANEL OF ADVISORS

**Linda Jonides** is a pediatric nurse practitioner in Ann Arbor, Michigan.

**Anne Price** is a former educational coordinator for the National Academy of Nannies, Inc. (NANI) in Denver.

**Bryan Shumaker, M.D.,** is a urologist at Michigan Institute of Urology in St. Claire Shores, Michigan.

# BELCHING
## 10 Steps to Squelch the Belch

Belching is often caused by *aerophagia*, a medical term for swallowing air. Everyone carries about a cup of air and other gases in the gastrointestinal tract. Yet the body is constantly acquiring air and other gases throughout the day—either through the mouth or by producing some of its own. In all, it works out to almost 10 cupfuls of gas in 24 hours. That's about 9 cupfuls more than your body can contain, so it constantly seeks ways to vent this excess.

One of those ways is by belching.

Soft drinks and beer are guaranteed to cause problems, but your saliva also contains tiny air bubbles that travel to your stomach with every swallow.

Those of us who swallow air along with our food are asking for trouble, but belching is a problem that seems infinitely curable right at home. Most of us can, with practice, control the amount of air we swallow and save the doctor for something more important. Here's how.

**Become aware of air.** "You can swallow up to 5 ounces of air every time you swallow," says André Dubois, M.D. People who are nervous will do this quite frequently.

Some people are compulsive swallowers and create a problem simply by swallowing too much saliva. "You can improve this by learning to control your swallowing reflexes," he says. "This is best done by simply becoming *aware* of it. Ask your friends or relatives to tell you if they notice you swallowing a lot. You probably won't notice it in yourself."

Once you're aware of an excessive swallowing habit, you will automatically curb it, says Dr. Dubois. There are also some personal habits you can change to help you take in less air.

- Avoid carbonated beverages.
- Eat slowly and chew your food completely before swallowing.
- Always eat with your mouth closed.
- Avoid chewing gum.

## Sometimes It's Better to Belch

Many physicians see no physiological need to stifle belching. They view it simply as a natural body function.

"Some societies think belching is good for you," says Richard Mc-Callum, M.D. "A couple of people from India and other Eastern countries tell me that it's perfectly normal to belch in public."

- Do not drink out of cans or bottles, and do not drink through a straw.
- Avoid foods with a high air content such as beer, ice cream, soufflés, omelets, and whipped cream.

**Nix a nervous belching habit.** Chronic air swallowers can belch forever, since belching tends to beget more belching. Yet even chronic swallowers can be helped.

Marvin Schuster, M.D., sometimes prescribes a pencil for those who swallow air and start bloating up during tense situations.

Clamping your teeth around a pencil, a cork, or your finger, keeps your mouth open and makes swallowing difficult, he says.

**Say good-bye to gassy goodies.** On occasion, all of us eat a little too much a little too quickly and burp, says Samuel Klein, M.D. But that's different than people who are chronic belchers, who belch hour after hour, day after day.

For those people, it may be useful to eat fewer foods that produce upper digestive system gas. Those foods include fats and oils such as salad oil, margarine, and sour cream.

**Smash bubbles with soothing simethicone.** To help alleviate a problem that already exists, digestive experts sometimes recommend over-the-counter antacids containing simethicone, such as Mylanta, Mylanta Supreme, Maalox Max, or Di-Gel.

"Simethicone breaks large bubbles into small bubbles in the stomach, which may decrease belching," says Dr. Klein. It does not reduce the amount of gas present, however.

### PANEL OF ADVISORS

**André Dubois, M.D.,** is a gastroenterologist in Bethesda, Maryland.

**Samuel Klein, M.D.,** is a William H. Danforth professor of medicine and nutritional science and director of the Center for Human Nutrition at Washington University School of Medicine in St. Louis.

**Richard McCallum, M.D.,** is a professor of medicine and chief of the gastroenterology and hepatology division at the University of Kansas Medical Center and the Kansas City Veterans Administration Medical Center in Kansas City, Kansas.
**Marvin Schuster, M.D.,** is director emeritus of the Marvin M. Schuster Center for Digestive and Motility Disorders at the Hopkins Bayview Medical Center, and professor emeritus of medicine and psychiatry at Johns Hopkins University School of Medicine, both in Baltimore.

# BITES, SCRATCHES, AND STINGS
## 50 Hints to Relieve the Pain

Most insect bites and stings are minor annoyances that itch like crazy and produce ugly, little welts that go away in a few days. Even love nips from Fifi and Fido are often more insult than real injury. But on those occasions when the bite is a little worse than the bark (or the buzz), doctors suggest the following.

### Flies and Mosquitoes

These pesky flying critters can make you pretty uncomfortable when they decide to munch on you. Here's what to do.

**Disinfect the bite.** Flies and mosquitoes can spread diseases. So wash the bite area thoroughly with soap and water, says Claude Frazier, M.D. Then apply an antiseptic.

**Rub in an aspirin.** Herbert Luscombe, M.D., recommends that you moisten your skin and rub an aspirin tablet over the bite as soon as possible after you're bitten. The aspirin helps control inflammation. Skip this tip if you're allergic to aspirin.

**Relieve the itching.** Fly and mosquito bites may produce swelling and intense itching that can last for 3 to 4 days. Dr. Frazier recommends the following to control these symptoms.

- An oral antihistamine (Choose an over-the-counter allergy or cold preparation.)
- Calamine lotion
- Ice packs
- Salt (Moisten it into a paste with water and apply it to the bite.)
- Baking soda (Dissolve 1 teaspoon in a glass of water. Dip a cloth into the solution and place on the bite for 15 to 20 minutes.)
- Epsom salts (Dissolve 1 tablespoon in 1 quart of hot water. Chill, then apply as above.)

**Practice prevention.** The hotter the weather is, the more active flies and mosquitoes seem to be. Mosquitoes, in particular, are at their worst in damp areas, such as near ponds or in marshes. Some species are especially pesky late in the day and are attracted to outdoor lighting after dark. So don't let your guard down at sunset. You may be able to avoid a bite in the first place by using the repellents below.

**DEET.** Dr. Frazier recommends any commercial repellent containing N,N-diethyl-m-toluamide (DEET). Apply generously over all exposed skin, but be careful around the eyes—it can sting badly if perspiration carries it into the eyes. Don't use insect repellents under clothing either. And make sure DEET-containing repellents used on children don't contain more than 10 percent DEET. The chemical, absorbed through the skin, can be harmful to children. Also, don't allow children to handle insect repellents, and don't apply repellent to a child's hands. Instead, apply it to your hands, then rub it on the child's skin.

**Chlorine bleach.** Dr. Luscombe recommends bathing in a very diluted solution of chlorine bleach before going outside. Mix two capfuls of bleach in a tub of warm water. Soak in it for 15 minutes. Be very careful not to get the solution near or in your eyes. The repellent effect should last several hours.

**Bath oil.** Certain bath oils, such as Alpha-Keri and Avon's Skin-So-Soft, have a repellent effect, Dr. Luscombe says.

**Vicks VapoRub.** Some people report success with this strong-smelling ointment, says Dr. Luscombe.

## Ticks

Because they transmit Lyme disease, ticks are Insect Public Enemy Number One. Named in 1977 after doctors discovered arthritis in a cluster of children in and near Lyme, Connecticut, the disease can trigger a rash, fever, fatigue, headache, muscle aches, and painful joints.

Here's what you need to know so you're prepared.

**Be vigilant.** Although June and July seem to mark the height of tick season, ticks are a danger from early spring until fall. If you're spending any time outdoors, especially in wooded or high-grass areas—even grassy dunes—take the following precautions.

- To discover if there are ticks in an area, tie a piece of white flannel to a string and drag it through the grass or underbrush. Examine it frequently. If ticks are present, they cling to the cloth, says Dr. Frazier.
- If you're in a tick area, leave as little skin exposed as possible, says Joseph Benforado, M.D. Wear long pants, high socks, and long sleeves.
- Consider a Lyme disease vaccination if you're sometimes or often exposed to tick-infested areas.
- Before going to bed at night, Dr. Benforado adds, inspect your body for any freeloading ticks. Certain species can be quite small, and you might otherwise overlook them.

**Ease it out.** Ticks pose a special problem because they dig into your skin and hold on for dear life. Trying to brush away a tick as you would a fly has no ef-

## When the Itsy Bitsy Spider Turns Nasty

Little Miss Muffet was no sissy—she was just savvy enough not to risk a spider bite. Basically, says paramedic Jeff Rusteen, all spiders are poisonous. It's just that most of them aren't big enough or powerful enough to penetrate the skin and do much harm.

If you do get bitten, follow this advice from Claude Frazier, M.D.

- Wash the wound and disinfect it with an antiseptic.
- Apply an ice pack to slow absorption of the venom.
- Neutralize some of the poison by moistening the bite with water and rubbing in an aspirin tablet, adds Herbert Luscombe, M.D. Skip this tip if you're allergic to aspirin.

Beware, a black widow spider bite can cause intense abdominal pain that could be confused with appendicitis. Let your doctor know you've been bitten so that she can administer injections of calcium gluconate, says Dr. Luscombe.

A bite from a brown recluse spider might also produce problems, he adds. If an intensely sore lump develops (sometimes weeks after the injury), consult your doctor.

fect. And forcefully plucking it out may leave its mouthparts embedded, setting the stage for infection. So use a gentler approach: Dr. Luscombe recommends taking a pair of tweezers and very slowly pulling the tick out. "Don't pull too fast," he cautions.

**Clean up.** Once you've removed the tick, wash the bite area with soap and water, says Dr. Frazier. Then apply iodine or another antiseptic to guard against infection.

## Dogs and Cats

When it comes to animal bites, anyone can become a victim. Between half a million to 1 million people seek medical attention for dog bites each year, and countless other bites go unreported and untreated, according to the American Veterinary Medical Association. Here's what to do if you are bitten.

**Assess the damage.** Seek medical help for all but the most minor wounds, say doctors.

**Thoroughly wash the bite.** Animal bites—especially from cats—may transmit infections, says public-health expert Stephen Rosenberg, M.D. He advises cleansing the wound thoroughly with soap and water to remove saliva and any other contamination. Wash for 5 full minutes.

**Control bleeding.** If there is any minor bleeding, cover the entire wound with thick sterile gauze or a clean cloth pad, says Dr. Rosenberg. If you have no appropriate bandage, thoroughly cleanse your hand and press it firmly against the wound. You may also put some ice against the pad (not directly on the skin) and elevate the wound above heart level to help stop bleeding.

**Bandage the area.** When the bleeding has stopped, says Dr. Rosenberg, cover the bite with a sterile bandage or clean cloth. Tie or tape it loosely in place.

**Reduce pain.** Use aspirin or acetaminophen to reduce pain, says paramedic Jeff Rusteen. This is appropriate even if the bite did not break the skin. Elevate the area and apply ice if there is any swelling.

**Get a tetanus shot.** Any animal bite can lead to tetanus, says Dr. Rosenberg. If you haven't had a booster shot within the last 5 to 8 years, get one now.

**Treat the wound.** Apply antibiotic ointment to the wound two times a day until it heals.

# WHEN TO CALL A DOCTOR

Any bite could develop complications. Stay alert for these potential problems.

*Infection.* Examine the wound periodically, says paramedic Jeff Rusteen. If it gets red, painful, or hot, infection has probably developed. Get professional help.

*Rabies.* All warm-blooded animals can carry rabies, says Stephen Rosenberg, M.D. If you're bitten, contact the animal's owner to see whether its rabies shots are up-to-date. Rabies treatment may be safely delayed as long as the animal shows no symptoms, he says, providing the bite was not too severe or too close to the head. Because of the danger of rabies, you may be required to report all bites to the authorities, he adds. Check with your state or local health department.

Bats are increasingly transmitters of rabies to people. The Centers for Disease Control recommend that you seek medical help if you awaken to find a bat in your room or have come into contact with a bat in any way, even if you can't see a bat bite or scratch.

*Rocky Mountain spotted fever.* If you're bitten by a tick, keep an eye out for a rash around your wrists or ankles that spreads to the rest of your body, says Herbert Luscombe, M.D. A high fever and terrible headaches can follow. These symptoms indicate Rocky Mountain spotted fever, which can be deadly. See a doctor immediately.

*Lyme disease.* The first sign of Lyme disease is often a characteristic bull's-eye rash accompanied by a fever. The time between a tick's bite and the first sign of symptoms is typically 7 to 14 days but may be as short as 3 days or as long as a month. Keep an eye on the area where you were bitten, Dr. Luscombe advises.

*Crush injury.* Sometimes a large dog, such as a German shepherd, will bite without breaking the skin. If you can see bite marks on both sides of an extremity, there may be internal damage, says Rusteen. If tingling develops or if the extremity changes color (turns blue, for instance), there may be structural damage. Get to a hospital or call the paramedics.

*Bites to the head, hand, or foot.* If a dog bites you in any of these places or if the wound is deep and gaping, call a doctor.

*Cat bites.* Cat bites are particularly prone to infection and warrant a call to the doctor. If you're just *scratched* by a cat, don't call a doctor unless you suspect that the wound is infected.

*Preexisting chronic disease.* If you have diabetes, lung disease, liver disease, cancer, AIDS, or any condition that makes it hard for you to fight infection, see a doctor.

# Insect Stings

Compared to insects, we're far outnumbered. If you happen to make one of them angry enough to sting you, here's what do to.

Bees, wasps, and their kin inject venom into the skin when they sting. That leads to pain, redness, and swelling at the site of the sting. Discomfort can last from several hours to a day, depending on what stings you and how many insects attack.

**Identify your attacker.** Knowing which insect did the damage can provide a clue to treatment—and help you avoid more stings. A honeybee, which has a fuzzy, golden-brown body, can sting only once. That's because its barbed stinger remains embedded in your skin. Without the stinger, the bee dies.

Bumblebees, wasps, hornets, and yellow jackets, on the other hand, have smooth stingers that can zap you repeatedly. So be prepared to flee.

Yellow jackets pose an additional problem. Smashing one of them can lead to a full-scale attack by its nest mates. That's because breaking its venom sac releases a chemical that incites other yellow jackets to attack.

**Act fast.** The key to effective treatment is quick action. The faster you apply some sort of first-aid treatment, the better your chances of controlling pain and swelling.

**Remove the stinger.** If it was a honeybee that got you, remove the stinger as soon as possible. Otherwise, the venom sac attached to it will continue to pump for 2 to 3 minutes, driving the stinger and its poison deeper into your skin. But be careful not to squeeze the stinger or the sac—doing so will release more poison into your system.

## WHEN TO CALL A DOCTOR

Bee stings cause more deaths than snakebites, says Herbert Luscombe, M.D. A normal bee sting produces pain for a brief time and swelling that usually lessens in a few hours. But more severe symptoms may indicate an allergy, which can lead to deadly anaphylactic shock. Be on the lookout for chest tightness, hives, nausea, vomiting, wheezing, hoarseness, dizziness, swollen tongue or face, fainting, or shock. The more rapidly symptoms appear, the more life-threatening they are.

If these symptoms appear, says Claude Frazier, M.D., use an insect sting kit as directed. Then rush the victim to the nearest hospital or physician. If no kit is available, apply an ice pack, if possible, and rush the victim to help.

"Scraping the stinger out is the best approach," says insect expert Edgar Raffensperger, Ph.D. Use your fingernail, a nail file, or even the edge of a credit card to gently scrape under the stinger and flip it out.

**Cleanse the area.** Bees and their brethren are scavengers, just like flies and mosquitoes, so they often carry undesirable bacteria in their venom, says Rusteen. Wash the sting well with soap and water or an antiseptic.

**Relieve the pain.** At this point, your wound is still throbbing, so you want to deaden the pain *fast*. The following substances are effective—but for them to work, you must act quickly after being stung.

*Cold.* An ice pack, or even just an ice cube, placed over the sting can cut down on swelling and keep the venom from spreading, says Dr. Luscombe.

*Heat.* Ironically, says Dr. Luscombe, heat can also make you feel better by neutralizing one of the chemicals that causes inflammation. Take a hair dryer and aim it at your sting.

*Aspirin.* One of the simplest, most effective things you can do, says Dr. Luscombe, is to apply aspirin. Moisten the sting, then rub an aspirin tablet into it. The aspirin neutralizes certain inflammatory agents in the venom. Don't try this if you're allergic to aspirin.

*Baking soda.* Dr. Frazier recommends applying a paste of baking soda and water.

*Meat tenderizer.* "An enzyme-based meat tenderizer, such as Adolph's or McCormick's, breaks down the proteins that make up insect venom," says David Golden, M.D. You have to use it right away for it to be effective, however.

*Activated charcoal.* "A paste of powdered activated charcoal will draw the poison out very quickly, so the sting won't swell or hurt," according to Richard Hansen, M.D. Carefully open a few charcoal capsules and remove the powder. Moisten it with water and apply it to the sting. The charcoal works best if it stays moist, so cover it with gauze or plastic wrap.

*Mud.* If you don't have anything else handy, says Dr. Hansen, you can mix a little clay soil and water into a mud paste. Apply as you would the charcoal, cover with a bandage or handkerchief, and leave it on until the mud dries.

**Take an antihistamine.** An over-the-counter oral antihistamine may help relieve pain. In classes he teaches, Rusteen often advises parents to give their children an antihistamine-containing cough syrup, such as Benylin. "The antihistamine helps sedate the child a little and also lessens the swelling, throbbing, and redness caused by the insect venom. Adults can benefit from this treatment, too," he says.

**Don't get stung in the first place.** A bit of prevention can save you a lot of anguish later. Here's how to minimize your chances of getting stung.

*Wear white.* Stinging insects prefer dark colors, says Dr. Raffensperger. That's why beekeepers generally wear khaki, white, or other light colors.

*Don't smell too good.* Avoid perfume, aftershave, or any other fragrance that will lead a bee to confuse you with a nectar-bearing flower, adds Dr. Raffensperger.

*Oil up.* Certain bath oils can repel stinging insects, says Dr. Luscombe. Skin-So-Soft from Avon and Alpha-Keri have helped a lot of people. Rub the oil onto exposed skin before going out.

*Run for shelter.* If you're being pursued by a buzzing horde, run indoors, jump into water, or head for the woods. Stinging insects have trouble following their prey through a thicket of woods, say researchers at the Cornell University Cooperative Extension Service.

*Take up painting.* As a last resort, you might become a painter. Housepainters rarely get stung, says Dr. Luscombe, because the turpentine they use repels stinging insects.

## PANEL OF ADVISORS

**Joseph Benforado, M.D.,** is a professor emeritus of medicine at the University of Wisconsin–Madison and past vice president of the U.S. Pharmacopoeia, which sets American drug standards.

**Claude Frazier, M.D.,** is an allergist in Asheville, North Carolina.

**David Golden, M.D.,** is an associate professor of medicine at Johns Hopkins University in Baltimore.

**Richard Hansen, M.D.,** is past medical director of the Poland Spring Health Institute in Poland Spring, Maine. He is the author of *Get Well at Home*.

**Herbert Luscombe, M.D.,** is a professor emeritus of dermatology at Jefferson Medical College of Thomas Jefferson University in Philadelphia. He is also formerly senior attending dermatologist at Thomas Jefferson University Hospital, also in Philadelphia.

**Edgar Raffensperger, Ph.D.,** is a professor emeritus of entomology in the department of entomology at Cornell University in Ithaca, New York.

**Stephen Rosenberg, M.D.,** is an associate professor of clinical public health at Columbia University School of Public Health in New York City. He is the author of *The Johnson & Johnson First-Aid Book.*

**Jeff Rusteen** is a firefighter-paramedic with the Piedmont Fire Department in Piedmont, California. He teaches emergency medical technology at Chabot College in Hayward.

**George Shambaugh Jr., M.D.,** is a professor emeritus of otolaryngology and head and neck surgery at Northwestern University Medical School in Chicago, a medical otologist and allergist in Hinsdale, and a member of the staff at Hinsdale Hospital. He writes a health and nutrition newsletter that he sends to his patients.

# BLACK EYE
## 8 Ways to Clear Up the Bruise

"Black eye" is somewhat of a misnomer. "Very dark blue eye" or "rainbow-of-color eye" would be better. Whether you've run into a door frame or gotten punched, blood instantly fills this plentiful space under your eye. Since the skin is so thin, the pooled blood beneath is readily seen as a very dark blue. Over the week most black eyes take to heal, the blood is slowly reabsorbed into the body, evolving into a kaleidoscope of colors that actually signifies healing.

Throughout the centuries, there have been a host of wild and sundry treatments for black eyes, ranging from leeches to liver to raw-steak compresses. They all share the same goal: to reduce swelling. But, it turns out, there are plenty of efficient ways to achieve that objective in a less disgusting manner. Here are some to try.

**Pack it in ice.** A cold pack keeps the swelling down and, by constricting the blood vessels, helps decrease the internal bleeding.

Jack Jeffers, M.D., recommends applying an ice pack for the first 24 to 48 hours. "If your eye is swollen shut, use it for 10 minutes every 2 hours the first day," he advises. To make an ice pack for the eye, put crushed ice in a plastic bag and tape it to the forehead. This keeps the ice from putting pressure on the eye.

## WHEN TO CALL A DOCTOR

Black eyes shouldn't be taken lightly, since they can involve serious internal eye injuries, including retinal detachment and internal hemorrhages that may not be evident at first.

"I think every patient with a black eye should be examined at an emergency room or by an ophthalmologist," says Anne Sumers, M.D. "Many times, serious complications will have no symptoms."

Dr. Sumers warns against trying to irrigate or rinse an injured eye or prying a swollen eye open.

Until you can see a doctor, she recommends applying ice packs, then protecting the eye by cutting off the bottom of a cup and taping the disk to uninjured skin, making sure that neither the disk nor the tape comes into contact with the eye itself.

If you have difficulty seeing, you need medical attention immediately, says Keith Sivertson, M.D. Here is his list of other red-alert symptoms: pain in the eye, sensitivity to light, blurred or double vision, or the sensation of objects floating through your field of vision.

**Try what boxers use.** When a professional fighter gets a shiner, trainers apply what looks like a small, metal iron, says David J. Smith, M.D. "It is extremely cold, and they use it to control the immediate hemorrhage so that the swelling is minimized. You can use the same sort of treatment by getting a cold soda can and holding it against the eye intermittently (5 to 10 minutes of every 15 minutes) until you can get some ice on it," he says. "Make sure the can is clean and then hold it lightly against your cheek, not your eye. Do not put any pressure on your eyeball."

**Go for green ice.** Parsley, an old gypsy remedy for bruising, has anti-inflammatory and anesthetic properties. And doctors recommend ice for treating bruises, because it causes blood vessels to narrow, which reduces swelling. To make this remedy, combine a cup of fresh parsley with about 2 tablespoons of water, whisk it into a fine slurry in the blender, and freeze the mixture in an ice cube tray. Wrap the cubes in a soft cloth before applying them to your eye socket for 15 to 20 minutes.

**Apply vitamin K.** Applied to moistened skin, 1 to 5 percent vitamin K cream can speed healing, promote blood clotting, and reduce the swelling of a bruise, says Melvin Elson, M.D. Use it twice a day or once at night. It's available in most drugstores.

**Turn to a botanical.** Herbal experts recommend both creams and gels made from the bright flowers of the arnica plant, and bromelain tablets, made from an enzyme found in pineapple, as remedies for bruises. You can find these products in health food stores.

**Be patient.** Once the eye bruises, there's not a whole lot you can do except control the swelling. Even makeup can't disguise it totally, although a good foundation will help once any cuts heal, says Anne Sumers, M.D.

**Avoid aspirin.** Aspirin is bad news for black eyes. "Aspirin is an anticoagulant, meaning the blood won't clot as well. You'll have a harder time stopping the bleeding that causes the discoloration," says Dr. Jeffers. "You may wind up with a bigger bruise." If, for some reason, you need to take a pain reliever, take acetaminophen.

**Don't blow your nose.** If a severe blow caused your black eye (something more than just bumping into a door), blowing your nose could cause your whole face to swell. "Sometimes the injury fractures the bone of the eye socket, and blowing your nose can force air out of your sinus adjacent to the socket," says Dr. Jeffers. "The air gets injected under your skin and makes the eyelids swell even more. It also can increase the chance of infection."

## PANEL OF ADVISORS

**Melvin Elson, M.D.,** is a dermatologist and president of Integrative Aesthetics in Nashville.

**Jack Jeffers, M.D.,** is an ophthalmologist and director of emergency services at the Sports Center for Vision at Wills Eye Hospital in Philadelphia.

**Keith Sivertson, M.D.,** is director of the department of emergency medicine at Johns Hopkins Hospital in Baltimore.

**David J. Smith, M.D.,** is an ophthalmologist in Ventnor City, New Jersey, and a member of the Medical Advisory Council of the State Athletic Control Board of the State of New Jersey. He is also on the medical team at the Sports Center for Vision at Wills Eye Hospital in Philadelphia. He has examined more than 300 boxers for eye injuries.

**Anne Sumers, M.D.,** is team ophthalmologist for the New York Giants and the New Jersey Nets in addition to operating an ophthalmology practice in Ridgewood, New Jersey. She serves as spokesperson for the American Academy of Ophthalmology.

# BLISTERS
## 18 Hints to Stop the Hurt

Blisters are your body's way of saying it's had enough. Be it too much friction or too much ambition, a blister—much like a muscle cramp or a side stitch—is designed to slow you down and make you better prepared for physical activity.

Though the following remedies concentrate on blisters of the feet, many of these recommendations can be applied to friction blisters on the hands or any other part of the anatomy where your body has said "slow down."

### Blister Treatment

Here's how experts recommend you deal with the discomfort of blisters you already have.

**Make a decision.** Once you have a blister, you have to decide what's best to do with it. That is, should you protect it and leave it alone, or should you prick it and drain the fluid?

"I think it depends on the size of the blister," says Suzanne Tanner, M.D. "A

---

### WHEN TO CALL A DOCTOR

"Head to the doctor at the first sign of infection," warns Nancy Lu Conrad, D.P.M.

"A good rule of thumb is that most wounds, no matter what they are, should get better each day," adds Clare Starrett, D.P.M. That rule holds for blisters as well, she says, noting that the classical signs of infection are redness, swelling, heat, and increased pain.

"A blister is definitely infected when the fluid coming from it is not clear like water or when it has some odor to it," adds Dr. Starrett. "That's the time to seek professional help."

"If a blister gives me pain," says Joseph Ellis, D.P.M., "I just go ahead and pop it." Use a sterilized needle and stick it in the side of the blister, he says. "Just make sure the hole's big enough so you can squeeze out all the fluid."

purist will probably tell you not to prick it, because then you don't run any risk of infection. But I think for most people that's just not very practical."

While purists do indeed exist, our experts say that you should prick large, painful blisters while leaving smaller, painless blisters intact. "When you have a big blister that's in a weight-bearing area, you almost have to drain it," says podiatrist Clare Starrett, D.P.M. "They can get so full that they get like a balloon."

Also, blisters likely to break on their own should be drained, our experts say. That way, you can control when and how the blister is opened, instead of leaving it to chance.

**Make a moleskin doughnut.** If you decide not to drain the blister, one way to protect it is to cut a moleskin pad into a doughnut shape and place it over the blister. "Leave the central area open where the blister is," says Dr. Tanner. The surrounding moleskin will absorb most of the shock and friction of everyday activity. As long as the skin is clean and dry, the moleskin will adhere by itself.

**Be wise and sterilize.** If you choose to drain a blister, first clean the blister and surrounding skin and sterilize your "instrument," be it a needle or razor blade. "I recommend alcohol to clean both," says podiatrist Nancy Lu Conrad, D.P.M.

Other doctors advise sterilizing your instrument by flame instead of alcohol. Simply heat the needle or razor blade with a match until it glows red. Then let it cool before touching it to your skin. Either method seems equally able to kill germs, and each is equally recommended.

**Keep the roof on.** Once you drain your blister, experts recommend leaving on the roof—the skin that goes over the top of the blister. "I think the biggest mistake most people make when treating their own blisters is that after they drain it, they pull off the roof. This is a terrible mistake," says Richard Cowin, D.P.M. Think of the roof as nature's bandage.

"If you remove it, you're going to end up with a very red, raw, sore area," says Dr. Cowin. "But if you leave it on, it'll eventually harden up and fall off by itself, significantly reducing your recovery time."

**Try a triple whammy for germs.** Research finds that triple antibiotics (such as Neosporin) can eliminate bacterial contamination from blisters after only two treatments, whereas old standbys such as iodine and camphor-phenol actually delay healing. Iodine and camphor-phenol are so good at killing germs that when used in high concentrations they can even kill the cells you are trying to heal, says Dr. Starrett.

**Keep the dressing simple.** After you've treated the blister, you'll need to keep it covered and protected while it heals. Though gauze pads and special bandages may be the first thing you'd expect a podiatrist to reach for, our experts suggest a much simpler approach.

"My first choice is a simple adhesive bandage," says Dr. Cowin.

Gauze pads, however, are recommended for blisters that are just too big for an adhesive bandage to cover. Keep them in place with waterproof adhesive tape.

**Use Second Skin for a second wind.** If you've treated and covered your blister and find that you just can't wait for it to completely heal before returning to an active lifestyle, then you'll need to know about Spenco's Second Skin dressing, a spongy material that absorbs pressure and reduces friction against blisters and surrounding skin.

"That's a good product," says Dr. Conrad, noting that a number of athletes (weekend and otherwise) apply petroleum jelly to a blister before covering it with Second Skin and taping it in place.

**Give it some air.** Most doctors suggest removing the dressing nightly to let the blister get some air. "Air and water are very good for healing," says Dr. Cowin, "so soaking it in water and keeping it open to the air at night is helpful."

**Change wet dressings.** Though some physicians say that you can leave a dressing on for 2 days without worry, all agree that if a dressing becomes wet for any reason, it should be replaced. That means you may need to change it quite often if your feet perspire heavily or if you engage in activities that will lead to sweating and damp dressings.

## Blister Prevention

Prevention is always the best option, so here's what experts recommend to keep blisters from developing in the first place.

**Try a heel lift.** Blisters that appear on the back of the foot usually result from the shoe's heel counter hitting the back of the heel in the wrong area, says Dr. Cowin. The fix? "All you usually have to do is put in a heel lift at the back of the shoe," he says.

# Cotton Up to Acrylic Socks

There's a major debate raging in the sock world that could have far-reaching consequences for millions of blister-footed Americans—weekend walkers and Olympic marathoners alike. The cause of the "friction" among foot care specialists is a study showing that acrylic socks may actually be better at preventing blisters than socks made of cotton or other natural fibers.

For years, most podiatrists recommended natural fibers and materials (think cotton socks and leather shoes).

But research now shows that cotton socks produce twice as many blisters in runners as acrylic socks and that the blisters formed by cotton socks are usually three times as big as those produced by their acrylic counterparts.

"As a veteran long-distance runner and someone who treats runners for blisters every day, the results don't surprise me in the least," says study author Douglas Richie Jr., D.P.M. "I'm well aware that cotton fiber becomes abrasive with repeated use and that it also loses its shape when wet. The shape of a sock is critical when it's inside a shoe."

"Many people equate acrylic with a silky, nylonlike fiber," he says, "yet spun acrylic feels exactly like cotton and maintains its soft, bouncy feeling even when wet."

According to Dr. Richie, other synthetic fibers, such as polypropylene and polyester, can work as well as acrylic fibers in keeping the foot warm and dry.

And the nonblistering property of synthetic fiber holds true for any type of sporting activity, be it walking, running, tennis, and so forth, he says.

**Keep your socks on.** As a general rule, avoid sock-free fashions. "The people who do this suffer blisters on the back of their heels all the time," says Dr. Cowin. He recommends that those who want to flash some ankle without suffering the consequences invest in "footie-type socks that only go around the foot area."

**Powder daily.** "Powder should be everybody's friend," says Dr. Conrad. "Make powdering your feet part of a daily routine."

"When people come in with shoes that fit but that still give them blisters," says Dr. Cowin, "I simply tell them to start off by applying baby powder to their feet before putting on their socks. This helps the sock to glide over the foot a little more and prevent blisters."

**Coat to protect.** If you're planning a long walk, run, tennis match, or whatever, one way to guard against blistered feet in new shoes is to coat blister-prone areas with petroleum jelly. "That will cut down on friction," says Dr. Conrad.

Joseph Ellis, D.P.M., says that A&D Ointment (typically used for diaper rash) is actually thicker than petroleum jelly. "The thicker the better," he says. For walkers or runners who insist on going without socks, greasing up blister-prone areas is highly recommended.

**Try new socks for new shoes.** "If you have a new pair of shoes that are rubbing up blisters, the first thing I'd do is change to different socks," says Dr. Ellis. "I recommend acrylic socks (available in sporting goods stores) because they're made in layers designed to absorb friction so your foot doesn't."

**Treat your feet to treated insoles.** Our experts agree that many of the products made by Spenco are excellent for preventing blisters. One of the best is a chemically treated insole "that has bubbled-in nitrogen," explains Dr. Cowin. "What that does is add some cushioning to the bottom of the foot and help it glide over the bottom of the shoe better, instead of sticking in places and causing a blister."

**Beware the terrible tube.** While tube socks, those unformed heelless wonders you can slip into without thinking, can be tempting to wear, our experts advise against them. "I personally don't believe in tube socks," says Dr. Cowin. "I don't think they ever fit properly. You need a regular, fitted sock to help prevent blisters."

## PANEL OF ADVISORS

**Nancy Lu Conrad, D.P.M.,** is a private practitioner in Circleville, Ohio. She specializes in footwear for children as well as in sports medicine and orthopedics.

**Richard M. Cowin, D.P.M.,** is a private practitioner and director of Advanced Foot Surgery in Lady Lake, Florida, where he specializes in the practice of minimal incision and laser foot and ankle surgery. He is a diplomate of the American Board of Podiatric Surgery and the American Board of Ambulatory Foot Surgery.

**Joseph Ellis, D.P.M.,** is a private practitioner in La Jolla, California. He is a consultant for the University of California, San Diego, and is the sports medicine consultant for the Asics-Tiger running shoe company.

**Douglas Richie Jr., D.P.M.,** is a sports podiatrist in Seal Beach, California, where he studies the function of socks and their effect on sporting activities. He also is a director of the American Academy of Podiatric Sports Medicine.

**Clare Starrett, D.P.M.,** is a professor at the Temple University School of Podiatric Medicine in Philadelphia.

**Suzanne Tanner, M.D.,** is a private practitioner in Denver, who specializes in sports medicine.

# BODY ODOR
## 10 Ways to Feel Fresh and Clean

Some scientists believe that body odor is a vestige of our evolution. That is, the smells we give off from certain areas of our bodies, primarily our armpits and groin, may have once served to advertise our sexuality, says Nathan Howe, M.D., Ph.D. "Of course," he adds, "whatever purpose was served by body odor then is plain objectionable now."

About this last point there is little disagreement. If you want people to want to be around you, don't stink.

Easier said than done? Actually, there are quite a few ways to take on body odor and come up smelling like a rose.

**Scrub-a-dub-dub.** The most basic way to hold body odor at bay is to scrub yourself with soap and water, particularly in those areas of the body most likely to smell, such as the armpits and groin, says Kenzo Sato, M.D.

Body odor is most often caused by a combination of perspiration and bacteria, he says. Scrubbing with soap and water washes both culprits away.

The best type of soap for a body odor problem is a deodorant soap because it hinders the return of bacteria. How often you need to scrub depends on your individual body chemistry, your activities, your mood, and the time of year. If you're not sure if you're washing enough, ask a friend. Remember that perspiration glands and bacteria work night as well as day shifts, which could mean you need to shower both morning and night.

## WHEN TO CALL A DOCTOR

Frequent, heavy sweating can be more than embarrassing. It can be a sign that you have an overactive thyroid or low blood sugar. You may also have an abnormality in the part of the nervous system that controls sweating. In any case, check with your doctor.

**Wash more than your body.** You can wash till your skin puckers like a prune, but you'll still smell bad if your clothes aren't clean. Seven days in the same undershirt is a sure way to give offense to others, says Lenise Banse, M.D. How often do you need to change into a fresh shirt? It depends on you as an individual. A daily change should suffice for most. On hot summer days, more than once a day might be in order.

**Choose natural fabrics.** Natural fabrics such as cotton absorb perspiration better than synthetic materials. The absorbed sweat is then free to evaporate from the fabric.

**Play doctor.** Sometimes, if you perspire a lot and have a tendency to smell bad, regular old deodorant soap may not be good enough. In this case, try an antibacterial surgical scrub, sold over the counter in most drugstores, says Dr. Howe.

**Antiperspirants attack best.** Commercial deodorants are effective at masking underarm odor in most people, says Hridaya Bhargava, Ph.D. They leave chemicals on the skin that kill odor-causing bacteria, but they don't control perspiration. So if you have a strong body odor, you may need an antiperspirant. They're basically drugs, he says, that reduce the amount of perspiration the body produces. Most commercial antiperspirants combine antiperspirant with deodorant.

**Don't get irritated.** If you can't use commercial deodorants or antiperspirants without developing a rash, try a topical antibiotic cream, sold in any drugstore. "It does the same thing as deodorants do, without any irritating perfumes," says Randall Hrabko, M.D.

**Make the French connection.** Another option if you can't tolerate common deodorants and antiperspirants is a product from France called Le Crystal Naturel, says Dr. Hrabko. It's a chunk of mineral salts, formed into a crystal, which helps keep bacteria under control without irritating the skin. Le Crystal Naturel, a product of the Burlingame, California–based French Transit company, is available in many cosmetic departments and health food stores.

**Take a walk on the wild side.** Forget the latest perfumes and take a cue instead from hunters. The name of the game in hunting, according to some, is to mask all trace of body odor lest the deer or bear being stalked catch wind of trouble and flee for cover.

How do hunters do it? One popular odor mask is pine soap, available in most hunting supply stores, says Dave Petzal, a veteran hunter and the managing editor of *Field and Stream* magazine. Pine soap not only masks human odor but also leaves you smelling like a pine forest, he says. If pine forest isn't your style, some hunters use plain old glycerin soap.

**Watch what you eat.** Extracts of proteins and oils from certain foods and spices remain in your body's excretions and secretions for hours after eating them and can impart an odor. Fish, cumin, curry, and garlic lead the list, says Dr. Banse.

**Keep calm.** "Getting sexually excited or feeling anxious and nervous will make you perspire more," says Dr. Bhargava. If you anticipate a situation that is likely to upset you, no matter how much you're meditating or practicing deep breathing, consider using an extra dose of deodorant that morning.

## PANEL OF ADVISORS

**Lenise Banse, M.D.,** is a dermatologist in Clinton Township, Michigan, where she is director of the Northeast Family Dermatology Center. She has special expertise in cutaneous oncology as well as cosmetic dermatology.

**Hridaya Bhargava, Ph.D.,** is a professor of industrial pharmacy at the Massachusetts College of Pharmacy in Boston. He is a consultant to groups such as the World Health Organization and UNICEF.

**Nathan Howe, M.D., Ph.D.,** is formerly a physician in the department of dermatology at the Medical University of South Carolina College of Medicine in Charleston. He was also a zoologist with a special interest in how animals communicate using chemical smells.

**Randall Hrabko, M.D.,** is a dermatologist in Los Angeles.

**Dave Petzal** is a veteran hunter and the managing editor of *Field and Stream* magazine.

**Kenzo Sato, M.D.,** is a professor emeritus of dermatology at the University of Iowa in Iowa City.

# BOILS
## 8 Tips to Stop an Infection

A boil, also called an abscess, is an infection deep inside the skin that produces redness, pain, swelling, and pus.

Boils generally develop when staphylococcus bacteria invade the body through a break in the skin, a blocked sweat gland, or an ingrown hair. The body's immune system sends in white blood cells, which collect as pus, to fight the bacteria. A pus-filled abscess begins to grow beneath the skin surface, rising up red with pain. Sometimes the body reabsorbs the boil; other times the boil swells to an eruption before it drains and subsides.

Boils are uncomfortable and unsightly. Sometimes they leave scars. Occasionally, they can even be dangerous. But for the most part, you can treat them safely at home. Here's how.

## WHEN TO CALL A DOCTOR

Some boils warrant medical care. If bacteria from a boil get into your bloodstream, it can cause blood poisoning. Don't squeeze a boil around your lips or nose because the infection can be carried to the brain. Other danger zones are the armpits, groin, and the breast of a nursing woman.

See your doctor if you are prone to recurrent boils in your armpit or groin. These abscesses may need to be treated with antibiotics.

Also, if the boil is extremely tender or under thick skin like that on your back or if the person with the boil is very young, very old, or sick, have a doctor treat it, says Rodney Basler, M.D. If there are any red lines radiating from it or if you feel any symptoms like fever and chills or swelling of lymph nodes, he adds, see a doctor because the infection may have spread.

People with diabetes are especially prone to such dangerous boils, Adrian Connolly, M.D., says, and may need a course of antibiotics. Sometimes recurrent boils can be symptoms of more serious diseases.

**Apply heat.** "Applying a warm compress is the very best thing you can do for a boil," says Rodney Basler, M.D. The heat will cause the boil to form a head, drain, and heal a lot faster.

At the first sign of a boil, place a warm, wet washcloth over it for 20 to 30 minutes three or four times a day. Change it a few times during each session to keep it warm. It's not uncommon for it to take 5 to 7 days until the boil breaks on its own, he says.

**Prevent a recurrence.** It's important to continue the warm compresses for 3 days after the boil breaks, Dr. Basler says. You have to drain all that pus out of the tissues. You may also want to bandage it to keep it clean, but it's not critical. "A bandage is mainly to keep the drainage off your clothes," he adds.

**Lance the lesion.** When the boil has come to a pus-filled head, if it's a small boil with no sign of spreading infection, you may want to break it on your own so that you can choose when and where it breaks. Letting the boil break on its own can create more of a mess, because it often breaks while you're sleeping. To lance the boil, simply sterilize a needle with a flame, make a small nick in the head, and squeeze gently.

While some doctors worry that squeezing can drive the infection deeper into the skin, thus spreading it through the lymph system, in reality that rarely happens, says Dr. Basler. "In the office, we just squeeze the dickens out of them."

> ## Cures from the Kitchen
>
> Folklore has it that home remedies for boils are as close as your vegetable bin. All the following, recommended by Michael Blate, cofounder of the G-Jo Institute, are variations of the warm-washcloth compress described in the beginning of the chapter. They should be wrapped in a thin cloth and changed every few hours.
>
> - A heated slice of tomato
> - A raw onion slice
> - Mashed garlic
> - The outer leaves of cabbage
> - A bag of black tea

**Use antiseptic if you want.** It's not really necessary to treat an opened boil with an antiseptic, because the infection is localized, Dr. Basler says. "The important thing is to keep it draining."

But Adrian Connolly, M.D., recommends an over-the-counter antibiotic ointment like Polysporin or Neosporin as insurance against spreading the infection.

**Keep it localized.** When a boil is draining, keep the skin around it clean, Dr. Connolly says. Take showers instead of baths to reduce the rare chance of spreading the infection to other parts of the body. After treating a boil, wash your hands well before preparing food because staph bacteria can cause food poisoning.

**Set the stage for prevention.** If you're prone to boils, you may be able to reduce their frequency, Dr. Connolly says, by cleaning your skin with an antiseptic cleanser like Betadine to keep the staph population down.

**Ignore cysts.** Boils are usually cysts (uninfected, fluid-filled mass) that have become infected. "Monkeying with a cyst is the surest way to get a boil," Dr. Basler says. Leave cysts alone or have them excised by a doctor.

## PANEL OF ADVISORS

**Rodney Basler, M.D.,** is a dermatologist and assistant professor of internal medicine at the University of Nebraska College of Medicine in Lincoln.

**Michael Blate** is founder and executive director of the G-Jo Institute of Columbus, North Carolina, a natural health organization that promotes acupressure and oriental traditional medicine.

**Adrian Connolly, M.D.,** is a dermatologist/Mohs surgeon in private practice in West Orange, New Jersey, and a member of the American Academy of Dermatology.

# BREAST DISCOMFORT
## 18 Hints to Reduce Soreness

Benign breast changes may be as bewildering as they are uncomfortable, but they are not unusual. An estimated 70 percent of North American women experience breast discomfort at some point in their lives, often during pregnancy and before menstruation.

This tenderness occurs because of the natural cycles of the reproductive hormones, estrogen and progesterone. These hormones trigger cell growth in the milk-producing glands, which requires nourishment from blood and other fluids that fill the surrounding areas. These fluid-logged tissues can stretch nerve fibers, causing pain and tenderness.

## WHEN TO CALL A DOCTOR

Whenever you find a lump during your monthly self-examination, consult your physician—whether or not a previous lump was diagnosed as benign. Your doctor may order a biopsy of the lump or use a needle to draw fluid out of a fluid-filled cyst.

About 90 percent of breast lumps are found not by doctors, nurses, or mammograms, but by women during their own breast self-exams, says Kerry McGinn, R.N.

The best time to do a self-exam is 1 week after your menstrual period begins. That's because lumps that sometimes surface just prior to menstruation can disappear just as quickly when your period is over.

Another cause of breast pain is fibrocystic changes, which include lumps and cysts. These changes usually affect the nonworking areas of your breasts: the fat cells, fibrous tissues, and other parts not involved in the making or transporting of milk.

In either case, the following strategies provide relief and promote healing, our experts say.

**Switch your diet.** Change to one low in fat and high in fiber by eating more whole grains, vegetables, and beans. A study at Tufts University School of Medicine in Boston found that women who maintained this kind of diet metabolized estrogen differently. More estrogen was excreted in the stool, leaving less to circulate, says Christiane Northrup, M.D. And that means less hormonal stimulation of the breasts.

**Stay slim.** Keep your weight within the proper range for your height. For seriously overweight women, losing weight can help relieve breast pain and lumpiness, says Kerry McGinn, R.N.

In women, fat acts like an extra gland, producing and storing estrogen. If you have too much body fat, you may have more estrogen circulating in your system than is good for you. And breast tissue, says Gregory Radio, M.D., is very responsive to hormones.

**Get your vitamins.** Be sure to eat plenty of foods rich in vitamin C, calcium, magnesium, and B vitamins, says Dr. Northrup. These vitamins and minerals help regulate the production of prostaglandin E, which in turn reigns in prolactin, a hormone that activates breast tissue.

**Pass on the margarine and other hydrogenated fats.** Hydrogenated fats interfere with your body's ability to convert essential fatty acids from the diet into gamma linoleic acid, says Dr. Northrup. This acid is important because it contributes to the production of prostaglandin E. And prostaglandin E may help keep prolactin, a breast tissue activator, in line.

**Keep calm.** Epinephrine, a substance produced by the adrenal glands during stress, also interferes with gamma linoleic acid conversion, says Dr. Northrup.

**Cut out all caffeine.** Caffeine's role in contributing to breast discomfort is not proven. Some studies say it does, other studies are inconclusive. Still, Thomas J. Smith, M.D., strongly recommends cutting out caffeine.

"I've seen women with pain and other symptoms of benign breast changes get markedly better after abstaining," he says. But just cutting the java isn't enough. "You really have to cut out all caffeine," he says. That means forgoing soft drinks, chocolate, ice cream products, tea, and over-the-counter pain relievers that contain caffeine, like Excedrin.

**Skip the pepperoni pizza.** Highly salted foods make you bloated, says Yvonne Thornton, M.D. Restricting your salt is particularly important to do 7 to 10 days before your menstrual period, before the monthly hormonal changes occur.

**Stay away from diuretics.** It's true that diuretics can help flush fluid from your system. And that can help reduce the swelling in your breasts. But the immediate relief will cost you, says Dr. Thornton. Overuse of diuretics can cause an imbalance in your electrolyte system and lead to dehydration and muscle weakness.

**Reach for over-the-counter relief.** Sandra Swain, M.D., recommends ibuprofen to alleviate painful breasts. "Avoid topical, steroidal anti-inflammatories," she cautions. Pregnant women, of course, shouldn't use any drug without a doctor's okay.

**Take the primrose path.** Evening primrose oil is an anti-inflammatory that can soothe pain and shrink lumps. Experts suggest taking one or two capsules (either 500 or 1,000 milligrams; many often prefer 1,000 milligrams) of evening primrose oil three times a day for several months.

**Apply cold.** McGinn says that some women find relief by dipping their hands in cold water and cupping their breasts.

**Try heat.** Other women, says McGinn, find relief by using a heating pad or hot-water bottle or by taking a warm bath or shower. And still others find that alternating heat and cold works best.

**Find a good support bra.** A sturdy bra, like those made for joggers, can help prevent nerve fibers in the breast, already stretched by waterlogged tissue, from stretching farther. Some women find that wearing the bra to bed at night helps, says Dr. Radio.

**Consider reconsidering the Pill.** The estrogen level in your oral contraceptive could help or hurt your attempt to manage benign breast changes, depending upon what your particular condition is, says Dr. Radio. In general, a low-estrogen pill may help a true fibrocystic condition but aggravate fibroadenoma, a condition in which a solid but often movable lump is present.

**Try massage to ease fluid accumulation.** McGinn says that some women find relief with a gentle breast self-massage that helps ease extra breast fluids back into the lymph passageways. A technique developed by masseuse Carolyn Gale Anderson involves soaping the breasts, rotating the fingers along the surface in coin-size circles, and then using your hands to press your breasts in and then up.

**Discover the emotional message behind your physical symptoms.** "This is absolutely the first thing I look at," says Dr. Northrup. "When I ask my patients 'what's going on in your life around the issue of nurturing or being nurtured?' I often see tears."

"Breasts as the symbol of nurturance are highly charged for women," she adds. "You know that tingling feeling that accompanies the letdown of milk? Some women who have gone through menopause still feel

## Cures from the Kitchen

To get relief from breast inflammation, try this castor oil compress recommended by Christiane Northrup, M.D. She says it helps heal minor breast infections, too.

You'll need cold-pressed castor oil, a wool flannel cloth, a piece of plastic, and a heating pad.

Fold the cloth into four layers and saturate it with the oil, but make sure it's not so wet that it will drip on the breast. Put the cloth on the breast, cover with plastic, and then apply the heating pad. Turn the setting on the pad up to moderate, then to hot if you can stand it, says Dr. Northrup. Leave it on for an hour.

Cold-pressed castor oil contains a substance that increases T11 lymphocyte function, says Dr. Northrup. This helps speed healing of any infection.

You may need to use the compress for 3 to 7 days to really see results. "This can often be extremely beneficial for taking away pain," she says.

## Pine Relief

Native Americans used poultices made with pine to relieve pain and inflammation. To try a modern version of this time-honored remedy, wash your breasts with pine tar soap, suggests Ellen Kamhi, R.N., Ph.D.

You can buy pine soap at some drugstores or your local health food store.

that when they hear a baby cry. That's how closely linked breasts are to the emotions."

## PANEL OF ADVISORS

**Ellen Kamhi, R.N., Ph.D.,** of Oyster Bay, New York, is the author of *The Natural Medicine Chest, Arthritis: An Alternative Medicine Definitive Guide,* and *Cycles of Life.* She hosts radio and TV shows nationally.

**Kerry McGinn, R.N., N.P.,** is a staff nurse at Kaiser Permanente South San Francisco; the author of *The Informed Woman's Guide to Breast Health;* and coauthor of *Women's Cancers.*

**Christiane Northrup, M.D.,** is an assistant clinical professor of obstetrics and gynecology at the University of Vermont College of Medicine in Burlington and a former president of the American Holistic Medical Association. She practices medicine at Women to Women, a health care center in Yarmouth, Maine.

**Gregory Radio, M.D.,** is a practicing obstetrician-gynecologist and chairman of primary care and the department of obstetrics and gynecology at Lehigh Valley Hospital in Allentown, Pennsylvania.

**Thomas J. Smith, M.D.,** is a chief of surgical oncology and director of the Breast Health Center at New England Medical Center in Boston. He is also associate professor of surgery at Tufts University School of Medicine, also in Boston.

**Sandra Swain, M.D.,** is a former assistant professor of medicine at Georgetown University and former director of the Comprehensive Breast Service of the Vincent Lombardi Cancer Center at Georgetown University School of Medicine in Washington, D.C.

**Yvonne S. Thornton, M.D.,** is a maternal fetal medicine specialist and associate clinical professor of obstetrics and gynecology at Columbia University College of Physicians and Surgeons in New York City. She is also director of the Perinatal Center at St. Luke's Hospital, also in New York City.

# BREASTFEEDING
## 21 Problem-Free Nursing Ideas

Breastfeeding is a wonderful way for mother and child to bond, and breast milk is nature's nearly perfect food. It not only contains all the nutrients that your baby needs, it also helps protect your infant against infections.

Some studies show that breastfeeding significantly reduces the risk of stomach upsets and pneumonia during a child's first year, as well as allergies, ear infections, and other illnesses even beyond the first year.

Less than an hour after birth, a full-term baby is physically able to nurse. With a little practice and sometimes a bit of help, both mom and baby can learn the age-old art of breastfeeding.

Breastfeeding *is* easy once you know how, says breastfeeding expert Julie Stock. And it's often easier than using bottles. For instance, while you feed your baby more often than infants given formula, you don't have to prepare the bottles or buy the formula. And even if you ran out of the house *sans* diaper bag, you always have a ready supply of milk on board.

Here's what our experts advise to make breastfeeding trouble-free.

## WHEN TO CALL A DOCTOR

If your breast feels inflamed, you're running a fever, or you have flu-like symptoms, call your doctor. You could have mastitis, a breast infection.

Mastitis is usually treated with antibiotics. If that's what your doctor prescribes, be sure to finish all the medication even if symptoms have already disappeared. This helps prevent recurrent infections.

Meanwhile, you can help speed healing on your own by going to bed, drinking lots of clear fluids, and nursing more frequently, says Carolyn Rawlins, M.D. Don't stop nursing. The milk isn't infected, and if you stop nursing while you have mastitis, it could trigger a breast abscess.

**Establish your milk supply.** To get your baby accustomed to nursing and establish your milk supply, breastfeed your baby exclusively for the first 3 to 4 weeks. Avoid giving bottles if possible, and don't give your baby a pacifier unless he has a very strong sucking reflex.

**Respect your body.** "It's unnecessary for a nursing mother to have breast pain while nursing," says Stock. Seek help if you do.

**Interrupt baby until he gets it right.** Be sure your baby's mouth is open wide before putting him to your breast; he should latch onto the nipple so that at least an inch of the areola is in his mouth.

Leave the baby on a breast as long as he is sucking effectively, which means swallowing every suck or two. If you see him drifting to sleep, wake him up, burp him, and switch sides. Let him nurse on the second side as long as he wants. In general, feeding time varies from 20 to 30 minutes, Stock says.

**Nurse from both breasts during each feeding.** Nurse on one side until it appears that the baby is losing interest, says Stock. Then offer your baby the other side. Next time you feed, start with the side you ended with the time before. To avoid confusion between feedings, put a safety pin on the side of the bra where you need to start the next feeding.

# Do just 1 thing

Position baby right. Our experts were unanimous that this is the key to problem-free feeding. Nurse practitioner Kittie Frantz, R.N., explains it this way: "The baby should face you entirely: head, chest, genitals, knees. Hold the baby so that the buttocks are in one hand and the head is in the bend of your elbow. Let your other hand slip under your breast, with all four fingers supporting your breast. But don't put your fingers on the areola (the darker area around the nipple).

"Now tickle the baby's lower lip with your nipple to get the mouth open wide. When the mouth opens wide, pull the baby's body straight in quickly so that the mouth fixes on the areola."

The nipple should be deep in the baby's mouth, adds Carolyn Rawlins, M.D. "This way there is no movement of the nipple when the baby sucks."

If the baby is sucking incorrectly, put your finger in the corner of his mouth to break the suction and reposition him.

**Nurse often.** "For women, there's often shock at how often a baby wants to nurse. Most doctors give instructions more appropriate to bottle-feeding," says Stock. You'll probably find yourself nursing 8 to 12 times a day in the early weeks.

Human milk is easily digested, so a baby needs to nurse frequently. That creates better bonding between mother and child, says Carolyn Rawlins, M.D.

**Don't toughen the nipples.** Exercises or manipulation to toughen the nipples won't help and could even do some damage, Dr. Rawlins says. "If you get the baby placed correctly, you won't have any soreness at all."

**Use a breast shell for inverted nipples.** It's best to start using these during the sixth or seventh month of pregnancy. Gentle suction from the device helps pull inverted nipples out. But don't use it for more than 15 to 20 minutes a day, says Dr. Rawlins.

**Don't soap your nipples.** "Use absolutely no soap on the nipples, because it dries them out," cautions Dr. Rawlins. The little bumps around the areola are glands that produce an antiseptic oil. So you don't need soap.

**Let your nipples air-dry.** Be sure to air-dry the nipples before you cover them, says Stock. And don't use any breast pads that retain moisture, such as those with plastic.

**Use your milk to help heal sore nipples.** "Truly, 95 percent of the problem with nipple soreness comes from the position in which the baby sucks," says Stock. Pain stops after you correct the problem, though the damage may take a little more time to heal. To speed healing, air-dry your nipples when you finish a feeding, express a little bit of milk, and rub it in your skin. Milk left at the end of the feeding is very high in lubricants and contains a natural antibiotic, she says.

**Wear the right nursing bra.** The best way to pick out a nursing bra is to go a cup size larger and a bra size bigger than your pregnancy bra, says Stock.

"I wouldn't overbuy bras in the beginning," she says. "It's best to wait and see. By the third or fourth day, you may be able to wear your pregnancy bras."

Here are other tips for selecting a good bra.

- Choose all-cotton versus nylon.
- Check to see that the opening for nursing is wide enough so that it doesn't compress the breast. That could lead to clogged ducts.
- Make sure that you can easily open and close the bra with one hand. That will help you be discreet.
- Be sure that the straps are comfortable and the bra isn't tight across the chest.

**Stay alert for plugged ducts.** Binding clothes, your own anatomy, fatigue, or prolonged periods without nursing can cause clogged milk ducts. A plugged duct can lead to an infection if not dealt with promptly.

"If you feel a hard, painful-to-touch spot anywhere on the breast, get rid of it by using warmth," says Stock. Massage the breast, starting at the chest wall and working your way down with a circular motion.

Most important, however, allow your baby to nurse on that side frequently, she says. "Baby's sucking will help clear out that duct faster than anything else. Usually within 24 hours, it will clear up."

**Try warm compresses to help with overproduction.** If your baby is not keeping up your milk production and you get overly full, put some warm, wet compresses on your breasts, says Kittie Frantz, R.N. This opens the ducts so that the milk flows more freely. Nurse the baby more often and longer, and take in enough fluids so that you urinate every hour.

**Chill out with a common cabbage.** Some breastfeeding experts recommend using raw green cabbage leaves to soothe engorged breasts. Apply clean, chilled, or room-temperature inner leaves of the cabbage as compresses, changing them every 2 hours as needed, or when they wilt. Use only until swelling subsides. Overuse can lead to reduction in milk supply, according to some reports.

**Control leaking.** If you feel milk leaking from your breasts, take the heel of your hand and press the nipple into the chest. If you leak a lot, find some reusable breast pads that you can launder yourself. All-cotton pads work well.

**Fill up on fenugreek.** An ancient treatment for increasing milk production, fenugreek seeds have an oxytocin-like effect on the body, stimulating milk production and contracting the uterus. The typical dosage that herbalists recommend is $\frac{1}{2}$ to $1\frac{1}{2}$ teaspoons of seeds per day, or up to 600 to 700 milligrams in capsule form a day. Start with a low dose and slowly increase it if necessary.

## PANEL OF ADVISORS

**Kittie Frantz, R.N., C.P.N.P.,** is director of the Breast-Feeding Infant Clinic at the University of Southern California Medical Center in Los Angeles and a pediatric nurse practitioner. She has been working with nursing mothers since 1963. She also spent 20 years as a leader for La Leche League International.

**Carolyn Rawlins, M.D.,** is an obstetrician in Munster, Indiana, and a former member of La Leche League International board of directors.

**Julie Stock** is medical information liaison for La Leche League International, a support group for breastfeeding mothers.

# BRONCHITIS
## 8 Tips to Stop the Cough

Murphy's Law being what it is, bronchitis can trigger a stubborn cough when coughs are least welcome: in the middle of a long sermon at church or synagogue, during a solo in a pricey Broadway show, in the middle of the night as a sleep-deprived spouse skids into despair.

Bronchitis is an infection and inflammation of the lining of the bronchial passages, the airways that connect the windpipe to the lungs. It is often triggered by an upper respiratory infection, and if it doesn't improve, bronchitis can lead to pneumonia.

In many ways, bronchitis is a lot like a cold. It's usually caused by a virus, says Barbara Phillips, M.D. "So antibiotics won't do much good. Sometimes, though, bronchitis is caused by bacteria, and in that case antibiotics will work."

Acute bronchitis most often goes away by itself in a week or two, she says. But people with chronic bronchitis can cough and wheeze for months. Although you have to let bronchitis take its course, there are things that you can do to breathe easier while you have it.

## WHEN TO CALL A DOCTOR

Bronchitis requires a doctor's attention when:

- Your cough is getting worse, not better, after a week.
- You have a fever or are coughing up blood.
- You are older and get a hacking cough on top of another illness.
- You are short of breath and have a very profuse cough.
- You are elderly.
- You have heart or lung disease.

# Antibiotics Generally Aren't the Answer

At the first sign of a nasty cough, fatigue, wheezing, sore throat, chest discomfort, and low-grade fever that characterize bronchitis, many people ask their doctors for antibiotics. Generally, though, antibiotics are a waste of time because up to 95 percent of all cases are caused by viruses, which antibiotics won't touch. Bacteria trigger only a small portion of acute bronchitis infections.

Doctors are often reluctant to prescribe antibiotics because there's scant evidence that they shorten the course of the illness or ease symptoms. There is some evidence, however, that bronchodilators—asthma drugs that open the airways—can relieve symptoms. Patients who use bronchodilators are more likely to stop coughing within a week of starting the medicines compared to those who took a placebo. The patients who used bronchodilators also returned to work sooner than patients taking a sugar pill. Doctors caution, however, that bronchodilators are most likely to work in patients whose bronchial passages are inflamed. Bronchodilators such as albuterol (Ventolin) usually come in the form of inhalers.

**Stop smoking.** It's the most important thing to do, especially if you're a chronic sufferer. Quit smoking, and your chances of ridding yourself of bronchitis go up dramatically. "Ninety to 95 percent of chronic bronchitis is due directly to smoking," says Daniel Simmons, M.D.

If you've smoked for a long time, some of the damage to your lungs may be irreversible, but the fewer years you've been smoking, the more likely it is that you will have a complete recovery, says Gordon L. Snider, M.D.

**Get active about passive smoking.** Avoid those who smoke, and if your spouse smokes, get him or her to stop. Other people's smoking could be causing *your* bronchitis. Exposure to secondhand smoke (called passive smoking) can result in bronchitis.

**Keep the fluids flowing.** "Drinking fluids helps the mucus become more watery and easier to cough up," says Dr. Phillips. "Four to six glasses of fluid a day will do a good job of breaking it up."

Warm liquids or just plain water is best. "Avoid caffeine or alcoholic beverages," says Dr. Phillips. "They are diuretics; they make you urinate more, and you actually lose more fluids than you gain."

**Breathe in warm, moist air.** Warm, moist air helps vaporize the mucus. If you have mucus that is thick or difficult to cough up, a vaporizer will help to loosen the secretions. You could also stand in your bathroom, close the door, and then run your shower, breathing in the warm mist that steams up your bathroom.

**Don't throw in the towel.** Drape it over the sink. "Steam inhalation from the bathroom sink is very helpful," says Dr. Snider. "Fill the sink with hot water, put a towel over your head and the sink, creating a tent, and then inhale the steam for 5 to 10 minutes every couple of hours."

**Don't expect too much from expectorants.** "There is no scientific evidence that there is any medicine that works to dry up mucus," says Dr. Phillips. Drinking fluids is the best way to loosen secretions.

**Listen to your cough.** "If you have a productive cough, one in which you cough up sputum, you don't really want to suppress it completely, because you won't be coughing up the stuff your lungs want to rid themselves of," says Dr. Simmons. His advice: Endure it as best you can.

On the other hand, "If your cough is nonproductive—that is, you're not coughing anything up—then it's good to take a cough medicine designed to suppress a cough. Look for those containing the active ingredient dextromethorphan," he suggests.

**Focus on prevention.** Infants, young children, smokers, people with heart or lung disease, and the elderly are more likely to develop bronchitis. They are, in turn, more likely to have a case of bronchitis balloon into pneumonia. People who are vulnerable should avoid strenuous outdoor work and exercising on days when air pollution is high.

## PANEL OF ADVISORS

**Barbara Phillips, M.D.,** is a pulmonologist and associate professor of pulmonary medicine at the University of Kentucky College of Medicine in Lexington.

**Daniel Simmons, M.D.,** is a pulmonologist and professor of medicine in the division of pulmonary disease at the UCLA School of Medicine in Los Angeles.

**Gordon L. Snider, M.D.,** is a professor of medicine at Boston University School of Medicine and Tufts University School of Medicine in Boston. He is also a pulmonologist and chief of medicinal service at the Boston Veterans Administration Medical Center.

# BRUISES
## 7 Healing Ideas

Unless you wrap yourself in cotton wool, you'll never be bruise-proof. But you can lessen the likelihood of large bruises and shrink and heal the ones you occasionally incur. Here's how.

**Put the chill on bruises.** Use an ice pack to treat any injury that might lead to a bruise, advises emergency room physician Hugh Macaulay, M.D. Apply an ice pack, wrapped in a thin cloth to protect your skin, as quickly as possible following the injury. Keep the ice in place for 15 minutes. If you suspect the bump will blossom into a severe bruise, continue this ice treatment every couple of hours for the first 24 hours. Allow your skin to warm naturally and don't apply heat between ice packs.

Cooling constricts the blood vessels, and that means less blood spills into the tissues to create a bruise. A cold pack also minimizes the swelling and numbs the area, so it won't hurt as much as a bruise left unchilled.

**Follow ice with heat.** After 24 hours, use heat to dilate the blood vessels and improve circulation in the area, says dermatologist Sheldon V. Pollack, M.D.

**Prop your feet up.** Bruises are little reservoirs of blood. Blood, like any liquid, runs downhill. If you do a lot of standing, blood that has collected in a bruise will seep down through your soft tissues and find other places to puddle.

## WHEN TO CALL A DOCTOR

Sometimes bruises are a sign of illness. So if you bruise easily and can't figure out the cause, talk with your doctor. Some blood disorders can cause unexplained bruises. Also, AIDS can cause purplish bumps that seem to be bruises but that won't go away.

**Add vitamin C to your daily diet.** Studies at Duke University Medical Center in Durham, North Carolina, show that people who lack vitamin C in their diets tend to bruise more easily.

Vitamin C helps build protective collagen tissue around blood vessels in the skin, says Dr. Pollack. Your face, hands, or feet contain less collagen than, say, your thighs, so bruises in those areas are often darker, says Dr. Macaulay.

If you bruise easily, Dr. Pollack suggests 500 milligrams of vitamin C three times a day to help build your collagen.

**Watch those medications.** People who take aspirin to protect against heart disease and those taking blood thinners will find that a bump turns into a bruise very easily. Other drugs such as anti-inflammatories, antidepressants, or asthma medicines can inhibit clotting under the skin and cause larger bruises. Alcoholics and drug abusers tend to bruise easily, too. If you're taking medicine that might cause easy bruising, talk to your doctor about the problem.

**Treat belated bruises.** You don't have to bump to bruise. If you notice bruises a day or two after exercising, use heat to begin the healing process.

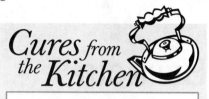

## Cures from the Kitchen

Keep parsley-packed ice cubes in your freezer for an instant bruise remedy. Herbalist Sharleen Andrews-Miller suggests putting a handful of parsley and ¼ cup of water in a blender or food processor. Whirl until it becomes the consistency of slush. Then fill an ice cube tray half full with the mixture and freeze. When needed, wrap the ice cubes in gauze or a thin cloth and apply them to the bruise. Parsley is a cooling herb that decreases inflammation and reduces pain, she says.

As a bonus, you can grab a parsley cube out of the freezer when you're cooking if you need a little parsley in a soup or sauce.

## PANEL OF ADVISORS

**Sharleen Andrews-Miller** is an herbalist and a faculty member at the National College of Naturopathic Medicine in Portland, Oregon, and medicinary botanical educator at the college's public clinic, where she teaches medicinary practicum and Northwest herbs.

**Hugh Macaulay, M.D.,** is an emergency room physician at Aspen Valley Hospital in Aspen.

**Sheldon V. Pollack, M.D.,** is a dermatologist and former associate professor of medicine in the division of dermatology at Duke University School of Medicine in Durham, North Carolina.

# BURNOUT
## 18 Paths to Renewal

Burnout starts insidiously: the feeling that the work will never be done, relationships at work aren't what they used to be, the job isn't fun anymore. Burnout's symptoms may be both emotional and physical, and they evolve so gradually that they're often hard to recognize at first. Loved ones and colleagues may be the first to notice.

Feelings of excessive responsibility and lack of a sense of control contribute to burnout, which in turn can contribute to serious medical problems, including high blood pressure, gastrointestinal problems, coronary artery disease, and sleep problems, says Peter S. Moskowitz, M.D.

The emotional signs often start first. "You may feel irritable, finding that you have less ability to deal with minor problems at home and at work," he notes. People under stress may begin to squabble with coworkers, experience road rage on the drive home, or reach for an extra cocktail before dinner. They may show signs of depression—struggling to get out of bed in the morning—or symptoms of anxiety—lying awake at night.

Later, physical signs appear, such as headache, abdominal pain, back pain, chronic fatigue, and a general I've-just-been-run-over-by-a-Mack-truck feeling.

Who's at greatest risk for burnout? Surprisingly, workers who burn out are often the most highly motivated, dedicated people on the job. "You can't burn out unless there's been a fire in the first place," explains Dr. Moskowitz. Some people may experience burnout as disillusionment with a job that no longer seems as challenging as it once did.

Other people at risk for burnout are those who tend to worry excessively or put work before self or family. "These people don't manage stress well, and they don't have a well-thought-out plan for taking care of themselves and balancing their lives," says Dr. Moskowitz. "They don't realize that lifestyle balance is the most potent form of stress management available."

Burnout costs companies a tremendous amount of money. "This is a $200-billion-a-year problem when you factor in medical claims, absenteeism, and lost productivity," reports Jack N. Singer, Ph.D.

Fortunately, burnout isn't inevitable. You can take steps to revitalize your outlook on your job, relationships, and life in general. Here are a few strategies that our experts recommend.

**Develop a goal.** If you're not satisfied in your job, view it as a stepping-stone to something better. "If you're in a bad position but you're on the road to a goal that really means something to you, it will be much easier to endure," says Karen Bierman, Ph.D. She encourages people to think about where they're headed in life and then make a plan to get there.

**Keep your perspective.** Many people who get burned out simply take their jobs and bosses too seriously, adds Dr. Bierman. "What the boss says or does carries far more weight than it should." To combat this tendency in yourself, try to be your own compass. Listen to your boss, but use your own judgment about how you can best do your job.

**Reframe your thoughts.** You can't always control what happens around you, but you can control how you respond to those events, says Dr. Singer. If layoffs in your company have led to a heavy workload for you, remind yourself that you were valuable enough to keep in the first place. Give yourself credit for being able to handle more work than you used to. Feel good about doing the best job you can.

**Dig into your work.** "Don't sit there fretting about how much there is to do, procrastinating out of fear that you'll never get it done," Dr. Singer adds. Get organized and set goals at the beginning of each day, doing the toughest tasks first and crossing off items on a list as you complete them. Build small rewards into your day, such as enjoying a cup of tea or a walk around the building, as you accomplish what you set out to do.

**Forget work-ethic clichés.** Many people have a message in their heads that repeats, "If a job's worth doing, it's worth doing right" or "Don't do anything halfway." Push the Stop button, Dr. Bierman says. "Let's face it. Some tasks aren't worth 100 percent of your effort." Take paperwork, for instance. "Paperwork often deserves to be done halfway at *most*," she says. Give yourself the right to differentiate between what is worth doing well and what is worth doing well *enough*. Some tasks aren't worth doing at all.

**Make your work space a place you like to be.** Hang cartoons that make you laugh, display pictures of people you love, or tack up photos of places you enjoy.

**Laugh.** Humor and laughter lower blood pressure and boost immunity, says Dr. Singer. "Every time you laugh, it's like exercising your internal organs."

He recommends putting a "fun quotient" into every office. Give a frozen ice pop to the customer service representative who puts up with the most heat from a customer, or keep a funny book next to your phone to flip through when you're on hold. Dr. Singer recommends *Chicken Poop in My Bowl* by John M. Irvin.

**Practice time management.** Melissa Stöppler, M.D., encourages people to learn "double-tasking" to save time and ease burnout. Sort mail while waiting on the phone, or fold clothes while catching up on the news. Save time by combining errands and never doing just one thing when you leave the house. Always have on hand stamps, greeting cards, and ingredients for a quick supper. Minimize waiting time by scheduling appointments first thing in the morning.

**Just say no.** People sometimes feel burned out because they are simply too overloaded. Dr. Stöppler recommends examining all of your "extra" responsibilities, such as coaching the soccer team, serving on the church board, or participating on a task force at work. Dump those that have become mere obligations. Don't take on new duties without first asking yourself, "Will this activity or event bring me joy?" Make your first answer to new requests, "I'll think about it," buying time to do just that.

**Tell a friend.** Find a sympathetic ear and talk about your feelings, says Dr. Bierman. Explaining your situation and getting some social support can relieve pressure.

**Have an annual checkup.** Burnout takes a physical toll on people, so if you live a stressful life, make sure that your body is in good shape. Your doctor can help you develop a program of self-care designed to make you feel better by exercising, eating right, and getting the sleep you need. Knowing you're taking care of your body also helps you feel more in control of your life.

**Exercise often.** Regular exercise combats burnout by reducing stress. It also boosts your resistance to disease, lowers your blood pressure, improves your cholesterol profile, helps control body weight, and helps lift depression. Exercising at least 3 days a week for 30 to 60 minutes is especially important for people who feel frazzled and burned out, so make this a priority, recommends Dr. Moskowitz.

**Eat well.** You don't have control over all of the stresses making you feel burned out, but you do have control over what you eat. Eat a low-fat, high-fiber diet. You'll gain a sense of satisfaction knowing that you're doing right by your body, and you may even lose some weight to boot.

**Get restful sleep.** Let go of the day's worries and unfinished business. Tell yourself that you will make decisions tomorrow, after a good night's rest. Visualize one of your favorite vacations or a serene scene from a movie. Imagine yourself in that place as you drift off to sleep. Avoid alcohol, tobacco, and exercise for at least 1 hour prior to sleep. "Invest in a firm comfortable mattress," says Dr. Moskowitz.

**Develop self-awareness.** For those who want to take care of themselves, Dr. Moskowitz recommends some form of calm reflection daily. Relaxation techniques that foster health, healing, and self-awareness include prayer, meditation, yoga, tai chi, breathing exercises, journaling, and self-hypnosis. Psychotherapy and career coaching are additional pathways to greater self-awareness.

Try different approaches until you find the best relaxation program for your needs, interests, and abilities, suggests Dr. Stöppler. Some, such as tai chi, involve both physical and mental exercises, while others, like meditation, chiefly rely upon mental discipline.

One way to begin, she says, is to set aside quiet moments every day in a place free of distraction where you can breathe deeply, relax your muscles, and reflect on a simple message such as "I am calm and relaxed."

Practicing a relaxation technique should never become a chore forced into a packed schedule but, rather, be a respite to which you look forward, Dr. Stöppler stresses.

**Deepen your relationships.** People who feel burned out often take out their frustration on those who love them most. That's like shooting yourself in the foot, because time devoted to enriching relationships with family and friends will help to ease feelings of burnout, says Dr. Moskowitz.

**Get a life and a community.** Seek out a community of like-minded people to share your life, whether it's pursuing a hobby, finding a place of worship, or doing community service. "Connecting with people will give you a wonderful source of support and encouragement and make you more resilient to stress," Dr. Moskowitz notes.

**Be brave—take risks and move on.** If you've determined that your unhappiness is coming from your job and you can't change or delegate the tasks that trouble you most, have the courage to find another job that better suits you. "It's scary, and it requires risk, but your risk will be rewarded tenfold over," promises Dr. Moskowitz. "Nothing changes without some pain. With risk comes personal growth and renewal."

## PANEL OF ADVISORS

**Karen Bierman, Ph.D.,** is a psychologist in Beverly Hills, California.

**Peter S. Moskowitz, M.D.,** is the director of the Center for Professional and Personal Renewal in Palo Alto, California. He conducts workshops and lectures and provides career/life coaching for physicians and other professionals on stress management and related life-balance issues.

**Jack N. Singer, Ph.D.,** is an industrial/organizational and consulting psychologist and a professional speaker who specializes in burnout. He is the author of *Conquering Your Internal Critic So You Can Sing Your Own Song.* He lives in Laguna Niguel, California.

**Melissa Stöppler, M.D.,** writes the stress-management column for the Web site About.com. A consultant on stress and health issues, she is a pathologist at the University of Marburg in Germany.

# BURNS
## 10 Treatments for Minor Accidents

When you accidentally catch your hand on the broiler, splash battery acid on your chest, or take a face full of steam upon opening a microwave dish, you need to put the fire out—*fast!* Here's how.

**Douse that flame.** "The first and most important thing is to stop the burning process," says emergency medicine expert William P. Burdick, M.D. Flush your burns with lots and lots of cold water—15 to 30 minutes' worth or until the burning stops. But *don't* use ice or ice water—they can make your burn worse.

"If it's a contact burn, run the injured part under cold water," says Dr. Burdick. "If it's hot grease or splattered hot material like battery acid or soup, remove the clothing that's saturated first, wash the grease off your skin, then soak the burn in cold water." If the clothing sticks to the burn, rinse over the clothing, then go to the doctor. Do not attempt to pull the clothing off yourself.

Once you've put the fire out, you're halfway to healing. The coolness stops the burning from spreading through your tissue and works as a temporary painkiller.

## WHEN TO CALL A DOCTOR

You can usually self-treat first- and second-degree burns smaller than a silver dollar. See a doctor for larger burns or for burns on people over 60. Third-degree burns are metaphorically too hot to handle on your own and need medical attention. Here's how to tell the difference between first-, second-, and third-degree burns.

- First-degree burns, like most sunburns and scalds, are red and painful.
- Second-degree burns, including severe sunburns or burns caused by brief contact with oven coils, tend to blister and ooze and are painful.
- Third-degree burns are charred and white or creamy colored. They can be caused by chemicals, electricity, or prolonged contact with hot surfaces. Usually, they are not painful because nerve endings have been destroyed, but they always require a doctor's care.

Other burns that demand a doctor's immediate attention include:

- Burns on the face, hands, feet, pelvic and pubic areas, or in the eyes.
- Any burn you aren't sure is first- or second-degree.
- Burns that show signs of infection, including a blister filled with greenish or brownish fluid, or a burn that becomes hot again or turns red.
- Any burn that doesn't heal in 10 days to 2 weeks.
- Chemical or electric burns. Corrosive chemical burns can burn through several layers of skin and tissue. If you are burned this way, immediately flush cool running water over the burned area for 15 to 20 minutes.

If you plan to see a doctor about a burn, wash it, but don't use any ointments, antiseptics, or sprays, advises emergency medical technician John Gillies. You may, however, wrap the affected area in a dry, sterile dressing.

For severe burns that damage several layers of skin or destroy underlying blood vessels or nerves, call 911 immediately. While you wait for help, elevate burned areas above the heart and cover with a clean sheet to reduce any loss of body heat.

**Leave the butter for your bread.** You wouldn't try to smother a fire with a giant slab of butter, would you? The same goes for a burn. Food on a burn can hold the heat in your tissue and make the burn worse. It also might cause an infection. Don't use other old-time folk remedies either. Vinegar, potato scrapings, and honey don't help.

**Reach for water.** If you burn your mouth sipping a scalding cup of coffee or other hot food or drink, rinse your mouth and gargle with cool water for 5 to 10 minutes. Avoid hot foods and drinks for several days.

**Cover the burn.** After you cool and clean the burn, gently wrap the burn in a clean, dry cloth, such as a thick gauze pad.

**Then do nothing.** At least for the first 24 hours, leave the burn alone. Burns should be allowed to begin the healing process on their own.

**Help it heal.** Starting 24 hours after you burn yourself, wash your injury gently with soap and water or a mild Betadine solution once a day, suggests emergency medical technician John Gillies. Keep it covered, dry, and clean between washings.

**Soothe with aloe.** Two to 3 days after you burn, break off a fresh piece of aloe and use the plant's natural healing moisture, or squeeze on an over-the-counter aloe cream. Both have an analgesic action that will make your wound feel better.

**Make soothing solutions.** When your burn starts to heal, break open a capsule of vitamin E and rub the liquid onto your irritated skin. It feels good and may prevent scarring. Or reach for an over-the-counter remedy such as the sunburn-cooler Solarcaine.

**Dab on an antimicrobial cream.** An over-the-counter antibiotic ointment containing the active ingredients polymyxin B sulfate or bacitracin discourage infection and speed your healing. (For a list comparing the effectiveness of various over-the-counter ointments, see page 151.)

**Leave blisters intact.** Those bubbles of skin are nature's own best bandages, says Gillies. So leave them alone. If a blister pops, clean the area with soap and water, then smooth on a little antibiotic ointment and cover.

## PANEL OF ADVISORS

**William P. Burdick, M.D.,** is a professor of emergency medicine at MCP Hahnemann University School of Medicine in Philadelphia.

**John Gillies, E.M.T.,** is a former emergency medical technician and program director for health services at the Colorado Outward Bound School in Denver.

# BURSITIS
## 10 Ways to Ease Your Pain

Bursitis is an inflammation of the fluid-filled sacs in the joints, called bursae, that ensure the body's movements are smooth and friction-free. You have more than 150 of them nestled in your shoulders, knees, and other joints. Bursitis pain flares whenever repeated movement stresses a specific joint, such as a long day of tennis or golf causing intense shoulder pain.

Bursitis strikes, it retreats, it strikes again. The acutely painful stage of bursitis lasts 4 to 5 days, sometimes even longer. The on-again, off-again nature of acute bursitis is aggravating for people with the condition and frustrating for those trying to determine what type of treatments actually work.

Right now, there is no "cure" for bursitis. Until medicine comes up with one, here are some tried-and-true remedies that may bring temporary relief from this painful condition.

**Rest—it's best.** The first thing you do with any joint pain is rest, says Alan Bensman, M.D. "Stop the activity that's causing the pain and rest the joint. Forget that old sports adage about working through the pain."

**Immobilize and ice.** If the joint is hot, reach for ice, says Allan Tomson, D.C. "Alternate 10 minutes of ice, 10 of rest, 10 of ice, and so on. As long as it is hot, do not apply heat to it."

## WHEN TO CALL A DOCTOR

Though painful, bursitis may subside with just a little TLC. But if it's due to an infection or gout, you need to see a doctor. How can you tell? If the joint is tender, warm, and red, that's a definite sign. But sometimes those signs won't be present even if you have an infection, so it's best to get a doctor's advice when you have a flare-up of bursitis.

**Attract relief with opposites.** Once the joint cools down and if the pain or swelling is not terribly acute, Dr. Tomson sometimes recommends cold-and-hot combination treatments—10 minutes of ice, followed by 10 minutes of heat, followed by 10 minutes of ice, and so on.

**Count on some pain relievers.** Naproxen (such as Aleve) often provides significant relief of minor bursitis symptoms, and it has a longer half-life than most of the other over-the-counter medications, notes Dr. Bensman. Ibuprofen can also be very effective and is preferred by many people. It has a shorter half-life, though, so you may need to take it more frequently.

For those who can tolerate it, aspirin is still considered to be a very effective anti-inflammatory medication, says Dr. Bensman. Enteric-coated aspirin (such as Ecotrin) is absorbed through the intestines and is therefore less likely to cause gastric ulcers.

Acetaminophen is also an effective pain reliever, and while there are some reports that acetaminophen may have some anti-inflammatory qualities, that's not been fully documented. If you're not sure which medication is right for you, talk over the options with your physician. And as with all medications, follow label instructions carefully.

**Calm the pain with castor oil.** When the pain is no longer acute, Dr. Tomson recommends a castor oil pack, which is as simple to make as it is effective. Spread castor oil over the afflicted joint. Put cotton or wool flannel over that and then apply a heating pad.

**Apply soothing balm.** Alternative remedies can speed relief when used with standard treatments, explains Alison Lee, M.D. One remedy worth trying is Tiger Balm, a Chinese massage cream containing menthol, which may ease bursitis pain when used one or two times a day. If you can't find Tiger Balm in your local health food store, you can make a homemade balm by mixing water and turmeric powder (a spice used in curry recipes) into a paste. Apply one or two times daily.

**Gently move the joint.** Once the pain is no longer acute, gentle exercises are in order. If elbow or shoulder pain is the problem, doctors recommend swinging the arm freely to relieve the ache. Exercise for only a couple of minutes at first, but do it often during the day.

"You want to maintain range of motion," says Edward Resnick, M.D. "You don't want to get a stiff shoulder, but you don't want to overstretch it either."

He recommends bending forward and supporting yourself with your good arm and hand on a chair. Allow the painful arm to drop downward, then swing this arm back and forth, side to side, and finally in circles both clockwise and counterclockwise.

Some experts recommend performing soothing exercises in a hot tub, bathtub, whirlpool, or swimming pool. Float your limb on the surface of the water, then move it gently, without pushing it along.

**Stretch.** The importance of exercise following a bursitis attack cannot be overemphasized. Our experts all recommend stretching techniques to return full, normal movement to the joint.

One effective primary stretching motion for stiff shoulder joints is called the cat stretch. Get down on your hands and knees. Put your hands slightly forward of your head, then keep your elbows stiff as you stretch backward and come down on your heels.

Another stretching motion is to stand facing a corner and walk your fingers up the wall in the corner, Dr. Resnick says. "The object is to try and get your armpit in the corner. That way you know you're getting effective exercise."

**Try a natural anti-inflammatory remedy.** Flaxseed oil, which contains omega-3 fatty acids known to reduce inflammation, is sometimes recommended for people with recurrent bursitis. Add 1 to 2 tablespoons to your salad dressing.

**Be patient.** Bursitis generally takes about 10 days to heal—sometimes more, sometimes less. If all else fails, say doctors, time will heal the wound.

## PANEL OF ADVISORS

**Alan Bensman, M.D.,** is a physiatrist at Rehabilitative Health Services, P.A., in Golden Valley, Minnesota.

**Alison Lee, M.D.,** is medical director of the Barefoot Doctors in Ann Arbor, Michigan, and a specialist in acupuncture and pain management.

**Edward Resnick, M.D.,** is an orthopedic surgeon and director of the Pain Control Center at Temple University Hospital in Philadelphia.

**Allan Tomson, D.C.,** is a chiropractor with the Natural Horizons Wellness Center in Fairfax, Virginia.

# CALLUSES AND CORNS
## 18 Ways to Smooth and Soothe

Those little bumps and lumps that give your feet that "ugly look" are a trash heap of discarded dead skin cells—calluses and corns formed by friction and irritation from the everyday wear and tear from shoes, or adjacent bones on the same foot.

Not only are they unsightly, they can be quite painful.

"Calluses are your body's way of protecting you from pressure," says Neal Kramer, D.P.M. "When the pressure gets extreme, the callus gets thicker and thicker. If it develops a hard core, it becomes a corn. Soft corns, which form between toes and remain soft from foot perspiration, happen when two bones from adjacent toes become overly friendly. The skin between them thickens in an attempt to protect you from the constant pressure."

"People can live with calluses more easily than with corns," says Richard Cowin, D.P.M. "If you get painful corns on your toes, it's like having a bad toothache. It can ruin your day."

So, to start *your* day—every day—on the right foot, heed these tips.

## WHEN TO CALL A DOCTOR

People with diabetes or any kind of reduced feeling in their feet should never treat themselves, says Neal Kramer, D.P.M. Diabetes affects tiny blood vessels throughout the body, including those in the feet. That leads to decreased circulation, which reduces the ability of wounds to heal and resist infection.

"Anyone with a circulation disorder is okay if his skin remains intact," says Dr. Kramer. "But if he gets any kind of cut or opening in the skin, it becomes very dangerous. And anyone who can't feel pressure or pain very well may not know he cut himself or may not realize the full severity of an injury and could wind up with a nasty infection."

**Stay away from sharp instruments.** First and foremost, say the experts, don't play surgeon. Resist the temptation to pare down calluses and corns with razor blades, scissors, or other sharp instruments.

"Bathroom surgery is extremely dangerous," says Nancy Lu Conrad, D.P.M. "It can lead to infections and worse. I've seen so many horrible things happen to people who thought they could be their own surgeons." And people with diabetes should *never* treat their own foot problems.

**Pad the area.** It's best to take action against a callus *before* it has the chance to become a corn. An easy way to take pressure off a callus, says Elizabeth H. Roberts, D.P.M., is to place a little gauze or absorbent cotton over the area, then cover it with a thin piece of moleskin. She recommends removing the covering each night, as well as when bathing, so that the skin can breathe and excessive moisture doesn't accumulate under the pad.

When you remove the moleskin, be sure to hold the skin of the sole of your foot taut while you *slowly* pull the moleskin back toward the heel. If you pull quickly or in the opposite direction, you risk tearing the skin.

**Customize your insoles.** Mark D. Sussman, D.P.M., recommends this easy way to modify insoles to relieve pressure on calluses: Buy a pair of foam-rubber insoles and wear them for a week. Your calluses will leave impressions, indicating the areas of greatest stress and showing you the areas *around which* each insole needs to be built up to even out the pressure.

If the callus is in the middle of the ball of your foot, cut $\frac{1}{8}$-inch-thick foam or felt into two strips (each $\frac{1}{2}$ inch wide by 2 inches long). Glue them on either side of the depression. Take another strip (2 inches wide by 2 inches long), and position it behind the depression. If the callus is off to one side, use appropriate combinations of strips. When you wear the insoles, the pads will redistribute weight away from the callus and provide relief.

**Be a little abrasive.** Before treating a callus, soak your foot in comfortably hot water for several minutes. Then, says Dr. Cowin, use a callus file or pumice stone to lightly abrade the area and rub off the top layers of skin. Finish by applying some hand cream, such as Carmol 20, which contains 20 percent urea and helps dissolve hard skin. If you have bad calluses, make this part of your daily routine after showering or bathing.

But, he cautions, don't use abrasive action on hard corns, because that makes the area very tender and more painful than it was before.

**Take five.** Here's another way to soften stubborn calluses. Crush five or six aspirin tablets into a powder. Mix into a paste with $\frac{1}{2}$ teaspoon each of water and lemon juice. Apply to the hard-skin spots on your foot, then put your foot into a plastic bag and wrap a warm towel around everything. The combination of the plastic and the warm towel will help the paste penetrate the hard skin. Sit still for at least 10 minutes. Then unwrap your foot and scrub the area with a pumice stone. All that dead, hard, callused skin should come loose and flake away easily. Because of the remote chance of a reaction, if you're allergic or sensitive to aspirin, don't use it on your skin.

**Leave some calluses alone.** Sometimes a little callus is good. "People who go barefoot a lot develop calluses across their soles," says Frederick Hass, M.D. "And that's desirable. They protect the skin from rough terrain or ground heat. If sufficiently developed and toughened, they can even ward off cutting by sharp objects. These calluses are rarely painful."

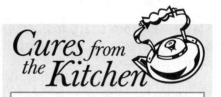

## Cures from the Kitchen

If you have a lot of callused tissue, Suzanne M. Levine, D.P.M., recommends soaking your feet in very diluted chamomile tea. The tea will both soothe and soften hard skin. The brew will stain your feet, but it comes off easily with soap and water.

Sometimes a callus develops as a safeguard against an ingrowing toenail. As the sharp-edged nail bites into the adjoining tissue, the skin thickens and hardens to prevent further intrusion.

Should you develop this kind of callus, you must leave it in peace, says Dr. Hass. If it proves painful, get temporary relief by soaking your foot in warm, soapy water, but don't ever attempt to hone it. If it becomes too painful, consult a doctor to have the ingrowing nail fixed.

**Work fast.** If your callus treatment has been unsuccessful and the pressure is extreme, the callus will get thicker and thicker. Once it develops a hard core, it becomes a corn. It's best to take action when a corn first takes shape, says Dr. Hass. At that point, your corn is a hardening small circle of skin that produces little or no pain. You should immediately massage the area gently with lanolin to soften the corn and make it less responsive to pressure, then pad the area to relieve pressure.

**Avoid medicated pads.** "I don't recommend corn plasters or any other over-the-counter medications," says Dr. Kramer. "Those things are nothing more than acid, which doesn't know the difference between corns and calluses and normal skin. So although they may work on your corn or callus, they will also eat away normal skin, causing burning or even ulcers."

If you *must* use corn plasters or other over-the-counter salicylic acid products, which come in liquid, salve, and disk form, religiously follow the advice of Suzanne M. Levine, D.P.M.: Apply *only* to the problem area, not surrounding skin. If treating a corn, first put a doughnut-shaped nonmedicated pad around the corn to shield adjacent skin. Never use such a product more than twice a week, and see a doctor if there's no sign of improvement after 2 weeks.

**Enjoy a good soak.** "Your corn pain may be coming from a bursa, a fluid-filled sac that becomes inflamed and enlarged at the site between the bone and the corn," says Dr. Levine. "For temporary relief of the pain, soak your feet in a solution of Epsom salts and warm water. This will diminish the size of the bursa sac and take some pressure off the nearby sensory nerves. But be aware that if you put your feet back into tight shoes, the bursa will soon swell up again to its painful size."

**Make horseshoes.** To cushion corns, says Dr. Roberts, don't use corn pads with an oval opening. The oval will cause pressure on the surrounding area, making the corn or callus bulge into the opening. If you have that type of pad, cut a wedge out of it to make a horseshoe shape. Position the pad far enough behind the corn so that as you walk—if your foot slides forward in your shoe—the pad won't rub against the corn it is supposed to protect.

**Get spot relief.** Even better than a corn pad, says Dr. Roberts, is a spot-shaped adhesive bandage, which also has the advantage of a sterile gauze center. But avoid bandages that must be wrapped completely around the toe. The bulk may lead to irritation and discomfort.

**Give soft corns space.** Soft corns—the ones that form between two toes—require different care than regular corns. Because soft corns are caused by bones from two adjacent toes rubbing together, says Dr. Cowin, "you need to put something soft there to separate the toes. You can buy toe separators or toe spacers, which are simply little pieces of foam that you place between the toes."

**Be a lamb.** Instead of foam pieces, you could use good-quality lamb's wool between toes, suggests Dr. Roberts. But don't get the coarse type found in beauty parlors. Your local drugstore probably stocks lamb's wool along with its other foot-care items. Draw the strands into a thin, even layer, and wrap it loosely around one of the toes. Remove the wool before bathing.

Since the shoes that you wear are often the culprits that caused your calluses and corns, making some simple adjustments to your shoes may help ease your pain.

**Stretch your shoes.** Sometimes relief of a painful, hard corn can be had by stretching your shoes to remove the pressure that caused the friction. Your shoe-maker can do the stretching, or you can take this home approach from Marvin Sandler, D.P.M. Apply Meltonian Shoe Stretch or another leather-stretching solution to your shoes. This allows the leather fibers to stretch while you are walking. Apply the solution many times, and walk in the shoes (while the leather is still wet) until the shoe becomes comfortable.

**Go to a bar.** For calluses at the base of the foot, you can modify your shoes by getting your shoemaker to attach a rubber or leather metatarsal bar to the sole of the shoe, says Dr. Sandler. It's placed so that the ball of your foot rocks over the bar without pressing on the bones in that area. Be sure to replace the bar when it becomes worn down.

Be careful though—these bars can catch on stairs, carpets, or curbs and cause you to trip. For this reason, they may not be suitable for older people. The elderly may be better off with a safer but less effective bar that is flat and continuous with the sole. Remember, however, that these bars do not prevent the metatarsal bones from pressing painfully against the *inside* of your shoe, so you may need a removable inlay there.

**Be well-heeled.** "I see a lot of problems in women because of high heels," says Dr. Conrad. "I've heard good shoe fitters say that any pump has to be fit short and narrow to keep it on. And that's true. Oxfords, on the other hand, have a tie that holds the shoe on and keeps the back of the foot firmly in the shoe. That keeps the foot from slipping forward and putting pressure on your forefoot as you walk. With a pump, your foot slides right to the forepart of the shoe, jamming everything together in a space that is too small."

To avoid problems, says Dr. Cowin, wear well-fitting shoes that don't have exceptionally high heels. "For special occasions, high heels won't hurt," he says, "but for everyday situations, lower shoes are better."

"If you must wear high heels," adds Dr. Levine, "look for ones with extra cushioning in the forefoot area, or have your shoemaker put extra foam cushioning there. And if you have bad calluses on the backs of your heels, avoid open-backed shoes until the area heals."

**Get a proper fit.** "The most important thing when buying a shoe is fit," says Terry L. Spilken, D.P.M. "Whether a shoe costs $20 or $200, if it doesn't fit correctly, it's going to give you problems. Make sure it's the proper length; you want a thumb's-width distance from the end of your longest toe to the end of your shoe. (And your longest toe isn't necessarily the big toe.) You should have enough width across the ball of the foot and enough room in the toebox so that there's no pressure across the toes."

"Look for natural materials, like leather, that breathe. And remember that it's just as harmful for the foot to get a shoe that's too big as one that's too small," he says. "If the shoe's too big, the foot will slide in it and cause friction. And the friction of the skin rubbing can cause a callus or corn just as easily as a tight shoe that pinches."

## PANEL OF ADVISORS

**Nancy Lu Conrad, D.P.M.,** is a private practitioner in Circleville, Ohio. She specializes in footwear for children as well as in sports medicine and orthopedics.

**Richard M. Cowin, D.P.M.,** is a private practitioner and director of Advanced Foot Surgery in Lady Lake, Florida, where he specializes in the practice of minimal incision and laser foot and ankle surgery. He is a diplomate of the American Board of Podiatric Surgery and the American Board of Ambulatory Foot Surgery.

**Frederick Hass, M.D.,** is a general practitioner in San Rafael, California. He is on the staff of Marin General Hospital in Greenbrae.

**Neal Kramer, D.P.M.,** is a podiatrist in Bethlehem, Pennsylvania.

**Suzanne M. Levine, D.P.M., P.C.,** is a podiatrist and a podiatric attending physician at New York–Presbyterian Hospital. She is the author of *Your Feet Don't Have to Hurt.*

**Elizabeth H. Roberts, D.P.M.,** has spent more than 30 years as a prominent podiatrist in New York City, where she is professor emeritus at the New York College of Podiatric Medicine.

**Marvin Sandler, D.P.M.,** is a podiatrist in Allentown, Pennsylvania. He was formerly chief of podiatric surgery at Sacred Heart Hospital in Allentown.

**Terry L. Spilken, D.P.M.,** is a podiatrist in New York City and Edison, New Jersey. He is on the adjunct faculty of the New York College of Podiatric Medicine in New York City.

**Mark D. Sussman, D.P.M.,** is a retired podiatrist who formerly practiced in Wheaton, Maryland.

# CANKER SORES
## 13 Ways to Ease the Sting

No one knows for sure why some people get canker sores and others don't. For most people, a hot pizza burn heals in 2 to 3 days with little or no pain, but for others it can lead to a lesion that won't heal for 2 weeks. Heredity, certain foods, overly aggressive toothbrushing, ill-fitting dentures, chewing on the inside of your mouth, and emotional stress can all lead to painful, craterlike canker sores.

Whatever the cause, medicating a canker sore is a difficult task, says Robert Goepp, D.D.S., Ph.D. Nothing sticks well to the skin in your mouth, and it's one of the most bacteria-laden places in the body. Remedies have a double-barreled aim: to protect the sore, thus minimizing pain and to kill the organisms.

The good news is that canker sores tend to be more prevalent in young people, becoming much less frequent with age. But meanwhile, a mouthful of sores can make you miserable. Here are a few escape routes.

## WHEN TO CALL A DOCTOR

A canker sore should heal within 2 weeks. "If the sores last a long time or you are unable to eat, speak, or sleep properly, you should see a doctor or dentist," advises Robert Goepp, D.D.S., Ph.D. He will probably prescribe topical steroids or oral antibiotics.

**Use a bubbly rinse.** Carbamide peroxide is the generic form of an over-the-counter (OTC) medication that combines glycerin and peroxide, such as Gly-Oxide. "The peroxide releases oxygen and cleans up the bacteria," Dr. Goepp says. "The bubbles get into the tiniest crevices. The glycerin puts on a coating and helps protect the sore."

**Read labels.** Look for over-the-counter canker sore medications that contain benzocaine, menthol, camphor, eucalyptol, or alcohol in a liquid or gel. They often sting at first, and most need repeated application because they don't stick, but they're also effective.

**Apply a paste coating.** Some OTC pastes form a protective "bandage" over the sore. To get pastes like Orabase to work, dry the sore with one end of a cotton swab, then immediately apply the paste with the other end. It works only on beginning sores, however.

**Draw tannin from a wet tea bag.** Several experts, among them dermatologist Jerome Z. Litt, M.D., recommend applying a wet, black tea bag to the ulcer. Black tea contains tannin, an astringent that "may pleasantly surprise you" with its pain-relieving ability, he says. Tanac is an OTC medication that contains tannin.

**Disinfect your mouth.** Dilute 1 tablespoon of hydrogen peroxide in a glass of water and swish it around in your mouth to disinfect the sore and speed healing, says Dr. Goepp.

**Attack with alum.** Alum is the active ingredient in a styptic pencil, an old-fashioned medicine cabinet standby for cuts and shaving nicks. It's an antiseptic and pain reliever that can prevent the infection from getting worse, say doctors, but it won't truly abort a canker sore.

**Use Mylanta as a mouth rinse.** Don't swallow your Mylanta or milk of magnesia. Instead, swish it around your mouth and allow it to protectively coat the sore before spitting it out. It may also have some antibacterial effect, Dr. Goepp says.

**Try goldenseal.** Make a strong tea of goldenseal root (available at health food stores) and use it as a mouthwash. Or you can make a paste with a bit of water and apply it directly. "It's antiseptic and astringent and is probably modestly effective," says Varro E. Tyler, Ph.D.

**Apply an alternative antiseptic.** Propolis, used by bees to construct their hives, and tea tree oil have antiseptic properties and can be dabbed on a canker sore with a moist cotton swab, says Andrew Weil, M.D. Both products are available in health food stores.

**Avoid food irritants.** Coffee, spices, citrus fruits, nuts high in the amino acid arginine (especially walnuts), chocolate, and strawberries irritate canker sores and can even cause them in some people, Dr. Goepp says.

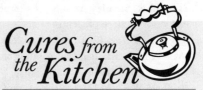

## Cures from the Kitchen

Eating 4 tablespoons of unflavored yogurt a day may help prevent canker sores by sending in helpful bacteria to counter the "bad" bacteria in your mouth, says Jerome Z. Litt, M.D. Look for yogurt that contains active cultures of *Lactobacillus acidophilus.*

**Brush carefully.** It is important to keep your mouth and teeth clean while a canker sore heals, but be cautious. You don't want to jab a healing sore with a toothbrush or toothpick and reinjure it. Also, read toothpaste labels if you're prone to canker sores. Sodium lauryl sulfate, used as a detergent in some toothpastes, may trigger canker sores in some people. Other toothpastes contain triclosan, an antimicrobial ingredient that may help canker sores heal.

**Rely on vitamins.** Craig Zunka, D.D.S., recommends squeezing vitamin E oil from a capsule onto your canker sore. Repeat several times a day to keep the tissue well-oiled. Also, at the first tingle of a canker sore, take 1,000 milligrams of vitamin C with bioflavonoids and then take 500 milligrams three times a day for the next 3 days. It's very important that you use vitamin C with bioflavonoids, he says, because vitamin C by itself doesn't work for canker sores. For those who chronically get canker sores, 500 milligrams of lysine (an amino acid) once a day is very effective. The homeopathic remedy Borax 12X may also help.

## PANEL OF ADVISORS

**Robert Goepp, D.D.S., Ph.D.,** is a professor emeritus in the departments of surgery and pathology, specializing in oral pathology at the University of Chicago Medical Center and hospital in Illinois.

Jerome Z. Litt, M.D., is a dermatologist and assistant clinical professor of dermatology at Case Western Reserve University School of Medicine in Cleveland. He is the author of *Your Skin: From Acne to Zits.*

Harold R. Stanley, D.D.S., is a professor emeritus of dentistry at the University of Florida College of Dentistry in Gainesville.

Varro E. Tyler, Ph.D., was a professor of pharmacognosy at Purdue University in West Lafayette, Indiana, and author of *The Honest Herbal.* He also served as a *Prevention* magazine advisor.

Andrew Weil, M.D., is a clinical professor of medicine and director of the program in integrative medicine at the University of Arizona in Tucson. He is the author of several books, including *8 Weeks to Optimum Health.*

Craig Zunka, D.D.S., is a dentist in Front Royal, Virginia, and is past president and advisor to the Board of the Holistic Dental Association. He also is a diplomate of the Board of Dental Homeopathy.

# CARPAL TUNNEL SYNDROME
## 14 Coping Techniques

The bane of office workers, restaurant servers, carpenters, and journalists, carpal tunnel syndrome is a painful reminder of how much many of us depend on our hands to earn a living. At first, symptoms include numbness, tingling, loss of strength or flexibility, and pain. Yet carpal tunnel can progress over time, with a very small percentage of patients developing permanent injury. That's why it's best to address symptoms head- (or hand-) on.

The good news is that most people with carpal tunnel syndrome recover completely and avoid injuring themselves again by changing the way they work. What's more, those with carpal tunnel can make other changes that ease the pain.

Carpal tunnel syndrome isn't something that happens overnight. It's a cumulative trauma disorder that develops over time when your hands and wrists perform repetitive movements.

Think of New York City's Holland Tunnel. Imagine what a pain it is to try to get through it during rush hour as multiple lanes of traffic fight to squeeze into two-lane tubes. Your wrist, known as the carpal tunnel, is a lot like the tunnel under the Hudson River during rush hour. When you use your hand in repeated motions—like writing, typing, or hammering—the tendons, which run

## WHEN TO CALL A DOCTOR

Wrist and hand pain is not always the result of carpal tunnel syndrome and could actually be the sign of a more serious illness, cautions physical therapist Susan Isernhagen. "If you get a crackly or crunchy feeling in your wrist when you exercise it, that's not a sign of carpal tunnel syndrome," she says. "It may be a symptom of osteoarthritis." Ask your doctor to check it out.

like lanes through your wrist, swell and compress the median nerve that runs to your hand.

Women are twice as likely as men to experience carpal tunnel syndrome. Symptoms normally affect one hand but can be present in both, says Colin Hall, M.D. "Sometimes the affected hand will feel numb or tingle, or feel like it's 'fallen asleep.'"

When the feeling comes, it's time to look for relief. Here's how.

**Go round in circles.** "When the tingling begins, it's time to do some hand exercises," says physical therapist Susan Isernhagen.

One of these is a simple circle exercise that rotates the wrist. Move your hands around in gentle circles for about 2 minutes. "This exercises all the muscles of the wrist, restores circulation, and gets your wrist out of the bent position that normally brings on the symptoms of carpal tunnel syndrome," Isernhagen says.

**Raise your hand.** Get those hands off the keyboard and up into the air. "Raise your arm above your head and rotate your arm while rotating your wrist at the same time," says Isernhagen. This gets your shoulder, neck, and upper back in a better position and relieves the stress and tension.

**Go on R and R.** Take a break from what you're doing. "Rest your hands on a desk or a table and then rotate your head for about 2 minutes. Bend your neck backward and forward," recommends Isernhagen, "then tip your head to either side. Also do some neck turns, looking over your right shoulder, then your left."

**Make exercise as routine as eating.** It's important to exercise and relax all the muscles that are giving you problems every day, even when you're not in pain, Isernhagen says. Practice motion exercises such as the ones described above at least four times a day.

**Reach for the aspirin.** "To reduce pain and inflammation, take a nonsteroidal anti-inflammatory medication like aspirin or ibuprofen," says orthopedic sur-

# The Vitamin B₆ Debate

Doctors first recommended vitamin B₆ for carpal tunnel syndrome 30 years ago. Yet as the years passed, the debate over the vitamin's usefulness intensified.

Several books recommend taking 100 to 200 milligrams of vitamin B₆ every day to ease symptoms, with some studies suggesting that low levels of vitamin B₆ may increase the risk of carpal tunnel syndrome.

Yet critics say that large doses of vitamin B₆ are not only useless in the treatment of carpal tunnel syndrome, they can be dangerous. The National Institutes of Health also takes a dim view of B₆ as a treatment for carpal tunnel syndrome. Its experts say that scientific studies don't show that vitamin B₆ is effective.

Because vitamin B₆ can be toxic at high levels, it should be used only under the supervision of a physician. The Daily Value is 2 milligrams. An excess can lead to nerve damage.

---

geon Stephen Cash, M.D. Don't take acetaminophen, though. "Acetaminophen reduces pain," he says, "but it doesn't do anything for inflammation."

**Put the pain on ice.** "Cold packs will work to bring the swelling down," Isernhagen says. Don't wrap your wrist in a heating pad. That just increases the swelling.

**Rise to the occasion.** "Avoid having your hand lower than your shoulder when you take a break from work," says Isernhagen. "Sit with your elbows supported on your desk or propped on the arms of your chair. Keep your hands pointed upward. That's a good relief position."

**Put the squeeze on your pain.** "Squeezing motions of the fingers will help relieve the tingling feeling," Isernhagen says. Press your fingers into your palm, then stretch them way back and hold. Repeat.

**Stay topside at night.** Keep your arms close to your body and your wrists straight while sleeping. "If you let your hand drop over the side of the bed, it can increase the pressure," Isernhagen says.

If you find yourself waking up because of the pain in your hands, Isernhagen recommends doing the same exercises at night that you do during the day.

**Go for splint second relief.** To relieve symptoms of carpal tunnel syndrome, use a wrist splint to keep your wrist straight. "The splints help take pressure off the nerve," says Dr. Cash. He recommends a splint that has a metal insert and Velcro fasteners. It gives support without being totally rigid.

"The ones made out of plastic usually are hard and are also hot and sticky," notes Isernhagen. "Whatever kind of splint you get, it should fit into the palm of your hand, leaving the thumb and fingers free."

You may want to consider having the splint tailor-made. "You should really have a professional like a physical therapist or occupational therapist fit you to make sure it fits your hand exactly," notes Isernhagen.

**Don't get too tight.** You don't want to completely tie up traffic in your wrist. Don't wrap your wrist with an elastic bandage, because you could wrap it too tight and cut off the circulation, says Isernhagen.

**Use the right grip.** If you have to carry anything with a handle, be sure the grip fits your hand. If the grip is too small, build it up with tape or rubberized tubing. If it's too large, get another handle, says Isernhagen.

**Handle with care.** "Don't concentrate pressure at the base of the wrist when using hand tools. Use your elbow and shoulder as much as possible," recommends Isernhagen.

## PANEL OF ADVISORS

**Stephen Cash, M.D.,** is an assistant clinical professor of orthopedic surgery in the division of hand surgery at Jefferson Medical College of Thomas Jefferson University in Philadelphia and a staff member of the Hand Rehabilitation Center there.

**Colin Hall, M.D.,** is a professor of neurology and medicine and director of the neuromuscular unit in the department of neurology at the University of North Carolina at Chapel Hill School of Medicine.

**Susan Isernhagen** is a physical therapist and president of Isernhagen Work Systems in Duluth, Minnesota. She acts as a consultant to industries to help reduce work injuries and rehabilitate injured workers.

# CHAFING
## 10 Ways to Rub It Out

For years, the varsity wrestling team at Ohio State University practiced while wearing gray shirts made of 100 percent cotton.

Then the team's training uniform changed. Wrestlers were given a 50 percent polyester, 50 percent cotton practice shirt. The shirt was thick and durable. A good buy, it seemed, since they'd last season after season.

But the wrestlers complained. The shirts rubbed against their faces and necks, leaving their skin sore and chafed. And even though the shirts were washed daily, the fabric stayed harsh and abrasive. Abrasions increase the chances of infection, and over time, 8 of the 42 team members reported a herpes simplex infection on their faces or necks.

The next year, team members again wore all-cotton shirts. Wrestlers noted few rashes. Herpes infections dropped.

The moral? When something rubs you the wrong way—and leaves a rash—find alternatives. For instance, try these strategies.

**Get on the natural fibers team.** Doctors at Ohio State University College of Medicine and Public Health pointed to the heavy-duty, synthetic-blend shirt as the culprit in the wrestlers' rash problem. When the team switched back to 100 percent cotton, the problem cleared up.

**Wash before you wear.** Wash any new exercise clothes before you wear them, says Richard H. Strauss, M.D. Washing sometimes softens the fabric enough to lessen abrasion.

**Wrap it up.** People who are overweight or who have big thighs, which makes chafing more likely, may find relief using elastic bandages around the portions of their legs that rub, says Tom Barringer, M.D. The bandages shield the skin when your thighs rub together, and instead of skin against skin, the rubbing will be fabric against fabric. Be sure the elastic bandage is secure so that it doesn't move across the skin.

| **What the Doctor Does ...** | Tom Barringer, M.D., finds that the coarser the cloth in an outfit, the more likely it will chafe. "I've run up to 50 miles a week at times, depending on my schedule. And I've found that when something chafes, sometimes the best thing to do is just toss it out and try something else," he says. |
|---|---|

**Keep it tight.** A pair of athletic tights or Lycra cycling shorts are snug, yet they stretch and cause no friction against the skin, says Dr. Barringer.

**Put cotton first.** When your exercise outfit is made of a possibly abrasive fabric, wear cotton undies to separate the fabric from your delicate skin, says Dr. Strauss. "Lots of male athletes will put on cotton underwear and put their supporters on top of that," he suggests.

**Grease your body.** Petroleum jelly between your thighs, around your toes, under your arms—anywhere you chafe—acts as a lubricant, helping the rubbing skin glide instead of chafe, says Robert Boyce, Ph.D.

**Find powder power.** Your mother may have used this remedy when you were a child. An old standby for chafing, talcum powder works as a lubricant, just the way petroleum jelly does. It helps the skin slip past other skin without catching and rubbing.

If you don't like powdery floors, sprinkle the powder into the middle of a large, soft, white handkerchief. Bind the edges together. Then, use the sack of powder like a powder puff. It will leave powder on you—not on the floor.

**Block it with a bandage.** Simply block the rub with an adhesive bandage. Runners, for instance, use a bandage over irritated nipples to prevent further rubbing.

**Try another sport.** Overweight exercisers may find chafing a regular problem until they lose a little excess girth, says Dr. Boyce. His advice: Switch sports while your skin heals. If you have sore spots from walking, try the stationary bicycle. If the bicycle causes problems, try swimming, a virtually chafe-free sport.

## PANEL OF ADVISORS

**Tom Barringer, M.D.,** is a family physician in Charlotte, North Carolina.

**Robert Boyce, Ph.D.,** is an expert in exercise physiology and owner of Robert Boyce Health Promotion in Charlotte, North Carolina.

**Richard H. Strauss, M.D.,** is formerly a sports medicine doctor at Ohio State University College of Medicine and Public Health in Columbus.

# Chapped Hands
## 24 Soothing Tips

Sometimes it seems there's nothing more painful—or unattractive—than chapped hands. Blame it on aging and the weather. As you age, your body produces less of the oil you need to keep skin smooth and supple. Add in the low humidity of fall and winter, and you have a mess of dry and irritated skin. Fortunately, there are many soothing solutions for turning rough, dry hands into something soft enough to hold.

Here's what the experts recommend.

**Don't go near the water.** "The basic plan for dealing with chapped hands is to avoid water at all costs," says Joseph Bark, M.D. "Consider water to be just like acid on your hands, because it is the worst influence for chapped hands that

### WHEN TO CALL A DOCTOR

"If you have splits and cracks on your hands, or if what you consider to be chapped hands starts as little blisters along the sides of the fingers, you have hand eczema, and it's a sign that you should see a dermatologist," advises Joseph Bark, M.D.

Other signs may indicate that what you have is more than a case of chapped hands. If after 2 weeks of self-treatment your hands don't clear up, see a dermatologist, says Dr. Bark. You may have a fungal infection or even psoriasis of the hands.

Diana Bihova, M.D., cautions that people (such as doctors, nurses, chefs, and housewives) whose occupations require them to immerse their hands for prolonged periods of time can easily contract monilial parony-chia, an annoying fungal infection involving the skin around the cuticle. "Bartenders and waitresses who handle beer, which is yeasty, are particu-larly susceptible. When the infection strikes the finger's protective nail fold, it becomes red, swollen, and painful."

we know of. Repeated washing removes the skin's natural oil layer, which allows moisture within the skin to evaporate. And that's extremely drying." Always think twice about washing your hands unnecessarily.

**Go palm up.** "When you must wash your hands often, try to do just the palms," recommends Diana Bihova, M.D. "You can wash the palms much more often than the backs of the hands, which have thinner skin and dry out easily."

**Use the lotion potion.** "Instead of using soap, clean your hands with an oil-free skin cleanser such as Cetaphil," says Dr. Bark. "Rub it on the skin, work it into a lather, then wipe it off with a tissue. It's a wonderful way to wash skin without any irritation whatsoever."

**Try the bath oil treatment.** Taking the no-soap concept one step further, Rodney Basler, M.D., recommends washing your hands with bath oil. "They may not *feel* really clean like they might with soap, but they won't get dried out either."

**Get topical.** Use some type of topical emollient every time you wash your hands and at bedtime. "Its strength should depend on the severity of your chapping," says Dr. Basler. "Lotions are the least moisturizing, followed by creams and then ointments. Try a lotion first. If that's not enough to carry you through the winter, step up to a cream, then an ointment."

**Don't throw in the towel.** "If your workplace bathroom has a hot-air blower instead of hand towels, bring in a towel from home," advises Dr. Bihova. "Hot-air blowers have been associated with chapped hands. If you must use one, keep your hands at least 6 inches from the nozzle and dry them thoroughly."

**Go soak your hand.** Although in general you should keep your hands

## Cures from the Kitchen

"If you want the cheapest home remedy going, use Crisco," says Dr. Bark. "It's a wonderful moisturizer that covers the skin and keeps water locked in. The key is to use very little and rub it in well so that your hands don't feel greasy. Your skin needs only two molecules' worth of barrier thickness to protect it from water loss. They used to call Crisco 'Cream C' at Duke University, where doctors dispensed it freely. It really works."

"You don't have to purchase expensive creams to get good results," agrees Howard Donsky, M.D. "Inexpensive substitutes for people with dry and normal skin include cocoa butter, lanolin, petroleum jelly, and light mineral oil."

out of water, sometimes a therapeutic soak is in order. "For an inexpensive way to achieve the same moisturizing effects produced by skin creams, simply soak your hands in warm water for a few minutes. Then pat off excess water and apply vegetable or mineral oil to the damp surface to seal in moisture," says Howard Donsky, M.D.

In the same vein, Dr. Basler recommends soaking in a water-and-oil solution. "Use 4 capfuls of a bath oil that disperses well (Alpha-Keri is the best) in 1 pint of water. At the end of the day, soak for 20 minutes to get oil back into the skin. That alone will help chapped hands."

**Double up.** "When applying any type of lotion or cream, use what I call Bark's double-layer application technique," says Dr. Bark. "Put on a very thin layer and let it soak in for a few minutes. Then apply another thin layer. Two thin ones work much better than one heavy one."

**Try lemon oil.** "To smooth and soothe irritated hands, mix a few drops of glycerin with a few drops of lemon essential oil (both are available at drugstores or health food stores). Massage this into your hands at bedtime," says skin-care specialist Lia Schorr.

**Dress to kill.** A lot of unsuspected things around the home can act as irritants for chapped hands. "I recommend wearing plain white cotton gloves for doing any kind of dry work," says Dr. Bihova. "That includes reading the newspaper and even unloading groceries. Any time you have friction against skin that's already dry, cracked, or red, you aggravate it. The advantage of cotton gloves is that they allow the skin to breathe and at the same time absorb any moisture that accumulates so it won't irritate your skin."

"In addition, cotton gloves keep the skin clean so you don't have to wash your hands so often and risk perpetuating the problem," according to Nelson Lee Novick, M.D.

"If you need to get an extra-good grip on something, use leather gloves," says hand model Trisha Webster.

**Mix rubber and cotton.** "For wet work, it's extremely important to use cotton gloves under vinyl ones," says

## Cures from the Kitchen

To remove the top layer of dead skin cells from chapped hands, skin-care specialist Lia Schorr recommends a weekly sloughing treatment. "Process 1 cup of uncooked, old-fashioned (not instant) rolled oats in a blender until you have a very fine powder. Place it in a large bowl, then rub your hands in the powder, gently removing dry skin. Rinse with cool water, pat dry, and lavish on hand cream. Wait 2 minutes and apply more cream."

## Model Your Hands after Hers

When your fingers are your fortune, you take darned good care of them. Ask Trisha Webster. She's a top hand model formerly with the Wilhelmina agency in New York City. You've seen her hands in many high-fashion jewelry and cosmetic ads. So how does she keep her hands looking young? The same way you can.

**Stop problems before they start.** "I try to keep my hands out of water at all costs," says Webster, "which is why I always let someone else do the dishes (well, it's *one* of the reasons!). When I can't avoid getting my hands wet, such as during bathing, I always moisturize them immediately afterward. It takes just a few minutes for the moisture that's accumulated in the skin to evaporate. When that happens, your hands are drier than they were before."

**Get protection.** "I never go outdoors in the winter without protecting my hands. That means putting on a good layer of moisturizer and then gloves."

**Use sun sense.** "A long time ago, I stopped going out in the sun, because it dries and ages hands just as surely as it does your face."

If you're not ready to give up the sun, Diana Bihova, M.D., suggests using a moisturizing sunscreen on your hands. "Sunscreens moisturize hands and keep them looking younger, so make their use an everyday habit," she says. "Just stay away from gels and alcohol-based sunscreens, because alcohol is drying. Also, products containing the active ingredient PABA can be irritating if you have sensitive skin."

Dr. Novick. That's because perspiration, lotions, and medications on your hands accumulate inside the gloves and may become irritating rather quickly. If the cotton gloves get wet, change them immediately. Otherwise, every 20 minutes is time enough to replace them with a fresh pair. "I don't recommend rubber gloves with built-in cotton linings, because it's very difficult to launder them," he says. "But you can launder separate cotton gloves in a mild detergent like Ivory Snow or Ivory Flakes."

Dr. Bihova agrees. "The biggest mistake women make when they have hand problems is wearing just rubber gloves. That only makes the hands worse. The rubber traps moisture, keeps the skin from breathing, and creates too much friction."

"Sometimes you can avoid gloves altogether," says Thomas Goodman Jr., M.D. "When you're doing dishes, for instance, a long-handled dish brush keeps your hands entirely out of water."

**Go elegantly into the night.** Dr. Goodman recommends occasionally wearing cotton gloves to bed for an extra-soothing treatment. "Moisten the fabric with about a teaspoon of petroleum jelly so that the gloves won't absorb the cream from your hands. Then apply hand cream at bedtime and slip on the gloves. Leave them on overnight. Your hands remain bandaged, in a sense, and can heal."

"The important thing," adds Dr. Bark, "is not to automatically run to the sink in the morning and wash off the cream. Also, I don't recommend sleeping in plastic gloves. They make your hands sweat too much overnight so that by morning you have the most incredible case of dishpan hands you've ever seen."

**Call on hydrocortisone.** Over-the-counter hydrocortisone creams and ointments are of value in treating chapped hands. Use Cortaid or any other 0.5 percent cream several times a day, says Dr. Goodman. Then put a heavier, greasier product on top of that. These hydrocortisone creams don't substitute for good hand care, but they are a boost. Every time you wash your hands, reapply them.

**Get a salon treatment.** "Believe it or not, even shampoo can make your tender hands feel worse," says Stephen Schleicher, M.D. "Either let someone else shampoo your hair or wear plastic gloves."

**Hire a cook.** "The juices of raw meat and vegetables—like potatoes, onions, tomatoes, even carrots—are sometimes very toxic to skin, especially if it's already

---

# Prevention Is Your Best Solution

Chapped hands are always easier to prevent than to treat, says Diana Bihova, M.D. Here are some ways to do that.

**Stay out of hot water.** "A good rule of thumb is to avoid hot water, detergents, and strong household solvents," says Dr. Bihova.

**Avoid soaping.** "Because chapped hands occur when oil is taken from the skin, you should not use a terribly harsh or alkaline soap. You're better off with a mild soap, preferably with a little cold cream in it. I often recommend Dove because it's virtually the mildest soap there is," says Joseph Bark, M.D.

**Put moisture in the air.** "Skin moisturizes itself from the inside out," notes Rodney Basler, M.D. "If there's moisture in the air, not as much will be drawn out through the skin. Therefore, it's a good idea to use a home humidifier."

**Pamper your hands.** "When you apply moisturizer to your face in the morning, immediately apply some to the hands. At night do the same," advises Dr. Bihova. "That keeps them supple and helps resist chapping. I'd say twice a day is a must. In addition, do it after each washing."

irritated. So you can either hire a cook to do all your kitchen work," quips Dr. Goodman, "or wear tissue-thin plastic gloves when handling food."

"You particularly don't want to squeeze acidic fruits like oranges, lemons, or grapefruit with your bare hands," adds Dr. Schleicher. "They're terribly irritating and will dry your hands further."

## PANEL OF ADVISORS

**Joseph Bark, M.D.,** is a dermatologist in Lexington, Kentucky, and the author of *Your Skin . . . An Owner's Guide.*

**Rodney Basler, M.D.,** is a dermatologist and assistant professor of internal medicine at the University of Nebraska College of Medicine in Lincoln.

**Diana Bihova, M.D.,** is a dermatologist affiliated with the dermatology department at the Columbia University College of Physicians and Surgeons in New York City.

**Howard Donsky, M.D.,** is a clinical instructor of dermatology at the University of Rochester and a dermatologist at the Dermatology and Cosmetic Center of Rochester in New York.

**Thomas Goodman Jr., M.D.,** is a dermatologist and former assistant professor of dermatology at the University of Tennessee Health Science Center in Memphis. He is the author of *Smart Face.*

**Nelson Lee Novick, M.D.,** is an associate clinical professor of dermatology at the Mount Sinai–New York University Medical Center in New York City.

**Stephen Schleicher, M.D.,** is medical director of DERM DX Centers for Dermatology, Inc. in Hazleton, Pennsylvania, with offices throughout eastern Pennsylvania. He is also an advisor for dermatological training to physician assistant students at Arcadia University in Glenside and at King's College in Wilkes-Barre.

**Lia Schorr** is a skin-care specialist and director of Lia Schorr Institute of Cosmetics Skin-Care Training in New York City.

**Trisha Webster** is a top New York City hand model formerly with the Wilhelmina, Inc. modeling agency. She has almost 20 years of experience in the business.

# CHAPPED LIPS
## 12 Tips to Stop the Dryness

Chapped lips give new meaning to the expression "crack a smile." Cold, dry weather; the sun's unrelenting rays; even allergic reactions to lipstick, toothpaste, food, or drink can make your lips peel. Doctors have a term for lip inflammation, *cheilitis*, and those who have chapped lips know they can quickly turn a smile into a scowl.

**Try the palm or balm solution.** "The best way to deal with chapped lips is to avoid the dry, cold weather that can cause them in the first place," says Joseph Bark, M.D. "But since heading for the tropics is not too practical for most people, you can head for the drugstore instead."

Pick up some lip balm. Then, before you go outside—and several times while you're out—coat your lips with it. Since lips don't hold anything on them very well, reapply it every time you eat or drink anything or wipe your lips.

**Use a sunscreen.** "Remember, too, that the sun fries lips—any time of the year," says Dr. Bark. So you're well-advised to choose a product with built-in sunscreen such as PreSun Ultra or Chap Stick Sun Zone, both of which have a sun protection factor (SPF) of 15.

Nelson Lee Novick, M.D., concurs: "Sun damage to the lips can cause dryness and scaliness, the same way sun can damage the rest of your skin. In its simplest form, it can harm the lower lip, which takes the brunt of ultraviolet rays."

**Wear lipstick.** A creamy lipstick helps soothe lips that are already chapped, says makeup expert Glenn Roberts. "In fact, just wearing lipstick gives some protection and may help prevent chapping in the first place."

"In addition, I believe use of lipstick is one of the reasons women seldom get lip cancer. In my 14 years of practice, I've treated maybe one or two women for lip cancer but literally hundreds of men," says Dr. Bark.

**Soothe and heal.** "The danger with chapped lips is that they can become infected," says Diana Bihova, M.D. "To prevent infection, apply an over-the-counter antibiotic ointment such as Bacitracin or Polysporin. Over-the-counter hydrocortisone ointments can also help with chapped lips, but they would not prevent infection. If your lips are severely chapped, you may want to use both. Apply one in the morning and one at night."

**Be wise.** "Nutritional deficiencies—such as those of B-complex vitamins and iron—can play a part in scaling of the lips. So make sure you're okay on that front with a multivitamin supplement," says Dr. Novick.

**Drink up.** Moisturize your lips from the inside out by drinking additional fluids in the winter. "I recommend several ounces of water every few hours," says Dr. Bihova. "As you age, the ability of your cells to retain moisture decreases, so your dryness problem may actually increase each winter. Another way to help counter wintertime dry lips is to humidify the air in your home and office."

**Mind your own beeswax.** "To my mind, the single best product for chapped lips is Carmex," says Rodney Basler, M.D. "It's an old-fashioned product that comes in a little tin and contains, among other things, beeswax and phenol. No prescription medication is better than that."

**Stop licking.** "Chapped lips are a dehydration problem," according to Dr. Basler. "When you lick them, you momentarily apply moisture, which then evaporates and leaves your lips feeling drier than before. Besides, saliva contains digestive enzymes. Granted they're not very strong, but they don't do your sore lips any good."

"Licking chapped lips can lead to something called lip-licker's dermatitis," cautions Dr. Bark. "It's usually seen in kids but can occur in adults, too." What happens when you lick your lips is that you scrape off any oil that might be on them from surrounding areas. (The lips themselves don't have any oil glands.) Pretty soon, you're licking not just the lips but also the area around them. Eventually, you end up with a red ring of dermatitis around the mouth. The moral: Don't start licking in the first place.

If you *are* tempted to lick your lips, remember what Dr. Basler laughingly calls the old Nebraska treatment: chicken manure applied to the lips. "It doesn't make your lips better, but it sure keeps you from licking them," he says.

**Give toothpaste the brush-off.** "Allergy and sensitivity to flavoring agents in toothpaste, candy, chewing gum, and mouthwash can cause chapped lips in some people," says Thomas Goodman Jr., M.D. "My dentist says that the new tartar-control toothpastes are even worse at drying lips than the regular ones. So I tell people to stop using toothpaste. Just use a toothbrush alone or a brush with baking soda on it."

**Think zinc.** "Some people have a tendency to drool in their sleep, which can dry out lips or aggravate ones that are already chapped," says Dr. Novick. If that's a problem, apply zinc oxide ointment every night before bed. It acts as a barrier to protect lips.

**Lay a finger alongside your nose.** "Here's what I tell farmers, who may be working outside and may not have anything else handy," says Dr. Bark. "Put your finger on the side of your nose. Then rub your finger around your lips. It picks up a little of the oil that's naturally there. It's the kind of oil the lips are looking for anyway, and they usually get it from contact with adjacent skin. You couldn't get any more of a home remedy than that."

**Opt for the udder alternative.** Here's another idea from down on the farm. "There's a product called Bag Balm that farmers use on cows' udders when they're sore. You can use that on your lips, too," says Dr. Bihova. "It's a petroleum-based product and is available in farm supply stores, vet supply stores, and some pharmacies and health food stores."

## PANEL OF ADVISORS

**Joseph Bark, M.D.,** is a dermatologist in Lexington, Kentucky, and the author of *Your Skin . . . An Owner's Guide.*

**Rodney Basler, M.D.,** is a dermatologist and assistant professor of internal medicine at the University of Nebraska College of Medicine in Lincoln.

**Diana Bihova, M.D.,** is a dermatologist affiliated with the dermatology department at the Columbia University College of Physicians and Surgeons in New York City.

**Thomas Goodman Jr., M.D.,** is a dermatologist and former assistant professor of dermatology at the University of Tennessee Health Science Center in Memphis. He is the author of *Smart Face.*

**Nelson Lee Novick, M.D.,** is an associate clinical professor of dermatology at the Mount Sinai–New York University Medical Center in New York City.

**Glenn Roberts** is director of creative beauty at Elizabeth Arden in New York City.

# COLDS
## 29 Remedies to Win the Battle

If colds are so common, why isn't there a cure? The answer has to do with simple mathematics. As many as 200 viruses are responsible for the 1 billion colds Americans get each year, stymieing scientists' ability to concoct a "cure" that will work against them all.

It's clear that antibiotics, highly effective at knocking out bacterial infections, are useless against colds, which are caused by viruses. So most people live with the sniffles and aches, maybe take an over-the-counter remedy or two, and hope the symptoms will disappear in the customary week or so.

But there's much more you can do to ease your way through a cold more comfortably, doctors say. Some remedies may even help you overcome a cold more quickly. Here's how.

## WHEN TO CALL A DOCTOR

If your cold is accompanied by one or more of the following symptoms, see your doctor. Your problem may be more serious than the common cold.

- A fever that remains above 101°F for more than 3 days, or any fever above 103°F
- Any hot, extreme pain, such as earache, swollen tonsils, sinus pain, or aching lungs or chest
- Excessively large amounts of sputum, or sputum that is greenish or bloody
- Extreme difficulty swallowing
- Excessive loss of appetite
- Wheezing
- Shortness of breath

**See if vitamin C works for you.** "Vitamin C works in the body as a scavenger, picking up all sorts of trash—including virus trash," says Keith W. Sehnert, M.D.

Vitamin C may also cut back on coughing, sneezing, and other symptoms, although scientific studies produce mixed results when the vitamin is put to the test. One summary of 30 studies, published in 2000, found "a consistently beneficial but generally modest therapeutic effect on duration of cold symptoms." On average, vitamin C reduced the number of days people experienced cold symptoms by 8 to 9 percent.

If you're going to take vitamin C, experts recommend that you take 100 to 500 milligrams a day. To help maintain levels of vitamin C throughout the day, take half of the recommended dose in the morning and half at night.

**Zap it with zinc.** Sucking on zinc lozenges can cut colds short, from an average of 8 days to an average of 4, report researchers at the Cleveland Clinic. Study subjects sucked on four to eight lozenges a day, each containing 13.3 milligrams of zinc. Zinc can also dramatically reduce symptoms such as a dry, irritated throat, says Elson Haas, M.D. "It doesn't work for everyone, but when it works, it works," he says.

The downside is that zinc has an unpleasant taste. Fortunately, there are many brands of zinc lozenges available that come in a variety of flavors. But before choosing a brand, remember to check the label. Some lozenges have more zinc content than others. Always follow the directions on the package, and don't take more than the amount recommended. Also, don't take vitamin C and zinc at the same time, since the two bind together, making zinc less effective. Either take the vitamin first or wait ½ hour after your zinc lozenge has disappeared to take it.

Taking more than 40 milligrams a day can cause nausea, dizziness, or vomiting. High doses over an extended period of time can hinder your ability to absorb copper, another vital mineral.

**Eat your Wheaties.** Really, any well-rounded breakfast may go a long way in helping to keep colds at bay, according to a current study in the United Kingdom. Researchers there found that people who regularly eat breakfast report having the fewest number of colds and illnesses, perhaps because breakfast is an indicator of healthy lifestyles.

**Be positive.** A positive attitude about your body's ability to heal itself can actually mobilize immune system forces, says Martin Rossman, M.D. He teaches this theory by getting his patients to practice imagery techniques to combat colds. After bringing yourself into a deeply relaxed state, "imagine a white tornado decongesting your stuffed-up sinuses," he suggests, "or an army of microscopic maids cleaning up germs with buckets of disinfectant."

# The Cold Truth

So you have a cold that won't let go, and want to know who to blame? Elliot Dick, Ph.D., who has conducted research for more than 30 years on how colds are transmitted, says a lot of suspects have been taking a bum rap. They include:

- Sharing food or beverages with someone who has a cold

- Kissing someone with a cold
- Stepping outside with a wet head

The *real* culprit, of course, is a virus transmitted through the air, says Dr. Dick. You can catch it, he says, when someone with a cold coughs, sneezes, or does a sloppy job of blowing his nose, sending the virus floating into your path.

**Rest and relax.** Extra rest enables you to put all your energy into getting well. It can also help you avoid complications like bronchitis and pneumonia, says Samuel Caughron, M.D.

Take a day or two off from work if you're feeling really bad, he advises. At the very least, slow down in your everyday activities and reschedule your time. "Trying to keep up with your regular routine can be draining because when you're not feeling well, your concentration is down, and you'll probably need to double the amount of time it takes you to do things," he says.

**Be a homebody.** When you're sick, parties and other good times can wear you out physically, compromising your immune system and causing your cold to linger, says Timothy Van Ert, M.D. Stay home and snuggle up.

**Warm up.** Bundle up against the cold, advises Dr. Sehnert. This keeps your immune system focused on fighting your cold infection instead of displacing energy to protect you from the cold.

**Take a walk.** Mild exercise improves your circulation, helping your immune system circulate infection-fighting antibodies, says Dr. Sehnert. Do gentle exercises indoors or take a brisk ½-hour walk, he suggests. But refrain from strenuous exercise, he warns, which could wear you out.

**Feed a cold—lightly.** The very fact that you have a cold in the first place may indicate that your diet is putting a strain on your body's immune system, says Dr. Haas. Counteract the problem, he advises, by eating fewer fatty foods, meat and milk products, and more fresh fruit and vegetables.

**Load up on liquids.** Drinking six to eight glasses of water, juice, tea, and other mostly clear liquids daily helps replace important fluids lost during a cold and helps flush out impurities that may be preying on your system. "Remember: Dilution is the solution to pollution," says Dr. Haas.

**Stop smoking.** Smoking aggravates a throat that may already feel irritated from a cold, says Dr. Caughron. It also interferes with the infection-fighting activity of cilia, the microscopic "fingers" that sweep bacteria out of your lungs and throat. So if you can't kick the habit for good, at least do it while you have a cold.

**Ease a sore throat.** Gargle morning, noon, and night—or whenever it hurts most—with salt water, Dr. Van Ert advises. Fill an 8-ounce glass with warm water and mix in 1 teaspoon of salt. The salt water soothes a sore throat.

**Take goldenseal and echinacea.** Goldenseal stimulates your liver, whose job includes clearing up infections. It also strengthens the ailing mucous membranes in your nose, mouth, and throat. Echinacea cleans your blood and lymph glands, which help circulate infection-fighting antibodies and remove toxic substances. You can buy these herbs separately or in combination capsules. "I recommend these herbs at the early onset of a cold," says Dr. Haas. Whichever you choose, take them following the directions on the bottle for up to 2 weeks.

**Sip a hot toddy.** Clear your stuffed-up nose and help yourself to a good night's sleep by drinking a "hot toddy"—a hot drink consisting of liquor like rum, water, sugar, and spices—or half a glass of wine before bedtime, suggests Dr. Caughron. Don't imbibe any more than that, however, since too much can stress your system, making recovery more difficult.

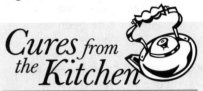

### Cures from the Kitchen

A longtime folk remedy is now a proven fact. A cup of hot chicken soup can help unclog your nasal passages. Researchers at Mount Sinai Medical Center in Miami Beach, Florida, found that hot chicken soup increases the flow of nasal mucus. Nasal secretions serve as a first line of defense in removing germs from your system, the scientists say.

It's also known that garlic and onions have antiviral properties, so adding some spice in the form of cayenne or chili peppers will further help unclog nasal passages.

**Drink tea at bedtime.** For a good night's sleep, brew a cup of hops, valerian herb tea, or Celestial Seasonings Sleepytime Herbal Tea, all of which have a natural tranquilizing effect. For even better results, Dr. Van Ert suggests adding a teaspoon of honey, a simple carbohydrate that has a sedative effect.

**Soothe your throat with licorice root.** Licorice root tea has an anesthetizing effect that soothes irritated throats and relieves coughs, says Dr. Van Ert. Although licorice root is available in tea bag form, he prefers making his own. Just put the root in a nonmetallic tea ball and steep in hot water for the desired amount of time. Drink it daily.

**Breathe steam.** Taking a steamy shower can help clear congestion, says Kenneth Peters, M.D. Or heat a teakettle or pot of water to boiling on your stove; turn off the flame; drape a towel over your head and the kettle, creating a tent; and inhale the steam until it subsides. This also relieves your cough by moistening your dry throat, he says.

You may also find comfort using a humidifier close to your bed at night, adds Dr. Van Ert.

**Use petroleum jelly on a sore nose.** Relieve a nose raw from blowing by applying with a cotton swab a lubricating layer of petroleum jelly around and slightly inside your nostrils, suggests Dr. Peters.

**Medicate at night.** Don't let your cold symptoms keep you from getting a healing night's sleep. Numerous medications for colds are available without a prescription. Some treat specific symptoms. Others, like NyQuil and Contac, contain a combination of drugs—plus alcohol, in some cases—aimed at treating a wide range of symptoms. These combination drugs, however, can have many uncomfortable side effects like nausea and drowsiness, says Dr. Van Ert. "I recommend only taking these at night, since you won't feel the side effects while you're sleeping."

If you need to take medications during the day, he suggests taking those that treat just the symptoms you're experiencing. Be sure to follow the instructions carefully, he advises. Here's what to reach for.

- For relief of the body aches or fever that can accompany a cold, take *aspirin* or *acetaminophen*.

- To stop sneezing and dry up your runny nose and watery eyes, take an *antihistamine*, which blocks your body's release of histamine, a chemical that causes these symptoms. Look for products, like Chlor-Trimeton, that are available over-the-counter, advises Diane Casdorph, R.Ph. Warning: Antihistamines frequently cause drowsiness, so save these for bedtime or at least for when you won't be driving or doing anything that requires coordination. If drowsiness is a problem, talk with your doctor about nondrowsy antihistamines, which are available by prescription.

- To unstuff your nose, take a *decongestant*. First, check your medicine cabinet and make sure you aren't taking an old product that contains phenylpropanolamine, which was voluntarily withdrawn by manufacturers when the FDA warned that it was associated with an increased risk of stroke, especially in women. Products currently on the market that do not contain phenyl-propanolamine include Sudafed, Actifed, Dristan, and Contac. Before taking a nonprescription antihistamine or decongestant, contact your doctor or pharmacist.

- *Nasal sprays and drops*, such as Afrin and Neo-Synephrine, are also effective decongestants. But they shouldn't be used for longer than 3 days, says Dr. Peters. Overuse can result in a "rebound effect," meaning your nose becomes more congested than ever, requiring more medication.

- To relieve a cough, try *cough drops and syrups*. Look for a product that contains cough-suppressing antitussives such as dextromethorphan, says Casdorph. These include Vicks cough drops and Robitussin DM cough syrup, which also contains an expectorant to loosen phlegm.

- *Lozenges* can also combat coughs. Many of them contain topical anesthetics that slightly numb your sore throat, says Dr. Van Ert, which relieves your need to cough. Sucrets, Cepacol, or Cepastat sore throat decongestant lozenges are among them.

- *Menthol or camphor rubs* have a soothing, cooling effect and may relieve congestion and help you breathe more easily, especially at bedtime. Apply Vicks VapoRub or a similar product to your bare chest, cover up, and get a good night's sleep, recommends Dr. Van Ert.

**Don't spread your germs.** When you need to cough, go ahead and cough. When you need to blow your nose, go ahead and blow. But cough and sneeze into disposable tissues instead of setting germs free in the environment, Dr. Van Ert advises, then promptly throw the tissue away and wash your hands. Your healthy friends and family who want to stay that way will appreciate it.

## PANEL OF ADVISORS

**Diane Casdorph, R.Ph.,** is an assistant clinical professor and assistant director of the Drug Information Center of the West Virginia University School of Pharmacy in Morgantown.

**Samuel Caughron, M.D.,** is an assistant clinical professor in family medicine at the University of Virginia in Charlottesville and a member of the Albemarle Medical Association.

**Elliot Dick, Ph.D.,** is a retired virologist and professor of preventive medicine at the University of Wisconsin–Madison. He has conducted research on the common cold for more than 30 years.

**Elson Haas, M.D.,** is the director of the Preventive Medical Center of Marin, an integrated health-care facility in San Rafael, California, and author of seven books on health and nutrition, including *The False Fat Diet* and *Staying Healthy with Nutrition*.

**Kenneth Peters, M.D.,** is medical director of the Northern California Headache Clinic in Mountain View. He also practices general internal medicine at El Camino

Hospital, also in Mountain View. He has published numerous articles on effective headache management and has done extensive clinical research in the area of new headache medications.

**Martin Rossman, M.D.,** is a general practitioner in Mill Valley, California, and author of *Guided Imagery for Self-Healing*.

**Keith W. Sehnert, M.D.,** was a physician with Trinity Health Care in Minneapolis and author of several books, including *The Garden Within* and *How to Be Your Own Doctor (Sometimes)*.

**Timothy Van Ert, M.D.,** is a staff physician at Western Oregon University in Monmouth, Oregon, where he specializes in self-care and preventive medicine.

# COLD SORES
## 18 Tips to Heal Herpes Simplex

Most people—some researchers estimate up to *90 percent*—get an unsightly cold sore at least once during their lives. Generally, they were exposed during childhood to the highly contagious virus that causes cold sores, called herpes simplex virus 1, a different strain of herpes virus from the one that causes genital herpes.

Normally, after an initial outbreak the virus lies dormant in nerve cells, but occasionally it becomes reactivated. When that happens, you may experience a telltale sensation of numbness, tingling, burning, or itching on your lip or the skin around your mouth before a cold sore appears.

Fortunately, there are a number of steps you can take to minimize the pain of a cold sore and speed its healing.

**Let it be.** "If the cold sore isn't really bothersome, just leave it alone," says James F. Rooney, M.D. "Make sure to keep the sore clean and dry."

## WHEN TO CALL A DOCTOR

If a cold sore develops pus, seek medical attention, advises James F. Rooney, M.D. You probably have a bacterial infection, which can benefit from antibiotic treatment.

**Replace your toothbrush.** Your toothbrush can harbor the herpes virus for days, reinfecting you after the present cold sore heals.

Researchers at the University of Oklahoma exposed a sterile toothbrush to the virus for 10 minutes. Seven days later, half of the disease-producing viruses remained, says Richard T. Glass, D.D.S., Ph.D.

Dr. Glass recommends that you throw away your toothbrush when you notice you're just beginning to get the virus. If you still develop the cold sore, throw your toothbrush away after the blister develops. That can prevent you from developing multiple sores. And once the sore has healed completely, replace your toothbrush again. He says that patients who tried this method found it significantly reduced the number of cold sores they typically experienced in a year.

**Don't keep your toothbrush in the bathroom.** A damp toothbrush in a moist environment like your bathroom is a perfect environment for herpes simplex virus. That moisture helps prolong the life of the herpes virus on your toothbrush. That's why Dr. Glass recommends storing your toothbrush in a dry spot.

**Use small tubes of toothpaste.** Toothpaste can transmit disease, too, says Dr. Glass. Buy small tubes so that you replace them regularly.

**Protect with petroleum jelly.** You can protect your cold sore by covering it with petroleum jelly, says Dr. Glass. Be sure not to dip back into the jelly with the same finger you used to touch your sore. Better yet, use a fresh cotton swab.

**Zap it with zinc.** Several studies show that a water-based zinc solution, applied the minute you feel that tingling, helps speed healing time.

In a Boston study of 200 patients who were followed over a 6-year period, a 0.025 percent solution of zinc sulfate in camphorated water was found very effective. Sores healed in an average of 5.3 days. The solution was applied every 30 to 60 minutes during the onset of the cold sore.

Researchers in Israel also found a 2 percent water-based zinc solution, applied several times a day, to be very helpful, says Milos Chvapil, M.D., Ph.D.

How does zinc help? The zinc ions crosslink with the DNA molecule of the herpes virus and prevent the DNA from replicating, reducing the number of viruses produced, he says.

Zinc gluconate is kinder to the skin than zinc sulfate, says Dr. Chvapil. The mineral is available at health food stores.

**Rely on lysine.** Mark A. McCune, M.D., advises patients who have more than three cold sores a year to supplement their daily diets with 2,000 to 3,000 milligrams of the amino acid lysine. He also recommends that they double up on the dosage when they feel the itching and tingling that signals the development of another cold sore. Don't take amino acids without your doctor's guidance, however.

Not all studies have found lysine helpful for people with cold sores. But in one study of 41 patients, Dr. McCune and his colleagues found that a daily dose of 1,248 milligrams of lysine helped subjects reduce the number of cold sores they have in a year.

Good food sources of lysine include dairy products, potatoes, and brewer's yeast.

**Identify the pattern.** What was going on in your life just before you got your last cold sore? What about the cold sore prior to that? If you do some sleuthing, you may figure out what triggers a cold sore for you. If you can find a trigger, take additional lysine when you're most prone to cold sores, says Dr. McCune. Common triggers include stress and a variety of foods.

**Freeze it.** Some of Dr. Rooney's patients reach for ice when they first feel the tingling. "I'm not sure that it works, but if I were to speculate, I'd say that ice decreases inflammation," he says. "And if inflammatory substances aid the re-activation process, this could help."

**Dab on witch hazel.** "Some patients claim that breaking a sore and using witch hazel or alcohol to dry it really helps," says Dr. Rooney.

**Form a barrier.** Abreva, an over-the-counter medication containing docosanol, works by protecting healthy cells from the infected cells. The cold sore infection is less likely to penetrate the healthy cells.

Use the cream five times a day, beginning when you experience the first symptoms, says David H. Emmert, M.D. This can help your cold sore heal 1 to 2 days quicker.

**Numb it.** Most over-the-counter products contain some emollient to reduce cracking and soften scabs, and a numbing agent like phenol or camphor.

Phenol may have some antiviral properties, says Dr. Rooney. "Theoretically, it is possible that phenol is capable of killing the virus."

**Block sun and wind.** Protecting your lips from trauma like sunburn or wind exposure was cited by all our experts as a key to preventing cold sores.

**Avoid arginine-rich foods.** The herpes virus needs arginine as an essential amino acid for its metabolism. So cut out arginine-rich foods such as chocolate, cola, peas, grain cereals, peanuts, gelatin, cashews, and beer.

**Perfect your coping skills.** Studies have shown that stress can trigger recurrences of the herpes simplex virus. High levels of stress are not necessarily the culprit, says Cal Vanderplate, Ph.D. "How you cope with the stress—how you perceive it—is what's important."

His number one stress deflator is maintaining a loving social support system. "A sense of control is also very important. If you take a positive attitude toward your health, you'll be better able to influence your symptoms."

**Relax.** "By the time symptoms appear, it's too late to intervene in stress reduction," says Dr. Vanderplate. "But you may be able to reduce the severity by doing some relaxation exercises." He favors deep muscle relaxation techniques, biofeedback, visualization, and meditation.

**Exercise.** "There is some evidence that exercise actually helps bolster the immune system," says Dr. Vanderplate. The stronger your immune system, the better able it is to defend you against viruses. Exercise is also a super way to relax, he says.

**Correct your perception.** No one likes getting a cold sore. But if you have one, focusing on it and worrying about how you look can make it worse. "Minimize any negative perceptions you have about it," says Dr. Vanderplate. "Tell yourself that it is just like a pimple and it won't interfere in your life in any way."

## PANEL OF ADVISORS

**Milos Chvapil, M.D., Ph.D.,** is a professor emeritus of surgery in the surgical biology section of the University of Arizona College of Medicine in Tucson.

**David H. Emmert, M.D.,** is a family physician in Millersville, Pennsylvania, who, in 2000, summarized cold sore treatments for the medical journal *American Family Physician.*

**Richard T. Glass, D.D.S., Ph.D.,** is director of the forensic graduate program and professor of oral pathology at Oklahoma State University, College of Osteopathic Medicine in Tulsa, Oklahoma. He is professor emeritus from the University of Oklahoma, Colleges of Dentistry, Graduate, and Medicine where he was professor and chairman of the department of oral and maxillofacial pathology and professor of pathology.

**Mark A. McCune, M.D.,** is a dermatologist in Overland Park, Kansas. He is chief of dermatology at Humana Hospital in Overland Park.

**James F. Rooney, M.D.,** is a clinical virologist and formerly a special expert in the Laboratory of Oral Medicine at the National Institutes of Health in Bethesda, Maryland.

**Cal Vanderplate, Ph.D.,** is a clinical faculty member at Emory University School of Medicine in Atlanta and a clinical psychologist specializing in stress-related disorders.

# COLIC
## 10 Ideas to Quell the Cries

When writer Thomas Paine penned his famous line, "These are the times that try men's souls," he was referring to America's struggle for independence. Yet any parent who tries to soothe an inconsolable infant at the witching hour just before dinner will tell you the truly trying times come when a baby careens into screams due to colic.

Ancient scholars first described infantile colic in the 6th century. Modern parents have no trouble describing it today. The baby cries wrenching sobs, pulls her knees up to her abdomen, and appears to be in great pain. She may become gassy, then quiet, then scream again.

Nothing much seems to have changed over the centuries, and nothing much seems to help. Colicky babies cannot generally be quieted with feeding or a change of diapers, and episodes may last for several hours. Colic tends to be most severe at 4 to 6 weeks of age and gradually subsides by 3 to 4 months.

Though none of the remedies offered below will cure colic, most have brought some relief to suffering parents, so you may want to give them a try. And remember that this, too, shall pass. Colic disappears as mysteriously as it begins.

**Try the colic carry.** "I'm a big believer in the colic carry," says child-care expert Anne Price.

Extend your forearm with your palm up, then place the baby on your arm chest down, with her head in your hand and her legs on either side of your elbow. Support the baby with your other hand and walk around the house with her in this position, Price says. "It definitely helps."

**Burp that babe.** "My experience is that at least some colicky babies do have more abdominal gas than the norm and may be more difficult to burp," says pediatric nurse practitioner Linda Jonides.

Her recommendation: Watch the position of the baby when feeding (upright is all right) and burp frequently. When bottle-feeding, burp after every ounce, and try a variety of nipple types (some parents swear by the Playtex disposable nurser).

**Cut the cow juice.** Some child-care specialists believe that colic is caused when cow's milk is transmitted from mother to infant through breast milk. Though some research casts doubt on this connection, experts agree that a maternal diet free of cow's milk may be worth a try, especially in families with a strong history of allergies.

"I firmly believe that milk in the mother's diet is a frequent cause of colic in breastfed babies," Price says. "I recommend mothers start by eliminating milk from their diets and see what happens. If that does it, you don't have to go any further, but if not, you may need to cut back other dairy products."

**Check out the diet connection.** "Occasionally, there may be some foods that set a baby off," says Morris Green, M.D. "The breastfeeding mother may try to notice if there's any correlation between what she eats and the onset of the colic." Some potential troublemakers include caffeine-containing drinks, chocolate, bananas, oranges, strawberries, and heavily spiced foods.

**Try a wrap session.** "I recommend holding and swaddling a colicky baby," Jonides says, "or using a backpack to hold the baby so you have your arms free to do other things."

For some reason, wrapping a baby snugly in a blanket has a calming effect. It's very popular in some cultures, and it does sometimes stop colic attacks. It does not spoil an infant.

**Use a vacuum instead of a lullaby.** Colicky babies seem to love the sounds a vacuum creates. Science has failed to explain this mystery.

"The noise of a vacuum cleaner running does seem to calm a colicky baby," says Dr. Green. Some parents tape-record the sound of a vacuum cleaner and play it back when baby gets fussy. Others simply start vacuuming the carpet and hope the child outgrows colic while there's still some rug left.

Price suggests a more aggressive approach: "If you put the baby in a front pack and vacuum at the same time, it's a double whammy. That colicky baby goes out like a light."

**Do the dryer dribble.** "Put the baby in an infant seat and rest it against the side of a running clothes dryer so the baby gets that buzzing sound and vibration through the seat," suggests pediatric nurse Helen Neville. "There's something about the vibration that really soothes a colicky baby."

Sound too far-fetched? Wait until the baby fusses for another 3 hours or so—you'll try anything.

**Warm that tummy.** "A hot-water bottle or heating pad *set on low* and placed on the baby's tummy sometimes helps," Jonides says. (Place a towel between the baby and the hot-water bottle to make sure she doesn't get burned.)

**Log it in.** "Keeping a log would be a very good idea," Neville says. "Often, when it seems like the baby was fussing for 2 hours straight, it was really only 45 minutes. A log will help you determine just how long the baby's crying, and—more important—what might be bringing it on."

**Swing into action.** "Motion-type things are good for colic," says Jonides. "Many babies will at least be quiet long enough to let you get through dinner when they're swinging."

## PANEL OF ADVISORS

**Morris Green, M.D.,** is chairman of the department of pediatrics at Indiana University School of Medicine in Indianapolis.

**Linda Jonides** is a pediatric nurse practitioner in Ann Arbor, Michigan.

**Helen Neville, R.N.,** is director of the Inborn Temperament Project at Kaiser Permanente Hospital in Oakland, California, and the author of *Temperament Tools*.

**Anne Price** is a former educational coordinator for the National Academy of Nannies, Inc. (NANI) in Denver.

# CONJUNCTIVITIS
## 7 Remedies for Pinkeye

Conjunctivitis is inflammation of the conjunctiva, a membrane that lines the inside of the eyelids and covers the white of the eye. Red and irritated, infected eyes feel as if they're bedeviled by stray grains of sand. There's often a discharge, too. The culprits behind all that itching? Viruses, bacteria, or allergies. While conjunctivitis won't threaten an adult's sight, it's unsightly. And it's no fun. Here's what you can do.

**Wash the red away.** "A warm compress applied to the eyes for 5 to 10 minutes three or four times a day will make you feel better," says pediatric ophthalmologist Robert Petersen, M.D.

**Keep eyes clean.** "A lot of times conjunctivitis gets better by itself," says Dr. Petersen. "To help the healing process along, keep your eyes and eyelids clean by using a cotton ball dipped in clean or sterile water to wipe the crusts away."

**WHEN TO CALL A DOCTOR**

Conjunctivitis is an easily treatable problem that will usually go away on its own in about a week. You should, however, avoid taking a wait-and-see attitude. See your doctor if:

- After 5 days the infection is getting worse, not better.
- You have a red eye that is associated with significant eye pain, change in vision, or a copious amount of yellow or greenish discharge.
- Redness is caused by an injury to your eye. "Sometimes infections can get in the eye if you've scratched the cornea, leading to an ulcer, loss of vision, or even loss of your eye," says Robert Petersen, M.D. Corneal infections aren't always triggered by injuries, though. Sometimes, the herpes simplex virus from a cold sore in the mouth can be spread if you touch your eye.

**Baby yourself.** A warm compress works well for children, but sometimes adults need a little something more. "Adults who have a lot of discharge should make a solution of 1 part baby shampoo to 10 parts warm water," says ophthalmologist Peter Hersh, M.D.

"Dip a sterile cotton ball into the solution and use it to clean off your eyelashes. It works very well. The warm water loosens the crust and the baby shampoo cleans off the junction of your eyelid and eyelash."

An over-the-counter solution called Eye-Scrub, used the same way, is just as effective.

**Throw in the towel.** Toss your towel, washcloth, and anything else that comes in contact with your eyes into the laundry. "This infection is highly contagious. Don't share a towel or washcloth with anyone, because it will easily spread the disease," says Dr. Petersen.

**Don't chlorinate your eyes.** Does swimming in a pool leave you seeing pink? "The chlorine in swimming pools can cause conjunctivitis, but without the chlorine, bacteria would grow—and that could cause it, too," says Dr. Petersen. "If you're going to go swimming and you're susceptible to conjunctivitis, wear tight-fitting goggles while in the water."

**Put allergic conjunctivitis on ice.** If you survive the summer swim but not the summer pollen, your conjunctivitis may be caused by allergies. "If your eye itches like a mosquito bite and you have stringy pus in your eye, most of the time that's the sign of allergic conjunctivitis," says ophthalmologist J. Daniel Nelson, M.D. "Taking an over-the-counter antihistamine will help that, and use cold, not warm, compresses. A cold compress will really relieve the itch."

**Get drugged at night.** "Germ-caused conjunctivitis intensifies when your eyes are closed. That's why it tends to get worse at night when you're asleep," says Dr. Petersen. "To combat that, put any prescribed antibiotic ointment in your eyes before you go to bed. That way it will prevent crusting."

## PANEL OF ADVISORS

**Peter Hersh, M.D.,** is an ophthalmologist and former assistant surgeon in the department of ophthalmology at Massachusetts Eye and Ear Infirmary in Boston. He is also a former instructor of ophthalmology at Harvard Medical School.

**J. Daniel Nelson, M.D.,** is an ophthalmologist at Regions Medical Center in St. Paul, Minnesota.

**Robert Petersen, M.D.,** is an assistant professor of ophthalmology at Harvard Medical School. He is also a pediatric ophthalmologist and director of the Eye Clinic at Children's Hospital in Boston.

# CONSTIPATION
## 17 Solutions to a Common Problem

Constipation is an uncomfortable, exceedingly common problem in the United States, affecting anywhere from 2 to 28 percent of the population and accounting for an estimated 2.5 million doctor visits each year. Women appear to experience more constipation than men, and older people more than younger people.

There are many causes of constipation, including a lack of fiber in the diet, insufficient liquid intake, stress, medications, lack of exercise, and bad bowel habits, says Paul Rousseau, M.D.

We take a look at all of these factors, as well as suggest ways to remedy the situation.

**Determine if you are *really* constipated.** Madison Avenue bombards us with laxative advertisements that give the impression that a daily bowel movement is essential to good health, and that just isn't so, says Marvin Schuster, M.D.

## WHEN TO CALL A DOCTOR

Constipation itself is usually not serious, says Marvin Schuster, M.D. You should call your doctor, however, when symptoms are severe, last longer than 3 weeks, or are disabling, or if you find blood in your stool, he says. Although it's rare, constipation can signal a serious underlying disorder.

In addition, contact your doctor if your constipation accompanies a distended abdomen, which may signal an intestinal obstruction, says Paul Rousseau, M.D.

Many Americans, he says, are subject to *perceived constipation*—they think they're constipated when they are not. In reality, the need to defecate varies greatly from individual to individual. For some, a bowel movement three times a day may be considered normal, for others three times a week may suffice.

**Fine-tune your fluid and fiber intake.** Our experts agree that the first thing you should do if you're constipated is check your diet. The foremost menu items for battling constipation are dietary fiber such as fruits, vegetables, beans and other legumes, and liquids, essential to keeping the stool soft and helping it pass through the colon.

How much liquid and how much fiber do you need? Let's start with the liquid. A minimum of six glasses of liquid, preferably eight, should be part of every adult's diet, says Patricia H. Harper, R.D. While any fluid will do the trick, the best is water, she says.

**Eat lots more fiber.** Most Americans don't get enough fiber in their diets, says Harper. The American Dietetic Association recommends a daily consumption of 20 to 35 grams of dietary fiber for all adults and at least 30 grams for those who experience constipation.

Whole grains, fruits, and vegetables are the best fiber sources, says Harper. It's not difficult to get 30 grams in your daily diet if you choose foods carefully. One-half cup of green peas, for instance, gives you 5 grams; one small apple supplies 3 grams, and a bowl of bran cereal can provide as much as 13 grams. Tops among the fiber heavyweights are cooked dried beans, prunes, figs, raisins, popcorn, oatmeal, pears, and nuts. One word of caution, though: Increase your fiber intake slowly to avoid gas attacks.

**Take time to go to the gym.** Exercise is good for your heart, but it's also good for your bowels. In general, regular exercise tends to combat constipation by moving food through the bowel faster, says Edward R. Eichner, M.D.

**Take a walk.** Any form of regular exercise tends to alleviate constipation, but the one mentioned most often by our experts is walking. Walking is particularly helpful for pregnant women, many of whom experience constipation as their inner workings are compressed to accommodate the growing fetus.

Anyone, including mothers-to-be, should walk a hearty 20 to 30 minutes a day, suggests Lewis R. Townsend, M.D. Pregnant women should take care not to get too winded as they walk.

**Learn new habits.** Throughout our lives, many of us condition ourselves to go to the bathroom not when nature calls but when it's convenient. Ignoring the urge to defecate, however, can eventually lead to constipation. It's never too late to improve your bowel habits, says Dr. Schuster. "The most natural time to go to the toilet is after a meal," he adds. So pick a meal, any meal, and every day following that meal sit on the toilet for 10 minutes. In time, says Dr. Schuster, you will condition your colon to act as nature intended.

**Slow down and take it easy.** When you're frightened or tense, your mouth dries, and your heart beats faster. Your bowels stop up as well. "It's part of the fight-or-flight mechanism," says John O. Lawder, M.D. If you suspect that tension is at the bottom of your constipation, take time to relax, perhaps by listening to relaxation tapes.

**Have a hearty laugh.** It may sound funny, but a good belly laugh can help with constipation in two ways. It has a massaging effect on the intestines, which helps foster digestion, and it's a great stress reliever, says Alison Crane, R.N.

**Reconsider laxative tablets.** Chemical laxatives often do what they're intended to do, but they're terribly addicting, warns Dr. Rousseau. Take too many of these chemical laxatives, and your bowel gets used to them, and your constipation can get worse. When should you take laxatives from a bottle? "Almost never," he says.

**Know that not all laxatives are the same.** In most drugstores, right next to the chemical laxatives, you'll find another category of laxatives, often marked "natural" or "vegetable" laxatives, whose main ingredient is generally crushed psyllium seed. This is a super-concentrated form of fiber, which, unlike the chemical laxatives, is nonaddictive and generally safe, even if taken over long periods, says Dr. Rousseau. He cautions, however, that these must be taken with lots of water (read the instructions on the package), or they can gum up inside you.

**Try one doctor's special recipe.** Psyllium-based laxatives can be expensive. So make your own by buying psyllium seeds in a health food store and crushing them yourself. Grind 2 parts psyllium with 1 part flax and 1 part oat bran (also available in health food stores) for a super-high-fiber concoction. "Mix the ingredients up with water, and have it as a little mash every night around 9 o'-clock," says Dr. Lawder.

**Review your medications and supplements.** There are a number of medications that can bring on or exacerbate constipation, says Dr. Rousseau. Among the common culprits are antacids containing aluminum or calcium, antihistamines, anti-Parkinsonism drugs, calcium supplements, diuretics, narcotics, phenothiazines, sedatives, and tricyclic antidepressants.

**Beware of certain foods.** Some things may constipate one person but not another. Milk, for instance, can be extremely constipating to some, while causing diarrhea in others. Foods that tend to produce gas, such as beans, cauliflower, and cabbage, can be problematic for people whose constipation is the result of a spastic colon, says Dr. Schuster. You should suspect a spastic colon and avoid gas-producing foods if your constipation is sharply painful.

**Use dietary oils sparingly.** By avoiding dietary oils, such as liquid vegetable, olive, or soy oil, you may be less constipated, says Grady Deal, D.C., Ph.D. "It's not oil per se, but eating it in its free state causes constipation and many other digestive problems," says Dr. Deal. He bases his theory on the work of turn-of-the-century health reformer John Henry Kellogg, M.D. (brother of the breakfast cereal magnate).

The problem with these oils, he explains, is that they form a film in the stomach, which makes it difficult to digest carbohydrates and proteins there and in the small intestine. Adequate digestion is delayed up to 20 hours, causing putrefaction, gas, and toxins, which back up the colon and large intestine, he says. But oils eaten in their natural form within whole nuts, avocados, and corn are released slowly into the body, so no oil slicks occur to block digestion and create constipation problems. These oils, as opposed to the separated kind, are "a wholesome and nutritious element of food," he says.

**Be cautious about herbs.** Herbal remedies for dealing with constipation abound. Among those touted are aloe juice, senna, medicinal rhubarb, cascara sagrada, dandelion root, and plantain seeds. Some, such as cascara sagrada, can be very effective, says Dr. Lawder, but you need to be careful. Herbal laxatives, just as chemical ones, should be carefully chosen and not overused.

**Don't strain.** Forcing a bowel movement is unwise. You risk giving yourself hemorrhoids and anal fissures, which are painful and can also aggravate your constipation by narrowing the anal opening. Straining can also raise your blood pressure and lower your heartbeat, which can be dangerous, especially in the elderly.

**Get fast relief—once in a while.** If you're really miserable, nothing works faster to move your bowels than an enema or a suppository. For occasional use, they are perfectly all right, says Dr. Rousseau. Use them too often, however, and you risk creating a lazy colon, exacerbating your constipation problem.

Use only clear water or saline-solution enemas, *never* soapsuds, which can be irritating, says Dr. Rousseau. And when shopping for a suppository, stick with glycerin, avoiding the harsher chemical selections on the market.

## PANEL OF ADVISORS

**Alison Crane, R.N.,** is the founder of the American Association for Therapeutic Humor.

**Grady Deal, D.C., Ph.D.,** is a nutritional chiropractor in Koloa, Kauai, Hawaii. He is also the founder and owner of Dr. Deal's Hawaiian Wellness Holiday health spa in Koloa.

**Edward R. Eichner, M.D.,** is an expert in the effects of exercise on the human body, a professor of medicine, and team internist at the University of Oklahoma Health Sciences Center in Oklahoma City.

**Patricia H. Harper, M.S., R.D.,** is a research nutritionist at the University of Pittsburgh School of Medicine. She also coordinates diabetes and weight-loss programs there.

**John O. Lawder, M.D.,** is a family practitioner specializing in nutrition and preventive medicine in Torrance, California.

**Paul Rousseau, M.D.,** is associate chief of the department of geriatrics and extended care at the Phoenix Veterans Affairs Medical Center in Phoenix.

**Marvin Schuster, M.D.,** is director emeritus of the Marvin M. Schuster Center for Digestive and Motility Disorders at the Hopkins Bayview Medical Center, and professor emeritus of medicine and psychiatry at Johns Hopkins University School of Medicine, both in Baltimore.

**Lewis R. Townsend, M.D.,** is a clinical instructor of obstetrics and gynecology at Georgetown University Hospital and former director of the physicians' group at the Columbia Hospital for Women Medical Center, both in Washington, D.C.

# COUGH
## 19 Throat-Soothing Strategies

It's no accident that the wracking coughs that accompany allergies, colds, and other respiratory problems never seem to go away. Coughing is the body's way of removing irritating substances from the airways. Too much coughing, though, can make it impossible to sleep or even relax. Some people have even broken ribs during severe coughing fits.

Mucus-filled "productive" coughs are usually caused by allergies, colds, or other respiratory tract infections. Buildup of mucus in the airways makes it hard to breathe, and the body responds by trying to remove it. "Dry" coughs, on the other hand, are caused by irritation due to smoking, for example, or from inhaling fumes, dust, or other airborne irritants.

Most coughs clear up on their own within a week to 10 days. In the meantime, here are a few ways to reduce the discomfort and help the cough pass more quickly.

### WHEN TO CALL A DOCTOR

If you cough up blood or if your cough lasts more than 2 weeks, see a doctor, especially if it doesn't seem to be getting better, says Anne Davis, M.D.

Cancer and heartburn are both common causes of persistent coughs, she warns. So are asthma, chronic obstructive pulmonary disease (COPD), and other respiratory diseases.

"You have to worry about pneumonia, especially if the cough is accompanied by sharp chest pains, chills, or a fever higher than 101 degrees," says Dr. Davis.

Other warning signs include wheezing, shortness of breath, or leg swelling. When accompanied by a persistent cough, these symptoms could be a sign of heart failure, which requires immediate medical attention.

**Enjoy slippery elm lozenges.** Available in drugstores and health food stores, slippery elm is loaded with a substance that soothes the throat and helps reduce coughing. These lozenges even taste pretty good, says Stuart Ditchek, M.D. Take a maximum of five or six lozenges per day.

**Try this slippery solution.** The next time you have a wracking cough, try this helpful formula. Add 1 teaspoon of slippery elm powder or liquid to 2 cups of hot water. Stir in 1 tablespoon of a sugar, add a sprinkling of cinnamon, and drink it down, suggests Dr. Ditchek.

**Sip ginger tea.** Ginger acts as a potent natural anti-inflammatory herbal agent. Most people use a ginger tea as a way to soothe their painful throats, although fresh ginger from the produce section of your local supermarket is also good. Always ensure that a throat culture is done in order to rule out strep throat, in which case an antibiotic should be taken simultaneously, says Dr. Ditchek.

**Try zinc lozenges.** The research isn't conclusive, but some studies suggest that sucking on zinc lozenges can reduce the discomfort of a scratchy throat. Most zinc lozenges contain 22 milligrams of zinc, but not all of it is absorbed, says Dr. Ditchek. Don't take more than the amount recommended by your doctor. Zinc can be toxic in large doses.

**Drink all the water you can hold.** The body naturally loses fluids when you have a cold or flu. In addition, the accompanying congestion forces mouth breathing, which increases throat dryness and coughing, says Anne Davis, M.D. Try to drink at least eight 8-ounce glasses of water each day. This will moisturize tissues and help calm the cough.

Here's another reason to drink more water. Mucous membranes kept moist are better able to resist cold-causing viruses, says Dr. Davis. "If mucus is too thick, it doesn't work as well."

---

## Do just 1 thing

Most coughs are the body's way of getting rid of debris and mucous secretions. You don't want to interrupt that normal process. What you do want to do is reduce the discomfort.

For productive coughs, blowing your nose frequently helps eliminate mucus before it has a chance to stimulate the cough reflex, says Stuart Ditchek, M.D.

For "dry" coughs, drink plenty of broth, tea, or other warm fluids, which soothes the throat and reduces irritation.

**Take vitamin C.** Nothing prevents the occasional cold, but studies have shown that taking vitamin C at the first sign of infection can cut the severity of symptoms, including cough, about 50 percent, says Dr. Ditchek. Megadoses like those used in years past are no longer commonly advised, he adds. While the Daily Value for vitamin C is 60 milligrams, doses between 100 and 500 milligrams per day can be beneficial.

**Add some echinacea.** Available in health food stores and most drugstores, echinacea helps the immune system battle cold viruses. It's also a very effective way to reduce the duration and severity of coughs and other cold symptoms, says Dr. Ditchek.

Take 12 drops of echinacea tincture four times a day. In capsule form, take one or two capsules three or four times per day for 10 days to 2 weeks. People with allergies and autoimmune diseases are discouraged from using this remedy, advises Dr. Ditchek.

**Drink something hot.** A cup of chamomile tea works well, especially if it's flavored with honey and lemon. "Hot liquids are soothing when you have a cough," says Dr. Davis. Adding honey to the tea may provide additional relief because the thick sweetener soothes irritated tissues and cough receptors in the throat, she says.

**Eat raw or lightly cooked garlic.** It's rich in chemical compounds that help inhibit cough-causing viruses in the respiratory tract, says Dr. Ditchek. Garlic is a wonderful natural antibiotic that can assist in fighting off colds and common upper respiratory infections.

Try to eat two to four garlic cloves each daily, Dr. Ditchek suggests. Or use garlic supplements, following the directions on the label.

**Swig chicken soup.** And be sure to add lots of hot, pungent spices like pepper, garlic, and curry powder. The warm fluid and the pungent spices will help break up stagnant mucus in your beleaguered lungs, and these natural expectorants will aid in getting rid of the mucus.

**Humidify the airways.** Once or twice a day, take a long, hot shower or bath. Or plug in a vaporizer or humidifier. Breathing steam reduces airway irritation and makes mucus easier to cough up.

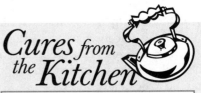

*Cures from the Kitchen*

"One thing that can trigger coughs is throat irritation," says Anne Davis, M.D. Sucking on hard candy increases saliva flow. The combination of saliva and juices from the candy soothes irritated tissues, she explains.

Humidifying the air is also a good way to prevent cough-causing colds and other infections, says Dr. Ditchek. Air that's too dry removes moisture from the nose, throat, and lungs, making it easier for viruses to take hold.

**Stay away from cigarette smoke.** Even if you don't smoke yourself, breathing secondhand smoke almost guarantees that you'll have an irritated throat. Smokers often have persistent coughs because the body responds to the irritation by producing enormous amounts of mucus, says Dr. Davis.

If you're currently a smoker, the best thing that you can do is quit. Insist that friends or family members who smoke do so away from you.

**Consider a cough suppressant.** Over-the-counter medicines that contain dextromethorphan (like Triaminic DM) aren't a cure for coughs, but they will help blunt the "cough reflex" in the brain. Doctors usually recommend these products only for temporary relief—when a cough keeps you up at night, for example.

Cough suppressants should be used only if you have a dry cough, Dr. Davis adds. Productive coughs should be encouraged, not suppressed, for it is important to clear secretions from the airways.

**Use an expectorant.** One way to make productive coughs even more productive is to take an over-the-counter expectorant that contains guaifenesin (such as Robitussin). Expectorants make mucus thinner and easier to expel, says Dr. Davis.

**Don't put up with heartburn.** It's a common cause of persistent coughs, says Dr. Ditchek. The same stomach acids that cause heartburn (also called gastroesophageal reflux) can also trigger coughing fits when the acids irritate the esophagus or airways. If you mainly cough at night, after meals, or while lying down, there's a good chance that stomach acids are to blame.

One of the easiest strategies to keep stomach acids where they belong is to elevate the head of your bed a few inches by putting wood blocks under the legs. It's also helpful to eat four or five small meals a day instead of two or three large meals. Finally, stay on your feet—or at least sit upright in a chair—for at least 2 hours after eating. Avoid food triggers, such as dairy, that aggravate symptoms.

If you want to try an herbal heartburn remedy, suck on licorice lozenges. Always use the deglycyrrhizinated form (DGL) which does not generally cause any elevation of blood pressure. DGL licorice lozenges are available standardized to 380 milligrams of licorice. Some taste better than others. Take two lozenges before meals. Always check your blood pressure if using this remedy for more than a few days, says Dr. Ditchek.

If the coughing persists and you are taking an ACE inhibitor, talk to your doctor about a possible trial of a different antihypertensive medication, says Dr. Davis. ACE inhibitors can cause cough.

**Get allergies under control.** If you're sensitive to pollen, mold, or other allergens, even a brief exposure can stimulate mucous production—followed by days or weeks of coughing as your body tries to remove it, says Dr. Ditchek.

Once you know what you're allergic to, avoidance is the best approach. If you get hay fever, for example, avoid pollen by staying indoors during the morning and evening hours, when pollen concentrations are highest. For quick relief from symptoms, take an over-the-counter antihistamine, such as diphenhydramine (Benadryl) or loratadine (Claritin).

"The rapid relief from antihistamines is helpful when you're having bad days," says Dr. Ditchek. "I actually love recommending stinging nettles. It is often as or more effective than medications with no drowsy or behavioral side effects. It simply takes longer to achieve therapeutic effect."

**Get some rest.** It's the oldest—and probably the most ignored—advice for combating cold symptoms like coughing. "People want to keep going, but you have to try to get some rest," Dr. Davis says. Otherwise, that "minor" cold and cough might progress to something a lot more serious, like pneumonia.

## PANEL OF ADVISORS

**Anne Davis, M.D.,** is an associate professor of clinical medicine at New York University School of Medicine and attending physician at the Chest Service at Bellevue Hospital Center, both in New York City.

**Stuart Ditchek, M.D.,** is a pediatrician and assistant professor of pediatrics at New York University School of Medicine in New York City and coauthor of *Healthy Child, Whole Child.*

# CUTS AND SCRAPES

## 15 Ways to Soothe a Sore

Mix one pair of roller skates with a sidewalk that boasts more cracks than Death Valley and voilà—a recipe for scraped knees and small cuts that seem anything but small to a frightened and hurting child.

While boys and girls seem to have a monopoly on boo-boos, adults trip and fall into their share of cuts and scrapes, too.

A finger gets in the way of a knife slicing bagels. A backpack carelessly tossed in the front hall sets the stage for a nasty fall. And every winter, ice lurks like a sinister prankster waiting for victims who fall, tearing their pants and skin at the same time.

Life is rife with mishaps. Luckily, your kitchen and medicine cabinet are filled with the tools to manage them. Here's a crash course—pardon the pun—on what to do.

**Stop the bleeding.** The fastest way to stop bleeding is to apply direct pressure. Place a clean, absorbent cloth over the cut, then firmly press your hand

## WHEN TO CALL A DOCTOR

First aid isn't always enough. See a doctor when:

- Bleeding is bright red and spurting. You may have punctured an artery.
- You can't wash all the debris out of the wound.
- The cut or scrape is on your face or any other area where you want to minimize scarring.
- Your wound develops any red streaks or weeps pus, or the redness extends more than a finger's width beyond the cut.
- The wound is large, and you can see way down inside. You may need stitches. Never try to stitch a wound closed yourself, even if you are stranded far from medical help.

# Why Are Little Paper Cuts Such a Big Pain?

Office workers know it. Paper pushers of any kind can testify to it, too. Even though they're small, paper cuts pack a real pain punch. What is it about them that prompts normally demure professionals to utter words that would make an ex-con blush? In a word, particles.

If a woman cuts herself shaving her legs, the razor makes a clean cut, leaving behind few, if any, particles that trigger pain. A paper cut, on the other hand, leaves paper fibers coated with chemicals from the papermaking process. These fibers and bacteria remain in the wound and stimulate pain receptors in the skin. What to do?

- If you can see the particles, remove them with a clean pair of tweezers.

- Crazy as it sounds, consider Krazy Glue. The glue binds the outer skin together, allowing inner layers to heal faster. Fill your cut with a tiny amount of Krazy Glue using a toothpick or the rod portion of a cotton swab. Apply the glue so that it's flat and smooth, with no bumps. Take care not to stick your fingers to each other or to objects. Don't use Krazy Glue for anything but paper cuts and small cracks in the skin. Stay alert for the sign of an allergic reaction: red, inflamed skin.

against it. If you don't have a cloth, use your fingers. If blood soaks through your first bandage, add a second one and press steadily. Add new bandages over old ones because removing a cloth may tear off coagulating blood cells.

If applying pressure doesn't stop the bleeding, elevate the limb to heart level to reduce the pressure of blood on the cut. Continue applying pressure. This should stem bleeding.

**Strap it up.** When the bleeding stops or slows, tie the wound firmly with a cloth or wrap it with an elastic bandage so there is pressure against the cut, *but do not cut off circulation,* says emergency medical technician John Gillies.

**Go for extra pressure.** If the cut continues to bleed, it is more serious than you thought, and you probably need to see a doctor immediately. Until you get medical help, find the pressure point nearest the cut between the wound and your heart. Pressure points are places you might think of when taking a pulse: inside your wrists, inside your upper arm about halfway between the elbow and armpit, and in the groin where your legs attach to your torso. Press the artery against the bone. Stop pressing about a minute after the bleeding stops. If bleeding starts again, reapply pressure.

**Don't use a tourniquet.** With most everyday cuts and scrapes, first aid is plenty. Tourniquets can be dangerous. "Once you apply a tourniquet, the person may end up losing that limb because you cut off all circulation," cautions Gillies.

**Clean the wound twice a day.** This is important to prevent infection and to decrease the chance of permanent discoloration. Wash the area with soap and water or just water, says Hugh Macaulay, M.D. The idea is to dilute the bacteria in the wound and remove debris. If you don't remove stones or sand from the cut, they can leave pigment under the skin.

**Smear on an over-the-counter antibiotic ointment.** Broad-spectrum antibacterial ointments work best, according to James J. Leyden, M.D. (See "Choosing an Over-the-Counter Ointment" below.)

People who use a triple-antibiotic ointment and the right kind of bandage heal 30 percent faster, says wound researcher Patricia Mertz.

Still, Mertz warns, be wary of over-the-counter drugs that contain neomycin or ointments that contain a lot of preservatives. They can cause allergic reactions. If you have an allergic reaction to the ointment, your scrape will get red and itchy and may become infected.

---

## Choosing an Over-the-Counter Ointment

Confused about choosing the best product for your boo-boo? In one study, James J. Leyden, M.D., compared the effectiveness of nine over-the-counter products on wound healing. He found that some products mend minor cuts, scrapes, and burns faster than others. Here's what his research uncovered.

- Polysporin (active ingredients: polymyxin B, bacitracin ointment): 8.2 days

- Neosporin (active ingredients: neomycin, polymyxin B, bacitracin ointment): 9.2 days

- Johnson & Johnson First Aid Cream (wound protectant with no antibiotic agent): 9.8 days

- Mercurochrome (active ingredient: merbromin): 13.1 days

- No treatment: 13.3 days

- Bactine spray (active ingredient: benzalkonium chloride): 14.2 days

- Merthiolate (active ingredient: thimerosol): 14.2 days

- Hydrogen peroxide (3 percent): 14.3 days

- Campho-Phenique (active ingredients: camphor, phenol): 15.4 days

- Tincture of iodine: 15.7 days

**Try a sweet treatment.** Got a cut or wound? You can speed up the healing process with a little table sugar, says orthopedic surgeon Richard A. Knutson, M.D. He's treated serious wounds with a mixture of tamed iodine and sugar, healing a variety of mishaps from cuts, scrapes, and burns to amputated fingertips. (Raw iodine will burn the skin.) Sugar, he says, leaves bacteria without the nutrients necessary to grow or multiply. Wounds usually heal quickly, without a scab and often with little scarring. Keloids (irregular, large scars) are kept to a minimum.

To make Dr. Knutson's ointment, mix 1 tablespoon of first-aid antibiotic solution (such as Betadine Antiseptic Cleaner Solution) with 10 tablespoons of white table sugar and 3 tablespoons first-aid antibiotic ointment (Betadine Antibiotic Ointment, for example). Both solution and ointment are available in drugstores. Pack a cleaned wound with the homemade ointment and cover carefully with gauze. Four times a day, rinse the area gently with water and hydrogen peroxide and pack on fresh ointment. Taper off as healing progresses.

Make sure the wound is clean and the bleeding has stopped before applying the mixture. Sugar makes a bleeding wound bleed more.

**Keep it undercover.** When exposed to air, cuts form scabs, which slow down new cell growth, says Mertz. She recommends a plastic bandage similar to food wrap. They come in all sizes. Or look for gauze impregnated with petroleum jelly. Both types of bandages trap healing moisture in the wound but allow only a little air to pass through. Cells regenerate more rapidly when moist.

**Top it off with a tetanus shot.** If you haven't had a tetanus shot in the past 5 years, you need a booster, says Dr. Macaulay. Local health departments usu-

## Bandage Busters

Got a boo-boo but dread taking off the bandage? Follow these tips for painless removal.

- Use a tiny pair of scissors to separate the bandage part from the adhesive sections. Pull it gently away from your scrape. Then remove the adhesive strips.

- If your scab is stuck to the bandage, soak the area in a mixture of warm water and salt—about a tea-spoon of salt to a gallon of water. Have patience. The dressing will eventually let go.

- If the bandage is stuck on your forearm, leg, or chest hair, pull in the direction of hair growth. Use a cotton swab saturated in baby oil or rubbing alcohol to moisten the adhesive fully before pulling away from the skin.

ally give them for a minimal fee or for free, he adds. If you don't remember when you had your last booster, it's a good idea to have one within 24 hours of the injury.

## PANEL OF ADVISORS

**John Gillies, E.M.T.,** is a former emergency medical technician and program director for health services at the Colorado Outward Bound School in Denver.

**Richard A. Knutson, M.D.,** is an orthopedic surgeon at Delta Medical Center in Greenville, Mississippi.

**James J. Leyden, M.D.,** is a professor of dermatology at the University of Pennsylvania in Philadelphia.

**Hugh Macaulay, M.D.,** is an emergency room physician at Aspen Valley Hospital in Aspen.

**Patricia Mertz** is a former research associate professor in the department of dermatology and cutaneous surgery at the University of Miami School of Medicine in Florida.

# DANDRUFF
## 16 Tips to Stop Flaking

Dandruff—the single most common scalp complaint among hairdressers' clients—plays no favorites. Dermatologists say that just about everyone has the problem to some degree, often leading to a scratch-and-itch cycle, says Maria Hordinsky, M.D. Ignoring the condition lets the scaling build up. That, in turn, can cause itching, which can lead to scratching. Scratching too vigorously can wound the scalp and leave it open to infection. This vicious cycle can be avoided, however, with some simple home remedies.

**Shampoo often.** The experts are unanimous on this point: Wash your hair often—every day if necessary. "Generally, the more frequently you shampoo, the easier it is to control the dandruff," says Patricia Farris, M.D.

**Start mild.** Often a mild, nonmedicated shampoo is enough to control the problem. Dandruff is frequently caused by an overly oily scalp, says hair-care specialist Philip Kingsley. Washing daily with a mild brand of shampoo, diluted

## WHEN TO CALL A DOCTOR

Severe dandruff is actually a disease known as seborrheic dermatitis, which requires prescription medications. So, see a doctor if you have:

- Scalp irritation
- Thick scale despite regular use of dandruff shampoos
- Yellowish crusting
- Red patches, especially along the neckline

with an equal amount of water, can control the oil without aggravating your scalp.

**Then get tough.** If regular shampoos aren't doing the job, switch to an anti-dandruff formula. Dandruff shampoos are classified by their active ingredients, which work in different ways. Those with selenium sulfide or zinc pyrithione work fastest, says Diana Bihova, M.D., retarding the rate at which scalp cells multiply. Those with salicylic acid and sulfur loosen flakes so that they can be washed away easily. Those with antibacterial agents reduce bacteria on the scalp—and, thus, the chance of infection. Those with tar retard cell growth.

**Beat the tar out of it.** "For very stubborn cases, I recommend tar-based formulas," says Dr. Farris. "Lather with the tar shampoo and then leave it on for 5 to 10 minutes so that the tar has a chance to work." Most people rinse dandruff shampoos off too quickly. Two brands to look for are Sebutone Tar Shampoo and MG 217 Medicated Tar Shampoo.

Today's newer tar formulas are much more fragrant than the smelly solutions of old.

**Don't be too harsh.** If tar-based shampoos—or any other dandruff preparations—are too harsh for everyday use, alternate them with your regular shampoo, says Dr. Farris.

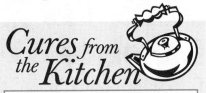

## Cures from the Kitchen

Thyme, a common kitchen herb, is reputed to have mild antiseptic properties that can help alleviate dandruff, says hairstylist Louis Gignac. Make an effective rinse by boiling 4 heaping tablespoons of dried thyme in 2 cups of water for 10 minutes. Strain the brew and allow it to cool. Pour half the mixture over clean, damp hair, making sure the liquid covers the scalp. Massage in gently. Do not rinse. Save the remainder for another day.

**Don't mix black with blond.** If you have light-colored hair, think twice about tar-based shampoos. In rare instances, they can give white, blond, bleached, or tinted hair a temporary brownish discoloration, says Dr. Farris.

**Lather twice.** Always lather twice with a dandruff shampoo, says R. Jeffrey Herten, M.D. Work up the first lather as soon as you step into the shower so that the shampoo has sufficient time to work. Leave it on until you're just about finished with your shower. Then rinse your hair very thoroughly. Follow that with a quick second lather and rinse. The second rinse will leave just a bit of the medication on your scalp so that it can work until your next shampoo.

**Cap it.** Dr. Bihova has still another approach to improving the effectiveness of medicated shampoos. After you lather up, put a shower cap on over your wet hair. Leave it on for an hour, then rinse as usual.

**Switch-hit.** If you've found a brand of shampoo that works well for you, keep using it, says Howard Donsky, M.D. Be aware, however, that your skin can adapt to a shampoo's ingredients, so it's a good idea to change your brand every few months to maintain its effectiveness.

**Massage it in.** When shampooing, says Dr. Farris, gently massage your scalp with your fingertips to help loosen scales and flakes. But don't scratch your scalp, she warns. That can lead to sores that are worse than the dandruff.

**Flake off.** Joseph F. Fowler Jr., M.D., recommends an over-the-counter product called Psoriasin Scalp Multi-Symptom Psoriasis Relief Liquid for people with particularly stubborn scaling and crusting. Apply it to your scalp at bedtime and cover your hair with a shower cap. Wash it out in the morning. Although you can use this preparation every night, Dr. Fowler recommends once-a-week treatments. "It's just too messy for daily use," he says.

## Cures from the Kitchen

Although excess scalp oil can cause problems, an occasional warm-oil treatment helps loosen and soften dandruff scales, says R. Jeffrey Herten, M.D. Heat a few ounces of olive oil on the stove until just warm. Wet your hair (otherwise the oil will soak into your hair instead of reaching your scalp), then apply the oil directly to your scalp with a brush or cotton ball. Section your hair as you go so that you treat just the scalp. Put on a shower cap and leave it on for 30 minutes. Then wash out the oil with a dandruff shampoo.

**Get into condition.** Although dandruff shampoos are effective on your scalp, they can be a little harsh on your hair, says Dr. Farris. So apply conditioner after every shampoo to counteract their effects.

**Let the sun shine.** "A little sun exposure is good for dandruff," says Dr. Fowler. That's because direct ultraviolet light has an anti-inflammatory effect on scaly skin conditions. And it may explain why dandruff tends to be less severe in summer.

But by all means, says Dr. Fowler, use sun sense. Don't sunbathe; just spend a little time outdoors. Limit sun exposure to 30 minutes or less per day. And wear your normal sunscreen on exposed skin. "You have to balance the sun's benefit to your scalp against its harmful effect on your skin in general," he advises.

**Calm down.** Don't overlook the role emotions play in triggering or worsening skin conditions such as dandruff and other forms of dermatitis. These conditions are often made worse by stress, says Dr. Fowler. So if your emotions are overtaxed, look for ways to counteract the stress. Exercise. Meditate. Get away from it all. And don't worry so much about your dandruff.

## PANEL OF ADVISORS

**Diana Bihova, M.D.,** is a dermatologist affiliated with the dermatology department at the Columbia University College of Physicians and Surgeons in New York City.

**Howard Donsky, M.D.,** is a clinical instructor of dermatology at the University of Rochester and a dermatologist at the Dermatology and Cosmetic Center of Rochester in New York.

**Patricia Farris, M.D.,** is an assistant clinical professor of dermatology at Tulane University School of Medicine in New Orleans and a dermatologist in Metairie, Louisiana.

**Joseph F. Fowler Jr., M.D.,** is an assistant professor of dermatology at the University of Louisville and a dermatologist in Louisville. In addition, he is a member of the North American Contact Dermatitis Group, an elite skin-allergy research group.

**Louis Gignac** is a hairstylist and the owner of the Stella Salons in New York City and Miami.

**R. Jeffrey Herten, M.D.,** is an assistant clinical professor of dermatology at the University of California, Irvine, College of Medicine.

**Maria Hordinsky, M.D.,** is an assistant professor of dermatology at the University of Minnesota Medical School–Minneapolis and a dermatologist in Minneapolis.

**Philip Kingsley** is a trained trichologist (hair-care specialist) who maintains salons in New York City and London. He's also the hair columnist for the style section of *The Times* of London and the author of *Hair: An Owner's Handbook*.

# DENTURE TROUBLES
## 13 Ideas for a More Secure Smile

The Etruscans of central Italy invented false teeth nearly 3,000 years ago. They made dentures out of ox teeth, held together with highly visible gold bands. For Etruscans, wearing dentures was nothing to be ashamed of—it was actually a status symbol.

False teeth have come a long way since Etruscan times. Today, with millions of Americans wearing at least partial dentures, choices in dental ware abound. There are partial and full dentures, those that can be removed, and those that are implanted into the bone and become like real teeth.

All dentures, like any artificial body part, take some getting used to, says prosthodontist George A. Murrell, D.D.S. He and other specialists have some suggestions.

**Look in the mirror.** Smile. Frown. Be happy. Be sad. Be serious. Practice moving your teeth and lips in private so that you'll be more confident in front of other people, says Dr. Murrell.

**Practice talking.** "Having dentures is like having a prosthetic limb," says Jerry F. Taintor, D.D.S. "You have to practice using it to use it well." Say your vowels. Recite your consonants. Read aloud to yourself, he says. Listen to your pronunciation and your diction and correct what doesn't sound right.

**Make a video.** Videos are valuable for several reasons, says Dr. Murrell. They give you a stranger's-eye view of how you look. Plus you can show the tape to a dentist, who can use the pictures to decipher problems in jaw muscles or lip movements.

**Watch out for toothpicks.** Those tiny wooden spikes are especially dangerous for denture wearers, says Dr. Taintor. "You lose a lot of your tactile sense with dentures. You bite into a toothpick, but you don't know it because you can't feel it. You can get it accidentally lodged in your throat."

**Use an adhesive.** If you feel that your new teeth are a less-than-perfect fit, there's nothing wrong with using a denture adhesive during the adjustment period, says Dr. Taintor. It's when you have to use the adhesive all the time that you need to have the denture refitted. You can find over-the-counter denture adhesives—a type of soft paste that forms a vacuum between your gums and your dentures to temporarily "glue" them together—in any drugstore.

**Start soft and slow.** No, you're not doomed to baby foods for the rest of your life, but start soft, says Dr. Taintor. Gradually increase the texture and hardness of your food so that your gums and your ability to use the dentures build on good experience.

**Scrub with soap and water.** When you're finished eating, take your dentures out and scrub them with plain soap and lukewarm water.

**Get those choppers clean.** If you wear implants, you'll need to set up a twice-daily cleaning ritual just like when you were caring for your original teeth, says Dr. Murrell. "We can do beautiful dentistry, but it won't last if it isn't taken care of."

**Baby your mouth.** "Babies are born with plaque in their mouths," says Eric Shapira, D.D.S. "Even if you have no teeth, you need to wash your gums to remove the plaque." Use a soft brush and gently whisk away at your gums. You shouldn't brush hard enough to make the inside of your mouth sore, however. A good cleaning lowers the possibility of bad breath and helps your gums stay healthier, he says.

**Try a lozenge.** One common complaint among denture wearers, says Dr. Murrell, is excess saliva during the first few weeks of wearing dentures. Solve this problem neatly by sucking on lozenges frequently for the first couple of days. This helps you swallow more frequently and gets rid of some of the excess saliva.

**Massage your gums.** Place your thumb and index finger over your gums (index on the outside) and massage them, says Richard Shepard, D.D.S. This promotes circulation and gives your gums a healthy firmness.

**Rinse with salty water.** To help clean your gums, rinse your mouth daily with a glass of warm water mixed with a teaspoon of salt, says Dr. Taintor.

**Give your gums a rest.** When you can, take out your teeth and let your gums do nothing for a while, says Dr. Taintor.

# DEPRESSION
## 28 Mood Lifters

It would be nice if blue moods came only once in a blue moon. But life happens. The breakup of a relationship, the loss of a job, and other bumps and knocks in the road of life can make a mood shift from rosy to blue.

"We have a range of emotions, and feeling depressed at times, for short periods, is very normal," says Bernard Vittone, M.D.

But for the more than 18 million Americans who experience depression, the blues just don't go away.

If you and your doctor agree that your depression is mild, experts offer many ways to boost your mood. Even if you're being treated for chronic or severe depression, the following strategies may help.

**Get educated.** Learn more about depression and look for signs of wellness. Read books, listen to tapes, or watch videos. Education helps you realize that you're not alone and that the condition you have is really very common, says Edward M. Hallowell, M.D.

**Express yourself.** The opposite of depression is expression. The blues often result from a pattern of suppressing and then repressing feelings, says Dr. Hallowell. Release your feelings through art, music, or anything creative.

## WHEN TO CALL A DOCTOR

See a doctor if you are depressed most of the time for 2 or more weeks, even though you haven't experienced a significant loss, such as the death of a loved one. Also seek help if you have experienced a loss and your depression continues for several months or if you have intermittent bouts of depression for more than 2 years. Be sure to get a physical to rule out other possible illnesses such as hypothyroidism or anemia.

Symptoms of depression include feeling hopeless, helpless, sad or blue; losing interest in previously enjoyable activities; or an inability to be cheered by normally happy events. Other signs include insomnia, changes in appetite, low energy, poor concentration, irritability, a negative attitude, and frequent guilty feelings. Know, too, that symptoms of depression and anxiety often overlap. (For more information on anxiety, see page 28.)

**Get out.** Of the house, that is. Aim for a few hours out every day, says Dr. Vittone. Being in the same place too long, particularly if you're alone, is a breeding ground for depressive thoughts and symptoms. Visit the library, go shopping, see a movie. Stimulation is important for people with depression, he says. Researchers speculate that stimulation keeps the brain's feel-good neurotransmitters, such as serotonin, flowing.

**Be with friends.** Socialize at least twice a week, Dr. Vittone says. Don't just schedule business meetings, client lunches, or telephone talks. Get together with people to talk, laugh, and relax. You'll be firing up those feel-good neurotransmitters. Although researchers aren't sure *how* socialization affects nerve chemicals, says Dr. Vittone, they do know that they are helpful.

**Get your chuckles.** Watch a comedy show on television, see a funny movie, or catch a comedian on stage. Happiness is contagious, says Dr. Vittone.

**Let it be.** It's okay to feel *anything*, says Dr. Hallowell. There are no "bad" feelings. Accepting how you feel helps you get past it. Similarly, remind yourself that feelings change and that you will survive.

**Take time to heal.** Be patient with yourself. Sometimes you'll take a step forward; other days you'll take two steps backward. Healing never occurs in a straight line. Remember that tomorrow is another day to try again.

**Stick to a schedule.** Alternating rest with activity brings healing by restoring the body's natural rhythms. For example, go to sleep at the same time and get up at the usual time every day. When your inner world is chaotic, maintaining a schedule gives you some sense of order, says Dr. Hallowell.

**Sleep.** Lack of sleep may cause depressive-like symptoms, such as lack of concentration and low energy, or exacerbate existing depression. Gauge how much sleep you need by how rested you feel.

**Be an optimist.** Be optimistic, even if you don't believe it at first, says Dr. Vittone. Your attitude is likely to become a self-fulfilling prophecy. If you expect a positive outcome, you're more likely to act in ways that make that happen, and other people are more inclined to respond favorably. The way we think directly affects our moods, he says.

**Stay current.** Tune in to the television or radio news. Pick up a newspaper or magazine. Keeping up with current events helps you feel more involved in life around you, says Dr. Vittone. One caveat: Limit viewing or reading about traumatic events, such as the September 11, 2001, terrorist attacks, to 30 minutes at a time. Viewing too much bad news, he says, isn't good.

## Do just 1 thing

Get going. Depression causes a huge amount of inertia. It makes it hard to get out of bed in the morning and may tempt you to become a couch potato. Don't, says Bernard Vittone, M.D. Rather, get moving. Exercise helps banish the blues.

Walk, jog, bicycle, swim, cross-country ski, or participate in other aerobic activities such as classes at a local fitness center. Aim for 20 to 30 minutes, four or five times a week. Or try yoga, tai chi, or stretching about three times a week to loosen your body, relieve stress, and get you smiling again. Even better, choose a mix.

Some doctors believe that exercise, especially aerobic, produces endorphins, the body's natural antidepressants. "We don't really know why exercise works," says Dr. Vittone. "We only know that it does."

**Don't decide now.** Keep decision making to a minimum when you're feeling low. Decisions are less clear when you're depressed than when you're feeling at your best.

**Forgive yourself.** Even with mild depression, temporary forgetfulness and clumsiness are common. You might misplace your keys or drop a glass. Try to laugh at silly mistakes and keep in mind that your nervous system is not at its best.

**Get a massage.** When you're feeling blue, you may feel as if your mind and body are disconnected. Healing touch—once a week if possible—helps reconnect mind, body, and spirit, says Dr. Hallowell.

**Reaffirm beliefs.** Research shows that spirituality can improve mood, whether you pray, attend services, or read uplifting materials. Spirituality restores hope.

**Don't lay blame.** No matter what mistakes you think you've made, forgive yourself. Treat yourself with kindness, and never give in to regret. Everybody has failures. Guilt is self-punishment that you don't deserve.

**Try shock therapy.** Consider taking a vacation, says Dr. Vittone. Even 3 days at the beach, for example, may be enough to jolt you out of a mild depression. Alternately, take mini-vacations throughout the day. When your mood is low, find a minute or two to picture where you'd like to be. Immerse yourself in the sights, sounds, feelings, and scents of that special locale. "It will give you a little lift," he says.

**Be thankful.** Remind yourself what's good in life. Each day, jot down five things for which you're grateful. "Try to find things, little or big, that you appreciate," says Dr. Vittone. When we feel blue, we tend to overlook the good things in life.

**Make someone's day.** One way to feel good about yourself is to make someone else feel good. Give a compliment, create a bond, or smile at a stranger. "You'll walk away feeling better," says Dr. Vittone, "and the other person will feel good, too."

**Look forward.** Try to have at least one substantial activity at the end of each week that you can anticipate with enthusiasm. Plan a day trip, a shopping excursion, or dinner at a favorite restaurant. When you feel blue, remind yourself of your plans.

**Eat healthfully.** Choose a balanced diet rich in complex carbohydrates (such as fruits, vegetables, and whole grains), lean protein, and some fat.

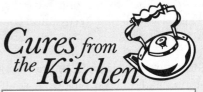

*Cures from the Kitchen*

Stock up on sardines, herring, mackerel, wild salmon, kippers, and other fish from cold northern waters, says Andrew Weil, M.D. These fish are high in omega-3 fatty acids. Some research shows that low levels of the fatty acids may underlie some psychiatric illnesses, such as depression. "In fact, there's some evidence suggesting that the rising levels of depression in the Western world in recent decades may be related to a low omega-3 intake," he says.

These foods provide the nutrients our bodies need to produce the necessary chemicals that help maintain normal mood states, says Dr. Vittone. Don't reach for too much or too little of anything. Moderation is the key.

**B diligent.** A lack of B vitamins is sometimes associated with depressive symptoms, such as fatigue, poor concentration, or moodiness. Take a multivitamin/mineral supplement that's high in the Bs, including folic acid, $B_6$, and $B_{12}$. Folic acid may even increase the effectiveness of antidepressant medications, says Andrew Weil, M.D. He recommends that your supplement contain about 400 micrograms of folic acid.

**Try St. John's wort.** Many studies show that this herbal remedy improves mild depression, says Dr. Weil. The recommended dosage is 300 milligrams of standardized extract of 0.125 percent hypericum, three times a day with meals. "Be prepared to wait several months before you see the full benefit," he adds.

**Sample SAM-e.** This dietary supplement, which is short for S-adenosylmethionine, helps regulate some hormones and the neurochemicals that are important to mood: serotonin, melatonin, dopamine, and adrenaline, Dr. Weil says. In Europe, where it is a prescription drug, SAM-e (pronounced "Sammy") is widely used to treat depression. Compared to antidepressant drugs, SAM-e works quickly, and patients often feel the effects within a week. But it's pricey and doesn't work for everyone, he notes. If you want to try SAM-e, take 1,600 milligrams of the butanedisulfonate form daily on an empty stomach. Because SAM-e may increase blood levels of homocysteine, a significant risk factor for cardiovascular disease, this supplement should be taken with folic acid and vitamins $B_6$ and $B_{12}$ to keep homocysteine levels down.

**Avoid alcohol.** Alcohol is a central-nervous-system depressant. After a drink, you may feel better at first. But later, depression may worsen, leading to a vicious cycle of drinking to chase away the blues, followed by more depressive feelings, followed by more drinking. Limit alcohol to one or two drinks at a time, Dr. Vittone says, "and definitely not every day."

**Spruce yourself up.** Spend time on grooming. Buy an outfit that enhances a positive outlook. "You'll feel better," Dr. Weil says.

## PANEL OF ADVISORS

**Edward M. Hallowell, M.D.,** is a psychiatrist and founder of the Hallowell Center for Cognitive and Emotional Health in Sudbury, Massachusetts. He is the author of *Worry: Hope and Help for a Common Condition* and *Connect: 12 Vital Ties That Open Your Heart, Lengthen Your Life, and Deepen Your Soul.*

**Bernard Vittone, M.D.,** is a psychiatrist and founder of the National Center for the Treatment of Phobias, Anxiety, and Depression in Washington, D.C.
**Andrew Weil, M.D.,** is a clinical professor of medicine and director of the program in integrative medicine at the University of Arizona in Tucson. He is the author of several books, including *8 Weeks to Optimum Health.*

# DERMATITIS AND ECZEMA
## 23 Clear-Skin Remedies

Eczema is sometimes called "the itch that rashes." That's because rather than a rash that itches, here the reverse is true: Scratching produces the rash. While eczema may look different from person to person, it usually shows up as dry, red, extremely itchy patches on the skin.

One of the most common forms of eczema is atopic dermatitis, which afflicts 10 to 20 percent of children and becomes a chronic disease of adulthood that waxes and wanes in an unlucky few.

Although scientists still do not fully understand what causes eczema, it ap-

### WHEN TO CALL A DOCTOR

When eczema is severe or widespread, and lotions, home remedies, and over-the-counter medications don't relieve the itching, a visit to a dermatologist is in order. Many prescription medicines can help. A physician will also be able to rule out other causes for your eczema. Lupus, an autoimmune disorder, is one such disease, leaving a patchy, red skin rash, roughly resembling a butterfly, on the cheeks or bridge of the nose. As one patch heals, a new one forms. These lesions itch and form scales. A person with lupus may experience severe arthritic joint pain, fever, and lung inflammation. Exposure to sunlight, certain drugs, or emotional crisis typically trigger lupus attacks. If you recognize these symptoms, contact your physician immediately.

Also, if oozing eczema, also known as weeping eczema, does not respond quickly to cold compresses applied several times a day, consult your physician, says John F. Romano, M.D.

pears to be an abnormal inflammatory response of the immune system in response to an irritant—anything from pet dander to rough fabrics to detergents. Some people can learn to avoid triggers, but for many the best strategy is to control the itching and dryness that typically accompany these physician-diagnosed skin conditions.

The experts tell us that, in general, the best way to treat the itching of eczema at home is to keep any patches of dry skin moist and well-lubricated. For that reason, many of the remedies offered in Dry Skin and Winter Itch, on page 205, may help with this problem as well.

**Beware of dry air.** Eczema is aggravated by dehumidified air, especially during winter months when forced-air heat circulates in the home.

"Forced-air heat is a bit more drying than other types of heat," says Howard Donsky, M.D. Since dry air tends to aggravate the itching of eczema or dermatitis, keeping indoor air moist should be a primary concern of sufferers and their families. "If you can counter dry air with a good humidifier, then forced-air heat is not as much of a problem," he notes.

But, the experts caution, don't expect a single-room humidifier to do it all. "People think that if they put a humidifier in their place, that'll take care of it," says Hillard H. Pearlstein, M.D. "But humidifiers are like air conditioners—you really need a big unit to do anything. If you sleep next to it, however, that's okay. Put it next to your bed."

**Make bathwater lukewarm.** A lukewarm bath helps to cleanse and moisturize your skin without overdrying. Baths or showers that are steamy or longer than 10 minutes will aggravate your condition. And always remember to use a moisturizer within 3 minutes of getting out of the tub.

**Moisturize.** You can use regular soap as long as you follow up with a moisturizer to keep the skin from drying out. "You can't bathe too frequently if you grease up afterward," says Dr. Pearlstein. "The grease is what holds the water in, and dry skin is a function of water loss, not of oil loss."

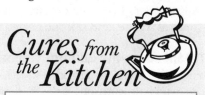

## Cures from the Kitchen

Cold, wet compresses can help soothe and relieve the itching associated with eczema that gets so bad that it begins to ooze. "I tell people to try cold milk instead of water," says John F. Romano, M.D. "It seems to be a lot more soothing."

His recommendation: Pour milk into a glass with ice cubes and let it sit for a few minutes. Then pour the milk onto a gauze pad or thin piece of cotton and apply it to the irritated skin for 2 to 3 minutes. Resoak the cloth and reapply, continuing the process for about 10 minutes.

Some favorite after-bath emollients include Complex-15, Eucerin, Keri, Lubriderm Lotion, or Moisturel Lotion. If your skin still seems dry after using one of those products, move up to creams such as Lubriderm, Purpose, or Moisturel, or ointments such as Aquaphor, Eucerin, or Nivea.

**Take an oatmeal bath.** For an additional soothing treat, Dr. Donsky recommends adding colloidal oatmeal products like Aveeno to the bath, and even using oatmeal as a soap substitute. For the bath, pour 2 cups of colloidal oatmeal (available at drugstores) into a tub of lukewarm water. The term *colloidal* simply means that the oatmeal has been ground to fine powder that will remain suspended in water. For use as a soap substitute, wrap colloidal oatmeal in a handkerchief, place a rubber band around the top, dunk it in water, and use as you would a washcloth.

**Avoid antiperspirants.** Metallic salts such as aluminum chloride, aluminum sulfate, and zirconium chlorohydrate are the active ingredients in many antiperspirants, and these can cause irritation in people with sensitive skin. "Usually it's the antiperspirant, as opposed to the deodorant, that's irritating," Dr. Donsky says. Look for products that contain aluminum zirconium, such as Tom's of Maine, and silicone-related moisturizers, like Secret Gentle Care.

**Try this over-the-counter cream.** Topical creams, ointments, and lotions containing cortisone are often used to alleviate the itching and inflammation of eczema. Hydrocortisone is the mildest member of the cortisone family of steroid hormones, and it is available at drugstores.

"Half-percent (0.5) hydrocortisone cream is available without a prescription," says Dr. Pearlstein, "and that can help." If that doesn't seem to help, he suggests trying 1 percent hydrocortisone cream, which is also available without a prescription.

---

## The Power of Prevention

Women who have atopic dermatitis may wish to protect their children from the same fate. An analysis by Israeli researchers of 18 scientific studies offers hope. The researchers found powerful evidence that, in families with a history of atopic dermatitis, exclusively breastfeeding in the first 3 months of life can protect infants from developing the condition during childhood.

The preventive role of breastfeeding was less powerful in the general population and "negligible" in babies with no first-degree relatives who had experienced atopic dermatitis.

**Cool with calamine.** "Calamine lotion is good for many types of rashes that ooze and may need to be dried out," says John F. Romano, M.D. "Also, calamine lotion with menthol or phenol added to it can be purchased over the counter at drugstores, and that seems to help itching better than calamine lotion alone."

**Take comfort in cotton.** Cotton clothing worn next to the skin is much better than polyester, and especially better than wool, says Dr. Romano. The bottom line: Avoid synthetics or itchy fabrics as well as tight- or ill-fitting clothes.

**Put your diet to the test.** "Food allergies can play a big role in atopic dermatitis during childhood," says Dr. Pearlstein. "They are intimately related before age 6, and you can manipulate an infant's diet and do well in helping his skin."

Traditionally, eggs, orange juice, and milk have been implicated as eczema aggravators in children. But, says Dr. Pearlstein, "I certainly wouldn't incriminate those foods wholesale." That means parents should consult their physicians about trying elimination diets, just to be sure. Such diets seem to work best in infants less than 2 years old, he says. "After age 6, we've found that food plays a minimal role in most people."

For adults, Dr. Pearlstein says that he leaves diet manipulation largely in the hands of his patients. If you think there's any food you eat that has an adverse effect on your skin, avoid it and see what happens, he says. If your problem clears up, you may have a food allergy.

**Try boosting your omega-3 intake.** Salmon, mackerel, and tuna contain omega-3s and other essential fatty acids that may help to prevent allergies and inflammation, both of which are associated with eczema.

**Avoid quick changes in air temperature.** "If you have eczema," says Dr. Donsky, "then rapid temperature changes can be a problem." Going from a warm room out into cold winter air, or even from an air-conditioned room to a hot shower, can trigger itching. Wearing layers of clothing—cotton clothing—and avoiding hot baths or showers are the best ways to protect yourself, says Dr. Donsky.

**Beware of baby lotions.** "Sometimes baby lotions aren't the best thing for childhood eczema," Dr. Romano says. "They have a high water content, and that can further dry and irritate the skin as evaporation takes place." Some of the fragrances and active ingredients in baby lotions (lanolin and mineral oil) are common causes of skin allergy.

"What you want instead are creams or ointments," he says. "Something like Eucerin cream, Aquaphor, or Vaseline Dermatology Formula."

# Got a Nickel Rash?

Eczema, or atopic dermatitis, is one type of skin rash, and doctors aren't quite sure what causes it. Another type, called contact dermatitis, is clearly caused by, you guessed it, contact with an irritant. One example of contact dermatitis is poison ivy. Another, increasingly common type is nickel rash.

"Nickel dermatitis is probably the most common contact dermatitis going," says Howard Donsky, M.D. "But people often don't suspect that that's the problem—they think they have a problem with gold."

Nickel dermatitis occurs 10 times more often in women than men and is often triggered by ear piercing. Strangely enough, having the ears pierced can cause rashes to occur in other areas of the body whenever the person comes in contact with nickel-containing metal. Suddenly, bracelets, necklaces, and other jewelry that the person has worn for years can bring on a contact rash.

If this sounds like what's happening to you, the following tips might help.

**Buy posts of stainless steel.** Newly pierced ears should be studded only with steel posts until the earlobes heal (about 3 weeks).

**Stay cool.** Since perspiration plays a big role in nickel dermatitis—it leaches out the nickel in nickel-plated jewelry—stay out of the heat if you're wearing this type of jewelry. Or don't wear it if you're going out in the heat.

**Go for the gold.** Buy only quality gold jewelry, says Dr. Donsky. "If it's less than 24-karat gold, there's some nickel in there," he says, "and the lower the karat, the higher the nickel."

**Consider dietary changes.** Some European dermatologists advise nickel-sensitive patients to watch what they eat. Having observed that nickel dermatitis can occur without any apparent contact with the metal, the doctors tell folks to avoid apricots, chocolate, coffee, beer, tea, nuts, and other foods high in nickel.

While intriguing, the theory hasn't garnered a great following on this side of the Atlantic. "The jury's still out on foods high in nickel causing a reaction," Dr. Donsky confirms. "But if you're highly sensitive to nickel, there might be some validity to it."

**Read labels for urea.** "Emollients that contain urea are pretty good for relieving the itch of eczema or dermatitis," says Dr. Pearlstein. "Urea is a sloughing agent, and it's a good product. We usually use it when the skin is a little thick from rubbing and scratching."

A couple of urea-containing products to try include Carmol 10 or 20 and Ultra Mide 25. Emollients that contain lactic acid (LactiCare 1 percent or 2 percent or Lac-Hydrin Five) are also recommended.

**Drink Oregon grape tea.** Oregon grape root, sold in health food stores, is known for its antihistamine, anti-inflammatory, antifungal properties. Add 1 tablespoon of the dried root to 1 cup of boiling water. Continue boiling for 10 minutes. Strain and drink every morning, adding dried chamomile for extra flavor. Herbalists say that this remedy may take more than a year, or as little as 3 months, to have a significant benefit for the skin.

**Use antihistamines for atopics.** Antihistamines block the release of histamine from mast cells, thereby reducing such classic allergy symptoms as headaches, runny nose, and itching. For that reason, "over-the-counter antihistamines such as Benadryl are good for eczema," says Dr. Romano.

Antihistamines reduce itching by preventing histamine from reaching and swelling sensitive skin cells. Follow label directions and be aware that antihistamines can cause drowsiness, leading to possible problems with driving a vehicle or handling dangerous machinery.

**Wash once, rinse twice.** When it comes to doing laundry for people with eczema or dermatitis, it's not the detergent so much as the rinse, says Dr. Romano.

"You have to make sure the detergent is washed out thoroughly," he says. "Don't use too much detergent when washing, and always use a second rinse cycle to get all the soap out."

**Get to know your eye doctor.** In a 20-year study of 492 people at the Mayo Clinic in Rochester, Minnesota, 13 percent of those with atopic dermatitis developed cataracts. "There is a higher incidence of cataracts in people with atopic dermatitis," Dr. Pearlstein confirms. So see your ophthalmologist regularly.

## PANEL OF ADVISORS

**Howard Donsky, M.D.,** is a clinical instructor of dermatology at the University of Rochester and a dermatologist at the Dermatology and Cosmetic Center of Rochester in New York.

**Hillard H. Pearlstein, M.D.,** is an assistant clinical professor of dermatology at the Mount Sinai School of Medicine of New York University in New York City.

**John F. Romano, M.D.,** is a dermatologist and an assistant clinical professor of dermatology at New York Hospital–Cornell University Medical Center in New York City.

# DIABETES
## 43 Ways to Steady Blood Sugar

Most people never give it a second thought—the food they eat is transformed into energy and that's that. Their bodies do all the work for them: digesting the food and converting carbohydrates into a type of sugar called glucose that enters the bloodstream. Next, the pancreas kicks out insulin, a hormone that travels through the body, attaching to receptors on the outside of cells. Once attached, insulin acts like a key that "unlocks" the cell so that glucose can enter it and be used for energy. If the body doesn't need the sugar for energy, it stores it as fat. Usually, this process hums along like a well-oiled machine. People only take notice when the process breaks down.

The monkey wrench that interrupts the flow is diabetes. Nearly 16 million people in the United States have this disease, a number that's tripled in the past 30 years—and may double again very soon.

Diabetes, also known as diabetes mellitus, comes in two forms. Type 1, previously called juvenile diabetes or insulin-dependent diabetes mellitus, is believed to be an autoimmune condition in which the pancreas fails to manufacture insulin. Though onset can occur at any age, patients are usually diagnosed in childhood or as young adults and require daily insulin injections throughout their lives.

People with the other form, type 2, usually develop the disease in adulthood, although unfortunately more and more children and young adults also are developing type 2 diabetes now. In this case, the pancreas *produces* insulin, but the body does not use it properly, and the pancreas kicks into overdrive to make up for this "resistance." In time, the pancreas cannot make enough insulin to make up for the insensitivity, and diabetes follows. Inactivity, aging, obesity, or a high-saturated-fat diet can all contribute to insulin resistance. Type 2 diabetes, also known as adult-onset diabetes or noninsulin-dependent diabetes mellitus, accounts for 90 to 95 percent of all cases. With either form of diabetes, glucose builds up in the bloodstream. Left untreated, this can lead to serious complications including kidney failure, limb amputation, heart disease, and blindness. But the good news is that type 2 diabetes often can be controlled through simple measures. Weight loss, proper nutrition, adequate exercise, and stress reduction

## WHEN TO CALL A DOCTOR

Diabetes is a serious illness that requires a doctor's care, even when it is controlled. Consult a health care professional before making any changes to your diet or exercise routines.

Three complications of diabetes require *prompt* medical attention: severe hyperglycemia, hypoglycemia, and ketoacidosis.

Hyperglycemia is when your blood sugar spikes high. Symptoms include frequent urination, fatigue, unexplainable weight loss, and increased thirst. "These are signs that your blood sugar is too high, and you should be in touch with a health care professional if you can't get it down," says Christopher D. Saudek, M.D.

Hypoglycemia is when blood sugar drops too low. Symptoms include shakiness, dizziness, headache, confusion, sudden mood changes, and a tingling sensation around the mouth. Many people with diabetes have periods of hypoglycemia, but you should call a doctor whenever symptoms are severe or occur frequently.

Self-treat mild hypoglycemia simply by taking three glucose tablets, eating five or six pieces of hard candy, or drinking a ½ cup of fruit juice. It's important to treat it immediately, since you can pass out if it gets worse.

Ketoacidosis is a serious, potentially fatal condition that occurs when ketones—acids that build up in the blood—become dangerously high and poison the body. Warning signs include increased thirst, nausea, frequent urination, fatigue, and vomiting. Ketoacidosis occurs in people with type 1 diabetes, not with type 2.

all can improve blood glucose levels. Some experts believe that dietary supplements may help, too. Even people with diabetes who require medication will maintain better glucose control if they adhere to a healthy lifestyle. Here's our experts' advice.

## Nurture Good Nutrition

No one nutrition prescription can apply to everyone with diabetes, explains Marion Franz, M.S., R.D. "Each person with diabetes deserves to have a meal plan that suits him or her individually." The American Diabetes Association (ADA) urges people to consider what ethnic and cultural foods they prefer, what other health concerns they may have (high cholesterol and high blood pressure, for example), and what changes they are realistically willing to make. Working within that framework, people should aim for the following nutrition goals.

**Count carbs.** The ADA emphasizes that carbohydrates are an important part of a healthful diet. This food group includes starches, such as whole grains, cereals, baked goods, legumes, fruits, vegetables, and low-fat milk.

Because carbohydrates have the biggest impact on blood sugar after eating, it's important to monitor the amount you eat at each meal. An average portion size consists of 15 grams of carbohydrates. That's equivalent to one slice of bread, $\frac{1}{3}$ cup of rice, a small piece of fruit, two small cookies, or $\frac{1}{2}$ cup of ice cream. Aim for three to four carbohydrate servings at each meal and one serving for snacks.

**Read labels.** The best way to figure out how many carbohydrates are in a meal is to look at food labels. Also, be sure to check the serving size. A serving of pasta, for example, is just $\frac{1}{2}$ cup, much less than most people typically eat at one time.

**Measure your food.** Don't guesstimate, says Carla Miller, Ph.D., R.D. Use a measuring cup for foods like rice and vegetables. For items like meats that are gauged in ounces, you'll need a kitchen scale, available at most department stores, says Dr. Miller. When you're without a scale, such as in restaurants, just remember that 3 ounces of meat is about the size of a deck of cards.

**Watch your sugars.** Sugars aren't as ominous as they would seem for people with diabetes. When eaten in equal amounts, starches and sugars have similar effects on blood sugar, Franz says. Still, foods containing sugars and sweets are often high in calories and low in nutritional value. If you do eat something high in sugar, it's important to substitute that for other carbohydrate foods in your menu.

# Do just 1 thing

Lose weight. The most effective thing that an overweight person with type 2 diabetes can do is to lose weight, says Christopher D. Saudek, M.D.

Shedding excess pounds is sometimes all it takes to bring blood sugar under control. How much weight to lose varies for each individual, but even small drops can yield big results.

"You don't have to be skinny-skinny, and you don't have to reach that ideal body weight," notes Carla Miller, Ph.D., R.D. Losing as little as 10 to 20 pounds, or just 5 to 10 percent of your body weight, may be enough to attain glucose control. Of course, you'll have to maintain that weight loss, or your blood sugar will rise again. That's why how you trim down is especially important.

Avoid fad diets, counsels Dr. Saudek. Most are difficult to sustain, and some are not healthy. Your best bet is to combine exercise with a low-calorie diet. Work with a health care professional or a registered dietitian to determine how many calories are right for you.

**Eat fewer fats.** Keeping fats to about 30 percent of your total calories can reduce your chance of developing high cholesterol and heart disease, both risk factors for diabetes.

**Eat even fewer saturated fats.** Saturated fats, from meats and cheeses, and polyunsaturated fats, like hydrogenated margarine, should account for only 10 percent of total daily calories. Switching to a diet higher in monounsaturated fats, found in olive oil and nuts, and lower in polyunsaturated fats may help reduce insulin resistance, according to Harry G. Preuss, M.D. Choose low-fat dairy products and lean meats, and avoid margarine and baked goods containing trans fatty acids, coconut oil, or palm oil.

**Pass on high-protein diets.** Because foods high in animal protein, such as meats and cheeses, also tend to be high in fat and cholesterol, limit proteins to between 10 and 20 percent of your diet. It's true that you might lose weight following popular high-protein, low-carb diets, but keeping it off can be a problem. You're better off adopting a balanced diet that you can live with for a long time, says Franz.

**Skimp on sodium.** Diabetes and high blood pressure sometimes go hand in hand, and people with diabetes can be more sensitive to the effects of excess sodium, says Franz. Limit sodium to less than 2,400 milligrams a day, which is the amount of sodium in 1 teaspoon of salt. The easiest way to do this is to eat less than 800 milligrams at each meal and no more than 400 milligrams in each food. Look for the amount of sodium on food labels.

**Feast on fiber.** One small study of 13 people who ate 25 grams each of soluble and insoluble fiber—a total of 50 grams a day—found that they were able to achieve a 10 percent drop in blood sugar levels.

While that's encouraging news, Franz cautions that, from a practical standpoint, 50 grams a day may be a bit tough to stomach. "We really don't know if, in the long term, people *can* eat enough fiber to influence blood glucose levels," she says.

Nevertheless, high-fiber diets have other health advantages. They slow the absorption of fats and carbohydrates into the system, reducing their adverse effects on the glucose-insulin system. Also, high-fiber foods tend to be very filling, so you eat less. Shoot for 25 to 35 grams a day by eating lots of whole grains, beans, lentils, and vegetables.

**Drink sparingly.** You needn't become a teetotaler the moment you're diagnosed with diabetes. Moderate drinking has been shown to lower the risk of heart disease and may actually improve insulin sensitivity, according to some studies. To realize such benefits, however, don't drink too much. Women should cork the bottle after one drink a day (or less), and men after two or less.

(One drink is 12 ounces of beer, 4 ounces of wine, or 1½ ounces of hard liquor.) If you choose beer, light is best since it contains fewer carbohydrates and calories.

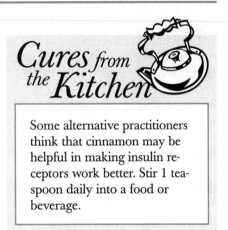

**Cures from the Kitchen**

Some alternative practitioners think that cinnamon may be helpful in making insulin receptors work better. Stir 1 teaspoon daily into a food or beverage.

**Enlist your spouse.** Dr. Miller studied the eating patterns and food choices of 45 men and women with type 2 diabetes for 1 year. She found that those with the best blood-sugar control were men whose wives prepared low-fat meals and walked with them. On the other hand, women without that level of support from another person didn't have good glucose control. Worst off were those women who prepared low-fat meals for themselves but made separate meals for their families. The moral: Persuade your family to get healthy along with you.

**Plan ahead.** Diabetes requires a pretty intensive lifestyle overhaul, acknowledges Dr. Miller. You need to exercise, eat healthy, and monitor your blood sugar, which requires an enormous amount of organization and time. In her study, Dr. Miller found that people most successful at controlling their blood sugar levels were those who did a lot of meal preplanning.

Decide at the beginning of the week what healthy foods you want to prepare. Then shop for those foods. If you make bag lunches and have healthy food on hand, you'll be less likely to rely on high-fat, fast-food meals or sugary snacks.

**Visit a dietitian.** A dietitian or nutritionist can design an individual nutrition plan just for you. That's especially important if you have multiple health issues, such as high cholesterol and high blood pressure, as well as diabetes, says Dr. Miller. Plan several sessions so that you can gradually incorporate changes.

## Get Your Heart Pumping

In addition to nutrition changes, experts recommend regular exercise for people with diabetes.

"Exercise acts just like medicine," explains diabetes educator Robert Hanisch. It lowers blood sugar as muscles turn glucose into energy.

According to the American College of Sports Medicine (ACSM), obese people with type 2 diabetes who exercise regularly achieve better glucose control. What's more, studies find that increased physical activity, including walking, can reduce the risk of heart attack, stroke, and other complications in people with diabetes.

Even people dependent on insulin or oral medicines can reap the benefits of exercise. "At the very least, they will take less medicine. And the results are immediate," says Hanisch. You should check your blood glucose immediately before and after exercise. There will be individual variations, but on average there is a 1 to 2 point drop in blood sugar for every minute you exercise. That means 10 minutes of aerobic exercise will usually cut blood sugar 10 to 20 points. The glucose will remain lower until the next meal or snack.

Check with your doctor before beginning any exercise program. Here are some tips to get you going.

**Start easy.** Not accustomed to exercise? Don't sweat it. Begin with a low-impact, low-intensity workout, such as walking. "Walk at a comfortable pace," advises Hanisch. If you push yourself too hard, you won't find it enjoyable, and you'll be less likely to continue. "Blood sugar can go down even when you are walking very slowly," he says.

**Join the 1,000 club.** ACSM recommends that people with type 2 diabetes burn a minimum of 1,000 calories a week through daily activity and that everyone with diabetes should do *at least* 3 nonconsecutive days of exercise each week for 10 to 15 minutes. Hanisch suggests a goal of gradually building up to a 30-minute workout on most days of the week. If you weigh about 150 pounds, you'll burn 166 calories in 30 minutes of brisk walking. Walk briskly for 30 minutes 5 days a week, and you'll come close to that goal. The rest of your daily activities will put you well over that minimum of 1,000 calories a week.

**Strive for five.** "Consistency is the key," notes Hanisch. Whether you hike, bike, swim, or jog, a routine you can manage five times a week will produce optimum results, producing a long-term change in your body. After 2 to 3 months of consistent exercise, you likely will become more sensitive to insulin, and you'll need less medicine, Hanisch says.

**Be a morning person.** An early workout will hold blood sugar down all day long. You will still see fluctuations in glucose levels after meals, but a 30-minute morning walk will keep levels 30 points lower than what they might otherwise be, says Hanisch.

**Drink up.** Dehydration can affect blood glucose levels, so staying well-hydrated during exercise is especially important for people with diabetes. Drink 16 ounces of fluid—two glasses of water—2 hours before exercising, and sip throughout your workout.

**Lift lightly.** Weight training can help build strength. But people with long-standing diabetes, and especially those with diabetes-related eye disease, need to limit themselves to many repetitions with very light resistance in the range of

1- to 5-pound weights. Heavy weights can injure weakened eye muscles, says Hanisch. To know that the weight is light enough, you should be able to perform the correct strengthening techniques with minimal effort. If in doubt, use the lighter weight.

**Take care of your toes.** People who have diabetes-related foot problems such as peripheral neuropathy (see "Take Care of Your Feet") should take special care before they go walking or jogging. "They may need to work with a podiatrist to get shoes that distribute the force differently when they land," says Hanisch.

## Stress Less

When something gets you stressed out, sending your emotions on a roller coaster, your blood sugar goes along for the ride. That's because stress hormones, such as adrenaline, increase blood glucose. "Stress hormones mobilize glycogen that has been stored in the liver and metabolize it to glucose," says Angele McGrady, Ph.D.

The adrenaline and extra sugar released into the bloodstream give you a boost of energy. If you were undergoing a physical stress, such as being chased by a pack of wild dogs, you'd respond by running away, and the extra blood sugar would be used up, Dr. McGrady points out. Today, however, most of our stressors are psychological. We sit and stew and don't use up the additional blood sugar.

Since their bodies don't metabolize glucose effectively, it's especially important for people with diabetes to try to decrease their stress levels. In a small study that Dr. McGrady conducted, 18 people with diabetes reduced their blood sugar levels 9 to 12 percent by practicing simple relaxation exercises. Those people who also had depression, however, did not benefit without additional treatment. Here are some stress busters worth trying.

**Breathe deeply.** "Deep breathing is a good way to start," says Dr. McGrady. Sit with your legs and arms uncrossed. Inhale deeply from your abdomen. Then breathe out as much air as possible, relaxing your muscles as you do. Continue this relaxed breathing for about 15 minutes.

**Purchase a relaxation tape.** Can't settle down? A relaxation tape can help. "Most of us aren't used to sitting quietly with no thoughts in our heads," says Dr. McGrady. "It's very helpful to have sound in the background." Recordings of gentle sounds from nature, such as ocean waves, enable you to pace your breathing and set a tone for you to relax. Or, choose a guided imagery tape, in which a soothing voice mentally shepherds you through a pleasant scene, such as a walk through a forest. Look for them wherever tapes or CDs are sold.

# Take Care of Your Feet

Peripheral neuropathy is a complication of diabetes in which high blood sugar damages nerve cells over time, leading to a lack of sensation. Because the nerves in the feet are the longest in the body, the feet are usually most affected by this condition, making them prone to injury and sores. Sores that don't heal properly can become ulcerated and infected and, in serious cases, may even require amputation. An estimated 6 out of every 1,000 people with diabetes have a limb amputated—the vast majority of these can be avoided. Here are some recommendations for protecting your feet.

**See a podiatrist.** Once you've been diagnosed with diabetes, have your feet checked frequently, recommends Marc A. Brenner, D.P.M. A podiatrist will determine if you have neuropathy and will help care for your feet if you do. Trimming toenails or self-treating calluses and corns, for example, can pose hazards for people with neuropathy and should be done by a podiatric physician.

**Keep them covered.** Wear a good pair of socks. The best are made of a combination of cotton and synthetic material. On very cold days, wear two pairs—a thin one next to your skin and a thick pair. "The more insulation you have between your foot and the ground, the better," says Dr. Brenner.

**Be sure the shoe fits.** Your shoe size should be determined by a certified pedorthist, a person specially trained to measure feet, says Dr. Brenner. Ask your podiatrist to recommend a shoe store that offers such services. Have your feet measured in the afternoon, when your feet are more likely to be swollen.

**Step out in sneaks.** You probably won't need custom shoes. A high-quality cross-trainer or running shoe will serve you well. Look for ones with a roomy toebox; a removable inlay to fit in a custom orthotic device; a padded, thick tongue; a cushioned heel; and cushioning on the ball of the foot.

**Wear an orthotic.** A diabetic orthotic is a custom-made device that fits into your shoe. It's important to wear one since it keeps pressure off certain spots on the foot or spreads pressure across the entire foot. Your podiatrist will advise you and measure you for an appropriate orthotic if indicated.

**Inspect daily.** Check for swelling or sores, using a large mirror to see all angles of the foot. Better yet, ask a family member to check for you, having him or her touch your foot to make sure it's not discolored or not too hot—signs of possible infection.

**Take them swimming.** If you have neuropathy, exercise is still important. "Swimming is safest," says Dr. Brenner, because you don't have to put pressure on your feet. Carefully dry your feet afterward and sprinkle them with foot powder to avoid fungus or yeast.

**Focus on something pleasant.** Guided imagery works because it uses your senses of recall and concentration to help you relax. You can achieve the same effect by examining an art book or an illustration that you find pleasant. "Look at the picture for several minutes, then close your eyes and recall as much as you can," explains Dr. McGrady. "If you do it enough, you can eventually do it without even having the book in front of you." You could put a peaceful scene on your screensaver, too, she suggests.

**Practice progressive relaxation.** Tensing and relaxing the muscles in your body allows you to consciously control muscle tension. First, lie on your back in a comfortable position. Then, begin deliberately tensing and releasing one muscle—the fist is a good place to start. Move upward along your arms, to the neck, and face, and then down the back and legs. Do not tense any muscle hard enough to produce pain, Dr. McGrady cautions. Scripts on tape are available to talk you through this process.

## Supplement Savvy

Some practitioners believe that dietary supplements can be helpful for people with diabetes. Consult your physician before trying them out. Here are a few that the experts recommend.

**Consider chromium.** Some people with diabetes can benefit from chromium supplements, especially if they have a deficiency of this mineral. Dr. Preuss suggests 400 to 600 micrograms of chromium a day for 1 to 2 months under the direction of a physician.

**Get some American ginseng.** One small Canadian study found that patients with type 2 diabetes who took 3 grams of American ginseng 2 hours before eating 25 grams of sugar reduced their after-meal blood sugar levels by 20 percent. Talk with your doctor about the right dose for you.

**Seek sight-saving herbs.** According to herbal experts, the herbs bilberry and ginkgo may improve circulation, thereby lowering the risk of eye damage for people with diabetes. Both are available freeze-dried or as a tincture. Follow the manufacturer's directions.

**Baby your arteries with baby aspirin.** Aspirin reduces heart attack risk by discouraging blood cells called platelets from sticking together in the arteries. Amazingly, it's even more effective for those with diabetes than for those without diabetes. That's good news, since the incidence of heart attack among women with diabetes has been on the rise in recent years. Ask your doctor how much aspirin is right for you, says Aaron Vinik, M.D., Ph.D.

**Try a multi.** Look for a good multivitamin/mineral supplement that provides at least 25 percent of the Daily Values of magnesium, zinc, vitamin E, and vitamin C. Magnesium deficiency is thought to increase insulin resistance, high blood pressure, and cardiovascular disease in people with diabetes. Zinc deficiency also can negatively impact glucose levels. Vitamin E helps sensitize insulin receptors. Vitamin C assists the immune system and enables tissue repair, says Dr. Preuss.

## Testing, Testing

Once diagnosed with diabetes, testing your blood sugar at home becomes an integral part of your life. Here are some techniques that experts advise.

**Look for patterns.** Monitor your glucose levels by recording your levels four times a day for several weeks, suggests Dr. Miller. That helps you discern patterns, she says. Check first thing in the morning, 1 to 2 hours after meals, and right before bed.

**Check out changes.** When making changes in your diet, test immediately before a meal, then 2 hours after. Before a meal, levels should range between 90 to 130 milligrams per deciliter (mg/dl). After a meal, levels should be no higher than 160 mg/dl.

**Test when you exercise.** When beginning a new exercise routine, test immediately before and immediately after your workout, says Hanisch. If your blood sugar is low before starting—100 to 120 mg/dl—eat a piece of fruit or drink half a cup (4 ounces) of juice. Both have about 15 grams of carbohydrates to elevate blood sugar about 25 points. Do the same if your levels drop after exercise.

**Do spot checks.** Most people with diabetes habitually monitor first thing in the morning. That's not enough, says Dr. Miller. Do an occasional test after lunch or in the evening to achieve a better picture of what influences your blood glucose. Blood sugar values should be 110 to 150 mg/dl on average at bedtime.

**Write it down.** Keep a written record of your levels, and note what and when you ate as well as when you exercised and for how long. "Use a spiral-bound notebook, or make up a spread sheet on your computer," suggests Dr. Miller. Show the log to your doctor so that he can better manage your care.

## PANEL OF ADVISORS

**Marc A. Brenner, D.P.M.,** is director of the Institute of Diabetic Foot Research in Glendale, New York; past president of the American Society of Podiatric Dermatology; and author and editor of various books.

**Marion Franz, M.S., R.D.,** is a nutrition consultant in Minneapolis and co-chairman of the American Diabetes Association's task force to revise nutrition principle recommendations.

**Robert Hanisch** is the senior medical exercise physiologist and certified diabetes educator with the Diabetes Treatment Center at Columbia–St. Mary's Hospital in Milwaukee.

**Angele McGrady, Ph.D.,** is a professor in the department of psychiatry and the director of the Complementary Medicine Center at the Medical College of Ohio in Toledo.

**Carla Miller, Ph.D., R.D.,** is an assistant professor in the department of nutrition and codirector of the Diet Assessment Center, both at Pennsylvania State University in University Park.

**Harry G. Preuss, M.D.,** is a diabetes researcher and professor of physiology, medicine, and pathology at Georgetown University Medical Center in Washington, D.C.

**Christopher D. Saudek, M.D.,** is president of the American Diabetes Association and director of Johns Hopkins Diabetes Center in Baltimore.

**Aaron I. Vinik, M.D., Ph.D.,** is a professor of internal medicine, pathology, and neurobiology at the Eastern Virginia Medical School and director of the Strelitz Diabetes Research Institute, both in Norfolk.

# DIAPER RASH
## 6 Easy Solutions

Diaper rash can interrupt the peaceful routine of an otherwise carefree baby, and it won't do much for a parent's quality of life either. Babies have a knack for making their problems their parents' problems, and if your baby has diaper rash, well, you'll know about it.

During the first 2 to 3 years of a baby's life, just about every parent shares in the diaper rash experience at least once. It's not surprising, given that the most common rash-triggering irritants come from what is typically found in baby's diaper: bowel movements and urine. Thankfully, nearly half of all diaper rashes go away by themselves within 1 day. But the other 50 percent can last 10 days or more (though it might seem longer).

Here's some other diaper rash trivia: In some babies, diaper rash may be a harbinger of future skin problems such as eczema or sensitive skin. Also, breastfed babies have less diaper rash than bottle-fed babies, and this resistance continues long after a baby is weaned.

Enough trivia. Here's some advice on how to help your little one feel better.

**Give 'em some air—or water.** The oldest advice is sometimes still the best. "Give that baby's bottom some air," says child-care expert Ann Price.

Simply take the baby's diaper off and lay her chest down, with her face turned to one side, on towels placed atop a waterproof sheet. Leave her resting on her chest as long as you're there to keep an eye on her. (An unwatched, undiapered baby is trouble waiting to happen.) Another option: Place the baby in a basin or tub of lukewarm water for several minutes every time you change her diaper. This keeps her bottom clean and may comfort her, too.

**Let super diapers come to the rescue.** Superabsorbent diapers are a lifesaver in your baby's battle for a dry bottom. "I think they're the best thing there is for preventing diaper rash," says Morris Green, M.D.

Studies confirm Dr. Green's observation. Diapers containing absorbent gelling material significantly reduce skin wetness and leave skin closer to its

## The "Bead Bottom" Mystery

A medical journal article tells of parents calling pediatricians to report a strange diaper rash that looks like "small, shiny beads" covering their babies' bottoms. Pediatricians investigating the mysterious outbreak of "bead bottom" noticed that the afflicted infants all wore superabsorbent disposable diapers. Was there a connection?

Yes. The "beads" are actually the gelling material that makes superabsorbent diapers "super." Apparently, small, loose quantities of the material may occasionally pass through a break in the top sheet of the diaper and transfer to the infant's skin. Doctors say the material is nontoxic and presents no reason for concern.

normal pH than earlier types of disposable diapers or cloth diapers. Make sure that you don't wait too long between changes, however. Some parents wait until disposable diapers are too saturated, which actually increases the baby's risk for diaper rash.

**Cleanse gently.** Don't use regular diaper wipes containing alcohol because they can burn irritated skin and worsen the condition. Instead, diapering experts recommend alcohol-free brands, or trying cotton balls dipped in baby oil. Another option is to use warm water in a squirt bottle to rinse the baby's bottom.

**Blow-dry that baby.** Keeping the diaper area clean promotes healing, but drying with a towel can irritate sensitive skin. Option? "Try a blow-dryer," says pediatric nurse practitioner Linda Jonides. Dry the diaper area with a hair dryer set on "low," which avoids abrasion to wet skin. After the area is dry, apply a zinc oxide ointment such as A&D Diaper Rash Ointment or Desitin. Petroleum jelly such as Vaseline also provides a protective coating, even on sore, red skin. Avoid sprinkling the baby's bottom with cornstarch or baby powder, because either one can trigger breathing problems in little ones.

**Give cloth diapers a vinegar rinse.** Diaper rash enzymes are most active in a high-pH environment, which often exists in cloth diapers after washing, says Price. To counter this, add 1 ounce of vinegar to 1 gallon of water during the final rinse to bring the pH of cloth diapers into line with the pH of baby's skin.

"Actually, I believe there's a lot to be said for diaper services," Price notes. "They go to a lot of trouble to get the pH balance right, and they're not all that expensive. If you're using cloth diapers and your baby has a bad rash, I recommend giving them a try."

**Make the cranberry connection.** When urine and feces mix in the diaper area, the result is a high pH that irritates the skin and promotes diaper rash.

Unorthodox as it may sound, Jonides notes that 2 to 3 ounces of cranberry juice given to older infants leaves an acid residue in the urine, helping lower pH and reduce irritation.

## PANEL OF ADVISORS

**Morris Green, M.D.,** is chairman of the department of pediatrics at Indiana University School of Medicine in Indianapolis.

**Linda Jonides** is a pediatric nurse practitioner in Ann Arbor, Michigan.

**Anne Price** is a former educational coordinator for the National Academy of Nannies, Inc. (NANI) in Denver.

# DIARRHEA
## 21 Strategies to Deal with It

In the past when someone had diarrhea, doctors whipped out their prescription pads and dispensed antidiarrheal medication. Today, they think the best medicine is to simply let diarrhea run its course, if you'll pardon the pun.

"Acute diarrhea is one of your body's best defense mechanisms," says Lynn V. McFarland, Ph.D. "It's your body's way of getting something nasty out of your system."

That thought may or may not be of comfort to you right now, but it explains why doctors today tell you to "tough it out" instead of automatically trying to stem the tide of this annoying, but hopefully short-lived, illness.

"I don't recommend antidiarrheal medications when a patient has acute diarrhea unless he has an urgent need for control—like a very important business meeting that just can't be missed," says David A. Lieberman, M.D. "Otherwise, I think the purge is probably beneficial and helps speed recovery," he says.

Heeding that approach, most of the tips below are designed to help you weather the discomfort of diarrhea and make a quick recovery, rather than try to halt the course of diarrhea and risk prolonging the illness. For those who may have "an urgent need for control" while stricken, we've listed some medications to help stem the tide while you take care of other business.

## WHEN TO CALL A DOCTOR

Diarrhea should normally leave you only slightly worse for wear. In infants, small children, elderly people, or those already sick or dehydrated from another illness, however, acute diarrhea can be particularly severe and demands prompt medical attention.

Medical help is also needed if diarrhea doesn't subside within 1 to 2 days, if it's accompanied by fever and severe abdominal cramps, or if it occurs with rashes, jaundice (yellowing of the skin and whites of the eyes), or extreme weakness. If blood, pus, or mucus is found in your stools, call your doctor.

"The most immediate risk associated with acute diarrhea is dehydration," says Harris Clearfield, M.D. "So if an individual is having a major bout of diarrhea and isn't taking in any food or drink during that time, you're looking at a medical emergency."

**Make the milk connection.** A leading cause of diarrhea in this country is lactose intolerance, says William Y. Chey, M.D.

"Lactose intolerance can have its onset when you're just a baby, or it can kick in suddenly during your adult years," says Dr. Chey. One day you could be drinking milk, and the next thing you know—bam!—you have gas, pain, and diarrhea.

The cure, of course, is to avoid lactose-containing foods, which means staying away from most dairy products, with the exception of yogurt, some aged cheeses like Cheddar and those specifically designed to be lactose-free, such as Lactaid.

**Take the tolerance test.** Given the dose-related nature of lactose intolerance, as well as its ability to kick in unexpectedly, how can you be sure that milk products are responsible for your tummy troubles?

First, completely abstain from milk products for a week or two and see if that helps, says Dr. Lieberman. If it does, then gradually add back milk products with the knowledge that at some point you may reach a level where the intolerance symptoms return. Once you know what that level is, you can avoid lactose-induced diarrhea by eating fewer dairy products.

**Think about your medications.** Our experts say there's a good possibility that the diarrhea you have now was caused by the heartburn you had earlier today. It's not because of a direct connection between stomach and bowel, but because of the antacid you may have taken to soothe your burning belly.

"Antacids are the most common cause of drug-related diarrhea," says Harris Clearfield, M.D. "Maalox and Mylanta both have magnesium hydroxide in them that acts exactly like milk of magnesia, which makes these antacids a common cause of diarrhea."

To avoid future bouts of heartburn-related diarrhea, he suggests trying antacids that contain aluminum hydroxide, with no magnesium added, such as Gaviscon or AlternaGel. "These are less likely to cause diarrhea," Dr. Clearfield says, "but they're less effective, too."

Antibiotics, quinidine, lactulose, and colchicine may also cause diarrhea. Consult your doctor if you suspect these or any other medications may be causing problems for you.

Large doses of vitamin C can be a culprit behind diarrhea, too. Amounts over the Daily Value (60 milligrams) may cause diarrhea in some people, but most are fine with up to 2,000 milligrams per day as long as they divide their doses over the course of the day.

**Consume a clear diet.** "Start with a clear-liquid diet," says Dr. Chey. "By 'clear' I mean chicken broth, Jell-O, or other foods and fluids you can look 'clear' through." This helps your bowel rest during the diarrhea, rather than forcing your system to handle more than it has to.

After you've tested the waters with broth and Jell-O, you can gradually introduce rice, bananas, applesauce, or yogurt into your diet as your symptoms improve.

**Keep liquid levels high.** "The type of food you eat doesn't really matter that much," says Dr. McFarland. "The most serious thing is to make sure your fluid intake is high." Though many folks don't feel like consuming large amounts of liquids during bouts of diarrhea, all our experts agree that increasing your fluid intake is vital to ward off dehydration.

Fluids that contain salt and small amounts of sugar are particularly beneficial, as they help the body replace glucose and minerals lost during diarrhea. A good "rehydration fluid" can be easily made by adding 1 teaspoon of sugar and a pinch of salt to 1 quart of water.

A more complex but tastier mix can be made by adding ½ teaspoon of honey or corn syrup and a pinch of table salt to 8 ounces of fruit juice. Stir well and drink often.

Or just buy Gatorade. It contains glucose and electrolytes in sufficient quantities to replace those your body is losing.

**Avoid these foods.** While eating may not be as important as drinking for riding out diarrhea, some foods should be avoided. Obvious ones to pass up include beans, cabbage, and Brussels sprouts.

# Traveler's Diarrhea: The Globetrotter's Curse

Montezuma's revenge, Delhi belly, Tiki trots. Whatever you call it, traveler's diarrhea—the official name is turista—can dampen one's spirits on even the best of vacations.

"If you're going to be abroad for any length of time, you'll probably have some episodes of diarrhea," says Stephen Bezruchka, M.D., a frequent traveler. "Conceptually, it is totally preventable. In reality, it's rare you don't get an occasional loose movement." In fact, you have up to a 50 percent chance of getting turista, even if you take the recommended precautions.

The most common cause is the *Escherichia coli* bacteria. This widespread little organism normally resides in your intestines and performs a role in digestion. But foreign versions of *E. coli*—and to a foreigner, the American version is foreign—can give you diarrhea by producing a toxin that prevents your intestines from absorbing the water you ingest in the form of fluid and food.

As the toxin prevents the absorption of water, you have all this extra water in there, and it's got to come out, Dr. Bezruchka says. "The toxin doesn't get absorbed. You don't usually feel sick, but you might feel you have to pass some gas. Only it isn't gas at all."

Shigella and salmonella bacteria can also produce turista, while a smaller number of cases are caused by rotavirus and the giardia parasite. Changes in diet, fatigue, jet lag, and altitude sickness have been blamed but without sufficient proof, and up to 50 percent of all turista cases are unexplained.

Luckily, there are ways to help your body fight turista. Here's what doctors suggest.

**Drink water, water anywhere.** When you have turista, your stools are mostly water. So why would the most important treatment be to drink plenty of the right fluids? Because dehydration, the loss of water and electrolytes, can kill.

"A lot of what you take in will be pumped right back out the other end," concedes Thomas Gossel, Ph.D. "But you'll reach a point where you stabilize and begin retaining it. If you didn't replace any fluids at all, you could become dehydrated in a day."

**Put your bladder to the test.** The yellower your urine, the more fluid you need. It should be clear or pale yellow.

**Use a rehydration solution.** An even better way to rehydrate is to drink an ORS, also known as an

Other foods containing large amounts of poorly absorbed carbohydrates can aggravate diarrhea. A short list includes bread, pasta, and other wheat products; apples, pears, peaches, and prunes; corn, oats, potatoes, and processed bran.

over-the-counter rehydration solution. These drinks contain sugar and salt and help replace important electrolytes that are lost through diarrhea. They also help your intestines absorb water better.

Over-the-counter rehydration solutions are readily available in the United States, so you can buy and take them with you. Brands include ReVital and Pedialyte.

**Choose a backup beverage.** If you didn't manage to pack an ORS, drink clear fruit juices, or weak tea with sugar.

**Get in the pink.** Pepto-Bismol, the well-known over-the-counter stomach medication, can be the traveler's friend. It makes stools bulkier and firmer, and it kills bacteria.

Don't worry if your tongue and diarrhea turn black. It's a natural side effect of Pepto-Bismol.

**Do a little coaxing.** Natural fiber-based laxatives for relieving constipation, such as Metamucil and Citrucel, also help with diarrhea. Some can absorb up to 60 times their weight in water to form a gel in the intestine. "You're still going to expel excess water," Dr. Gossel says, "but it won't be so runny." Other brands are Equalactin, FiberCon, and Konsyl.

Of course, it's best to not have to worry about traveler's diarrhea in the first place. Here's how to protect yourself.

- Avoid uncooked vegetables, especially salads, fruits you can't peel, undercooked meat, raw shellfish, ice cubes, and drinks made from impure water (the alcohol in drinks won't kill the turista bug).

- Ask if the dishes and silverware you use have been cleaned in purified water.

- Drink only water that's been carbonated and sealed in bottles or cans. Clean the part of the container that touches your mouth and purified water. Boiling water for 3 to 5 minutes purifies it, as does adding iodine liquid or tablets.

- Drink acidic drinks like colas and orange juice when possible. They help keep down the E. coli count, the bacteria most responsible for digestive distress.

- Drink acidophilus milk or eat yogurt before your trip. The bacterial colonies established in your digestive system before your trip and maintained during it reduce the chance of a turista invasion.

And, just in case you were reaching for that carton of ice cream, all our experts say that you should avoid dairy products (with the exception of yogurt) during a bout of diarrhea. Even if milk products didn't trigger diarrhea, they tend to aggravate diarrhea after you have it.

**Avoid soft drinks.** "I'd suggest avoiding carbonated beverages as well," says Dr. Clearfield. "The gas they contain may add additional explosiveness to a delicate situation."

**Stay out of the kitchen.** While we're still on the subject of food, you or any member of your family with diarrhea should not prepare food for other members of the household until the diarrhea subsides. Also, good hand-washing helps keep a parasitic infection from spreading. (If your job involves contact with large numbers of people or food handling, state law may require that you stay off the job until all symptoms subside.)

**If you must, take something to stem the tide.** Our experts insist that letting diarrhea "run its course" is the best medicine going. If, however, you absolutely must go someplace and be in control while you're there, an over-the-counter product called Imodium, available in capsule or liquid form, is probably your best bet for slowing the flow.

"Imodium is very effective," says Dr. Clearfield. "It works by causing the bowel to tighten up, and by doing so, prevents things from moving along."

Imodium isn't your only choice. Hydrophilic (*hydro* means water, and *phili* means love) products, such as Kaopectate and Pepto-Bismol, may also help treat mild diarrhea.

**Skip these food remedies.** Such things as pectin, acidophilus tablets, carob powder, barley, bananas, Swiss cheese, and a host of exotic foods, teas, and other folk remedies have been used by some as a treatment for diarrhea. "They work to bind the bowel and slow the course of the diarrhea," says Dr. McFarland. But in his opinion, that's not necessarily what you want to do. "You're just increasing the time that whatever is causing the problem will stay inside you. What you want to do is get it out."

## PANEL OF ADVISORS

**Stephen Bezruchka, M.D.,** is an emergency physician at Virginia Mason Hospital and Group Health Hospital in Seattle and an affiliate associate professor in the School of Public Health and Community Medicine at the University of Washington in Seattle.

**William Y. Chey, M.D.,** is director of the Rochester Institute for Digestive Diseases and Sciences and a physician in Rochester. He is a former professor of medicine at the University of Rochester School of Medicine and Dentistry in New York.

**Harris Clearfield, M.D.,** is a professor of medicine and section chief of the division of gastroenterology at Hahnemann University Hospital in Philadelphia.

**Thomas Gossel, Ph.D., R.Ph.,** is a professor of pharmacology and toxicology at Ohio Northern University in Ada. He is an expert on over-the-counter products.

**David A. Lieberman, M.D.,** is a gastroenterologist and associate professor of medicine at Oregon Health Sciences University School of Medicine in Portland.
**Lynn V. McFarland, Ph.D.,** is a former research associate with the department of medicinal chemistry at the University of Washington in Seattle and director of scientific affairs of Biocodex, Inc.

# DIVERTICULOSIS
## 23 Self-Care Techniques

Once upon a time–say, before 1900–diverticulosis was just another of the many "rare" medical conditions that doctors had heard about but seldom had seen. Even today, diverticulosis is rare in Third World countries.

But not in the United States, land of the Big Mac. Studies indicate that more than half of all Americans over the age of 60 have diverticulosis–characterized by tiny, grapelike pouches or sacs (diverticula) along the outer wall of the colon. Almost everyone over age 80 has the condition.

These pouches show up on x-rays, but many people never have this area x-rayed and don't even know that they have the condition, says Samuel Klein, M.D.

## WHEN TO CALL A DOCTOR

If you live long enough, chances are you will get diverticulosis. Even so, odds are you won't get *diverticulitis*—a painful inflammation that is potentially serious. Still, you should be aware of the warning signs.

Fever and severe pain in the lower left portion of the abdominal region are good indicators that diverticulosis has advanced to diverticulitis, says Marvin Schuster, M.D.

This change shouldn't be taken lightly.

"You can have rupturing or bleeding," says Albert J. Lauro, M.D. And while it doesn't happen often, people can die from diverticulitis.

So act on those warning signs and get to a doctor fast. And stay calm— the odds are still in your favor. "If it's just an infection," Dr. Lauro says, "it usually can be handled with rest, diet, and antibiotics. You'll be okay."

Of those who do have diverticulosis, Dr. Klein says, only about 10 percent will ever progress to diverticulitis—a painful inflammation that can become serious. So having diverticulosis does not mean that you're destined for severe pain or a hospital stay.

Fortunately, you can take an active role in treating and preventing diverticulosis, thus avoiding the pain of diverticulitis. Here's what our experts suggest.

**Bulk up on fiber.** "Diverticulosis is a problem that is acquired," says surgeon Paul Williamson, M.D. "It's come about with the advance of processed foods—foods that are low in fiber."

The average American gets about 16 grams of fiber daily, or only half of what we should be getting, says Marvin Schuster, M.D.

Fiber helps reduce tension on the colon and helps it expand when eliminating waste. Fiber also draws water into the stool, making bowel movements smoother. Whole wheat bread and all-bran cereals are excellent sources of bran fiber, which appears to be the most effective type of fiber in preventing diverticulosis. Sprinkling raw bran over foods is also an option.

Vegetables and fruits are other good sources of fiber, adds Dr. Klein. Fruit and vegetable juices contain hardly any fiber, however, so reach for an apple instead of its juice.

**Eat highly processed foods in moderation.** This is good general-health advice, but it also applies to treating diverticulosis. If you eat a lot of low-fiber processed foods, says Dr. Klein, you won't have room to eat the high-fiber foods you need.

**Don't say "so long" to seeds.** Until recently, many doctors told their patients to avoid tomatoes, strawberries, and other foods with small seeds. They believed that the seeds could lodge in the diverticula and trigger inflammation. Today, this is a controversial point among doctors. The National Institutes of Health says that there's no evidence to support the ban on seeds and that many of these foods are also good sources of fiber. So dig out that fresh tomato from your garden.

## Cures from the Kitchen

Internal medicine specialist Craig Rubin, M.D., generally recommends this homemade remedy for constipation, but it's useful to anyone who wants to add fiber to their diet: Mix $\frac{1}{2}$ cup of unprocessed bran and $\frac{1}{2}$ cup of applesauce with $\frac{1}{3}$ cup of prune juice. Refrigerate. Take 2 to 3 tablespoons of the mixture after dinner, then drink a full glass of water. If you need to, you can increase your dose to 3 to 4 tablespoons.

"Whole prunes, prune juice, and herbal teas are very effective natural laxatives," Dr. Schuster adds. Specially formulated teas can be found in most health food stores.

## Strive for 35

You know that getting enough fiber in your diet (30 to 35 grams daily) is the most important thing you can do to treat and prevent diverticulosis. But what you may not know is how much fiber is in the recommended high-fiber foods or how to inject more fiber into your diet without sitting down to a bowl of raw bran.

Here are some tips for making the transition to a high-fiber diet.

- Make a habit of eating whole grain bread instead of white bread.

- Answer your sweet tooth with fruit desserts—berries, bananas, peaches.

- Eat more vegetarian meals.

- Leave the skins on apples, peaches, and pears when you bake them.

- Add dried fruits, such as raisins and apricots, to your meals.

- Substitute beans for beef in chili or casseroles.

- Add barley to vegetable soups.

**Increase your fiber intake slowly.** Take 6 to 8 weeks to gradually increase your fiber intake up to the recommended 30 to 35 grams each day, Dr. Klein suggests. "You need time for your digestive system to adapt."

You can expect bloating and gas in the first few weeks, Dr. Schuster says. But most people will get over this.

**If you can't get enough fiber in your diet, take a supplement.** The best are psyllium seed supplements (such as Metamucil), says Dr. Schuster. "They're natural, too."

**Don't use suppositories.** While they may offer a quick fix to constipation, suppositories aren't the best choice for stimulating bowel movements.

"Your system can get addicted to them," Dr. Klein explains. "And then it becomes a vicious circle—you need more suppositories."

**Drink lots of liquids.** "Drink six to eight glasses of water a day," advises Dr. Klein, adding that the liquid is an important partner to fiber in combating constipation, which is associated with diverticulosis.

"If you have to strain a great deal when having a bowel movement," says Dr. Schuster, "you tend to expand those little diverticula through the muscle walls of the colon."

**Go when you have to go.** If you don't yield to nature's call, you defeat the purpose of adding more fiber to your diet and drinking more liquids. "Don't suppress the need to move your bowel," Dr. Williamson advises.

**Exercise.** It tones more than your legs and hips. Exercise also tones the muscles in your colon. "It helps bowel movements; you don't have to strain as much," says Dr. Klein.

**Soothe your pain with heat.** To relieve tenderness or cramping, hold a heating pad against the left side of your abdomen.

**Don't smoke.** Harmful in so many ways, smoking may also aggravate diverticulosis, says Albert J. Lauro, M.D.

**Drink in moderation.** "Alcohol in moderation—a drink or two a day—will actually relax spasm of the colon and could improve the situation a little bit," says Dr. Schuster.

**Avoid caffeine.** "Coffee, chocolate, teas, colas—all tend to irritate," Dr. Williamson says.

**Look for a pattern.** Certain foods may disrupt your bowel habits or cause loose stools, Dr. Williamson says. Try to identify those foods and avoid them.

**Take it easy with ibuprofen and acetaminophen.** Avoid high doses of ibuprofen, a common painkiller in the family of drugs known as nonsteroidal anti-inflammatory drugs (NSAIDs). Regular and consistent use of acetaminophen is also associated with increased symptoms of diverticular disease. One study of more than 35,000 men found that those who took NSAIDs or acetaminophen more than two times a week were twice as likely to develop diverticular disease than men who didn't take the drugs regularly. NSAIDs inhibit prostaglandins, fatty acids that protect the cells in the intestinal tract.

## PANEL OF ADVISORS

**Samuel Klein, M.D.,** is a William H. Danforth professor of medicine and nutritional science and director of the Center for Human Nutrition at Washington University School of Medicine in St. Louis.

**Albert J. Lauro, M.D.,** is director of emergency medical services at Charity Hospital in New Orleans.

**Craig Rubin, M.D.,** is a professor of internal medicine and chief of the geriatric section at the University of Texas Southwestern Medical Center at Dallas.

**Marvin Schuster, M.D.,** is director emeritus of the Marvin M. Schuster Center for Digestive and Motility Disorders at the Hopkins Bayview Medical Center, and professor emeritus of medicine and psychiatry at Johns Hopkins University School of Medicine, both in Baltimore.

**Paul Williamson, M.D.,** is an associate clinical professor of surgery at the University of Florida in Gainesville and a colon and rectal surgeon in Orlando.

# DIZZINESS
## 17 Tips to Stop the Spinning

Few sensations are more uncomfortable, and potentially dangerous, than dizziness. More than 2 million people visit a doctor for dizziness each year. Older people usually experience dizziness or balance disorders more frequently, but these problems can affect people of all ages.

The sensation that the world is spinning is a type of dizziness called vertigo. Inner-ear problems such as injury, viral infections, inflammation, debris in the inner ear, and bleeding can all cause vertigo, says Terry D. Fife, M.D.

But not all dizziness is due to inner-ear problems, Dr. Fife adds. Dizziness may also result from poor circulation, side effects from medications, and a condition called orthostatic hypotension, in which blood pressure temporarily drops when you're in the upright position or after you suddenly get up.

Dizziness often disappears on its own, but it can have long-term conse-

## WHEN TO CALL A DOCTOR

Everyone gets dizzy from time to time—when getting out of bed, for example, or standing up after working in the garden—and it isn't always a problem.

"If it is mild, occurs rarely, and was clearly provoked by a particular activity, it is probably harmless," says Terry D. Fife, M.D. Dizziness that occurs often, however, or is accompanied by other symptoms is potentially serious.

Dizziness that's followed by fainting, for example, could be a warning sign of heart disease. A stroke can also cause vertigo or dizziness, especially if you're also experiencing slurred speech, blurred or double vision, or numbness or tingling in the arms or legs.

If vertigo comes on completely out of the blue or is accompanied by any of these other symptoms, you need to see a doctor right away, Dr. Fife advises.

# Do just 1 thing

Know dizziness triggers. Dizziness and vertigo that occurs at predictable times—first thing in the morning when getting out of bed, for example, or when you suddenly change position—may indicate an easy-to-treat inner-ear disorder.

A sudden drop in blood pressure can trigger dizziness, and this can be caused by a variety of things, including sudden temperature changes, such as when you go from a hot car into an air-conditioned building. "Hunger is another trigger for some people, and having just eaten is a trigger for others. Hunger-related dizziness may be related to low blood sugar, while dizziness after a meal can be attributed to digestive processes that 'steal' blood from the brain," says Terry D. Fife, M.D.

If you've recently had a cold, don't be surprised if you start experiencing dizziness, he adds. Cold viruses sometimes travel to the inner ear and cause a condition called vestibular neuritis, which causes inflammation and injury to the inner-ear balance mechanism, resulting in vertigo. "It usually clears up within a few months," says Dr. Fife.

quences, especially when it leads to a loss of balance and falls. "People can become so frightened of falling that they stop being physically active," says Dr. Fife.

To get dizziness under control, here's what experts advise.

**Stop moving immediately.** If you feel an attack coming on, stay absolutely still for a few minutes. Don't move your head at all. Holding still allows your blood pressure to stabilize and helps the inner ear regain its normal equilibrium.

**Then sit down.** Dizziness and vertigo usually occur when you change position or stand. Sitting down right away often causes the symptoms to subside—and it's a lot safer than trying to stay on your feet when the world is spinning.

**Reach out and touch something.** When you feel an attack of dizziness or "spinning" coming on, lightly rest your fingers on objects around you—a bookcase, for example, or a table or the back of a chair.

Spinning sensations occur when the brain receives conflicting messages, Dr. Fife explains. Your eyes may be convinced that you're whirling, while your feet know very well that you're standing still. This conflict in sensations makes the vertigo worse. "If you make contact with enough objects, your sensory nerves start to adjust," he says.

**Flex your legs.** If you have orthostatic hypotension, the blood tends to pool in the legs and feet. This causes a reduction in brain bloodflow, which can result in dizziness. "Flexing your leg muscles before you stand up—by crossing and uncrossing your legs, for example—helps push blood back into circulation," says Joshua Hoffman, M.D.

**Get up in stages.** Don't leap out of bed in the morning. Instead, swing your legs over the side of the bed and rise to a sitting position. Wait for a minute or two, then slowly stand up. This gives your blood pressure time to adjust, which may prevent dizziness, says Dr. Hoffman.

**Keep moving.** It's normal for people who experience frequent dizziness to become increasingly afraid of falling. As a result, they become more and more sedentary. This reduces the ability of the brain to monitor and fine-tune the sense of balance—which will make falls even *more* likely.

It's important to stay physically active to maintain muscle strength as well as balance, says Dr. Hoffman. Take your usual walks. Go shopping. Jog or ride an exercise bike. As long as you move carefully at "high-risk" times—using handrails when walking down stairs, for example, or moving slowly after changing position—you're unlikely to lose your balance.

If you've already lost confidence in your balance, doctors advise consulting a balance specialist.

**Wear flat shoes.** Apart from the fact that walking on heels is hazardous when the world seems to be spinning, flat shoes provide more contact with the ground. More contact makes it easier for your brain to process information about your posture. This prevents some inner-ear "confusion" and can help prevent falls, says Dr. Fife.

**Use a night-light.** Darkness can be especially treacherous for those with inner-ear problems because the brain, which normally compensates for the lack of information from the ears by drawing on more information from the eyes, does not receive enough visual clues to help the body stay properly oriented. Simply using a night-light could help prevent dizziness or falls, says Dr. Fife.

"If you have significant inner-ear problems, never swim in the dark," Dr. Fife adds. "When underwater, some people have found themselves unable to tell what's up and what's down. We have had a few patients that nearly drowned because they could not perceive which way to come up for air and kept groping at the bottom of the swimming pool, convinced that the bottom was the direction to go to come up for air."

**Be careful walking on heavily padded carpeting.** Carpets with deep, soft padding may feel good on your feet, but the cushioning can make it harder for your body to stay properly oriented, says Dr. Fife. This is because the soft surface makes it harder for the nerves in the feet to detect changes in joint position used to maintain balance.

**Be cautious in bathrooms.** The bathroom is a high-risk area because the combination of slick surfaces and off-balance movements—bending over to brush your teeth, for example—make falls more likely. In addition, bathing or showering causes blood vessels to dilate and triggers a drop in blood pressure. If you move too quickly, your brain may not get enough oxygen, making you feel light-headed and dizzy, says Dr. Hoffman. So install grab bars in the bath, shower, and beside the toilet. Available in hardware stores, the bars give you something to hold on to should dizziness strike when you're standing or stepping out of the bath.

**Drink plenty of water.** The sense of thirst declines over time, which means older adults tend to run a little on the dry side. Even mild dehydration can cause drops in blood pressure that result in occasional dizziness, says Dr. Fife.

Try to drink 8 to 10 glasses (8 ounces each) of water daily. "Water is good, but when someone is dehydrated, sports drinks are even better," says Dr. Fife. They contain sodium and other electrolytes that help the body retain fluids.

**Consider motion-sickness medication.** If you experience dizziness associated with motion (carsickness, airsickness, seasickness), your doctor may recommend an over-the-counter medication called Dramamine or Bonine. These medications help reduce chemical signals from the inner ear to the brain's "vomiting center."

**Reduce your salt intake.** Vertigo is sometimes caused by a condition called Ménière's disease, which occurs when fluid accumulates in the inner ear. If you have been diagnosed with this condition, following a low-salt diet can help reduce fluid buildups that result in attacks of vertigo. Doctors usually advise no more than 2,000 milligrams of sodium daily.

When buying packaged foods, check the labels to see how much sodium they contain. Your best bet is to buy products that are labeled "low sodium" or "sodium-free." It's fine to add a little bit of salt to foods at the table, but don't use it during cooking. Some people find that adding salt to food during cooking imparts less flavor than when it is added at the table.

**Reduce stress.** Doctors aren't sure why, but emotional stress tends to

*Cures from the Kitchen*

Dizziness is often accompanied by nausea. Ginger, a traditional remedy for stomach upset, has been shown to ease this nausea, says Terry D. Fife, M.D. Fresh ginger, eaten by the slice or grated and used to make a tea, can be effective. Or try over-the-counter supplements, following the directions on the label.

make inner-ear disorders worse. If you're experiencing vertigo or dizziness more than you used to and your doctor has ruled out some of the physical causes, it may be a sign that you need to unwind. Set aside time to take some long walks. Practice deep breathing for a few minutes every day. Or simply permit yourself to relax and do nothing now and then.

**Make a list of medicines.** Then check it twice—first with your doctor, then with your pharmacist. Many prescription and over-the-counter drugs, including aspirin, antidepressants, and drugs for treating high blood pressure, cause dizziness. In some cases, switching drugs may be all that's needed to reduce or eliminate dizziness.

## PANEL OF ADVISORS

**Terry D. Fife, M.D.,** is an associate professor of clinical neurology at the University of Arizona in Tucson and director of the Balance Center at Barrow Neurological Institute in Phoenix.

**Joshua Hoffman, M.D.,** is an internist and medical director of Sutter Medical Group hospitalist program in Sacramento, California.

# DRY EYES
## 17 Moistening Ideas

Dry eye occurs when the eye doesn't produce enough tears to keep it moist and comfortable. This condition affects millions of Americans and is more common in women, especially after menopause, according to the National Eye Institute. As we age, the eyes usually produce fewer tears.

"Eye dryness is a common problem," says Anne Sumers, M.D. Half of all people over age 40 experience eye dryness in some form, whether it's an intermittent or a persistent problem. Dry eyes are a part of aging, she says. "It's rotten, unfortunate, but true."

Blinking your eye creates a three-layered film of water, oil, and mucus. Around age 40, the tear glands begin to slow down, producing less of this soothing eye liquid. The problem is even worse for women after menopause because hormonal shifts dry up secretions, including tears, says Dr. Sumers.

Dry eye is a simple name for a complex and irritating condition that is char-

# Do just 1 thing

Try artificial tears. Available over-the-counter, artificial tears help soothe tender, gritty eyes, says Anne Sumers, M.D. A mixture of saline and a film-forming substance such as polyvinyl alcohol or synthetic cellulose, artificial tears can be used throughout the day. They come in different thicknesses, so experiment to find the brand that's right for you, she says.

The thinner brands are less likely to blur your vision or leave a residue on your eyelashes, but they require more frequent application.

Choose a preservative-free brand, because some preservatives can be toxic and damage the surface of the eye, Dr. Sumers says.

Two good choices, according to Stephen C. Pflugfelder, M.D., are GenTeal and Refresh Tears.

Whichever type you choose, here's how to insert the eyedrops. Gently pull down the lower lid and squeeze the drops into the corner of your eye near your nose. Keep the eye closed for a minute to make sure the drops stay in the eye.

Use them anywhere from 1 to 10 times per day, depending on how severe your dryness problem is, says Dr. Sumers.

acterized by redness, burning, itching, scratchiness, tearing, and sensitivity to light. Although usually just another hazard of aging, dry eyes may also be caused by exposure to environmental conditions, injuries to the eye, or general health problems. Sun, wind, cold, indoor heating and air conditioning, staring at computer screens, and even high altitudes can cause further discomfort if you experience eye dryness.

In addition to postmenopausal women, those who are more prone to dry eye include contact lens wearers, people who have undergone LASIK surgery, and those with arthritis and diabetes. A wide variety of medications, including decongestants, antihistamines, diuretics, anesthetics, antidepressants, drugs for heart disease, ulcer remedies, chemotherapies, and drugs containing beta-blockers, can slow down your tear production and cause a case of dry eye, says Stephen C. Pflugfelder, M.D.

The good news? Whether your eyes are only slightly parched or as dry as your father's wit, it is possible to get those tears flowing again. Here's how.

**Apply a warm compress.** If your eyes become dry every now and then, place a warm compress on your eyelids for 5 to 10 minutes at a time, two or three times each day, suggests Dr. Pflugfelder. The warm compress can stimulate tear flow.

**Opt for ointment.** To combat cases in which eye dryness gets unbearable while you sleep, apply a tear-replacement/moisture-sealing ointment at

## WHEN TO CALL A DOCTOR

See your doctor if you've used artificial tears for a few days and made other changes in your environment but still don't notice any improvement in the dryness of your eyes, says Phillip J. Calenda, M.D.

Your doctor can insert a tiny collagen plug into your tear drainage canal, says Anne Sumers, M.D. The plug helps conserve the tears that you produce and also keeps any artificial tears in your eyes longer.

bedtime to help ease your pain, says Dr. Sumers. These extra-thick, over-the-counter eye ointments contain white petroleum jelly and mineral oil, and they last longer than drops.

To apply the ointment, pull the lower eyelid down, look up and squeeze a dab of ointment in the trough between your lid and eye. Blink to spread the ointment around. These thick ointments can blur your vision for a while, so they're best applied when you're already in bed, Dr. Sumers cautions.

**Pop out those contacts.** If your eyes are feeling dry and irritated, the last thing you need is something sitting in them, like contact lenses. A contact lens is basically a sponge, and it soaks up natural and artificial tears. When there are fewer tears in the eye, contacts can make the eyes even drier, more irritated, light sensitive, and red.

So, pop out those contact lenses, put on your glasses for the rest of the day, and apply artificial tears as frequently as needed, suggests Dr. Pflugfelder. You should notice quite an improvement.

**Wear wraparound shades.** Because wind and sun can further dry out your eyes, wear sunglasses for extra protection, preferably wraparound shades, which extend past the side of your eyes, suggests Dr. Sumers.

**Stay out of the direct line of fire.** A blast of heat or air conditioning may be just what the rest of your body needs to make the morning commute more bearable, but a direct flow of hot or cold air to your eyes can make them even more irritated. If you have dry eyes, point your car's air vents downward, says Dr. Sumers. That way, you'll get the relief you need from the outdoor elements without causing your dry eyes any more misery.

According to Dr. Sumers, the same principle applies in your home or when traveling on an airplane. In your home, point heating and cooling ducts away from areas where you spend a great deal of time. This is particularly important if you have forced-air heating in your home, which causes your eyes to dry out more quickly.

When traveling by plane, be sure that the overhead air vents aren't pointed directly at your eyes. "Airplanes are notoriously dry environments, so don't make matters worse on your eyes by having cool air blowing directly on your face," she says.

**Get fresh.** Open a window and let in some fresh air, suggests Dr. Sumers. This will allow some much-needed moisture into the room, which could do your dry eyes a world of good, says Dr. Sumers.

**Commune with nature.** Buy a houseplant or two and put them in rooms where you spend lots of time. They can increase the amount of humidity in a room, says Dr. Sumers.

**Avoid a common mistake.** Too many people notice that their eyes are getting dry and itchy and immediately head to their medicine cabinet for an antihistamine. That makes already dry eyes even drier, says Dr. Sumers.

**Blink a lot.** If part of your job description includes spending long hours in front of a computer screen, take occasional blink breaks, says Phillip J. Calenda, M.D. By constantly staring at the task at hand, you don't blink as much as you should, which causes eye moisture to evaporate more quickly. Taking a blink break will help restore the much-needed tear film over your eyes. Spending 5 minutes each hour looking off in the distance instead of reading or doing other close work will allow the eyes to blink more.

**Keep a level head.** Dr. Pflugfelder has another practical suggestion for people with dry eyes who spend a majority of their workday in front of a computer screen. "Position your computer so that it's directly at eye level or so that you're looking slightly down at the computer screen," he says. "If you're looking up at your computer screen, your eyes will be more wide open and will dry out more quickly."

The American Academy of Ophthalmology recommends the following changes in your workstation to minimize eye dryness and eyestrain while sitting in front of a computer all day.

- Screen distance: Sit about 20 inches from the computer monitor, a little farther away than reading distance, with the top of the screen at or below eye level.
- Equipment: Choose a monitor that tilts or swivels and has both contrast and brightness controls.
- Furniture: Make sure you have an adjustable chair.
- Reference material: Place papers on a document holder so that you don't have to keep looking back and forth, frequently refocusing your eyes and turning your neck.

- Lighting: Modify your lighting to eliminate reflections or glare. A micromesh filter for your screen may also help limit reflections and glare.
- Rest breaks: Take periodic rest breaks and blink often to keep your eyes from drying out.

## PANEL OF ADVISORS

**Phillip J. Calenda, M.D.,** is an ophthalmologist in Scarsdale, New York.
**Stephen C. Pflugfelder, M.D.,** is an ophthalmologist in Houston and a spokesman for the American Academy of Ophthalmology.
**Anne Sumers, M.D.,** is team ophthalmologist for the New York Giants and the New Jersey Nets in addition to operating an ophthalmology practice in Ridgewood, New Jersey. She serves as spokesperson for the American Academy of Ophthalmology.

# DRY MOUTH
## 17 Mouthwatering Solutions

For some people, the sensation of having a mouth as dry as the Sahara Desert is simply an infrequent nuisance. For others, it's quite a serious problem, says John J. Caimi, D.M.D.

Mouth dryness, officially known as xerostomia, can be really debilitating, he says. If left untreated, it can lead to painful mouth sores, rampant tooth decay, and other oral health problems. Your mouth needs adequate saliva flow in order to coat and lubricate oral tissues, which in turn helps prevent tooth decay and gum disease.

According to Dr. Caimi, dry mouth affects a wide variety of people, including older adults whose mouths naturally dry out over time, as well as people who have diabetes, depression, or an autoimmune disease known as Sjögren's syndrome. For cancer patients, dry mouth is often the result of chemotherapy or radiation therapy, and a consultation with both the oncologist and the dentist is advised.

Most often though, mouth dryness is a side effect of prescription drugs, says Dr. Caimi. Hundreds of prescription and over-the-counter medications cause mouth dryness, including 6 of the 20 most prescribed medications—fluoxetine (Prozac), amlodipine (Norvasc), sertraline (Zoloft), paroxetine (Paxil), lisinopril (Zestril), and enalapril (Vasotec).

## WHEN TO CALL A DOCTOR

Regular biyearly dental checkups are an important first line of defense against dry mouth syndrome, because your dentist will be better able to diagnose any problems in an earlier stage, when they can be easily corrected. Plus, your dentist may be able to recommend something like a fluoride mouth rinse or a fluoride gel as an extra safeguard for your teeth, says John J. Caimi, D.M.D.

If you notice a red, dry irritation in your mouth or a lack of saliva, see either a doctor or dentist, says Dr. Caimi. The sooner you get help, the better, because it's easier to correct the problem in an early stage.

If you think that your medication is causing dry mouth, tell your doctor immediately, says Dr. Caimi. In some cases, a different prescription or a simple adjustment in dosage may provide relief from mouth dryness and the oral difficulties that can come with it.

As the population ages and prescription drugs become more common, dry mouth is becoming more prevalent. Here are some suggestions to help relieve the dryness, preserve soft tissue, and help prevent the tooth decay that results from dry mouth.

**Chew sugarless gum.** Chewing stimulates the salivary glands. Try sugarless gum that contains xylitol, a sweetening agent that reduces cavity-causing bacteria, says Dan Peterson, D.D.S. He also recommends Trident Advantage gum, which contains Recaldent, a remineralizing agent that adds calcium and phosphate to the teeth.

**Sip away.** Take frequent sips of water throughout the day. Swirl it around in your mouth and through your teeth to battle the dry feeling, says Dr. Caimi.

Drink eight 8-ounce glasses of water each day, says dental hygienist Anne Bosy. The more active you are, the more water you need. If you're working out in the gym, take a water bottle along with you. Have an all-day meeting with a key client? Make sure to have pitchers of water at the table.

**Suck on some ice.** Ice chips are another source of water, suggests Dr. Caimi. But suck on the ice, don't chew it. Chomping on ice can damage your teeth.

**Rinse away the pain.** Chronic dryness will make your mouth more easily irritated and sore, because one of the primary chores of saliva is to neutralize the erosive acids from plaque, according to Dr. Caimi. Rinse your mouth with a mixture of ¼ teaspoon of baking soda, ⅛ teaspoon of salt, and 1 cup of warm water for some oral comfort. The soothing combination neutralizes acids and draws out infection from gum tissues.

**Give hard candy a try.** Suck a piece of sugarless hard candy to stimulate saliva flow, says Dr. Peterson, who recommends citrus- or mint-flavored candies. They can stimulate more saliva flow.

**Munch on some veggies.** Diets high in fiber and bulk also seem to stimulate salivary glands. Bosy suggests eating fibrous foods, such as raw carrots, celery, or apples at mealtimes and as snacks. These rough-textured foods also clean your tongue as you chew and swallow, which is good for overall oral hygiene.

**Say no to sweets.** Limit your intake of sweet, sticky, sugary foods if you're experiencing dry mouth. Your lack of saliva will keep these foods stuck to your teeth, increasing your risk of cavities, says Dr. Peterson.

**Avoid irritants.** Spicy or salty foods may cause pain in a dry mouth, says Dr. Caimi. Orange juice can be a common culprit because of its high acidic content. As an alternative, look for low-acid orange juice products, which have become more widely available.

**Choose your toothpaste wisely.** When saliva production is low, your risk of cavities and gum disease is high. Dr. Peterson recommends brushing at least twice a day with an extra-strength fluoride toothpaste approved by the American Dental Association.

If you have mouth dryness, do not use toothpaste that contains the foaming agent sodium lauryl sulfate, because it can irritate gum tissue, says Dr. Peterson. He recommends trying Rembrandt's Natural or Biotene's Dry Mouth Toothpaste.

Here's a fluoride-treatment program that Dr. Peterson recommends for extra tooth protection. After brushing your teeth and right before you go to bed, apply toothpaste with your toothbrush or a cotton swab to

## Cures from the Kitchen

Use sauces and gravies on foods to add more moisture to the foods you eat, suggests Dan Peterson, D.D.S. A dry mouth can make foods with little moisture taste like pencil shavings. A little moisture makes foods much more palatable. Drinking fluids frequently throughout the meal will increase the moisture content of your mouth, make food easier to swallow, and improve taste sensation.

gums and teeth. Let it sit for 1 minute, then swish for 1 minute to force the paste to cover all your teeth and gums. Then spit out all the excess paste, but don't rinse your mouth. Go to bed with the fluoride residue on these surfaces. Do this again in the morning, and don't eat or drink anything for 30 minutes after this routine. This procedure should be done one or two times a day for 4 to 6 weeks.

**Use mouthwash.** Use an antibacterial mouthwash like Periostat or Peridex, which doesn't contain alcohol or sugar, suggests Dr. Caimi. Alcohol further dries your mouth and can irritate the already sensitive gum tissues. And as most everyone knows, sugar can cause tooth decay and cavities, which will occur even more quickly if you have mouth dryness.

**Change your toothbrush frequently.** When your toothbrush has a buildup of toothpaste in between the bristles, it's time to make the investment in a new one, says Bosy. Over time, toothbrushes can harbor bacteria and infect your mouth with the bacteria that cause bad breath. Therefore, spending a few bucks for a new toothbrush every couple of months is a sound investment to keep bacteria and bad breath at bay.

**Brush diligently.** One of the primary tasks of saliva is to dislodge trapped food morsels in your mouth explains Bosy. So if you're lacking the normal amount of saliva, food particles can hang around longer in your mouth and cause bad breath. The solution? Brush your teeth after every meal, morsel, or midnight snack.

**Soak your dentures.** Dentures make people with dry mouth more susceptible to infection from yeast organisms, which adhere to the plastic. Soak your dentures overnight in 1 part chlorine beach to 10 parts water to prevent infection, says Dr. Peterson. Rinse thoroughly in the morning before putting them in.

**Moisturize the air.** Use a cool-air vaporizer in your bedroom to get some much-needed humidity in the air and to cut down on mouth dryness at night, says Dr. Peterson. If you're a mouth breather, make an effort to breathe through your nose at night to prevent saliva from evaporating while you sleep.

**Moisten up with a multivitamin.** A number of vitamin deficiencies, particularly riboflavin and vitamin A, can rob your mouth of moisture as well. Pernicious anemia from a vitamin $B_{12}$ deficiency can also cause mouth dryness. If that's the case, try a daily multivitamin/mineral supplement to battle the dryness, says Dr. Peterson.

**If all else fails, fake it.** For better overall comfort and lubrication of your mouth, Bosy suggests over-the-counter saliva substitutes in the form of rinses, gels, and sprays for people who have chronically dry mouth or little or no salivary action. These saliva substitutes include many of the same enzymes and minerals as real saliva and help keep mouth tissues lubricated. Use two or three times a day (one of those times being just before bedtime).

## PANEL OF ADVISORS

**Anne Bosy** is a dental hygienist and cofounder and clinical director at the Fresh Breath Clinic in Toronto. She is also a professor in the faculty of community services and health sciences at the George Brown College of Applied Arts and Technology in Toronto and a member of the International Society of Breath Odor Research. She has treated several thousand patients with dry mouth associated with bad breath.

**John J. Caimi, D.M.D.,** is a dentist from Ridgway, Pennsylvania. He has been in practice for more than 23 years.

**Dan Peterson, D.D.S.,** is a dentist from Gering, Nebraska. He has been in practice for more than 25 years and has treated hundreds of patients with dry mouth syndrome.

# DRY SKIN AND WINTER ITCH
## 10 Cold-Weather Options

Too often, the winter months are synonymous with dry, itchy skin. But it doesn't have to be. Even if you live in a cold, dry climate—or stay warm in a home with drying, forced-air heat—you can retain healthy skin that is soft and slightly moist. Because the dryness results from a lack of *water*, not oil, all you need to do is replenish that moisture.

Here's how.

**Don't try to drink dryness away.** Many beauty books and glamour magazines recommend drinking "at least seven or eight glasses of water per day" to keep your skin hydrated and prevent dryness. And while adequate water is essential for good health, don't believe the hype that you'll see results in your skin.

"If you're totally dehydrated, your skin will become dry," says Kenneth

Neldner, M.D. "But if you are normally hydrated, you cannot possibly counteract or correct dry skin by drinking water."

**Put water where it counts.** "The best way to get water into the skin is by soaking in it," says Hillard H. Pearlstein, M.D. He recommends a 15-minute soak in *lukewarm*, not hot, water. Forget the notion that you should bathe every day. The rule of thumb for dry skin is: Bathe less and use cooler water.

**Lubricate the skin.** "Follow each bath with a moisturizer," says Dr. Pearlstein. "The tendency is for all the moisture that soaked into the skin to evaporate. If you bathe frequently, a moisturizer is doubly important. The moisturizer is what holds the water in."

While many people think that moisturizer puts oil back into the skin, that's not totally true. Instead, he says, moisturizers applied after the bath help keep water in the skin and therefore prevent drying.

**Dry yourself damp—then stop.** "It's much more effective to apply moisturizer to damp skin immediately after bathing than to put it on totally dry skin," says Dr. Neldner.

That's not to say you have to hop from the tub or shower soaking wet and immediately apply lotion. "But a couple of pats with a towel will make you as dry as you want to be before you apply the lotion," he says. "You're trying to trap a little water in the skin, and that's the fundamental rule of fighting off dryness."

**Don't get greased by ad hype.** "Nothing beats plain petroleum jelly or mineral oil as a moisturizer," says Howard Donsky, M.D. In fact, if you don't mind the greasiness, virtually any vegetable oil (sunflower oil, peanut oil) or hydrogenated oil (Crisco) can be used to combat dry skin and winter itch. They're effective, safe, and pure skin lubricants—and inexpensive as well.

Those products do have one drawback, however. All tend to be greasy. "People like things that smell good, feel good, and don't make them feel like a greased pig," Dr. Pearlstein says. So if you prefer an over-the-counter moisturizer, go for it. Just know that they're all basically alike. "It all depends on how much you want to spend, what you want to smell like, and how you want to feel," he says. "There's no scientific way to prove that any one of the commercially available products is any better for you than another. It's strictly your personal decision."

**Use oatmeal to heal.** Some researchers believe that people first discovered the skin-soothing effects of oatmeal nearly 4,000 years ago. Many folks are still discovering it today. "Oatmeal can work in the bath as a soothing agent," says Dr. Donsky. Just pour 2 cups of colloidal oatmeal (like Aveeno, available at drugstores) into a tub of lukewarm water. The term *colloidal* simply means that the oatmeal has been ground to a fine powder that remains suspended in water.

"You can also use oatmeal as a soap substitute," he says. Tie some colloidal oatmeal in a handkerchief, dunk it in water, squeeze out the excess water, and use as you would a normal washcloth.

**Select superfatted soaps.** "Most soaps have lye in them, and while lye is great for cleaning, it's very irritating to dry skin," says Dr. Pearlstein. He recommends that people with dry skin reach instead for "superfatted" soaps like Basis, Neutrogena, or Dove. Superfatted soaps have extra amounts of fatty substances—cold cream, cocoa butter, coconut oil, or lanolin—added during the manufacturing process.

"A product like Dove, for instance, isn't really a soap at all," Dr. Pearlstein says. "It's more like a cold cream." But such are the trade-offs in the skin game. Though they don't clean as well, the superfatted soaps are less irritating to dry skin, and they do make a difference, he adds.

**Don't soap as often.** "There's nothing therapeutic about soap," says Dr. Pearlstein. "We in America are the great overwashed, overdeodorized society, and we as dermatologists see more problems from the overuse of soap than we ever do from the lack of it." His advice: If it's not dirty, don't wash it.

**Let a humidifier help.** "Part of the problem with dry skin and itching is dry heat in the wintertime," says Dr. Pearlstein. Furnace-heated air can reduce the humidity level inside your house to 10 percent or less, whereas 30 to 40 percent is closer to ideal for keeping moisture in your skin. For that reason, our experts all recommend the use of humidifiers during those dry winter months—but with a caution.

"People think that if they put a humidifier in their place, that'll take care of it," says Dr. Pearlstein. "But humidifiers are like air conditioners—you would really need a huge unit to do the whole house. If you put a smaller unit next to your bed, however, that can help."

If you do use a humidifier in your bedroom, Dr. Neldner adds, close the door to keep moisture in. It might also help to leave the bathroom door open when you take a shower. "Every little bit of humidity helps," he says.

**Keep it cool.** One good way to combat winter itch is as easy as reaching for your thermostat and turning it down. "Keeping your house on the cool side in the winter might help," says Dr. Pearlstein. "That's because cool air has an anesthetic effect—it makes your skin feel good." When you heat your house too much, it makes blood vessels dilate, and when blood vessels dilate, the itch/tingle cycle begins. "But when you cool the skin, either by cool water or cool air, it feels good," he explains.

## PANEL OF ADVISORS

**Howard Donsky, M.D.,** is a clinical instructor of dermatology at the University of Rochester and a dermatologist at the Dermatology and Cosmetic Center of Rochester in New York.

**Kenneth Neldner, M.D.,** is a professor emeritus in the department of dermatology at the Texas Tech University School of Medicine in Lubbock.

**Hillard H. Pearlstein, M.D.,** is an assistant clinical professor of dermatology at the Mount Sinai School of Medicine of New York University in New York City.

# EARACHE AND EAR INFECTION
## 25 Ways to Stop the Pain

Earaches can be very painful, and unfortunately, they most often strike at night. The explanation is a combination of anatomy and pressure.

Eustachian tubes lead from the back of the throat to the middle ear. Clogged tubes are the most common cause of earache for children and adults, explains Dudley J. Weider, M.D.

During the day, you hold your head up, and your eustachian tubes drain naturally into the back of your throat. Also, as you chew and swallow, the muscles of the eustachian tubes contract, opening them and allowing air into the middle ear.

But at night when you sleep and your head isn't upright, the tubes can't drain as easily. And you're not swallowing as often, so they aren't getting as much air. The air already in the middle ear is absorbed, and a vacuum occurs, sucking the eardrum inward. Several hours after you've fallen asleep, your eustachian tubes may plug, especially if you have a cold, sinus infection, or allergy.

Sometimes earache pain signifies a middle-ear infection, called otitis media. This condition is more common in children than adults, because as we grow, our eustachian tubes become narrower, longer, and less prone to plugging up. Another reason children get ear infections is that the nerves to the area may not be fully developed in some babies, which can affect the eustachian tubes. Also, children in day-care centers are exposed to more colds, which can lead to ear infections.

In adults, the stage is set for a middle-ear infection when sinuses get plugged as a result of allergies or a head cold, or when the eustachian tubes get clogged during an airplane descent.

## WHEN TO CALL A DOCTOR

If you have ear pain, you need to see a doctor. But you should also make an appointment if you have hearing loss or if your ears stay plugged up for more than a couple of days after a cold. You could already have an ear infection or fluid in the middle ear, says George W. Facer, M.D. Left untreated, an ear infection can cause a permanent hearing loss. Ten to 14 days of antibiotics is the usual treatment.

Even though the usual symptoms of a middle-ear infection are pain and hearing loss, adults and children can get ear infections without pain, says George W. Facer, M.D. Once infection hits, the best way to cure it is with antibiotics, although some infections clear up on their own, usually in a week to 10 days.

Other things cause earaches, too. Infections of the ear canal, known as external otitis or swimmer's ear, can trigger pain. Atmospheric pressure from airplane travel and deep-sea diving can cause ears to ache even if they aren't infected. Odd things, such as tiny clippings from a haircut, can fall into the ear canal and irritate your eardrum. Then there's referred pain—a problem that exists somewhere else—that makes your ears tingle. Those earaches can originate in your teeth, tonsils, throat, tongue, or jaw.

When your ears ache, you need to see a doctor. But until you get there, here are some quick pain stoppers.

**Try acetaminophen.** If you have an earache, acetaminophen is a doctor's first choice. A dose at bedtime may be enough to let you sleep.

**Sit up.** A few minutes upright decreases swelling and starts your eustachian tubes draining. Swallowing also helps ease the pain. If you can, prop your head up slightly while you sleep to get better drainage, says Dr. Weider.

**Take a drink.** Swallowing triggers the muscular action that helps your eustachian tubes open and drain, Dr. Weider adds. Open tubes mean less pain.

**Wiggle your ear.** Here's a test to help determine whether you have otitis externa (an external problem like swimmer's ear) or otitis media (an internal middle-ear infection). Grab your outer ear, says Donald B. Kamerer, M.D. If you can wiggle it without pain, the problem is probably in the middle ear. If moving your outer ear causes pain, then the infection is probably in the outer ear canal.

**Use warm drops.** Place a bottle of baby oil or mineral oil in a pan of body-temperature water, says Dr. Weider. Let the oil sit in the water until it, too, is

# An Ounce of Prevention

Ear infections are the most common cause of hearing loss in children, according to the American Academy of Otolaryngology/Head and Neck Surgery. While you can't really prevent ear infections, there are some things you can do that may help lower the chances of your child getting them.

**Choose child care carefully.** Children exposed to large groups of other children are more likely to come into contact with the bugs that cause ear infections. Parents who need day care for a child prone to ear infections may want to consider a small group setting, such as a family day-care home, until the child outgrows ear infections, says Dudley J. Weider, M.D.

**Breastfeed.** The American Academy of Pediatrics cites "strong evidence" from six major scientific studies that breastfeeding protects infants from otitis media.

In a study of 306 infants being seen in general pediatric practices, twice as many formula-fed infants as breastfed infants developed an ear infection between the ages of 6 months and 1 year. In fact, formula feeding was the most significant factor associated with ear infections, even more important than being in day care.

An earlier study of 237 infants in Helsinki, Finland, showed that 6 percent of breastfed babies and 19 percent of formula-fed babies had developed middle-ear infections by the end of their first year. By age 3, only 6 percent of those breastfed developed an infection compared with 26 percent of those fed formula.

Why the big difference? Researchers believe that breastfed infants have an enhanced immune response to respiratory infections.

If you bottle-feed your infant, experts advise holding her in your arms during feedings so that her head is above the stomach level, rather than laying her down with a bottle. This semi-upright position will help keep the eustachian tubes from becoming blocked and reduce the risk of ear infections.

**Quit smoking.** Smoking can push an adult with ear problems toward an infection by littering the air with irritants, which in turn leads to eustachian tube congestion, says Dr. Weider. Secondhand smoke, which is also pollutant-filled, can be just as hard on children prone to ear problems.

**Douse the fire in your wood-burning stove.** For the same clean-air reasons that you should quit smoking, put out the fire in your woodstove. Soot and smoke from the fire in your stove load the air with hard-to-breathe and hard-to-tolerate toxins.

**Be patient.** Some children outgrow ear infections by age 3, says George W. Facer, M.D.

at body temperature. Place a drop or two of oil in the offending ear to lessen the pain.

*Caution:* Never drop fluids into your ear if you think the eardrum may be ruptured or punctured.

**Take an herbal approach.** Herbalists commonly recommend garlic and mullein oils for ear infections. Mullein is antimicrobial, and garlic works like an antibiotic. The oils will also migrate past the eardrum and help prevent further infections. You can buy garlic oil, mullein oil, or a combination of the two in most health food stores or drugstores. Apply 2 to 4 drops in the affected ear. Cover the ear with a little wad of cotton to keep the oil from running out. Apply more drops every 6 to 8 hours as needed. Use fresh cotton with each application.

*Caution:* If you think the eardrum may be ruptured or punctured, never drop fluids into your ear.

**Chew gum.** Most people know this is one way to open their ears on an airplane flight, but have you considered it at midnight? The muscular action of chewing may open the eustachian tubes.

**Yawn.** Yawning moves the muscle that opens the eustachian tube even better than chewing gum or sucking on mints.

**Hold your nose.** If you're flying at 32,000 feet when your ears begin to ache, pinch your nostrils shut, suggests the American Academy of Otolaryngology/Head and Neck Surgery. Take a mouthful of air and then, using your cheek and throat muscles, force the air into the back of your nose as if you were trying to blow your fingers off the end of your nose. A pop will tell you when you have equalized the pressure inside and outside your ear.

**Don't sleep during an airplane descent.** If you must doze off while flying, close your eyes at the beginning, not at the end of the trip, the academy recommends. Rapid changes in air pressure occur during ascent as well, but ear pain is typically more acute during descent because atmospheric pressure increases as you move closer to the ground. You don't swallow as often when you're asleep, so your ears won't keep up with pressure changes during descent, and you might wake up in pain.

**Head off trouble.** Before you get into trouble, use an over-the-counter decongestant. For instance, if you have to fly and you know your sinuses are going to back up and block your ears, take a decongestant or use nose drops an hour before you land, Dr. Weider suggests. At home, if you have a stuffy head, use a decongestant at night before you climb in bed to help avoid the middle-of-the-night ache.

# Drying-Out Cures for Swimmer's Ear

All it takes to come down with a stubborn bout of swimmer's ear is a set of ears and unrelenting moisture. "It's like keeping your hands in dishwater. The skin gets macerated and leathery," says Brian W. Hands, M.D. "The ears are constantly bathed in water—swimming, showering, shampooing. Then people try to dry the ear with a cotton-tipped swab. That takes the top layer of skin off, along with protective bacteria. Then the bad bacteria win."

Swimmer's ear begins as an itchy ear. Left untreated, it can turn into a full-blown infection. The pain can be excruciating. Once infection sets in, you'll need a doctor's help and a round of antibiotics to squelch it. But there are plenty of things you can do to keep the pain from getting worse, and even more to stop it before it starts.

**Try an over-the-counter remedy.** Most drugstores carry ear drops that can help dry up swimmer's ear. If ear itchiness is still your only symptom, one of these preparations might snatch it back from the brink of infection, says Dan Drew, M.D. Use it each time your ears get wet.

**Plug up the problem.** Wear earplugs when you swim, shampoo, or shower to keep the water out, says John House, M.D. Wax or silicone plugs that can be softened and shaped to fit your ear are available at most drugstores.

**Swim on the surface.** Even if you're battling swimmer's ear, you can keep on swimming, says Dr. Drew. Swim on the surface of the water. It allows less water in the ear than when you break the surface.

**Soothe away pain with heat.** Warmth—a towel fresh from the dryer, a covered hot-water bottle, a heating pad set on low—also helps ease the pain.

**Leave your earwax alone.** Earwax serves several purposes, including harboring friendly bacteria, say Donald B. Kamerer, M.D. and Dr. House. Cooperate with your natural defenses by *not* swabbing the wax out. Wax coats the ear canal, protecting it from moisture.

**Avoid tight-fitting head gear.** Like people who fly, scuba divers must be able to equalize the pressure inside their ears with that of the water around them, or they can experience ear trouble. Shallow diving is more likely to cause an earache because the greatest changes in air volume occur in relatively shallow water, less than 33 feet. Avoid super-snug earplugs and wet suits with tight-fitting hoods, which prevent equalization of pressure during descent, recommends Gary D. Becker, M.D.

For recreational swimmers, swimming on the surface puts less pressure on the eardrums than swimming underwater, says Dan Drew, M.D. To avoid stress on your eardrums, don't dive deeper than 3 to 4 feet.

**Make substitute wax.** Since the irritation of swimmer's ear wears away earwax, you can manufacture your own version using petroleum jelly. Moisten a cotton ball with the jelly, says Dr. Hands, and tuck it gently, like a plug, just in the edge of your ear. It will absorb any moisture, keeping your ear warm and dry.

**Take a drop.** Several fluids are great for killing germs and drying your ears at the same time. If you're susceptible to swimmer's ear or if you spend a lot of time in the water, use a drying agent every time you get your head wet. Any of the following homemade solutions works well.

*A squirt of rubbing alcohol.* Put your head down, with the affected ear up. Pull your ear upward and backward (to help straighten the canal) and squeeze a dropperful of alcohol into the ear canal. Wiggle your ear to get the alcohol to the bottom of the canal. Then tilt your head to the other side and let the alcohol drain out.

*A kitchen solution.* Ear drops of white vinegar or equal parts of alcohol and white vinegar kill fungus and bacteria, says Dr. House. Use it the same way you would rubbing alcohol.

*Mineral oil, baby oil, or lanolin.* These can be preventive solutions before swimming. Apply as you would the alcohol.

**Choose your swimming hole with care.** You are less likely to pick up bacteria in a well-treated pool than you are in a pond, says Dr. Drew. Don't swim in dirty water.

**Take breaks from your hearing aid.** If you wear a hearing aid, you can get swimmer's ear without even going near the water. A hearing aid has an earplug effect, explains Dr. Hands. In addition to picking up sound, it also picks up moisture that lodges in the ear canal. And trapped moisture can breed the germs that brew an infection. The solution? Take your hearing aid out of your ear as often as possible to give your ear a chance to dry out.

**Avoid aggravating the situation.** If you're prone to ear problems when you have a cold or allergies, consider delaying air travel or avoid diving until your head clears.

## PANEL OF ADVISORS

**Gary D. Becker, M.D.,** is a staff physician at Kaiser Permanente Medical Center in Panorama City, California.

**Dan Drew, M.D.,** is a physician in Indianapolis. He is also an avid swimmer.

**George W. Facer, M.D.,** is an otolaryngologist at the Mayo Clinic in Scottsdale, Arizona.

**Brian W. Hands, M.D.,** is an ear, nose, and throat specialist in Toronto.

**John House, M.D.,** is a clinical professor of otolaryngology at the University of Southern California School of Medicine in Los Angeles. He serves as a national team physician for United States Swimming, the national governing association for competitive amateur swimming that selects the Olympic team.

**Donald B. Kamerer, M.D.,** is a professor in the department of otolaryngology at the University of Pittsburgh School of Medicine.

**Dudley J. Weider, M.D.,** is an otolaryngologist at Dartmouth-Hitchcock Medical Center in Lebanon, New Hampshire.

# EARWAX
## 4 Steps to Clean Ears

Earwax, also known as cerumen, protects your eardrum from dust and debris. Left alone, it does its job quite nicely, migrating harmlessly to the outer ear as it dries, only to be replaced by fresh wax that forms in the ear canal.

Occasionally, the wax forms a hard, little plug next to the eardrum that has to be removed by a doctor, says David Edelstein, M.D. Here's how to prevent that from happening.

**Stick nothing in your ear.** That old cliché, "Never put anything smaller than your elbow into your ear," is one that ear doctors swear by. Never stick anything sharp—a bobby pin, a pencil tip, a paper clip—into your ear, because you could tear your eardrum. Don't use a cotton-tipped swab or finger either, says George W. Facer, M.D. Even though you think you're cleaning out your ear, you are actually ramming the wax deeper so that it acts like a plug over your eardrum.

**Drop in a softening fluid.** A few drops of a liquid that you probably already have at home can soften your earwax. Try hydrogen peroxide, mineral oil, or glycerin for inexpensive cleaning, says Dr. Facer.

Or buy an over-the-counter cleaner such as Debrox or Murine Ear Drops, says Dr. Edelstein.

Add a drop or two of one of the liquids to each ear. Allow the excess to flow out of your ear. The liquid left inside will bubble away at the wax and soften it. Try this for a couple of days.

Once the wax is soft, you're ready to rinse. Fill a bowl with body-temperature water, says Dr. Facer. Then fill a rubber bulb syringe with the water and, holding your head over the bowl, squirt the water *gently* into your ear canal. The stream of water should be under very little pressure. Turn your head to the side and let the water run out.

**Blow-dry your ears.** Don't rub your ears dry, say doctors. Instead, dry your ears with a hair dryer or drop a little alcohol in each ear to complete the drying. Do this once you have rinsed your ears to clean them, as described above, and also every time you shower.

**Let nature do its work.** A once-a-month ear wash is plenty for anyone, says Dr. Edelstein. More than that, and you're washing away the protective layer of earwax that's supposed to be in there.

## PANEL OF ADVISORS

**David Edelstein, M.D.,** is a clinical professor of otolaryngology at the Joan and Sanford I. Weill Medical College of Cornell University in New York City.
**George W. Facer, M.D.,** is an otolaryngologist at the Mayo Clinic in Scottsdale, Arizona.

# EMPHYSEMA
## 23 Tips for Easy Breathing

Emphysema is a degenerative disease, developing gradually after many years of exposure to toxins or smoke, which destroy the alveoli or small air sacks in the lungs. Over time, the lungs lose their elasticity, making breathing difficult.

Although it develops slowly, the toll emphysema exacts on the lungs is anything but minor. The alveoli, which normally stretch as they transport oxygen from the air to the blood and then shrink as they force out carbon dioxide, lose their effectiveness. Patients with emphysema have difficulty exhaling because their damaged lungs trap air and cannot exchange the old air for fresh air.

While there is no cure for emphysema, there are plenty of steps you can take to ease symptoms, prevent progression of the disease, and enjoy life. Here's how to save your energy for the things you really want to do.

## WHEN TO CALL A DOCTOR

See a doctor if you experience any of the following symptoms:

- Feeling confused or disoriented during an acute respiratory infection
- Sleepiness or slurred speech during an acute respiratory infection
- Blood or any other change in color, thickness, odor, or the amount of mucus that you cough
- Shortness of breath, coughing, or wheezing that worsens
- Waking up short of breath more than once a night
- Fatigue that lasts more than one day
- Ankles that stay swollen even after a night of sleeping with your feet elevated
- Needing to use more pillows or sleep in a chair instead of a bed so that you don't get short of breath
- Morning headaches, restlessness, and dizzy spells

**Stop smoking now!** "It's never too late to stop," says Henry Gong, M.D. "Even if you stop in your fifties or sixties, you'll help slow down the deterioration of your lungs."

**Stay away from passive smoke.** If the smoke from your own cigarettes can harm you, so can the secondhand smoke from your spouse's cigarette or the air in a smoky bingo hall. A nonsmoking spouse can develop emphysema by inhaling the cigarette smoke from a smoking spouse after many decades of living together, says Dr. Gong.

**Avoid allergens.** If you have known allergies that affect your breathing, it's doubly important to stay away from what causes them when you have emphysema, says Dr. Gong. (For more on allergy control, see Allergies on page 15.)

**Control what you can.** You can't repair your airways. What you can do, says Robert Sandhaus, M.D., Ph.D., is increase how efficiently you breathe, use your muscles, and approach your work. You can rearrange your kitchen, for instance, so that you can do in 5 steps what used to take 10.

The American Lung Association suggests that you obtain a three-shelf utility cart to help with your housework. Small changes like these pay back with extra energy.

**Exercise.** All our experts agree that regular exercise is vitally important to people with emphysema. What kinds are best?

"Walking is probably the best overall exercise," says Robert B. Teague, M.D. "You should also exercise to tone the muscles in your upper extremities. Try using 1- or 2-pound hand weights, and work the muscles in your neck, upper shoulders, and chest." This is important, he says, because people with chronic lung diseases use their neck and upper respiratory chest muscles more than other people.

People who have asthma and emphysema seem to really benefit from swimming, because the activity allows them to breathe very humidified air, says Dr. Teague.

**Eat less—but more often.** As emphysema progresses and there is more obstruction to airflow, the lungs enlarge with trapped air. These enlarged lungs push down into the abdomen, leaving less room for the stomach to expand.

That's why six small meals will make you feel better than three large ones. Your best bet, says Dr. Teague, is to reach for foods that pack a lot of calories into a small volume, like high-protein selections.

Be aware, too, that prolonged digestion draws blood and oxygen to the stomach and away from other parts of the body, which may need them more.

**Maintain your ideal body weight.** Some people with emphysema gain a lot of weight and tend to retain fluid, says Dr. Teague. It takes more energy to carry extra body weight. The closer you are to your ideal weight, the better for your lungs.

Other emphysema patients tend to be very skinny, adds Dr. Teague. "Because they have to breathe harder, they expend more energy." If you're underweight, conscientiously add calories, says Dr. Teague. High-protein foods are a good source of calories.

**Become a champion breather.** There are several things you can do to get the maximum oomph from each breath you take. They include:

*Make your breathing uniform.* When Dr. Teague and his colleagues studied 20 patients with advanced emphysema, they found that even under normal conditions their subjects had very chaotic breathing patterns.

"Their breathing was all over the map—big breaths, little breaths. We taught them normal breathing patterns, and it helped, at least in the short term," Dr. Teague says.

*Breathe from your diaphragm.* This is the most efficient way to breathe. Babies do it naturally. If you watch them, you'll see their bellies rise and fall with each breath.

Not sure whether you're breathing from your diaphragm or your chest? Francisco Perez, Ph.D., tells his patients to lie down, put phone directories on their bellies, and watch what happens to them when they breathe. If you're breathing from your diaphragm, the directory will rise with each intake of breath.

***Keep those airways open.*** You can strengthen your breathing muscles by blowing out slowly through pursed lips for 30 minutes a day, says Dr. Gong. Try to exhale twice as long as it took you to breathe in. This will help you rid the lungs of stale air, so fresh air can get in.

You can also buy a device from the drugstore that offers resistance when you blow against it. "It looks like a little plastic mouthpiece with a ring on the end," says Dr. Sandhaus. "When you turn the ring, the opening at the mouthpiece changes size. You start with the largest opening, take a deep breath in and blow out. Once you master one setting, you move on to another one."

## Try vitamins C and E. 
Dr. Sandhaus advises his emphysema patients to take a minimum of 250 milligrams of vitamin C twice a day, and 500 IU of vitamin E twice a day. (Of course, don't practice this or any vitamin therapy without your doctor's okay and supervision.)

Dr. Sandhaus says that the vitamin therapy can't hurt. He thinks that vitamins C and E may be helpful because they're antioxidants. "We know that the oxidants in cigarette smoke are what damage the lungs," he says.

## Allow yourself to grieve. 
Your life with emphysema won't be the same as your life before emphysema. Allow yourself to move through each stage of the grieving process, says Dr. Perez. "There are some losses, but then you recognize that you have control over it."

## Relax. 
"If you cognitively view the disease as a threat, you'll arouse some physiological mechanisms that can make your emphysema worse," says Dr. Perez. "When you're in a constant state of alarm, you're demanding a lot of oxygen in the process. Alarm is created by the thought process, which you can control. That means you can also control the physiological mechanisms."

## Shift your focus to the present. 
When you find yourself feeling guilty that you brought on your disease, shift your orientation to the present and concentrate on what's happening now, says Dr. Perez. "You can't deal with events that happened in the past. You can only learn from them."

## Set small goals. 
One way to shift your focus from "emphysema is incapacitating" to "emphysema is something I have control over" is to set realistic small goals for yourself, says Dr. Perez.

Exercise is a great way to boost your confidence, he says. "Set some real objective goal based on the physical evidence. Use charts and graphs to measure your progress. This gives you a very objective measure of your ability to do something."

**Join a rehabilitation group.** Consider joining a pulmonary rehabilitation group, says Dr. Gong. If you can't find one locally, contact your nearby American Lung Association chapter. A group can educate you about your condition and provide social support. "Statistics show that these programs can decrease the number of hospitalizations," he says.

**Have a family member play "coach."** Have your significant other become your coach and help you through those times when you're short of breath, suggests Dr. Perez.

**Don't isolate yourself socially.** "You need to avoid generalizing about the shortness of breath," says Dr. Teague. "Some people with emphysema think, 'Well, I probably can't do this.' Because they're scared they might get out somewhere and get short of breath, they quit going places they'd normally enjoy." Don't let it isolate you.

**Pace yourself.** "The other thing people with emphysema have to learn to do is to take their own time," says Dr. Teague. "They really can do what they want to do, but they have to do it at their own pace. That is not an easy thing to do."

**Coordinate your breathing to your lifting.** According to the American Lung Association, lifting will be easier if you lift while you exhale through pursed lips. Inhale while you rest. Similarly, if you have to climb steps, climb while you exhale through pursed lips and inhale while you rest.

**Don't use unnecessary sprays.** You don't need to add to your respiratory problems by inhaling unknown substances, says the American Lung Association. Use liquid or gel-type hair products and roll-on or solid deodorants. Avoid aerosol-spray household cleaners.

**Let loose.** On your clothing, that is. Choose clothing that allows your chest and abdomen to expand freely. That means no tight belts, bras, or girdles, says the American Lung Association.

## PANEL OF ADVISORS

**Henry Gong, M.D.,** is a professor of medicine and preventive medicine at the University of Southern California in Los Angeles and chairman of the department of medicine at Rancho Los Amigos National Rehabilitation Center in Downey.
**Francisco Perez, Ph.D.,** is an associate clinical professor of neurology and physical medicine at Baylor College of Medicine in Houston.

**Robert Sandhaus, M.D., Ph.D.,** is a pulmonary specialist, a clinical professor at the University of Colorado Health Sciences Center, director of Alpha-1 Clinic at the National Jewish Medical and Research Center, and executive vice president and medical director of the Alpha-1 Foundation and AlphaNet, all in Denver.
**Robert B. Teague, M.D.,** is an associate professor of medicine at Baylor College of Medicine in Houston.

# EYESTRAIN
## 10 Tips to Avoid It

People who spend as little as 2 hours a day staring at a computer screen can experience "computer vision syndrome." The classic symptoms include eyestrain, blurred vision, headaches, and dry eyes. Our eyes just weren't designed to focus for hours on end at words on an illuminated background.

If you find your eyes straining to read your birthday cards or your vision blurring as you try to focus on your computer screen, here are some suggestions that may help.

**Rest your eyes.** Our experts say that it's the best way to relieve eyestrain. And that's easier than you may think. "You can do it while you're on the phone," says Samuel L. Guillory, M.D. "If you don't need to read or write, just close your eyes while you're talking. Depending on how much time you spend on the phone each day, you may be able to rest your eyes for almost an hour or two

## WHEN TO CALL A DOCTOR

Sometimes the cause of eyestrain is a lot more serious than just passing your 40th birthday. "Strain can also be caused by eye misalignment, where one eye starts to turn in or out," says David Guyton, M.D. "If that's the case, the problem needs to be treated by an ophthalmologist who can suggest specific exercises, prescribe special prism glasses, or, if necessary, even perform eye muscle surgery to realign the eyes."

All the experts agree that if you have pain in your eye or sensitivity to light, you need to see an ophthalmologist right away.

## Insight with Yoga

For Meir Schneider, Ph.D., yoga wasn't only the key to gaining spiritual insight. It also was the key to simply gaining sight. "Yoga helped cure my blindness," claims Dr. Schneider, who was born blind. He credits daily yoga exercises for helping bring back his vision, which he says is now 20/60. And it's still improving. While it might be straining science a bit to say it cures blindness, some of his techniques may be helpful in handling eyestrain.

**Try a different sort of eye/hand coordination.** If you want to help your eyes, Dr. Schneider says, you need to lend them a hand. "Take your hands and rub them together until they are warm. Then close your eyes and put your palms over your eye orbits. Don't press on your eyes; just cover them. Breathe deeply and slowly and visualize the color black. Do this for 20 minutes every day."

**Put your eyes "on the blink."** Your eyes have their own personal masseuse—the eyelids. "Make it a point to consciously blink your eyes 300 times every day and not squint," says Dr. Schneider. "Each blink cleanses your eyes and gives them a tiny little massage." And it's free.

daily. People who practice this technique say that their eyes really feel better, and it helps rid them of eyestrain."

**Pay attention to lighting.** "It doesn't hurt your eyes to read in dim light, but you can strain them if the light doesn't provide enough contrast," says Dr. Guillory. "Use a soft light that gives contrast, but not glare, when you read. And don't use any lamp that reflects light directly back into your eyes."

**Try reading glasses.** You can get them from your doctor or even from the drugstore. "If you have good distance vision in both eyes and just have trouble seeing up close, go to your local drugstore and buy the reading glasses they have on display there," says ophthalmologist David Guyton, M.D. They're commonly available, cost from $10 to $20, and are impact-resistant, good-quality glasses that will help you.

**Pick the right power.** You are the best judge of which reading glasses work best for you. "Pick the weakest, or least powerful, ones that will allow you to read at the distance you want," says Dr. Guyton. "If you buy ones that are too powerful, you will see fine up close, but things will be blurred beyond that distance."

**Interrupt your work.** Save and store what's on your computer every once in a while. "If you use the computer for 6 to 8 hours," says Dr. Guillory, "take a break every 2 to 3 hours. Do some other work, get coffee, go to the bathroom—just take your eyes off the screen for 10 to 15 minutes." Also, consider working from a printout instead of reading on the screen.

**Darken your screen.** Those aren't just letters and numbers on your screen. They're also tiny lightbulbs that send light directly into your eyes. You need to turn the wattage down, so to speak. "Don't make the screen too bright," advises Dr. Guillory. "Turn the brightness down to a dim level and then adjust the contrast to make up the difference."

**Work in the shade.** When it comes to relieving eyestrain, it's best to keep your computer in the dark. "Shade your screen by creating a hood over it," Dr. Guillory suggests. "Go to an art supply store and buy a sheet of heavy black cardboard. Put it on top of your terminal and fold both sides down over it. That will allow you to slide it back and forth. What you've done, essentially, is put your machine in a black box. So now you can turn the brightness down to a very low level."

**Brew a pot of eyebright tea.** Cool it slightly and then soak a towel in the still-warm tea, says Meir Schneider, Ph.D. Lie down and place the warm towel over your closed eyes, leaving it there for 10 to 15 minutes. It will make your eyestrain go away. Be very careful not to pour tea into your eyes, though.

## PANEL OF ADVISORS

**Samuel L. Guillory, M.D.,** is an ophthalmologist and associate clinical professor of ophthalmology at Mount Sinai School of Medicine of New York University in New York City.

**David Guyton, M.D.,** is the Krieger professor of pediatric ophthalmology and director of the Krieger Children's Eye Center at the Wilmer Institute at the Johns Hopkins University School of Medicine in Baltimore.

**Meir Schneider, Ph.D.,** is founder of the School for Self Healing in San Francisco. He is the author of *Self Healing: My Life and Vision* and coauthor of *The Handbook of Self-Healing.*

# FATIGUE

## 35 Hints for a High-Energy Life

Be honest. When you hear the words *energy crisis*, do you think of fuel-efficient cars or yourself?

Everyone, at one time or another, feels fatigued. And who wouldn't like to have more energy than they now have?

The broad prescription from doctors is still the same: Get plenty of rest, eat a balanced diet, and exercise. But here authorities on fatigue go beyond these generalities and offer more specific, high-octane suggestions.

So, ladies and gentlemen, start your engines.

**Warm up.** "Give yourself an extra 15 minutes in the morning before you start your day," says Vicky Young, M.D. "That way you don't start off feeling rushed and tired."

**Eat a three-piece breakfast.** The three components of a good breakfast are carbohydrates, proteins, and fats, advises Rick Ricer, M.D. You don't really need to *add* fat to your breakfast table. You will get plenty of fats, a good form of storable energy, in the proteins you eat.

But even cereal (a complex carbohydrate) with milk (a source of protein) can

---

### WHEN TO CALL A DOCTOR

Fatigue may be just a signal that you need to manage your life better or that a cold or the flu is coming on.

But it also can be a warning sign of serious illness. "Anything that's chronic—diabetes, lung disease, anemia—will cause fatigue," says Rick Ricer, M.D.

Fatigue is also a symptom of many other illnesses, including hepatitis, mononucleosis, thyroid disease, and cancer. So if your tiredness persists, don't try to diagnose yourself. See a doctor.

get your day off to a good start. Wheat toast and muffins are also good complex-carbohydrate options. For protein, you may want to consider low-fat yogurt or scrambled egg whites.

Meanwhile, Dr. Ricer warns not to eat an ultra-high-carbohydrate breakfast laden with simple sugars. "You can actually overactivate your insulin, and your blood sugar will drop. That can leave you jittery." So avoid the doughnut shop between home and the office.

**Know where you're going.** If you don't, you'll probably be too tired to get there. "Take time each morning to set specific goals for the day," says David Sheridan, M.D. "Determine what you want to do; don't let the routine control you."

**Arrest the energy robbers.** "If it's a problem on the job, or if it's a family feud, you have to resolve it," says M. F. Graham, M.D.

But if you can't resolve your problem, at least take a vacation from the situation, Dr. Ricer suggests. So if you're trying to hold down a second job, quit it or take a leave of absence. And if relatives have overstayed their welcome, politely suggest they visit again—in about 3 years.

**Turn off to turn on.** Television is famous—make that infamous—for lulling human beings into lethargy. "Try reading instead," Dr. Ricer says. It's more energizing.

**Work out to rev up.** "Exercise actually gives you energy," Dr. Young says. Study after study supports those words, including one by NASA. More than 200 federal employees were placed on a moderate, regular exercise program. The results: 90 percent said they had never felt better. Almost half said they felt less stress, and almost one-third reported that they slept better.

Dr. Young recommends giving yourself a dose of energetic exercise—brisk walking is enough—three to five times a week for 20 to 30 minutes each time, and no later than 2 hours before bedtime.

**Remember—honesty is the best policy.** For all the good that exercise can do, it can be addictive. And you can overdose if you're not honest about what your body is telling you.

"I have to work at telling myself that it will be good for me, that I will gain by taking time off," says endurance athlete Mary Trafton.

**Tackle one thing at a time.** "Make lists," Dr. Sheridan says. "Many times, people feel fatigued because they think, 'I have so much to do, and I don't know where to start.'" By setting priorities and charting your progress as you make your way through the list, you can remain focused and energetic.

**Take one a day.** If you're guilty of missing meals, dieting, and not eating properly, Dr. Young says, taking one multivitamin/mineral supplement a day is a good idea.

"A lack of good nutrition can cause fatigue, and a supplement can help make up for the missing nutrients. But don't look to a vitamin to give you instant energy," says Dr. Ricer.

**Teach your body to tell time.** Circadian rhythms act as our bodies' internal clocks, raising and lowering blood pressure and body temperature at different times throughout the day. This chemical action causes the "swings" we experience—from feeling alert to feeling mentally and physically fogged in.

So why are some people's natural peak times so inconvenient—like late at night? "I think sometimes people, perhaps without even knowing it, work themselves into a particular time cycle," says exercise physiologist William Fink.

Fink suggests changing your schedule as much as practically possible to complement your circadian rhythms. Start by getting up a little earlier or a little later—say, 15 minutes—until you feel comfortable. Keep it up until you reach your desired schedule.

**Put out the fire.** Doctors always advise giving up smoking, but add this to the list of reasons: Smoking reduces the amount of oxygen available in your body. The result is fatigue.

When you first quit, however, don't expect an immediate energy boost. Nicotine acts as a stimulant, and withdrawal may cause some temporary tiredness.

**Make exercise an all-day activity.** Whether you work out early, at lunchtime, or in the evening, don't save all your exercising for one block of time. "Get up and move around at least every couple of hours," Dr. Sheridan says.

The options are limitless: the executive who rides a stationary bicycle in the privacy of his office, the medical resident who runs hospital stairs, and the researcher who does isometric exercises while sitting at her desk.

**Just say no.** "Learn to delegate," Dr. Sheridan says. If too many obligations or commitments are wearing you out, learn to say, "No, thank you."

**Shed.** As in pounds. "If you're obese—if you need to drop 20 percent of your weight or more—losing weight will be a great help," Fink says. Of course, make sure you follow a sensible diet in combination with exercise. Losing more than 2 pounds a week isn't healthy and will wear you down.

**Get fewer Zzzs.** You can get too much of a good thing, even sleep. "If you oversleep, you tend to be groggy all day," Fink says. "Usually, 6 to 8 hours of sleep per night is enough for most people."

**Blow out the candle.** Burning the candle at both ends—not going to bed until 2:00 A.M. and getting up at 5:00 A.M., for example—will leave you feeling burned out. Don't shortchange yourself on sleep.

**Get 20 winks.** Naps aren't for everybody, but they might help recharge older people who aren't sleeping as soundly as they used to, Dr. Ricer says. Younger people with very hectic schedules and short nights also might consider taking naps. If you do decide to take naps, try taking them at the same time each day and for no more than an hour.

**Breathe deeply.** It's one of the best ways to relax and energize at the same time, according to doctors and athletes.

**Have just one.** Alcohol is a depressant, notes Dr. Ricer, and will calm you down, not rev you up. Limit your alcohol intake to one drink, Dr. Ricer suggests, or don't drink at all.

---

## Open Your Mind to Energy

When your mind goes, your body follows. That the mind can influence the body is now generally accepted. Here are some beneficial attitudes that can affect your energy level.

**Think positive.** Championship athletes do it, successful chief executive officers do it, and you should do it, too.

"It's important to think positively," says Mary Trafton, an avid hiker and marathoner. "If I step in a huge puddle while hiking, I don't think, 'Ah, I'm going to be cold and tired.' I think about the wool socks I have on for protection and warmth."

**Be motivated.** When you think about it, it's pretty hard to do much of anything if you're not motivated. But it's next to impossible to accomplish tasks that require mega-energy if your spirit just isn't in it.

Take E. Drummond King, for example. He has participated in the grueling Ironman competitions in Hawaii—where competitors swim, bicycle, and run long distances for hours on end. He says that when he's too far behind to win his age group, he finishes the race by walking instead of running. Yet when there's a chance to win or a bet riding on how long it takes him, he somehow finds the energy to continue running.

**Be confident.** Chances are, if you feel you can do it, you will have the energy to do it. And once you've proven to yourself that you have the energy, you'll become even more confident.

**Eat a light lunch.** Some doctors advise a light lunch to avoid a severe case of the post-lunch I-want-to-crawl-under-my-desk-and-take-a-nap blues. If you're too tired too often, this advice is worth trying. Soup and salad and a piece of fruit is a light but nutritious meal.

**Make lunch your big meal of the day.** If a light lunch doesn't satisfy you, Dr. Young suggests eating your largest meal of the day at lunch and following it up with a 20-minute walk. Eating most of your calories early in the day gives you the fuel you need to keep perking. But you have to be selective in the type of fuel you choose. Carbohydrate, for example, is a fast burner. Fat, on the other hand, burns slowly, so it'll slow you down.

**Go visit Mickey Mouse.** "In a lot of cases, taking a vacation is almost mandatory," Dr. Ricer says. "If you haven't had a vacation in a long time, it can be the perfect energy booster." That's *really* good advice.

**Divert your energy.** Strong emotion is mentally draining, but it can be physically draining, too, says Dr. Young. Redirect strong emotions, such as anger, and apply that energy to your job or a workout.

**Color your world.** "If you live in a dark, dark house, you're going to feel fatigued," Dr. Ricer says. He suggests a little sunshine—literally or figuratively. Several studies have shown that lots of color and variety are important in keeping energy levels high. Red, for example, is good for short-term, high-energy stimulation, while green is good at eliminating distractions and maintaining focus for long periods of time.

**Tune in.** Music can light your fire, Dr. Ricer says. Listen to U2, Willie Nelson, Frank Sinatra—whatever and whoever peps you up.

**Give yourself a target.** Some people simply need deadlines to keep moving forward, Dr. Sheridan says. If you're like that, give yourself both short and long deadlines—so neither becomes too routine.

**Make a splash.** When fatigue starts to drop one New York stockbroker, he doesn't buy or sell. He stops—long enough to hit himself in the face with splashes of cold water.

But if he were home, a cold shower might restore his energy even better. Cascading water emits negative ions in the air, which surround the body. Negative ions are thought to make some people feel happier and more energetic.

**Drink up.** Dehydration can cause fatigue. Drink at least eight 8-ounce glasses of water each day, even more when you're active. If you know you're going to be active, really fill up the day before. The day before you're going to be physically active and out in the hot sun—say, a day at Disney World with your kids—doctors advise drinking plenty of water and continuing to do so the day of the activity.

E. Drummond King, an over-50 triathlete, learned the hard way that it's best to start drinking a lot of fluids the day before his body is going to need them.

"The major problem is dehydration and the fatigue that comes with it," he says. "Now I spend the day before walking around with a water bottle in my hand."

**Rethink your medications.** Do you really need to take all those prescription and over-the-counter medicines? If not, you may be shocked at what eliminating or reducing dosages of certain medications may do for you.

Sleeping pills, for example, are notorious for their next-day hangover effects. But also among the villains, according to doctors, are high blood pressure medicines and cough and cold medicines.

If you suspect a medication is guilty of grand theft energy, discuss it with your doctor. Maybe you can get a new prescription or, better yet, quit the medicine altogether. But never stop taking a prescription medication without your doctor's approval.

**If it feels good, do it.** There's no denying the pleasures of massages, whirlpools, and steam baths. "It's hard to study scientifically whether or not they lessen fatigue," says Fink. "But there are those who swear by them. I'm convinced, too—if people feel better, they'll perform better."

**Change and explore.** Sometimes fatigue can be caused by a rut. Even the simplest of changes, says Dr. Ricer, can make the difference. If you always start your day reading the paper, for example, try reading something inspirational. If you always eat fish for Monday dinner, reel in chicken next Monday instead. If you're a daily runner, try interspersing some scenic bicycle rides.

**Curb your caffeine.** One or two cups of coffee can kick you into gear in the morning, says Dr. Ricer, but the benefits usually end there. Too much caffeine is just as bad as too much of anything. Drinking it throughout the day for an energy boost can actually backfire.

Caffeine is a magician, Dr. Ricer says. "It makes you feel like you have more energy, but you really don't."

## PANEL OF ADVISORS

**William Fink** was formerly an exercise physiologist and assistant to the director of the Human Performance Laboratory at Ball State University in Muncie, Indiana.

**M. F. Graham, M.D.,** is a pediatrician in Dallas and a former consultant to the American Running Association.

**E. Drummond King** is a triathlete and a lawyer in Allentown, Pennsylvania.

**Rick Ricer, M.D.,** is the vice chairman for educational affairs and a professor of family medicine at the University of Cincinnati in Ohio.

**David Sheridan, M.D.,** is the medical director at Palmetto Government Benefits Administrators in Columbia, South Carolina.

**Mary Trafton** is a hiker, marathoner, and skier and a former information specialist for the Appalachian Mountain Club in Boston.

**Vicky Young, M.D.,** is an occupational health doctor at the TriCity Medical Center Work Partners in Vista, California.

# FEVER
## 22 Cooling Tactics

Think of fever not so much as a menace, but as your body's early-warning system. It's the way your body protects itself against infection and injury—and a tool it uses to enhance its natural defense mechanisms.

The mechanics are rather simple. Your brain tells your body to move blood from the surface of your skin to the interior of the body. With blood so far away

## WHEN TO CALL A DOCTOR

See a doctor for:

- Fever associated with a stiff neck
- Fever above 101°F that lasts more than 3 days or fails to respond at least partly to treatment
- Fever above 103°F under any condition

Adults with chronic illnesses, such as heart or respiratory disease, may not be able to tolerate prolonged high fevers.

from the skin, the body loses less heat and your temperature rises. Voilà! You have a fever.

Before you take steps to douse the fire, listen to what doctors say.

**Make sure you have a fever.** Although 98.6°F is considered the norm, that number is not etched in stone. "Normal" temperature varies from person to person and fluctuates widely throughout the day. Food, excess clothing, emotional excitement, and vigorous exercise can all elevate temperature, says Thomas Gossel, Ph.D., R.Ph. "In fact, vigorous exercise can raise body temperature to as high as 103°F. Furthermore, children tend to have higher temperatures than adults and greater daily variations. So here's a general rule: If your temperature is 99° to 100°F, start thinking about the possibility of fever. If it is 100°F or above, it is a fever," he says.

Dr. Gossel adds that often a person's appearance is a better indicator of his condition than hard-and-fast numbers. "A person with a raised temperature who looks ill needs attention sooner than one who looks and acts well."

**Don't fight it.** If you do have a fever, remember this: Fever itself is not an illness—it's a symptom of one. When your body senses a bacterial or viral invasion, it releases substances that tell your brain to raise your internal temperature, causing a fever. An elevated body temperature makes it harder for bacteria and viruses to reproduce and spread. So, in essence, your body's natural defenses can actually shorten an illness with its quick response and increase the power of antibiotics. These possibilities should be weighed against the discomfort involved in letting a slight fever run its course, says public-health authority Stephen Rosenberg, M.D.

If you feel the need for extra relief, try the following steps.

**Liquefy your assets.** When you're hot, your body perspires to cool you down. But if you lose too much water—as you might with a high fever—your body turns off its sweat ducts to forestall further water loss. That makes it more difficult for you to cope with your fever. The moral of this story: Drink up. In addition to plain water, doctors favor the following:

*Fruit and vegetable juices.* They're high in vitamins and minerals, says nutrition counselor Eleonore Blaurock-Busch, Ph.D., and that's exactly what you need to build up your strength. She particularly favors nutrient-dense beet juice and carrot juice.

*One doctor's botanical tea.* Although any tea will provide needed fluid, several are particularly suited for fever, says Dr. Blaurock-Busch. (Look for the following botanicals in health food stores.) One mixture she likes combines equal parts dried thyme, linden flowers, and chamomile

# Thermometer Ins and Outs

Mothers are famous for the skill in gauging temperatures just by feeling their children's foreheads. If you didn't inherit the knack, you'll need to rely on thermometer readings. Here's how to get the safest, most accurate results.

- First, consider the many types available. Some of the options are digital thermometers, ear thermometers, and glass galinstan thermometers, which are very similar to mercury thermometers except they contain gallium, indium, and tin.

- All of these are very good alternatives to old-fashioned mercury thermometers, which can cause neurological problems if the glass breaks and the mercury vapor is inhaled. In fact, the concern about mercury thermometers is so great that several cities in the United States have banned the sale of mercury thermometers altogether. (One important environmental note: If you do have mercury thermometers at home, don't rush to toss them in the trash can. Instead, ask your local poison control center to provide tips on safe disposal.)

- Wait at least 15 minutes after eating or drinking anything hot or cold or after smoking before taking an oral reading. These activities alter mouth temperature and will cause inaccurate readings. Hot baths can also lead to inaccurate readings.

- Before using a glass thermometer, hold it by the top end (not the bulb) and shake it with a quick snap of the wrist until the colored dye is below 96°F. If you're concerned about dropping and breaking the thermometer, do this over a bed, suggests Stephen Rosenberg, M.D.

- Place the thermometer under your tongue in one of the "pockets" located on either side of your mouth rather than right up front. These pockets are closer to blood vessels that reflect the body's core temperature.

- Hold the thermometer in place with your lips, not your teeth. Breathe through your nose rather than your mouth so that the room temperature doesn't affect the reading. Leave the thermometer in place for at least 3 minutes (some experts favor 5 to 7 minutes).

- After use, wash a glass thermometer in cool, soapy water. Never use hot water. And never store it near heat.

flowers. Thyme has antiseptic properties, chamomile reduces inflammation, and linden promotes sweating, she says. Steep 1 teaspoon of the mixture in 1 cup of boiling water for 5 minutes. Strain and drink warm several times a day.

***Linden tea.*** This tea by itself is also good, she says, and can induce sweating to break a fever. Use 1 tablespoon of the flowers in 1 cup of boiling water. Prepare as above and drink hot often.

***Willow bark.*** This bark is rich in salicylates (aspirin-related compounds) and is considered "nature's fever medication," says Dr. Blaurock-Busch. Brew into a tea and drink in small doses.

***Ice.*** If you're too nauseated to drink, you can suck on ice. For variety, freeze fruit juice in an ice-cube tray.

**Get compressed relief.** Wet compresses help reduce the body's temperature output, says Dr. Blaurock-Busch. Ironically, she says, hot, moist compresses can do the job. If you start to feel uncomfortably hot, remove those compresses and apply cool ones to the forehead, wrists, and calves. Keep the rest of the body covered.

But if the fever rises above 103°F, she says, don't use hot compresses at all. Instead, apply cool ones to prevent the fever from getting any higher. Change them as they warm to body temperature and continue until the fever drops.

**Sponge off.** Evaporation also has a cooling effect on body temperature. Mary Ann Pane, R.N., recommends cool tap water to help the skin dissipate excess heat. Although you can sponge the whole body, she says, pay particular attention to spots where heat is generally greatest, such as the armpits and groin area. Wring out a sponge and wipe one section at a time, keeping the rest of the body covered. Body heat will evaporate the moisture, so you don't need to towel off.

**Don't suffer.** If you're very uncomfortable, take an over-the-counter pain reliever. For adults, Dr. Gossel recommends aspirin, acetaminophen, or ibuprofen taken according to package directions. The advantage of acetaminophen and ibuprofen over aspirin, he adds, is that fewer people experience side effects.

So which one should you take? All are effective, but some work better for particular ailments. For example, aspirin and ibuprofen are common nonsteroidal anti-inflammatory drugs (NSAIDs), so they're effective at reducing muscle pain and inflamed areas. Acetaminophen is recommended if you have

| What the Doctor Does ... | "Often when I have a fever, I really start to shiver," says pharmacology expert Thomas Gossel, Ph.D., R.Ph. "At that point, I'm most comfortable getting into a warm shower." |
|---|---|

gastrointestinal sensitivity or are allergic to aspirin. It doesn't work as well as NSAIDs for inflammation and muscle aches; however, it's a safer drug to use and has minimal side effects.

**Dress the part.** Use common sense as far as clothing and blankets go, says Pane. If you're very hot, take off extra covers and clothes so that body heat can evaporate into the air. But if you have a chill, bundle up until you're just comfortable.

**Create a healing atmosphere.** Do your best to make the sickroom conducive to healing, says Dr. Blaurock-Busch. Don't overheat it—German doctors generally recommend that the temperature not exceed 65°F, she says. Allow just enough fresh air to promote recuperation but not to create a draft. And keep the lighting subdued so that it's properly relaxing.

**Eat—if you want to.** Don't fret over whether you should *feed* a fever or *starve* one. Some doctors, like Dr. Blaurock-Busch, prefer juice fasting until the fever is reduced nearly to normal. Others feel that you should eat during a fever because the body's increased heat uses up calories. Ultimately, of course, the choice is yours and hinges on your appetite. Just remember to keep up your fluid intake.

## PANEL OF ADVISORS

**Eleonore Blaurock-Busch, Ph.D.,** is associate laboratory director of King James Medical Laboratory and Trace Minerals International, both in Cleveland. She is also the director of Micro Trace Minerals in Hersbruck, Germany; cochairman of the International Association of Trace Elements and Cancer; and the author of several books.

**Thomas Gossel, Ph.D., R.Ph.,** is a professor of pharmacology and toxicology at Ohio Northern University in Ada. He is an expert on over-the-counter products.

**Mary Ann Pane, R.N.,** is a nurse clinician in Philadelphia. She was formerly affiliated with Community Home Health Services, an agency catering to people who require skilled health care in their homes.

**Stephen Rosenberg, M.D.,** is associate professor of clinical public health at Columbia University School of Public Health in New York City. He is the author of *The Johnson & Johnson First-Aid Book.*

# FLATULENCE
## 8 Gas-Reducing Ideas

It's tough to be serious about flatulence, though we promise to try. It's tough because even the scientists who study the subject poke fun at their own research, writing of failed experiments that ended "without even a whiff of success."

Yes, the pun was intended, and, yes, it was in very bad taste, but such is the nature of this science—even at the highest levels. Consider Michael D. Levitt, M.D., one of the top researchers in the field. His peers know him as "the man who brought status to flatus and class to gas." In his own words, Dr. Levitt describes his work as "an attempt to pump some data into the field filled largely with hot air."

Hot air, perhaps, and a colorful history as well. Hippocrates investigated flatulence extensively, and ancient physicians who specialized in it became known as "pneumatists." In early American history, such great men as Benjamin Franklin taxed their minds seeking a cure for "escaped wind."

Yes, it's tough to be serious about flatulence, but we promise to try. Read on.

**Lay off the lactose.** "If you are lactose intolerant, you could have flatulence problems from eating dairy foods," says Dennis Savaiano, Ph.D. (For more tips, see Lactose Intolerance on page 366.) Lactose-intolerant people have a low intestinal level of the enzyme lactase, which is needed to digest lactose, the type of sugar found in many dairy foods.

But you don't necessarily need to

*Cures from the Kitchen*

Integrative medicine specialist Andrew Weil, M.D., notes that sugar-coated fennel seeds are served after meals in India just as Americans would have an after-dinner mint. Fennel is known as a carminative—an agent that can disperse gas from the intestinal tract, he says. The seeds can also be brewed as tea.

## Bean Cuisine: Getting the Gas Out

If you love beans and legumes but hate living with the consequences, there is a solution.

Clearly, beans and legumes cause flatulence, although the better they're cooked, the less the problem. Indeed, beans seem to lose a lot of their gas-producing properties in water. Studies show that soaking beans for 12 hours or germinating them on damp paper towels for 24 hours can significantly reduce the amount of gas-producing compounds. In fact, soaking followed by 30 minutes of pressure cooking at 15 pounds per square inch reduced the compounds by up to 90 percent in one study.

be diagnosed as lactose intolerant to have unwanted repercussions. Some people can handle only certain amounts and different kinds of milk products with comfort. If you or your doctor suspects that your favorite dairy product is causing your problem, try eating it in smaller servings or along with a meal for a day or two until you notice where gas begins to be a problem.

**Avoid gas-promoting foods.** The primary cause of flatulence is the digestive system's inability to absorb certain carbohydrates, says Samuel Klein, M.D.

Though you probably know that beans are surefire flatus producers, many people don't realize that cabbage, broccoli, Brussels sprouts, onions, cauliflower, whole wheat flour, radishes, bananas, apricots, pretzels, and many more foods can also be highly flatugenic.

**Fight off fiber-induced flatus.** "Although we often encourage fiber in the diet for digestive health, some high-fiber vegetables and fruits may increase gas," says Richard McCallum, M.D.

If you're adding fiber to your diet for health reasons, start with a small dose so that the bowel gets used to it. That lessens the increase of flatus, and doctors have found that most people's flatus production returns to normal within a few weeks of adding fiber.

**Use charcoal to help you reach your goal.** Some studies have found that activated charcoal tablets are effective in eliminating excessive gas. "Charcoal absorbs gases and may be useful for flatulence," says Dr. Klein. "It's probably the best available treatment—after appropriate dietary changes have been made and other gastroenterological diseases have been treated or ruled out." Check with your doctor if you're taking any medication, because charcoal can soak up medicine as well as gas.

**Get quick relief from popular products.** While many physicians recommend activated charcoal for relief of intestinal gas, pharmacists say that simethicone-containing products are still the most popular with consumers. Among the over-the-counter favorites: Gas-X, Extra Strength Maalox, and Maximum Strength Mylanta.

Unlike activated charcoal's absorbent action, simethicone's defoaming action relieves flatulence by dispersing and preventing the formation of mucus-surrounded gas pockets in the stomach and intestines.

**Buy Beano.** Andrew Weil, M.D., cites the food enzyme dietary supplement Beano. Available in tablets or drops, take this plant enzyme at the beginning of meals to help break down the gas-producing elements of foods such as bean, broccoli, and grains.

## PANEL OF ADVISORS

**Samuel Klein, M.D.,** is a William H. Danforth professor of medicine and nutritional science and director of the Center for Human Nutrition at Washington University School of Medicine in St. Louis.

**Richard McCallum, M.D.,** is a professor of medicine and chief of the gastroenterology and hepatology division at the University of Kansas Medical Center and the Kansas City Veterans Administration Medical Center in Kansas City, Kansas.

**Dennis Savaiano, Ph.D.,** is a professor of foods and nutrition and dean of the School of Consumer and Family Sciences at Purdue University in West Lafayette, Indiana.

**Andrew Weil, M.D.,** is a clinical professor of medicine and director of the program in integrative medicine at the University of Arizona in Tucson. He is the author of several books, including *8 Weeks to Optimum Health*.

# FLU
## 20 Remedies to Beat the Bug

Getting the flu is sort of like taking a multiple-choice quiz. That's because there are three main types of influenza: A, B, and C. Within these types, though, the pesky viruses have unlimited ability to mutate into many forms.

Because the flu is a viral infection, antibiotics are powerless against it. But if you get to your doctor within the first 48 hours of symptoms, prescription antiviral drugs, such as zanamivir (Relenza) or oseltamivir (Tamiflu), may help you recover quicker. Still, the best defense is avoidance. (See "Outsmart the Flu Bug" on page 240.)

If avoidance didn't work, and you've succumbed to the bug, take these steps to help ease the symptoms.

**Stay home.** The flu is a very infectious disease that spreads like wildfire, says Thomas Gossel, Ph.D., R.Ph. So don't be a workaholic or a martyr. Stay home from

---

## WHEN TO CALL A DOCTOR

Influenza can be as deadly today as it was in 1918, when the Spanish flu killed more than 20 million people worldwide. So, says Thomas Gossel, Ph.D., R.Ph., see a doctor if:

- Your voice becomes hoarse.
- You develop pains in your chest.
- You have difficulty breathing.
- You start bringing up yellow- or green-colored phlegm.

Also be aware that prolonged vomiting can lead to dehydration, which is especially serious in the very young and in elderly people, says Mary Ann Pane, R.N. Abdominal pain may be a sign of another problem, such as appendicitis. If the pain or vomiting doesn't subside after a day, see a doctor.

# Is It Really the Flu?

How can you tell a cold from the flu? This isn't a riddle. Or maybe it is. Although similarities exist between the two illnesses—and their treatment—they're caused by entirely different viruses. The worst part of a cold might last longer, but the flu generally causes more discomfort. Here, according to Thomas Gossel, Ph.D., R.Ph., is a comparison of common symptoms and the differences between them, depending on whether they are caused by a cold or the flu.

*Fever.* Prominent with flu, coming on suddenly; rare with a cold.

*Headache.* Prominent with flu; rare with a cold.

*General aches.* Prominent and often severe with flu; slight with a cold.

*Fatigue.* Extreme with flu, lasting 2 to 3 weeks; mild with a cold.

*Runny nose.* Occasional with the flu; common with a cold.

*Sore throat.* Occasional with the flu; common with a cold.

*Cough.* Common and possibly severe with the flu; mild to moderate hacking cough with a cold.

work—and anywhere else—until at least 1 day after your temperature returns to normal. And keep your children home from school until they have fully recovered.

**Get some rest.** You shouldn't have much trouble following this advice, since you're probably too sick to do much else. Bed rest is essential, says Dr. Gossel, because it lets your body put its energy into combating the flu infection. Being active while you're still quite ill weakens your defenses and leaves you open to complications.

**Drink up.** Liquids are especially important to prevent dehydration if you have a fever. In addition, fluids can provide needed nutrients when you're too sick to eat. Thin soups are good, as are fruit and vegetable juices. Nutrition counselor Eleonore Blaurock-Busch, Ph.D., advises drinking juices that are rich in vitamins and minerals.

Jay Swedberg, M.D., recommends diluting fruit juice with water. "A little sugar provides necessary glucose, but too much can cause diarrhea when you're ill," he says. "Also dilute ginger ale and other sugar-sweetened soft drinks. And allow them to go flat before drinking, because their bubbles can create gas in the stomach and make you more nauseated."

**Reach for pain relief.** Aspirin, acetaminophen, or ibuprofen can reduce the fever, headache, and body aches that so often accompany the flu. Follow label instructions. Because symptoms are often most pronounced in the afternoon and evening, take the medication regularly over this period says Dr. Gossel.

Children and teenagers should not take aspirin without their doctor's consent first, he warns.

**Think twice about what you take.** Over-the-counter cold medicines may give you some temporary relief of symptoms, says Dr. Gossel. Those with antihistamines, for instance, can dry up a runny nose. But be careful—these drugs may suppress your symptoms to the point where you feel better. Prematurely resuming your normal activities can bring on a relapse or trigger serious complications.

**Do something sweet.** Sucking on hard candy and lozenges keeps your throat moist so it feels better, says Mary Ann Pane, R.N. If you're concerned about the calories these products contain, look for sugar-free brands. They're just as effective.

**Humidify the air.** Raising the humidity in your bedroom also helps reduce the discomfort of a cough, sore throat, or dry nasal passages. "A humidifier or vaporizer may also be helpful if there is chest congestion or nasal stuffiness," says Calvin Thrash, M.D.

**Pamper your nose.** If you've been blowing your nose a lot, it's probably pretty sore. So lubricate your nostrils frequently to decrease irritation, says Pane. A product such as K-Y Jelly is preferable to petroleum jelly, which dries out quickly.

**Take some heat.** One characteristic of the flu is tired, achy muscles. Warm them and ease their pain with a warm bath or heating pad, says Pane.

**Warm your feet.** Soaking your feet in hot water may help if you have a headache or nasal congestion, says Dr. Thrash. The warm water helps widen blood vessels, thereby diverting blood-flow from your head to your feet, which relieves congestion.

**Breathe fresh air.** Make sure your sickroom has a good supply of fresh air at all times, says Dr. Thrash. But avoid a draft. Prevent chills by using warm, close-fitting bedclothes.

**Get rubbed the right way.** A back rub may help activate your immune system to fight the flu, says Dr. Thrash. And it's very comforting.

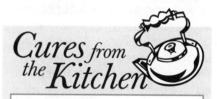

## Cures from the Kitchen

A sore or scratchy throat is apt to accompany the flu. Get some relief—and wash out any secretions collecting in your throat—by gargling with a salt-water solution, says Mary Ann Pane, R.N. Dissolve 1 teaspoon of salt in 1 cup of warm water. This concentration approximates the pH level of body tissues and is very soothing, she says. Use as often as needed, but do not swallow the liquid because it's very high in sodium.

**Eat lightly and wisely.** During the worst phase of the flu, you probably won't have an appetite at all. But when you're ready to make the transition from liquids to more substantial fare, put the emphasis on bland, starchy foods, says Dr. Swedberg. "Dry toast is fine. So are bananas, applesauce, boiled rice, rice pud-

## Outsmart the Flu Bug

Individual immunity and the particular strain of flu virus circulating in a given year play a large role in determining who will knuckle under to the flu. Still, there are steps you can take to reduce your susceptibility to this virulent bug.

**Get a flu shot.** Every year, scientists develop a vaccine against the most recently circulating strain of the virus. So the best thing you can do to protect yourself against flu is to be vaccinated in October or earlier if you're at high risk, says epidemiologist Suzanne Gaventa. She particularly advises shots for residents of nursing homes; those with chronic conditions such as heart or kidney disease, asthma or other ongoing lung problems, or a weakened immune system; anyone over 65; and most medical personnel. All other groups, including household members of high-risk persons, healthy persons ages 50 to 64, and others who wish to decrease their risk of influenza infection, should begin vaccination in November.

In cases where the shot doesn't prevent the flu, it considerably lessens the disease's severity. Don't wait until the flu's in town before acting, because the vaccine takes about 2 weeks to work. And don't get a flu shot at all if you're allergic to eggs—the vaccine is made from them.

**Avoid crowds.** Because the virus spreads easily, stay away from movies, theaters, shopping centers, and other crowded places during an epidemic, says Thomas Gossel, Ph.D., R.Ph. And keep your distance from sneezing or coughing people, even if it means getting off an elevator or giving up a seat on the bus.

**Come in from the cold.** Prolonged exposure to wet and cold weather lowers your resistance and increases your risk of infection.

**Give up bad habits.** Smoking and alcohol can also impair your resistance. Smoking, in particular, injures the respiratory tract and makes you more susceptible to the flu, Dr. Gossel says.

**Kiss at your own risk.** Kissing is an efficient way for the flu to spread, says Dr. Gossel. Just sleeping in the same room with a sick spouse is asking for trouble. So, if possible, move to another room for the duration.

**Keep up your strength.** Don't get tired or run-down. Paint the living room, clean the attic, or build a basement playroom *some other time*, not during flu season.

ding, cooked cereal, and baked potatoes, which can be topped with yogurt." For a refreshing dessert, peel and freeze very ripe bananas, then puree them in a food processor.

## PANEL OF ADVISORS

**Eleonore Blaurock-Busch, Ph.D.,** is associate laboratory director of King James Medical Laboratory and Trace Minerals International, both in Cleveland. She is also the director of Micro Trace Minerals in Hersbruck, Germany, cochairman of the International Association of Trace Elements and Cancer, and author of several books.

**Suzanne Gaventa** is an epidemiologist formerly in the division of viral diseases at the Centers for Disease Control and Prevention in Atlanta.

**Thomas Gossel, Ph.D., R.Ph.,** is a professor of pharmacology and toxicology at Ohio Northern University in Ada. He is an expert on over-the-counter products.

**Mary Ann Pane, R.N.,** is a nurse clinician in Philadelphia. She was formerly affiliated with Community Home Health Services, an agency catering to people who require skilled health care in their homes.

**Jay Swedberg, M.D.,** is a family practitioner at the Family Health Care, P.C., in Casper, Wyoming.

**Calvin Thrash, M.D.,** was the founder of Uchee Pines Institute, a nonprofit health education facility in Seale, Alabama. He was also coauthor of *Breast Cancer: Causes, Prevention, and Treatment.*

**Donald Vickery, M.D.,** is president of the Center for Corporate Health Promotion in Reston, Virginia. He is also assistant clinical professor of family medicine and community medicine at Georgetown University School of Medicine in Washington, D.C., and associate clinical professor of family medicine at Virginia Commonwealth University School of Medicine in Richmond. He is the coauthor of *Take Care of Yourself.*

# FOOD POISONING
## 25 Solutions for Food Flu

With frequent headlines to remind us of *Campylobacter* bacteria lurking in meat, *Escherichia coli* outbreaks from unpasteurized cider, and salmonella poisoning from eggs, it's hard to think of food as safe.

Raw or undercooked meat or poultry, improperly washed fruits and vegetables, sun-warmed potato salad, and a host of other foods can harbor microscopic organisms capable of triggering potentially life-threatening cases of food poisoning. Despite well-publicized guidelines about food safety and inspections at restaurants and food-processing centers, government researchers estimate that Americans have 76 million foodborne illnesses each year, sending 325,000 people to the hospital and killing 5,000 in the United States.

Even non-life-threatening cases of food poisoning can make you feel miserable, resulting in dizziness, queasiness, diarrhea, vomiting, abdominal cramps, headache, and fever.

Toxic bacteria get into food in a variety of ways, generally as a result of inadequate cooking or processing.

In any case, once inside you, these bad bugs attack your intestines. For a day or so, you feel wretched as your body tries to battle back. Here's what the experts say to do to help your body fight a case of food "flu."

**Fill up on fluids.** The bacteria irritate your intestinal tract and trigger a great deal of fluid loss from diarrhea, vomiting, or both. Drink lots of fluids to prevent dehydration. Water is best, followed by other clear liquids such as apple juice, broth, or bouillon.

Soft drinks are okay, too, if you drink them flat, says Vincent F. Garagusi, M.D. Otherwise, the carbonation can further irritate your stomach. Defizzed Coca-Cola, for reasons yet to be determined, has an added bonus of settling your stomach. Get the bubbles out of soft drinks quickly by pouring the soda back and forth between two glasses, he suggests.

**Sip a little, slowly.** Trying to gulp down too much at once may trigger more vomiting, says Dr. Garagusi.

## WHEN TO CALL A DOCTOR

With a normal case of food poisoning, the symptoms—cramps, nausea, vomiting, diarrhea, and dizziness—disappear in a day or two. But for the very young, the elderly, or someone with a chronic health condition or immune disorder, food poisoning can be very serious. Those people should contact a doctor at the first signs of food poisoning.

Even if you don't fall into one of those categories, call a doctor immediately if your symptoms are also accompanied by:

- Difficulty swallowing, speaking, or breathing; changes in vision; muscle weakness or paralysis, particularly if this occurs after eating mushrooms, canned food, or shellfish
- Fever over 100°F
- Severe vomiting—meaning you can't hold down even any liquids
- Severe diarrhea for more than a day or two
- Persistent, localized abdominal pain
- Dehydration—you have extreme thirst, a dry mouth, or decreased urination, and when you pinch the back of your hand, the skin stays pinched
- Bloody diarrhea

**Replenish electrolytes.** Vomiting and diarrhea can flush out important electrolytes—potassium, sodium, and glucose. Experts suggest that you replace them by sipping commercially prepared electrolyte products like Gatorade. Or try this rehydration recipe: Mix fruit juice (for potassium) with ½ teaspoon of honey or corn syrup (for glucose) and a pinch of table salt (for sodium).

**Save the antacids for heartburn.** They can reduce the acids in your stomach and weaken your defense against bacteria. If you take an antacid, it's possible that the bacteria could multiply in greater numbers and more rapidly.

**Don't interfere with progress.** Your body is trying to flush the toxic organism out, explains Daniel Rodrigue, M.D. In some cases, taking antidiarrheal products (like Imodium, Kaopectate, or Lomotil) may interfere with your body's ability to fight the infection. So stay away from them and let nature take its course. If you feel it's necessary to take something, consult your doctor first.

**Reintroduce bland foods.** Usually within a few hours to a day after the diarrhea and vomiting have subsided, you'll be ready for some "real" food. But go easy. Your stomach has been attacked; it's weak and irritated. Experts suggest starting with easily digestible foods. Try cereal, pudding, soda crackers, or

*(continued on page 246)*

# Don't Let It Happen Again!

You can't always blame the diner across town for your stomach troubles. The truth is, says Daniel Rodrigue, M.D., many cases of food poisoning probably come from carelessness in your own home. Despite a 25 percent drop in the number of *Escherichia coli* infections and a 41 percent drop in shigella infections on account of improved government food-safety programs, foodborne illnesses demand consistent vigilance.

Follow these commonsense rules to significantly decrease your chances of poisoning yourself.

- Wash your hands with warm water and soap for at least 20 seconds before and after preparing food to avoid passing on bacteria such as staphylococcus. This is especially important before and after handling raw meat and eggs. If you have an infection or a cut on your hands, wear plastic or rubber gloves. Be sure to wash your gloved hands just as often as you would wash your bare hands.

- Heat or chill raw food. Bacteria can't multiply above 150°F or below 40°F.

- Don't leave food at room temperature for more than 2 hours, and avoid eating anything that you suspect may have been unrefrigerated for that long. Bacteria thrive in warm protein food made with meat or eggs, cream-filled pastries, dips, potato salad, and so forth.

- Raw food can harbor bacteria. Don't eat raw protein food like fish, fowl, meat, or eggs. Avoid sushi, oysters on the half shell, Caesar salad made with raw eggs, and unpasteurized eggnog. Don't use eggs if they have hairline cracks—harmful salmonella bacteria may have already set up shop. Don't sample raw cookie dough that you've made with eggs. (Commercially prepared cookie dough, however, is not a food hazard.)

- Don't buy cooked seafood, such as shrimp, if it's displayed in the same case as raw fish.

- Buy fresh seafood only from reputable dealers where the products are kept properly refrigerated or on ice.

- If you are a recreational fisher and you eat your catch, follow state and local government announcements about fishing areas and frequency of consumption.

- Cook meat until a meat thermometer inserted into the thickest part registers 160°F and the pink disappears, chicken with bone in until thermometer registers 170°F and there are no red joints, chicken without bone until thermometer registers 160°F, turkey breast until thermometer registers 170°F, other turkey (ground or whole) until thermometer registers 165°F, and fish until it flakes easily. Complete cooking is the only way to ensure that all potentially harmful bacteria have been killed.

- Don't taste-test foods before they're cooked, especially pork, fish, and eggs.

- Don't let raw meat juice drip onto other food. It can taint otherwise harmless food.

- Use a separate chopping board and utensils when handling raw meat, and sanitize them with hot, soapy water and bleach solution after use to prevent cross-contamination.

- Scrub fruits and vegetables thoroughly. Peel nonorganic produce like cucumbers and remove the outer leaves of leafy vegetables.

- Scrub can openers and countertops and always clean out crevices to prevent bacteria from hiding there. For all areas that come in contact with food, use hot water and soap then a bleach solution.

- Replace sponges often and use paper towels to wipe off counters.

- Thaw meat in the refrigerator. Or thaw it in the microwave and cook it immediately after it's thawed. Bacteria can multiply on food surfaces while the center is still frozen. When using the microwave to defrost, follow the instructions and leave at least 2 inches of space around the item to allow air to circulate.

- Immediately refrigerate leftovers, even if they are still hot. Cool down large stews faster by refrigerating in smaller portions.

- Never pick and eat wild mushrooms. Some carry toxins that attack the nervous system and can be deadly. Picking wild mushrooms should be left for the experts.

- Never taste home-canned food before boiling for 20 minutes. If not properly canned, food contains bacteria that can produce a dangerous toxin.

- Use common sense and don't taste any food that doesn't smell or look right. Avoid cracked jars or swollen, dented cans or lids, clear liquids that have turned milky, or cans or jars that spurt or have an "off" odor when opened. They could contain dangerous bacteria. Make sure you discard them carefully so that pets don't come in contact with them.

broth. Avoid high-fiber, spicy, acidic, greasy, sugary, or dairy foods that could further irritate the stomach. Do this for a day or two. After that, your stomach will be ready to get back to its routine.

## PANEL OF ADVISORS

**Vincent F. Garagusi, M.D.,** is professor emeritus of medicine and microbiology and former director of the Infectious Disease Service at Georgetown University Hospital in Washington, D.C.

**Daniel C. Rodrigue, M.D.,** is an infectious disease specialist at Lexington Infectious Disease Consultants in Lexington, Kentucky.

# FOOT ACHES
## 16 Feet Treats

The American Podiatric Medical Association reports that an overwhelming majority of Americans—75 percent—experience problems with their feet at some point during their lifetimes.

It's no wonder, considering the complexity of the foot. Each foot contains 26 bones, 33 joints, 107 ligaments, 19 muscles, and many tendons that hold the foot together and help it move in various directions. The average person takes 8,000 to 10,000 steps a day, at times putting so much pressure on the feet that it exceeds his or her body weight.

Amazingly, it's not really the workout that batters feet, it's most often a combination of ill-fitting shoes and neglect. Fortunately, much can be done to ease foot pain. Here's what our experts recommend.

**Elevate your feet.** The best thing you can do for your feet when you get home is to sit down, put your feet up, and exercise your toes to get the circulation going again, says Gilbert Wright, M.D. Elevate your feet at a 45-degree angle to your body and relax for 20 minutes.

**Soak them in salts.** A tried-and-true foot revitalizer is to soak your feet in a basin of warm water containing 1 to 2 tablespoons of Epsom salts, says Mark D. Sussman, D.P.M. Rinse with clear, cool water, then pat your feet dry and massage with a moisturizing gel or cream.

## WHEN TO CALL A DOCTOR

According to Mark D. Sussman, D.P.M., you should definitely see a doctor if:

- You have pain in your feet that continually increases during the day.
- Your feet get to the point where you can't keep your shoes on.
- You have trouble walking first thing in the morning.

Also be aware that painful burning in the feet can be a sign of poor circulation, athlete's foot, a pinched nerve, diabetes, anemia, thyroid disease, alcoholism, or other problems, and always warrants a call to the doctor.

**Run hot and cold.** Dr. Sussman recommends this treatment, popular at European spas. Sit on the edge of the bathtub and hold your feet under running water for several minutes. Alternate 1 minute of comfortably hot water with 1 minute of cold, repeating several times and ending with the cold. The contrasting bath will invigorate your whole system. If you have a shower-massage attachment, use it for an even more stimulating workout.

If you have diabetes or impaired circulation, however, don't expose your feet to extremes of temperature.

**Massage away your aches.** "A really nice thing is to have somebody massage your feet with baby oil," says Dr. Sussman.

If you can't find a willing partner, either before or during a soak, says aromatherapist Judith Jackson, give yourself a nice little foot massage. Work over the whole foot, squeezing the toes gently, then pressing in a circular motion over the bottom of your foot. One really effective movement is to slide your thumb as hard as you can in the arch of the foot.

**Get relief on ice.** Another way to refresh tired feet is to wrap a few ice cubes in a wet washcloth, then rub it over your feet and ankles for a few minutes. Ice acts to relieve any inflammation, and it also serves as a mild anesthetic, says Neal Kramer, D.P.M. Then dry your feet and swab them with witch hazel, cologne, alcohol, or vinegar for a cooling and drying effect.

**Exercise.** We don't mean aerobics or any other heavy-duty activity. But many doctors recommend that you exercise your feet and leg muscles throughout the day to ward off aches and keep the circulation going. Try these ideas from experts at the Kinney Shoe Corporation.

- If your feet feel tense and cramped anytime during the day, give them a good shake, as you would your hands if they felt cramped. Do one foot at a time, then relax and flex your toes up and down.

- If you must stand for long periods of time, walk in place whenever you can. Keep changing your stance, and try to rest one foot on a stool or step occasionally. If possible, stand on carpeting or a spongy rubber mat.

- To relieve stiffness, remove your shoes, sit in a chair, and stretch your feet out in front of you. Circle both feet from the ankles 10 times in one direction, then 10 times in the other. Point your toes down as far as possible, then flex them up as high as you can. Repeat 10 times. Now grasp your toes and gently pull them back and forth.

- For a nice mini-massage, remove your shoes and roll each foot over a golf ball, tennis ball, or rolling pin for a minute or two.

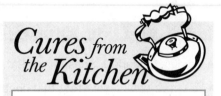

## Cures from the Kitchen

Pour a cup for yourself to drink if you'd like, but soaking your foot in tea can be very soothing. Aromatherapist Judith Jackson suggests brewing a strong peppermint or chamomile tea. Steep four tea bags in 2 cups of boiling water. Add the brew to 1 gallon of hot water. Soak your feet for 5 minutes. Slosh your feet in the water and let the tea's warm scent relax you. Then drain the water and pour some cold water over your feet. Follow that with hot water from the tap and then more cold.

**Save your soles.** Try wearing shoes with thick, shock-absorbing soles to shield your feet from rough surfaces and hard pavements. Don't let your soles become too thin or worn, because they won't do the job they're supposed to do. Women's thin-soled, pointy-toed high heels are classic villains, says Dr. Wright. If you must dress up for work, ease foot strain by wearing walking or athletic shoes to and from the job and switching to heels at the office.

**Change heel heights.** Wearing high heels tightens the calf muscles, which leads to foot fatigue, says John E. Waller Jr., M.D. So changing heel heights from high to low during the day is an excellent idea.

**Wear insoles.** High heels have the added disadvantage of causing your foot to pitch forward as you walk, putting painful pressure on the ball of your foot, says Dr. Waller. To prevent this discomfort, wear a half-insole to help keep your foot in place. And be sure to take the insoles with you to the shoe store to ensure that they'll fit comfortably in your new shoes.

**Shoe-shop in the afternoon.** Since your feet expand during the day, you should buy shoes with enough space to accommodate the slight swelling. Measure your feet while standing, and always try on both shoes. If one foot is a bit larger than the other, buy the pair that feels best on the bigger foot, advises the American Podiatric Medical Association.

**Stretch your shoes.** When you add insoles to shoes you already have, says Dr. Sussman, make sure they don't cramp your toes. If things are tight, you may be able to stretch the shoes to accommodate the insoles. Fill a sock with sand, stuff it into the shoe's toebox, and wrap the shoe with a wet towel. Let it dry out over the next 24 hours. Repeat once or twice, if needed.

## PANEL OF ADVISORS

**Judith Jackson** is a health and beauty consultant in Greenwich, Connecticut. She is also a certified aromatherapist with a degree in massage and aromatherapy.

**Neal Kramer, D.P.M.,** is a podiatrist in Bethlehem, Pennsylvania.

**Mark D. Sussman, D.P.M.,** is a retired podiatrist who formerly practiced in Wheaton, Maryland.

**John F. Waller Jr., M.D.,** is an orthopedic surgeon specializing in the foot and ankle. He is attending surgeon in orthopedic surgery at Lenox Hill Hospital in New York City.

**Gilbert Wright, M.D.,** was an orthopedic surgeon in Sacramento, California, and spokesman for the American Orthopedic Foot and Ankle Society. He was also director of the Sacramento Orthopedic Foot Clinic.

# Foot Odor
## 16 Deodorizing Secrets

Every parent who has chaperoned a trip to the ice-skating or roller rink recognizes it instantly. Twenty-five little boys and little girls take off their shoes to reveal socks that, ahem, should have been laundered two outfits ago. It's ripe, the smell of 50 little perspiring feet. Riper than that piece of Limburger that fell behind the sofa last month.

Doctors don't have to look far for the cause of foot odor. Bacteria feed on the dead skin beneath our socks, producing the characteristic stench. Exercising, wearing shoes that don't breathe—anything that makes the feet moist—can make the odor worse.

Canceling trips to the skating rink won't remedy the problem. The key to eliminating foot odor is good foot hygiene.

**Wash—often.** Keep your feet scrupulously clean. Use warm, soapy water and wash your feet as often as needed—several times a day if you perspire a lot or notice an odor. Scrub gently with a soft brush, even between your toes, and be sure to dry your feet thoroughly.

**Powder your toes.** After washing, apply foot powder, cornstarch, or an antifungal spray. Another good method for keeping feet cool and dry is to treat your shoes—sprinkle the insides with talcum powder or cornstarch, says Suzanne M. Levine, D.P.M.

**Use an antiperspirant.** The key to controlling odor is to use either an antiperspirant or a deodorant on your feet. You can buy foot deodorants or simply use your underarm brand. Keep in mind that deodorants eliminate odor, but they don't stop perspiration. Antiperspirants take care of both problems. Dr. Levine recommends products that contain aluminum chloride hexahydrate.

Don't use an antiperspirant if you have active athlete's foot lesions (see page 40 for signs and symptoms of athlete's foot), says Stephen Weinberg, D.P.M., because it will sting. "In addition, I recommend roll-on products rather than

## Do Your Feet Work Harder Than You Do?

Sometimes feet perspire a lot because they simply *work* harder than they should, says Neal Kramer, D.P.M. A structural defect (such as flat feet) or a job that keeps you hopping all day could be the underlying culprit. Either would increase the activity of your foot muscles. And the harder your feet work, the more they perspire in an attempt to cool themselves.

Although feet that perspire don't necessarily smell bad, the wetness is an open invitation for odor-producing bacteria.

"If you correct the underlying problem with an arch support or some other orthotic shoe insert," says Dr. Kramer, "you can actually cut down on the amount of sweat produced. If the muscles don't have to work as hard, they just don't give off as much heat."

sprays because most of a spray's antiperspirant action is lost in the air," he says. "Use the product two or three times a day in the beginning, then gradually cut back to once a day."

**Change your socks—often.** The answer to sweaty, smelly feet is to change socks as frequently as possible—even three or four times a day, says Glenn Copeland, D.P.M. Wear socks made of natural fibers, such as cotton, which are far more absorbent than socks made from synthetic materials.

**Show shoe sense.** "Closed shoes aggravate sweaty feet and set up a perfect environment for bacteria to grow, leading to more odor and more sweat," says Dr. Levine. Choose sandals and open-toed shoes when appropriate, but stay away from rubber and plastic shoes, which don't allow feet to breathe easily. And never wear the same shoes 2 days in a row. It takes at least 24 hours for shoes to dry out thoroughly.

**Sleep on it.** Mark D. Sussman, D.P.M., recommends this nighttime treatment to help dry feet: Wash your feet thoroughly with rubbing alcohol to dry and cool them. Then apply a heavy-duty deodorant such as Mitchum to the bottom of each foot. Cover the foot with plastic wrap to induce sweating so that the deodorant can penetrate the foot better. Pull a sock over the wrap and sleep with it on. In the morning, wash off the excess deodorant. Repeat every night for 1 week, then once or twice a week as needed.

**Take frequent soaks.** Various soaking agents can help keep the feet dry, which may also control odor.

***Tea.*** Tannin, which can be found in tea bags, is a drying agent. Boil three or four tea bags in 1 quart of water for about 10 minutes, then add enough cold water to make a comfortable soak, suggests Diana Bihova, M.D.

Soak your feet for 20 to 30 minutes, then dry them and apply foot powder. Do this twice a day until you get the problem under control. After that, repeat it twice a week to keep odor from recurring.

***Sodium bicarbonate.*** This makes the foot surface more acidic, thereby cutting down on the amount of odor produced, says Dr. Levine. Dissolve 1 tablespoon of baking soda in 1 quart of water. Soak twice a week for about 15 minutes a time.

***Vinegar.*** Another acid footbath that Dr. Levine recommends is ½ cup of vinegar in 1 quart of water. Soak for 15 minutes twice a week.

***Hot and cold water.*** Alternate hot and cold footbaths, says Dr. Levine. This procedure constricts the bloodflow to your feet, reducing perspiration. Then fix yourself a third footbath of ice cubes and lemon juice. Finally, rub your feet with alcohol to cool and dry them. In hot weather, when your feet perspire a lot, you could probably do this every day.

*Warning:* People with diabetes and those with impaired circulation should not use this treatment.

**Heed sage advice.** Europeans sometimes sprinkle the fragrant herb sage into their shoes to control odor, says Dr. Levine. Perhaps a dash of dry, crumbled sage leaves will do the trick.

**Try inserts.** Some shoe inserts, such as Odor-Eaters, contain activated charcoal, which absorbs moisture and helps control odor. Dr. Levine says that these products have helped some of her patients.

**Stay cool.** The sweat glands in your feet, similar to those in your armpits and palms, respond to emotions, says Richard L. Dobson, M.D. Stress can trigger excessive sweating. That, in turn, can increase bacterial activity in your shoes, leading to extra odor. So try not to get frazzled.

**Watch what you eat.** As bizarre as it may sound, says Dr. Levine, when you eat spicy or pungent foods (such as onions, peppers, garlic, or scallions), the essence of these odors can be excreted through the sweat glands on your feet. So, yes, your feet can end up smelling like your lunch.

## PANEL OF ADVISORS

**Diana Bihova, M.D.,** is a dermatologist affiliated with the dermatology department at the Columbia University College of Physicians and Surgeons in New York City.

**Glenn Copeland, D.P.M.,** is a podiatrist at the Women's College Hospital in Toronto. He is also consulting podiatrist for the Canadian Back Institute and podiatrist for the Toronto Blue Jays baseball team.

**Richard L. Dobson, M.D.,** is a professor emeritus of the department of dermatology at the Medical University of South Carolina College of Medicine in Charleston.

**Frederick Hass, M.D.,** is a general practitioner in San Rafael, California. He is on the staff of Marin General Hospital in Greenbrae.

**Neal Kramer, D.P.M.,** is a podiatrist in Bethlehem, Pennsylvania.

**Suzanne M. Levine, D.P.M., P.C.,** is a podiatrist and a podiatric attending physician at New York–Presbyterian Hospital. She is the author of *Your Feet Don't Have to Hurt.*

**Mark D. Sussman, D.P.M.,** is a retired podiatrist who formerly practiced in Wheaton, Maryland.

**Stephen Weinberg, D.P.M.,** is director of the running clinic at the Weil Foot and Ankle Institute in Des Plaines, Illinois, and director of podiatric services for the Chicago Marathon.

# FROSTBITE
## 19 Safeguards against the Cold

When Tod Schimelpfenig was 18, he and a friend wanted a winter adventure. So they went hiking and mountain climbing in the northern Vermont wilderness.

"We were out trying to be mountaineers and ended up going to the school of hard knocks," Schimelpfenig says now, 30 years later.

Schimelpfenig, in fact, took an advanced course in frostbite. The toes of his right foot turned white and hard. "They looked like a frozen steak," he recalls with a laugh.

Of course, he wasn't laughing then. Fortunately, he and his companion found a place to camp for the night, and he was able to stay off the frozen foot for a while. To prevent even more serious injury, he had to make sure that the foot didn't thaw and refreeze. So while keeping the rest of his body in a warm sleeping bag, he kept the frostbitten foot outside the bag and frozen. And he had to stay awake all night to do it.

## WHEN TO CALL A DOCTOR

Frostbite demands professional medical attention. Tissue is dying. And that opens the door to some dark possibilities—infection and loss of fingers or toes, and in extreme cases, loss of an arm or leg.

With deep frostbite, the skin is cold, hard, white, and numb. When rewarmed, the skin may turn blue or purple. It also may swell, and blisters might form. The idea, of course, is to treat frostbite quickly and effectively so none of that happens. Here's what you should do while you wait for medical attention.

**Do not allow a frostbitten part to refreeze.** "Never," emphasizes Ruth Uphold, M.D. "The water crystals are bigger when the part refreezes, which causes even more tissue damage."

**Use your head to save your foot.** It's not advisable to walk on frozen feet, but it's better than allowing a frozen foot to thaw and refreeze. If you think walking may be your only route to survival, leave your shoe or boot on the frostbitten foot, says Bruce Paton, M.D. "The foot could blister and swell if you take it off, and you wouldn't be able to get the boot back on."

"I walked out 8 miles the next morning, and I was fine," he says. "I still have all my toes."

Schimelpfenig, who is now safety and training manager for the National Outdoor Leadership School in Lander, Wyoming, and a volunteer emergency medical technician, admits he put himself in a dangerous situation. Yet less severe forms of frostbite can occur quickly in very cold weather when you're simply shoveling snow or changing a tire.

So here's what you need to know about frostbite—from treating mild pain on the tip of your nose to preventing it in the first place.

**Know the signs.** Frostnip is the least severe form of frostbite and typically leaves skin somewhat numb and white.

The cheeks, tip of the nose, and ears are most frequently frostnipped, says Bruce Paton, M.D. Peeling and blistering, he adds, are also possible after the affected area is warmed.

Peeling and blistering after warming are more likely with superficial frostbite, a more serious condition. Frostbite is an injury in which the tissues of the body freeze, causing damage to the tissue. The skin is also frozen harder than with frostnip, but not so deeply that all resiliency is lost.

"Frostbite is the body's way of trying to preserve heat by shutting down circulation to an extremity," says Ruth Uphold, M.D. "Unfortunately, as you develop frostbite," she warns, "you might not even know that you have it because of the numbness."

**Hide from the wind.** Obviously, getting out of the elements into a warm place is a good idea. But if that's impossible, at least get out of the wind—windchill factors contribute significantly to frostbite.

**Think before warming.** Don't use dry, radiant heat, such as a heat lamp or campfire, Dr. Paton says, if your skin appears to be frostbitten. Frostbitten skin is easily burned.

**Use yourself.** If you can't get inside, take advantage of your own body heat. To warm fingers and hands, for example, place them under your armpits. "Rolling yourself into a ball also makes you more energy efficient," Schimelpfenig says.

**Don't rub with snow.** "It just causes friction with the skin," Dr. Uphold says. "Plus, you lose more heat when you get extremely wet."

**Make Mom proud.** "Wear mittens instead of gloves—mittens are warmer—and wear a stocking cap to protect your ears," advises James Sturm, M.D.

**Avoid booze.** "You only *think* alcohol is warming you from the inside out. Alcohol actually causes more heat loss," says Dr. Uphold.

**Don't smoke.** Smoking decreases peripheral circulation and makes the extremities more vulnerable to frostbite, Dr. Uphold says.

**Hang loose.** To protect circulation, wear loose clothing and don't wear any jewelry on your fingers, says Schimelpfenig.

**Don't get wet.** Heat loss is greatly accelerated by contact with water, says Dr. Paton.

**Don't delay.** Schimelpfenig learned the hard, cold way. "You can get into a trap saying, 'Well, my feet or my hands are kind of cold, but I'm going to get inside in a little while anyway.' Now I make sure I can honestly say my feet and hands are still *warm.*"

**Use the "buddy system."** You watch a friend's face—specifically the ears, nose, and cheeks—for any noticeable change in color, and he does the same for you.

**Avoid contact with metal.** Just a few moments with your bare hand on a metal wrench can lead to frostbite in severe cold.

**Stay in your vehicle.** If you get stranded in your vehicle on a subfreezing night, it's best to stay put and not venture out into the unknown, says

# Another Cold-Weather Danger—Hypothermia

The human body was designed to operate at an internal temperature of 98.6°F. Just a 6.5°F drop could be enough to kill. Below 92°F, cardiac arrest can occur, says James Sturm, M.D.

Hypothermia, simply defined as low body temperature, begins in its mildest stage at about 96°F, Dr. Sturm says. Symptoms include shivering, slow pulse, lethargy, and a general decrease in alertness. If body temperature drops low enough, muscles turn rigid, and the person may lose consciousness.

Falling into an icy pond would bring on hypothermia in less than an hour, but most cases result from prolonged exposure to cold temperatures. Elderly people are at increased risk for hypothermia because their bodies regulate temperature less effectively.

If hypothermia occurs, follow these tips and get the victim to a doctor as soon as possible.

- Move the person to a warmer place.
- Wrap the person with blankets.
- Give the person warm liquids. But don't give any alcohol, Dr. Sturm says. "Alcohol just gives an artificial feeling of warmth."

Schimelpfenig. You risk developing hypothermia or an abnormal drop in body temperature. "Many of the people we've found who were stranded and tried to walk for help were dead," he says.

## PANEL OF ADVISORS

**Bruce Paton, M.D.,** is a former clinical professor of surgery at the University of Colorado in Denver.

**Tod Schimelpfenig** is director of the Rocky Mountain division of the National Outdoor Leadership School in Lander, Wyoming. He also is a volunteer emergency medical technician.

**James Sturm, M.D.,** is a former staff physician in the emergency medicine department of St. Paul–Ramsey Medical Center in Minnesota.

**Ruth Uphold, M.D.,** is medical director of the emergency department at Fletcher Allan Health Care in Burlington, Vermont.

# GENITAL HERPES
## 15 Managing Strategies

Genital herpes, herpes simplex 1 or 2, is a sexually transmitted disease that sounds dire but that, in fact, can be treated.

An attack of genital herpes looks like a red swelling on the genitals with groups of flat blisters. After the blisters burst, they develop into painful sores. Once the initial attack of herpes comes and goes (usually in 2 to 3 weeks), the virus lies dormant—a sleeping giant—most of the time. But, if the immune system is disturbed or taxed, as with an injury, fever, or even menstruation, the virus may reactivate. Subsequent attacks are usually infrequent and generally not nearly as severe as the first one. Although herpes is one of the most common sexually transmitted diseases (STDs), the blisters only recur in about 1 percent of infected people.

To limit outbreaks, try these doctor-recommended steps.

## WHEN TO CALL A DOCTOR

If you have a stubborn case of herpes or are experiencing many recurrences, you may want to consider seeing your doctor for a prescription of valacyclovir (Valtrex), a drug that reduces frequency of attacks, limits their severity, and speeds healing time. This drug, approved by the FDA in 2001, stays in the body longer than acyclovir (Zovirax), the drug doctors used to prescribe for herpes patients, so you only have to take one pill a day to fight off recurrences.

If you are having your first attack or your recurrences are frequent, or if you *believe* them to be frequent, talk to your doctor. If you are pregnant, make sure you tell your doctor that you have herpes, since the virus can infect newborns, says Stephen L. Sacks, M.D.

A strong link was once suspected between genital herpes and cervical cancer. That link is not as strong as once thought, but it's still important for women with herpes to get a yearly Pap test, says Will Whittington, M.D.

**Beef up your immune system.** Experts don't know exactly what causes the herpes virus to lie dormant for long periods and then abruptly awake to create havoc. But many think that a weakened immune system, like a drunken sheriff in an old western town, invites the little bandits to act up. However strong this connection may be, it's best for you to keep your immune system sober and armed with a well-rounded diet, lots of rest and relaxation, and regular exercise.

**Try an herbal approach.** Try echinacea to stimulate your immune system and burdock root as a gentle cleansing tonic. Here's a recipe by herbalist Aviva Romm. Toss 1 ounce of each dried herb into a quart jar. Fill it to the top with boiling water. Let the herbs steep for 4 to 8 hours, then strain the liquid. To treat an outbreak, drink 4 cups a day until the blisters disappear. To prevent recurrent outbreaks, drink ½ cup two to four times a day. You can use this infusion for up to 3 months. After that, take a 3-day break after each 27-day stretch.

**Use soap and water.** You may be inclined to bombard your newly discovered sores with everything in your medicine cabinet. As with any sores, you do need to be concerned about developing a secondary (bacterial) infection, but soap and water is all you need or want to keep the area sufficiently germ-free, says Will Whittington, M.D. You won't kill the virus with anything in your medicine cabinet anyway, and lots of things in there may make matters worse.

**Steer clear of ointments.** Genital sores need lots of air to heal. Petroleum jelly and antibiotic ointments can block this air and slow the healing process, says Stephen L. Sacks, M.D. *Never* use a cortisone cream, which can inhibit your immune system and actually encourage the virus to grow, he says.

**Warm the discomfort away.** During your primary attack or bad secondary attacks, taking a bath or shower to get warm water over the genital area three or four times a day may provide soothing relief. When you get out of the shower or bath, blow the genital area dry with a hair dryer set on low or cool, taking care not to burn yourself. The air from the dryer also proves soothing and may possibly speed up the healing process by helping the sores dry out, says Dr. Sacks.

**Wear loose-fitting cotton undies.** Since air is essential to healing, wear only underpants that allow your skin to breathe—that is, cotton, not synthetics, says Judith M. Hurst, R.N. If you wear nylon panty hose, make sure the crotch is made of cotton. If you want to wear a bathing suit without compromising fashion, consider cutting the cotton crotch out of a pair of undies and sewing it into the swimsuit, says Hurst.

**Ease painful urination.** Urination during a first herpes outbreak can bring intense pain as acidic urine passes over open sores. This is particularly true for

# The Mind/Body Connection

Why do some people carry the herpes virus for years without an attack, while others carrying the virus experience regular attacks?

The answer is largely in the mind, says Christopher W. Stout, Ph.D. "People who are more tense and depressed, carry more hostility, and are more easily aroused to anger, seem to suffer more frequent outbreaks," says Dr. Stout. "These kinds of attitudes are thought to suppress the body's immune system."

"I don't care how much research is done over the next 1,000 years, I'm convinced that stress will always be the number one factor," says Judith M. Hurst, R.N.

But if you weren't subject to stress *before* you learned you had herpes, you're certainly feeling stress now. This can create a situation in which your stress contributes to outbreaks, which contributes to stress, which . . . you get the picture.

The question is, how do you get off this roller coaster?

**Learn all that you can.** Read about herpes, speak with your doctor, try to make as much sense out of, and gain as much control over, your situation as you can, says Dr. Stout.

**Join a support group.** Every major city has one. Support groups offer camaraderie, emotional support, and a place to talk confidentially and share information, says Hurst. The American Social Health Association can help you find one in your area. Call (919) 361-8400, or look for them on the Web at www.ashastd.org.

**Consider short-term therapy.** Upon learning you have herpes, you may experience sadness, depression, anger, and guilt. A good professional psychotherapist, in only a few sessions, should be able to help you gain some perspective, says Dr. Stout.

**Learn relaxation techniques.** Find an approach that works for you, such as meditation, relaxation therapy, visualization, and biofeedback, says Dr. Stout.

women. Try directing the urine stream away from your sores with a bit of rolled-up toilet tissue, suggests Dr. Sacks.

**Don't touch.** Although the disease is called *genital* herpes, it is possible, though not very common, to pass the virus to other parts of the body by touching an open sore and then bringing your fingers into contact with, say, your mouth or eyes. For this reason, it's important to wash your hands if you touch a sore, says Mitch Herndon, program manager of the Herpes Resource Center and National Herpes Hotline at the American Social Health Association (ASHA). If you think you might scratch at night, cover your sores with protective, breathable material such as gauze, he says.

**Consider these supplements.** The amino acid lysine healed sores and prevented their recurrence in laboratory studies at UCLA in Los Angeles. Other potential supplements that may fight off herpes attacks include zinc, in ointment form or capsules, or the food additive butylated hydroxytoluene (BHT), taken as a supplement. But despite mixed studies on their effectiveness, these two are unproven remedies, say most doctors. If you decide to try either, know that high dosages may be dangerous and should only be taken under a doctor's supervision.

**Call for help.** If you have any questions regarding your condition, help is available, says Herndon. ASHA runs two hotlines that offer free advice to people with herpes. Call the National Herpes Hotline at (919) 361-8488, Monday through Friday, 9:00 A.M. to 7:00 P.M. (Eastern time); or the STD Hotline at (800) 227-8922, 24 hours a day and 7 days a week. ASHA also offers an e-mail response service, herpesnet@ashastd.org, where you can write in with your questions about herpes. Or just go to the ASHA Web site, www.ashastd.org.

**Don't do unto others.** Remember how you got herpes. You now have a responsibility to protect others. When you have sores, you are highly contagious—so avoid sex. When sores are not present, you probably will not pass the virus, but you may wish to use a condom for further protection and peace of mind. Incidentally, because you already have herpes doesn't mean you can't catch another form of it. Although this doesn't happen often, genital herpes can recur with more than one strain of virus, says Dr. Sacks.

## PANEL OF ADVISORS

**Mitch Herndon** is the program manager at the Herpes Resource Center and the National Herpes Hotline at the American Social Health Association (ASHA) in Research Triangle Park, North Carolina.

**Judith M. Hurst, R.N.,** is medical advisor to Toledo HELP, a support group for people with herpes in the Toledo, Ohio, area. She is also a retired obstetric nurse.

**Aviva Romm** is a certified professional midwife, herbalist and professional member of the American Herbalists Guild who practices in Bloomfield Hills, Michigan and is coauthor of *Naturally Healthy Babies & Children: A Commonsense Guide to Herbal Remedies.*

**Stephen L. Sacks, M.D.,** is a professor of medicine at the University of British Columbia and the founder and president of the Viridae Clinic, both in Vancouver. He is also the founder and former director of the UBC Herpes Clinic. A renowned expert on the management of genital herpes, he is the author of *The Truth about Herpes.*

**C. Norman Shealy, M.D., Ph.D.,** heads the Shealy Wellness Center in Springfield, Missouri. He is also a professor of energy medicine at Holos University Graduate Seminary, the founding president of the American Holistic Medical Association, and the author of such books as *Sacred Healing* and *Holy Water, Sacred Oil.*

**Christopher W. Stout, Ph.D.,** has a private practice near Denver and is a clinical psychologist specializing in psychoneuroimmunology (the study of the connection between the immune system and human emotions). He is also an industrial consultant.
**Will Whittington, M.D.,** was a research investigator with the division of sexually transmitted diseases at the Centers for Disease Control and Prevention in Atlanta.

# GINGIVITIS
## 21 Ways to Stop Gum Disease

A survey reported in the *Journal of the American Dental Association* found that a majority of adults have gingivitis, the first sign of periodontal disease and the major reason adults lose their teeth.

Gingivitis is simply inflammation of the gums. The gums' usual pale pink color turns bluish red. The tender gums swell between the teeth and bleed easily, especially during toothbrushing. Caused by plaque and tartar above and below the gumline, gingivitis, if left unchecked, can lead to periodontitis, in which pus collects in deep pockets of the gum, teeth become sensitive to pressure, loosen, and fall out.

But don't despair. Dentists have much to offer that will keep the false teeth away.

**Brush right.** If you want to get rid of gingivitis, you have to take time to floss and brush correctly. Block out 3 to 5 minutes two or three times a day for good oral hygiene, says Robert Schallhorn, D.D.S.

**Brush at the gumline.** The plaque-catching area around the gumline is where gingivitis starts, and it is the most neglected area when we brush, says Vincent Cali, D.D.S. Place your brush at a 45-degree angle to your teeth so that half of your brush cleans your gums while the other half cleans your teeth. Then shimmy your brush by moving it in a forward and backward motion.

**Have two toothbrushes.** Alternate between them, advises Dr. Cali. Allow one to dry while using the other.

**Choose your toothbrush.** Although studies show that using an electric toothbrush improves oral health, the American Dental Association reports that

## WHEN TO CALL A DOCTOR

You can risk more serious periodontal disease and the possible loss of your teeth if you ignore sore, bleeding gums. The warning signs to make an appointment with your dentist are:

- You have bad breath that doesn't go away within 24 hours.
- Your teeth look longer—a result of your gums shrinking away from your teeth.
- Your mouth feels out of alignment when you shut it because your teeth come together differently.
- Your partial dentures fit differently.
- Pus pockets form between your teeth and gums.
- Your teeth are loose or fall out.

Also, if your gums still bleed when you brush your teeth and continue to be sore and swollen despite your efforts at good oral hygiene, see your dentist again.

manual toothbrushes are just as effective. As long as you're brushing properly, it doesn't matter which toothbrush you use. Electric toothbrushes are advantageous for people who have limited manual dexterity or people with hand braces, since the rotating heads can clean hard-to-reach areas.

**Bank some bone.** Gingivitis is the beginning of what Dr. Cali calls periodontal osteoporosis. Just as the bones in the rest of your skeleton can shrink and become brittle, so, too, can your jawbone. Bolster your bones with plenty of calcium (found in dairy products, salmon, almonds, and dark leafy green vegetables such as kale and broccoli), exercise, and a no-smoking policy.

**Try a gum massage.** Grip your gums between your thumb and index finger (index on the outside) and rub, suggests Richard Shepard, D.D.S. This increases healthy blood circulation to your gums.

**Use a gum stimulator.** A rubber or specially designed triangular gum stimulator is better than a toothpick for massaging the gums, says Dr. Cali. It also cleans the surfaces between the teeth. Place the rubber point so that it rests between two teeth. Point the tip in the direction of the biting surface until the stimulator is at a 45-degree angle to the gumline. Apply a circular motion for 10 seconds, then move on to the next tooth.

**Stock up on vitamin C.** Vitamin C won't cure gingivitis, but it can help check bleeding gums, according to a study at the USDA Western Nutrition Research Center in San Francisco. The suggested daily intake is 100 to 500 milligrams.

**Brandish a proxa brush.** A proxa brush is a specially designed brush (available at most drugstores) that's shaped like a tiny bottle brush. It slides between your teeth or under your crown or bridge to get to those hard-to-reach places, says Roger P. Levin, D.D.S.

**Use Listerine.** In a study reported in the *Journal of Clinical Periodontology*, Listerine mouthwash inhibited the development of plaque and reduced gingivitis.

**Look at the label.** When buying generic mouthwash, look for the chemicals cetylpridinium chloride or domiphen bromide on the label. Research shows these are the active ingredients in mouthwash that reduce dental plaque.

**Examine your lifestyle.** Too much stress? Too little relaxation? Do you work around toxic chemicals? Any of those factors can adversely affect your gums. Examine every aspect of your lifestyle to see what you can change to make living more healthy, suggests Dr. Cali.

**Cut your vices.** Excessive smoking and drinking can drain your body of vitamins and minerals vital to a healthy mouth, says Dr. Cali.

**Scrape your tongue.** Remove the bacteria and toxins hiding there. It doesn't matter what you use to scrape with, as long as it isn't sharp, says Dr. Cali. He recommends a small spoon, a Popsicle stick, a tongue depressor, or your toothbrush. Scrape from back to front 10 to 15 times.

**Take an intermission.** Don't try to perform all these oral ablutions in one day. Massage your gums one day, and scrape your tongue the next, says Dr. Cali. If you do something different after you brush and floss, you won't bore yourself to death.

**Snuff it with $H_2O_2$.** Buy a 3 percent solution of hydrogen peroxide, mix it half-and-half with water, and swish it around your mouth for 30 seconds. Don't swallow. Use this wash three times a week to inhibit bacteria, says Dr. Cali.

**Wash with an oral irrigation unit.** Use an oral irrigation device to flush water around your teeth and gums, says Dr. Cali. To use it correctly, direct the stream of water between your teeth, not down into your gums.

**Pack a portable irrigator.** When you travel, carry an ear syringe (a rubber bulb with a long nose). Fill it with water, then flush your teeth, says Dr. Cali.

**Eat a raw vegetable a day.** It will keep gingivitis away, says Dr. Cali. Hard and fibrous foods clean and stimulate teeth and gums.

**Try the baking soda and water solution.** Take plain baking soda, mix it with a little bit of water, and apply it with your fingers along the gumline in a small section of your mouth. Then brush. You'll clean, polish, neutralize acidic bacterial wastes, and deodorize, all in one swoop, says Dr. Cali.

**Say "aloe" to your druggist.** Some people brush their gums with aloe gel, says Eric Shapira, D.D.S. "It's a healing agent, and it will reduce some of the plaque in your mouth."

## PANEL OF ADVISORS

**Vincent Cali, D.D.S.,** is a New York City dentist and author of *The New, Lower-Cost Way to End Gum Trouble without Surgery.* He also has a postgraduate degree in clinical nutrition from the Fordham Page Institute at the University of Pennsylvania in Philadelphia.

**Roger P. Levin, D.D.S.,** is the chief executive officer of the Levin Group, a dental practice in Baltimore.

**Robert Schallhorn, D.D.S.,** is a dentist in Aurora, Colorado, and past president of the American Academy of Periodontology.

**Eric Shapira, D.D.S.,** is an assistant clinical professor and lecturer at the University of the Pacific School of Dentistry in San Francisco and a dentist in Half Moon Bay, California.

**Richard Shepard, D.D.S.,** is a retired dentist in Durango, Colorado. He is also the executive director of the Holistic Dental Association.

# GOUT
## 15 Coping Ideas

Gout is an extremely painful form of arthritis—so painful that most patients can't even bear the weight of a bedsheet on the tender joint. Gout's throbbing pain often hits at night, turning the skin red-hot and leaving the affected joint swollen and tender for 5 to 10 days.

Once considered the domain of royalty, gout is actually a fairly common disorder, affecting more than 2 million Americans who happen to have excessive levels of uric acid, a waste product from body tissues. We all have uric acid in our blood, which carries it to the kidneys to be excreted in urine. But if you experience gout, either you produce too much uric acid or you produce a normal amount but don't excrete enough, says Branton Lachman, Pharm.D. Either way, the excess turns into tiny crystals that collect in joints, causing intense inflammation and pain.

Often the big toe is the prime target, but almost any joint can become a sore point. While any adult can fall prey to gout, the typical victim is a middle-aged male, who may be overweight and have a family history of the disease. If you're a current—or potential—sufferer, heed these dos and don'ts from the experts.

## WHEN TO CALL A DOCTOR

If you experience sudden and intense pain in a joint, call your doctor. Even if the pain goes away in a day or two, it is important to see your doctor, because gout left untreated can only lead to more pain and joint damage.

Your doctor can prescribe a number of prescription medications to help reduce inflammation and relieve pain during a gout attack, including corticosteroids such as prednisone.

Once an attack has passed, your doctor may prescribe a medication to lower your uric acid in an attempt to prevent future attacks. You also may receive colchicine, an anti-gout medicine used for thousands of years, now sold under the names allopurinol and probenecid.

**Get some R and R.** During an acute attack, rest and elevate the affected joint, says Agatha Thrash, M.D. You'll probably have little trouble following this advice because the pain will be so intense.

**Reach for ibuprofen.** It is the tremendous inflammation around the affected joint that causes the pain. So when you need a painkiller, make sure it's one that can reduce inflammation—namely ibuprofen, says Jeffrey R. Lisse, M.D. Follow label instructions. If those dosages don't give relief, he says, consult your doctor before increasing them.

**Avoid aspirin or acetaminophen.** All pain relievers are not created equal. Aspirin can actually make gout worse by inhibiting excretion of uric acid, says Dr. Lisse, and acetaminophen doesn't have enough inflammation-fighting capability to do much good.

**Apply ice.** If the affected joint is not too tender to touch, try applying a crushed-ice pack, says John Abruzzo, M.D. The ice has a soothing, numbing effect. Place the pack on the painful joint for about 10 minutes. Cushion it with a towel or sponge. Reapply as needed.

**Drink lots of water.** Large amounts of fluid can help flush excess uric acid from your system before it can do any harm. Robert H. Davis, Ph.D., recommends plain old $H_2O$. "Most people just don't drink enough water," he says. "For best results, have five or six glasses a day."

As a bonus, lots of water may also help discourage the kidney stones that also affect people with gout.

**Consider herbal teas.** Another good way to take in sufficient liquid is with herb teas. They're free of both caffeine and calories, so large amounts won't make you jittery or pile on unwanted pounds. Eleonore Blaurock-Busch, Ph.D., especially recommends sarsaparilla, yarrow, rose hip, and peppermint. Place two tablespoons of the dried herb in a pint of boiling water. Steep for 10 to 20 minutes, then strain before drinking.

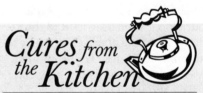

## Cures from the Kitchen

Cherries have long been a folk remedy for gout. Although there is no hard scientific evidence that cherries help relieve gout, many people find them beneficial. It doesn't seem to matter whether they use sweet or sour varieties or whether the cherries are canned or fresh. Reported amounts vary from a handful (about 10 cherries) a day up to $\frac{1}{2}$ pound. People have also reported success with 1 tablespoon of cherry concentrate a day, says Agatha Thrash, M.D.

**Avoid high-purine foods.** "Foods that are high in a substance called purine contribute to higher levels of uric acid," says Robert Wortmann, M.D. Avoiding such foods is prudent.

Those foods most likely to *induce* gout contain anywhere from 150 to 1,000 milligrams of purine in each 3½-ounce serving. They include high-protein animal products such as anchovies, brains, consommé, gravy, heart, herring, kidney, liver, meat extracts, meat-containing mincemeat, mussels, sardines, and sweetbreads.

**Limit other purine-containing foods.** Foods that may *contribute* to gout have a moderate amount of purines (from 50 to 150 milligrams in 3½ ounces). Limiting them to one serving daily is necessary for those with severe cases. These foods include asparagus, dry beans, cauliflower, lentils, mushrooms, oatmeal, dry peas, shellfish, spinach, whole grain cereals, whole grain breads, and yeast.

In the same category are fish, meat, and poultry. Limit them to one 3-ounce serving 5 days a week.

**Skip the beer.** Avoid alcohol if you have a history of gout, says Gary Stoehr, Pharm.D. Alcohol seems to increase uric acid production and inhibit its secretion, which can lead to gout attacks in some people. Beer may be particularly undesirable because it has a higher purine content than wine and other spirits, says Dr. Blaurock-Busch.

If you do tipple on special occasions, minimize your risk of a reaction by drinking slowly and buffering wine with readily absorbed carbohydrates such as crackers and fruit, suggests Felix O. Kolb, M.D.

**Control your blood pressure.** If you have high blood pressure in addition to gout, you have double trouble. That's because certain drugs prescribed to lower blood pressure, such as diuretics, actually raise uric acid levels, says Dr. Lachman. So taking steps to lower your blood pressure naturally is wise. Try decreasing your sodium intake, losing excess weight, and exercising. But never discontinue any prescribed medication without consulting your doctor.

**Beware of fad diets.** If you're overweight, slimming down is imperative. Heavier people tend to have high uric acid levels. But stay away from fad diets, which are notorious for triggering gout attacks, says Dr. Lisse. Such diets—including fasting—cause cells to break down and release uric acid. So work with your doctor to devise a gradual weight-loss program.

**Use a bowl of charcoal.** Charcoal draws toxins from the body, notes Dr. Thrash. She recommends mixing ½ cup of powdered activated charcoal with a few tablespoons flaxseed (ground to a meal in a blender) and enough very warm water to make a paste. Apply to the affected joint. Cover with a cloth or plastic to hold in place. Change every 4 hours or leave on overnight.

If you prefer a warm soak instead of a compress, use the same recipe (without the flaxseeds) and then gradually add enough hot water until you can comfortably submerge your foot in the mixture. Soak for 30 to 60 minutes. Just be careful to use an old basin and not to get any charcoal on clothes or bed linens because it stains.

Taken by mouth, activated charcoal can help reduce uric acid levels in the blood, says Dr. Thrash. Take ½ to 1 teaspoon four times a day at the following times: upon rising, at midmorning, at midafternoon, and at bedtime.

**Consult your doctor about supplements.** Be careful when taking vitamins, says Dr. Blaurock-Busch, because too much of certain nutrients can make gout worse. Excess niacin and vitamin A, in particular, may bring on an attack, she says. So always consult a physician before increasing your vitamin intake.

**Don't hurt yourself.** For some unknown reason, gout often strikes a joint that's been previously traumatized. "So try not to stub your toe or otherwise injure yourself," says Dr. Abruzzo. "Also don't wear tight shoes, which can also predispose your joints to minor injury."

## PANEL OF ADVISORS

**John Abruzzo, M.D.,** is director of the division of rheumatology and a professor of medicine at Thomas Jefferson University in Philadelphia.

**Eleonore Blaurock-Busch, Ph.D.,** is associate laboratory director of King James Medical Laboratory and Trace Minerals International, both in Cleveland. She is also the director of Micro Trace Minerals in Hersbruck, Germany; cochairman of the International Association of Trace Elements and Cancer; and author of several books.

**Robert H. Davis, Ph.D.,** was a professor of physiology at the Pennsylvania College of Podiatric Medicine in Philadelphia. He is now retired.

**Felix O. Kolb, M.D.,** is a clinical professor emeritus of medicine at the University of California, San Francisco, School of Medicine.

**Branton Lachman, Pharm.D., J.D.,** is a practicing attorney and consultant pharmacist in Corona, California. He has also taught at the University of Southern California School of Pharmacy, Western State College of Law, Southern California Law School, and within the California public school system.

**Jeffrey R. Lisse, M.D.,** is a professor of medicine, head of clinical osteoporosis research, and associate chief of the Arthritis Center at the University of Arizona in Tucson.

**Gary Stoehr, Pharm.D.,** is an associate professor of pharmacy and associate dean for student and academic affairs at the University of Pittsburgh School of Pharmacy.

**Agatha Thrash, M.D.,** is a pathologist who lectures worldwide. She is also co-founder of Uchee Pines Institute, a nonprofit health-training center in Seale, Alabama, and author of many books.

**Robert Wortmann, M.D.,** is a professor of medicine and chairman of the department of internal medicine at the University of Oklahoma College of Medicine in Tulsa.

# HAIR PROBLEMS
## 16 "Bad Hair Day" Fixes

While the average human head has 150,000 hairs, some people think they have too few, and others think they have too many—if not on their head then elsewhere on their bodies: their faces, bikini area, underarms, or legs.

Although a really bad hair day can *feel* like the end of the world, most hair problems are merely cosmetic and easily addressed.

Here's what our experts have to say about unwanted hair, hair loss, and dry, flyaway hair.

### Too Much Hair

Visible hair in spots where you'd rather look smooth can be embarrassing. There are numerous ways to eliminate unwanted hair, with the best method dependent on the type and location of hair you're trying to eliminate, says Victor Newcomer, M.D.

### WHEN TO CALL A DOCTOR

Excessive hair, hair loss, and hair texture problems can signal hormonal imbalances, illness, nutritional deficiencies, or stress. See a doctor if you notice a sudden change in your hair, just to rule out a serious underlying cause.

Even if your problem is cosmetic, doctors can offer a number of solutions that aren't available over the counter.

**Shave it.** Simple and quick, shaving works fine for hair in places where next-day stubble is okay, such as your legs. Contrary to what you may have heard, shaving doesn't make hair grow back faster or coarser, says Dr. Newcomer.

**Bleach it.** Hiding the hair rather than removing it is a painless option for light, fuzzy hair above the lip, but it doesn't work as well on thick or especially dark growth.

**Wax it.** Waxing is best for light fuzz, Dr. Newcomer believes. He says that the least painful waxing methods are prewaxed plastic strips and kits for sugaring, a process that coats hairs with a mixture of sugar and wax, then removes the hair when it is pulled off.

Don't use wax if you're taking the medication isotretinoin (Accutane) or using tretinoin (Retin-A or Renova) for fine facial lines. These medications make skin more sensitive. Sunburned or broken skin should never be waxed.

**Depilate it.** Chemical hair removers like Nair work by actually dissolving the hair, so they are too harsh to use on sensitive, sunburned, or broken skin. Dr. Newcomer suggests talking with your doctor about using prescription skin creams containing hair-growth inhibitors, so you don't have to use other, more irritating products too often.

If your skin becomes irritated after using a depilatory, soothe it with aloe.

## Too Little Hair

A normal person loses 100 scalp hairs each day, but you have to lose much more—over 50 percent of your scalp hair—before it becomes apparent, according to the American Academy of Dermatology.

More than half of men have heredity-driven male pattern hair loss by the age of 50. Women aren't immune either. About 40 percent of women notice that their hair is thinning by the time they reach menopause.

Because some medical conditions may be at play (thyroid imbalance, iron deficiency, anorexia), and even medications can cause hair loss, it's best to check in with your doctor if you notice your tresses thinning. In the meantime, here's what to do.

**Make a styling change.** Maximize the hair you have. If you have white hair, add some color so that it shows up better. If it's straight, a mild perm will help fill in the spaces. Consult your hairstylist for the newest, most gentle products, suggests Lenore S. Kakita, M.D.

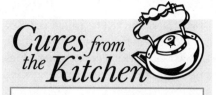

## Cures from the Kitchen

Try these expert-approved kitchen cures for dry hair.

**Go heavy on the mayo.** "Mayonnaise makes an excellent conditioner," says Steven Docherty, former senior art director at the Vidal Sassoon Salon. He recommends leaving the oily, white goo in your hair for anywhere from 5 minutes to an hour before washing it out.

**Try a sudsy solution.** "Beer is a wonderful setting lotion. It gives a crisp, healthy, shiny look, even to dry hair," says Docherty. The trick is to spray the brew onto your hair using a pump bottle after you've shampooed and towel-dried, but before you blow-dry or style. Don't worry about smelling like a lush—the odor of the beer quickly disappears, he adds.

**Go for natural nutrients.** Hairdresser Joanne Harris makes a nutrient-rich conditioner in her kitchen. "I take old bananas, rotten and black, and mash them together with mushy, rotten avocado," she says. Leave the tropical puree in your hair for 15 minutes, and then wash it out in the kitchen sink.

**Avoid pulling on your hair.** Don't use tight braids or rollers on thinning hair. These styling methods can break off thin hairs and make your situation worse.

**Use an over-the-counter solution.** Minoxidil (Rogaine) is a hair-restoring treatment available in different strengths for men and women. Applied twice a day, it has been shown to stop hair loss and regrow new hair in some people.

Be patient. Rogaine, like other solutions to thinning hair, takes a while to work. Expect it to take at least 6 months.

## Too Dry Hair

Dry, flyaway hair can be unattractive and unmanageable. Ironic as it may sound, too much water may be responsible for the hair's parched condition, particularly water of the salty, chlorinated, or sudsy variety.

Swimming and overshampooing are two common causes of arid, flyaway locks, says hairstylist Jack Myers. Other culprits, he says, include colorings, perms, curling irons, excessive blow-drying, and too much exposure to wind and sun.

Here's a quick rescue course for dried-out hair.

**Shampoo with care.** Shampooing doesn't only wash away dirt, it also washes out the hair's protective oils, says Thomas Goodman Jr., M.D. If your hair is dry from too much lather, give it a needed break by washing less often. Use only a mild shampoo, one labeled "for dry or damaged hair."

**Use a conditioner.** When hair becomes dry, the outer layers, called cuticles, peel off from the central shaft. Conditioners glue the cuticles back to the shaft, add lubricant to the hair, and prevent static electricity (which creates frizz). Pick a conditioner that works well for you and use it after every shampoo, says Dr. Goodman.

**Snip off those frayed ends.** Dry hair tends to suffer most at the ends. The answer? Snip 'em off, says hairstylist Anja Vaisanen. A trim once every 6 weeks or so should keep those frayed ends under control.

**Chill out.** Hot curling irons and electric curlers can both contribute to dried-out hair, says hairdresser Joanne Harris. She suggests that you rediscover those unheated, plastic cylinder rollers from years gone by. For straightening, wrap slightly moist hair under and around rollers (like a pageboy hairdo) for about 10 minutes. For curling or adding wave, try using sponge rollers overnight or sleeping with moist braids.

**Protect your hair from the elements.** "Whipping wind can fray your hair just like a piece of fabric," says Steven Docherty, former senior art director at the Vidal Sassoon Salon. Sun, too, takes a mighty toll. Solution: Wear a hat, both on breezy, balmy summer days and gusty, frosty winter days.

**Use a swim cap.** "Chlorine is one of the most destructive things to hair," says Docherty. So make a rubber cap part of your regular swim attire. For extra protection, he says, first rub a little olive oil into your hair.

## PANEL OF ADVISORS

**Steven Docherty** is the former senior art director of New York City's Vidal Sassoon Salon. He has cared for the hair of some of New York's top magazine and television models.

**Thomas Goodman Jr., M.D.,** is a dermatologist and former assistant professor of dermatology at the University of Tennessee Health Science Center in Memphis. He is the author of *Smart Face*.

**Joanne Harris** has created character hairstyles for some of Hollywood's top actors and actresses, including Richard Gere (in *Sommersby*) and Gwyneth Paltrow (in *Seven*). She operates the Joanne Harris Salon in Los Angeles.

**Lenore S. Kakita, M.D.,** is an assistant clinical professor of dermatology at UCLA School of Medicine in Los Angeles and a dermatologist in Glendale, California.

**Jack Myers,** a professional cosmetologist for more than 40 years, is a member of Hair America, the educational body of the National Cosmetology Association. He is also the owner and operator of Jack Myers Hair Styles in Owensboro, Kentucky.

**Victor Newcomer, M.D.,** is a professor of dermatology at the UCLA School of Medicine in Los Angeles.

**Anja Vaisanen** is a hairstylist at New York City. Trained in Finland, she's been a stylist for more than 10 years.

# HANGOVERS
## 17 Ways to Deal with the Day After

The best and only foolproof cure for a hangover is 24 hours. In the meantime, many of the symptoms—the headache, nausea, and fatigue—can be alleviated. Here's how.

**Get some pain relief.** A headache is invariably a part of the package that goes with a hangover, and good old-fashioned aspirin may be your best bet at relief. Watch out for nonaspirin pain relievers that contain acetaminophen. Combining these with the alcohol that's still in your system can wreak havoc on your liver. And if you regularly have more than three drinks a day, talk with your doctor to see which pain reliever is best for you. Aspirin may cause stomach bleeding in some people.

**Bark back.** Willow bark is a natural alternative if you'd like an organic pain reliever, according to Kenneth Blum, Ph.D. "It contains a natural form of salicylate, the active ingredient in aspirin," he says. He suggests taking it in capsule form.

**Replenish your water supply.** "Alcohol causes dehydration of your body cells," says John Brick, Ph.D. "Drinking plenty of water before you go to bed and again when you get up the morning after may help relieve discomfort caused by dehydration."

**Take B-complex vitamins.** Drinking drains the body of these valuable vitamins. Research shows your system turns to B vitamins when it is under stress—and overtaxing the body with too much booze, beer, or wine definitely qualifies

# How to Avoid a Hangover

A hangover once is a hangover never wanted again. But it doesn't mean that you have to give up alcohol altogether to have a fun night out turn into a feel-good day after.

"There's good evidence emerging that the chief cause of hangover is acute withdrawal from alcohol," says Mack Mitchell, M.D. "The cells in your brain physically change in response to the alcohol's presence, and when the alcohol's gone—when your body's burned it up—you go through withdrawal until those cells get used to doing without the alcohol."

Couple that with the effects alcohol has on the blood vessels in your head (they can swell significantly depending on the amount you drink), and you end up living through a day after that you'd rather forget. So how do you avoid it all?

**Drink slowly.** The slower you drink, the less alcohol actually reaches the brain—even though you may actually drink more over the long haul. The reason, according to Dr. Mitchell, is simple math: Your body burns alcohol at a fixed pace—about an ounce an hour. Give it more time to burn that alcohol, and less reaches your blood and brain.

**Drink on a full stomach.** "This is probably the single best thing you can do besides drinking less to reduce the severity of a hangover," Dr. Mitchell says. "Food slows the absorption of alcohol, and the slower you absorb it, the less alcohol actually reaches the brain." The kind of food you eat doesn't matter much.

**Drink the right drinks.** What you drink can play a major role in what your head feels like the next morning, according to Kenneth Blum, Ph.D. The chief villains are congeners.

as stress, says Dr. Blum. Replenishing your body with a B-complex vitamin can help shorten the duration of your hangover.

**Eat amino acids.** Amino acids are the building blocks of protein. Like vitamins and minerals, they can also be depleted by use of alcohol. Replenishing amino acids plays a role in repairing the ravages of a hangover, says Dr. Blum. Eating a small amount of carbohydrates will help get amino acids back in the bloodstream. Amino acids are also available in capsule form at most health food stores.

**Eat a good meal.** If you can tolerate it, that is. A balanced meal will replace the loss of essential nutrients, explains Dr. Blum. But keep the meal light—no fats or fried foods.

"Congeners are other kinds of alcohols (ethanol is what gets you drunk) found in essentially all alcoholic beverages," Dr. Blum says. "How they work isn't known, but they're closely related to the amount of pain you experience after drinking."

The least perilous concoction is vodka. The most perilous are cognacs, brandies, whiskeys, and champagnes of all kinds. Red wine is also bad, but for a different reason. It contains tyramine, a histamine-like substance that produces a killer headache. Anyone who's spent an evening entertained by a bottle of red wine knows what we're talking about.

**Avoid the bubbly.** That doesn't mean just champagne. Anything with bubbles in it—and a rum-and-Coke is just as bad as champagne—is a special hazard, say Drs. Blum and Mitchell. The bubbles move the booze into your bloodstream much more quickly. Your liver tries to keep up but can't, and the overflow of alcohol pours into your bloodstream.

**Be size sensitive.** With few exceptions, there's no way a 110-pounder can go one-on-one with a 250-pound drinker and wake up the winner. So scale down your drinks. To come out even, the 110-pounder can handle about half the alcohol of the 250-pounder.

**Have an Alka-Seltzer cocktail at bedtime.** "There's no hard scientific data on this, but my own clinical experience and that of a lot of others says that water and Alka-Seltzer before going to bed can make your hangover much less of a problem," says John Brick, Ph.D. Others claim that two aspirin tablets (which is really Alka-Seltzer without the fizz) can also help.

**Drink fruit juice.** "Fruit juice contains a form of sugar called fructose, which helps the body burn alcohol faster," explains Seymour Diamond, M.D. A large glass of orange juice or tomato juice will help accelerate removal of the alcohol still in your system the morning after.

**Try crackers and honey.** Honey is a very concentrated source of fructose, and eating a little the morning after is another way to help your body flush out whatever alcohol remains, says Dr. Diamond. The crackers are just the delivery system for the honey.

**Drink some broth.** A clear broth made from bouillon cubes or any homemade soup broth will help replace the salt and potassium that your body loses when you drink, Dr. Diamond says.

# Drinking Affects Next-Day Performance

After a night of drinking, *feeling* fine doesn't mean you're *really* fine, according to a study performed at Stanford University in cooperation with the U.S. Navy.

The Stanford team took a close look at Navy pilots who fly P-3 sub-chasers. Using P-3 simulators, they evaluated the pilots' flying skills when stone-cold sober and 14 hours after drinking enough to get legally drunk.

The result: "Pilots who said they felt absolutely fine and in whom we couldn't find even a trace of alcohol still couldn't fly as well as they did during times they were off alcohol completely," says Von Lierer, Ph.D.

The meaning for *your* life? Sand in the system is still sand in the system, even when you don't know it's there.

"If you have an important business meeting the next day, a key presentation you have to give—any situation where you need peak performance—I wouldn't drink the night before," Dr. Lierer says.

Pilots aren't the only ones in peril from hangover aftereffects. Ground-bound drivers suffer the same deterioration of performance, according to a Swedish study reported in the *Journal of the American Medical Association*.

Swedish researchers tested 22 volunteers on a pylon-marked test course using—what else?—a Volvo station wagon. At unpredictable intervals, they received a signal that meant they were to swerve the car right and left around the pylons. Braking time and number of pylons hit were used as measures of driving ability.

Nineteen of the 22 volunteers scored significantly worse while hung over.

**Coffee.** "Coffee acts as a vasoconstrictor—something that reduces the swelling of blood vessels that causes headache," Dr. Diamond says. "A couple of cups can do a great deal to relieve the headaches associated with hangovers." But don't drink too much. You don't need coffee jitters on top of the alcohol jitters.

**Let time heal.** Treat your symptoms as best you can. Get a good night's sleep, and the next day, hopefully, all will be forgotten.

## PANEL OF ADVISORS

**Kenneth Blum, Ph.D.,** is an adjunct research professor in the department of biological sciences at the University of North Texas in Denton and a retired professor of pharmacology at the University of Texas Health Sciences Center at San Antonio. He is also the president and chief executive officer of NutriGenomics Inc. in San Antonio.

**John Brick, Ph.D.,** is the former chief of research in the division of education and training at the Center of Alcohol Studies at Rutgers, the State University of New Jersey, in Piscataway. He is now the executive director of Intoxikon International in Yardley, Pennsylvania.

**Seymour Diamond, M.D.,** is director and founder of the Diamond Headache Clinic and the Inpatient Headache Unit at St. Joseph Hospital in Chicago. He also is executive chairman of the National Headache Foundation. He has written several books on headaches.

**Von Lierer, Ph.D.,** is a former cognitive psychologist at Stanford University.

**Mack Mitchell, M.D.,** is president of the Alcoholic Beverage Medical Research Foundation in Baltimore and chairman of medicine at the Carolinas Medical Center in Charlotte, North Carolina.

# HEADACHES
## 39 Hints to Head Off the Pain

"It's a very rare person indeed who has never experienced a headache," says headache expert Seymour Solomon, M.D.

About 90 percent of all headaches are classified as muscle contraction, or more commonly, "tension headaches," according to the National Headache Foundation. These are the head knockers that hit hardest with the onslaught of bills, work, and arguments.

The pain is typically generalized all over the head. You may feel a dull ache or a sense of tightness and perhaps experience a sense of not being clearheaded, says Fred Sheftell, M.D. "Most people will describe it as feeling like a band is wrapped around their head."

More than 45 million Americans not only get headaches, they get them time and time again. "Some people are born with biology that makes them headache prone," explains Joel Saper, M.D. For these people, headaches are a chronic problem. Further, an estimated 28 million of them experience migraines, which rightfully have an even uglier reputation than tension headaches.

Migraines are part of the vascular headache family and most often strike women. Seventy percent of those who get migraines are female.

"Migraines can be crippling," says Patricia Solbach, Ph.D. So much so that they cause a loss of more than 157 million workdays each year.

## Cluster, Cluster Go Away

But please don't come back another day. Unfortunately, cluster headaches do tend to come back, even after long periods of remission. These headaches, which afflict about 1 million people—90 percent of whom are men—hit the unfortunate person with heavy-duty pain, typically around or behind one eye.

Cluster attacks may occur every day for weeks, or even months. The cause is unknown, but "it's probably either hormonal or genetic," says Seymour Solomon, M.D. The male hormone testosterone is currently being studied for possible connections to cluster headaches.

Meanwhile, doctors have noticed a common denominator. "For reasons we don't completely understand, men who have cluster headaches are typically heavy smokers," says Dr. Solomon.

So quit smoking, or at least cut back drastically. And don't nap, advises Joel Saper, M.D. Then, maybe when the cluster headaches go away, they'll stay away.

Typically, migraines bring severe, one-sided throbbing pain. In 25 percent of cases, however, the pain occurs on both sides. Often nausea and vomiting, and perhaps tremor and dizziness, accompany these headaches. Some people also experience premigraine warning symptoms, including blurred vision, "floating" visual images, and numbness in an arm or leg.

Unfortunately, even the doctors who operate headache clinics can't guarantee that they can diagnose which kind of headache a patient has. "There's no laboratory test that can tell you this patient has migraine, this one has tension," says Jerome Goldstein, M.D. Diagnosis is usually based on the patient's history.

Thus, regardless of the name you give your headaches—tension, migraine, various obscenities—you are the one in the best position to recognize what habits and factors bring on your headaches. It's up to you to do everything within your control to prevent or treat them. So for a better chance of heading off pain tomorrow, read this today.

## Home Headache Prevention

People who get headaches know that an ounce of prevention is worth a pound of cure. Since many headaches are caused by tension, lots of these preventive measures focus on stress relief. Here's what our experts advise.

**Breathe deeply.** Deep breathing is a great tension reliever. "You're doing it right," Dr. Sheftell says, "if your stomach is moving more than your chest."

**Do the body scan.** Dr. Sheftell suggests checking yourself for signs that you are tensing up and inviting a headache: clenched teeth, clenched fists, hunched shoulders.

**Learn biofeedback.** Studies have proven it effective for both tension headaches and migraines, Dr. Solbach says. And learning this technique doesn't have to shift pain from your head to your wallet. "There are all kinds of free courses given at community centers or maybe even where you work," she says. To find a biofeedback center near you, visit the Biofeedback Certification Institute of America at www.bcia.org.

**Go with the flow.** Maybe older people are better at this. "We see more headaches in younger individuals," says Seymour Diamond, M.D. "And they're under more stress—trying to make a living, supporting a family. But it's important to not overdo."

Decreasing your expectations, both of yourself and others, wouldn't hurt either, adds Dr. Sheftell.

**Relax with imagery.** "Imagine the muscle fibers in your neck and head to be all scrunched up," says Dr. Sheftell. "Then begin to *smooth* them out in your mind."

**Have a sense of humor.** "If people take life too seriously—and you can see who those people are—they're likely to be walking around with their faces all scrunched up," says Dr. Sheftell. And probably wondering why they have another headache.

**Sleep straight.** Sleeping in an awkward position, or even on your stomach, can cause the muscles in your neck to contract and trigger a headache. "Sleeping on your back helps," says Dr. Diamond.

**Don't oversleep.** Sleeping in may *feel* relaxing, but it's not a good idea. So no matter how tempting, avoid sleeping in on the weekend, advises Ninan T. Mathew, M.D. "You're more likely to wake up with a headache." Same goes for napping.

**Exercise to prevent.** "Exercise is useful as a preventive measure," says Dr. Solomon. Moving your body is a great way to release stress.

**Say no to cologne.** "Strong perfume can set off migraine," says Dr. Solbach.

**Stand tall, sit straight.** Slouching can cause the muscles in your neck to contract and trigger head pain. Also avoid leaning or pushing your head in one direction, adds Dr. Diamond.

**Be gentle.** Believe it or not, even if you're headache-free and "in the mood," you might develop a headache during sex. "It's considered an 'exertional' type of headache," says Robert Kunkel, M.D. "It's more common in people with migraines than in those who just have tension headaches."

**Seek quiet.** Excessive noise is a common trigger for tension headaches.

**Protect your eyes.** Bright light—be it from the sun, fluorescent lighting, television, or a computer screen—can lead to squinting, eyestrain, and, finally, headache. Sunglasses are a good idea if you're going to be outside. If you're working inside, take some rest breaks from the computer screen and also wear some type of tinted glasses, Dr. Diamond suggests.

**Watch your caffeine intake.** If you don't get your daily dose of caffeine, your blood vessels will dilate, possibly giving you a headache, says Dr. Solbach. Too much caffeine will also give you a headache, so try to limit yourself to two cups (or one mug) of coffee a day.

**Don't chew gum.** The repetitive chewing motion can tighten muscles and bring on a tension headache, says Dr. Sheftell.

**Go easy on the salt.** High salt intake can trigger migraines in some people.

**Eat on time.** Skipping or delaying meals can cause headaches in two ways. A missed meal can cause muscle tension, and, when blood sugar drops from lack of food, the blood vessels of the brain tighten. When you eat again, they expand, leading to headache.

Nan Finkenaur, who used to experience chronic headaches, says, "I noticed I got headaches if I didn't eat frequently. Now I eat a lot of small meals, and it seems to help."

**Know your danger foods.** For Finkenaur, milk was a culprit. She cut back, and the headaches decreased. But there are other headache foods.

**Pass on the hot dog.** You're certainly not losing out on nutrition and you may spare yourself a headache. Hot dogs, like luncheon and other cured meats, contain nitrates. And nitrates dilate blood vessels, which can mean big-time head pain, says Dr. Mathew.

**Read the labels.** Some people who don't absorb monosodium glutamate (MSG) will say they get a throbbing headache from it. Many products are loaded with it, so read labels carefully for additives like hydrolyzed protein, glutamate, or caseinate, all MSG in disguise. Reactions to MSG have been reported after exposure to anything from soap to shampoo to soy sauce.

**Say no to chocolate.** It contains tyramine, a chief suspect in causing headaches. The good news is that many young people outgrow this chemical reaction. "The body appears to build up a tolerance," says Dr. Diamond.

**Don't go nuts.** And go easy on aged cheeses, too. Both contain tyramine.

**Don't smoke and drive.** You shouldn't smoke, period. But smoking with the car windows down when you're driving in heavy traffic gives you a double dip of carbon monoxide. This gas appears to adversely affect brain mechanisms that can spark a killer headache, according to Dr. Saper.

**Curtail the cocktails.** One alcoholic drink probably won't hurt, but don't hit your head on the rocks too many times. Also, some liquor contains tyramine.

**Don't be a conehead.** You probably can remember more than one occasion when you ate a big bite of ice cream and seconds later felt an intense rush of pain to your head.

Eat the ice cream slowly, Dr. Saper advises, "so your palate will cool gradually instead of receiving a shock of cold."

**Don't worry, "B" happy.** Fifty-two quarts of chocolate syrup. Nine hundred bowls of cornflakes. These might prevent a headache—if they weren't guaranteed to give you a stomachache first. They add up to a super-high dose of riboflavin, or vitamin $B_2$, which research hints may ward off headaches.

"I wouldn't use riboflavin as my first line of attack, because we have other agents with proven value," says Dr. Solomon. "But it would be worthwhile to explore riboflavin with patients who haven't responded well to standard therapy."

## Home Headache Relief

If, despite your best efforts, your brain is throbbing, here are some expert-recommended ways to get rid of the pain in your head.

**Take 2, not 10.** For that once-or-twice-a-month tension headache, aspirin or one of the many over-the-counter anti-inflammatory drugs may work well. Certainly a lot of us think so—we spend more than $4 billion annually on these pills.

But overuse of these drugs, more than 2 days a week on a regular basis, will just cause more pain. "It's like scratching a rash," Dr. Saper says. "The more you scratch, the more it itches."

**Don't delay.** If you do decide to use aspirin for a headache, take it right away—at the beginning of the headache, Dr. Solbach says. Otherwise, it may not do you much good.

# Give Your Face a Workout

All you need is your own handsome face and a mirror, and you're ready to do some face and scalp calisthenics, courtesy of Harry C. Ehrmantraut, Ph.D. The exercises are designed to relax the muscles of the face and scalp and teach you conscious control over these muscles so that you can go into action at the first sign of a headache.

Here, in summary, are 11 face and scalp calisthenics that Dr. Ehrmantraut recommends.

- Eyebrows up and return: Lift both eyebrows up quickly, then relax and let them drop down.
- Right eyebrow up and return: This move could be tough to do. Start by holding the other eyebrow in place and then move the right eyebrow up, as you did before.
- Left eyebrow up and return.

- Squint both eyes closed and release: Do this quickly, hold briefly, then relax.
- Squint right eye hard and release: Squeeze the right side of your face hard enough to raise the corner of your mouth.
- Squint left eye hard and release.
- Frown deeply and release: Squeeze eyebrows down and in toward the bridge of your nose.
- Yawn wide and close: Slowly open your mouth by lowering your jaw gradually to a wide position. Then close slowly.
- Open jaw, move right and left: Open mouth slightly and slide jaw from right to left, then from left to right.
- Wrinkle nose: Squeeze nose upward, as if smelling a foul odor.
- Make faces: Ad-lib this one, just like when you were a kid. And don't worry, your face won't get stuck.

**Exercise during.** "If the headache isn't too severe, I think exercise will work to make it better," Dr. Solbach says. "If you have a slight tension headache, I think you can probably end it if you exercise."

**Or not.** Don't exercise if it's severe. You'll just make your head hurt more, especially if you're experiencing a migraine.

**Sleep.** A lot of people sleep a headache off, says Dr. Mathew.

**Go cold.** "Some people like the feeling of cold against their foreheads or necks, and for them it seems to help," says Dr. Solbach.

**Or hot.** "But others," adds Dr. Solbach, "prefer hot showers or putting heat on their necks."

## WHEN TO CALL A DOCTOR

"The average person," says Seymour Diamond, M.D., "typically has a tension headache." No big deal, no danger. But occasionally headaches are warning symptoms for serious disease. Here are the red flags to signal you to call your doctor.

- You are over 40 and never had recurring headaches before.
- The headaches have changed locations.
- The headaches are getting stronger.
- The headaches are coming more frequently.
- The headaches do not fit a recognizable pattern; that is, there seems to be nothing in particular that triggers them.
- Headaches have begun to disrupt your life; you've missed work on several occasions.
- The headaches are accompanied by neurological symptoms, such as numbness, dizziness, blurred vision, or memory loss.
- The headaches coincide with other medical problems or pain.

**Use your hands.** Both self-massage and acupressure can help, according to Dr. Sheftell. Two key points for reducing pain with acupressure are the web between your forefinger and thumb (squeeze there until you feel pain) and under the bony ridges at the back of the neck (use both thumbs to apply pressure there).

**Pretend it's a rose.** "Put a pencil between your teeth, but don't bite," says Dr. Sheftell. "You *have* to relax to do that." The relaxation—and distraction—could help ease the headache.

**Wear a headband.** "This old business of Grandmother tying a tight cloth around her head has some merit to it," Dr. Solomon says. "It decreases blood-flow to the scalp and lessens the throbbing and pounding of a migraine."

## PANEL OF ADVISORS

**Seymour Diamond, M.D.,** is director and founder of the Diamond Headache Clinic and the Inpatient Headache Unit at St. Joseph Hospital in Chicago. He also is executive chairman of the National Headache Foundation. He has written several books on headaches.

**Harry C. Ehrmantraut, Ph.D.,** is the author of *Headaches: The Drugless Way to Lasting Relief.*

**Jerome Goldstein, M.D.,** is a private practitioner and director of the San Francisco Headache Clinic and the San Francisco Clinical Research Center.

**Robert Kunkel, M.D.,** is a consultant in the department of neurology at the Cleveland Clinic Headache Center in Ohio. He also is president of the National Headache Foundation.

**Ninan T. Mathew, M.D.,** is director of the Houston Headache Clinic in Texas. He also is president of the International Headache Society.

**Joel Saper, M.D.,** is director of the Michigan Head Pain and Neurological Institute in Ann Arbor. He also is the author of the *Handbook of Headache Management.*

**Fred Sheftell, M.D.,** is director of the New England Center for Headache in Stamford, Connecticut.

**Patricia Solbach, Ph.D.,** is a neuroscience scientific liaison for Ortho-McNeil Pharmaceutical, a division of Johnson & Johnson in Lawrence, Kansas, and former director of the Headache and Internal Medicine Research Center at the Menninger Clinic in Topeka.

**Seymour Solomon, M.D.,** is a professor of neurology at Albert Einstein College of Medicine at Yeshiva University and director of the Headache Unit at Montefiore Medical Center, both in Bronx.

# HEARTBURN
## 24 Ways to Put Out the Fire

Drop this book. Run to the fridge. Throw together two bologna sandwiches made with gobs of mayonnaise, plus tomatoes and hot peppers—lots of hot peppers. Drink some beer. Pull out that cold pizza from Friday night. Help yourself to some ice cream with chocolate sauce. Don't forget the coffee, extra cream. Now down it all as fast as you can.

All done?

Now we're ready to talk about heartburn.

What causes it? It could be a number of things, but in most cases, it's *acid reflux.* That is, some of the digestive juices normally found in the stomach back up into the esophagus, the pipe between the stomach and mouth. These juices include hydrochloric acid, the corrosive substance used in industry to clean metal.

The stomach has a protective lining that shields it from the acid, but the esophagus has no such lining. That's why upwardly mobile stomach acid burns, sometimes so badly that you may think you're having a heart attack.

If you're experiencing heartburn regularly for no apparent reason, it's time to call your doctor, says Samuel Klein, M.D.

How regularly? As a rule of thumb, two or three times a week for more than 4 weeks, says Francis S. Kleckner, M.D. Although heartburn is most usually caused by simple acid reflux, he cautions that it can also be a sign of an ulcer.

See a physician right away if any of the following symptoms accompany your heartburn, says Dr. Klein. It could mean you're having a heart attack or other serious disorder.

- Difficulty or pain when swallowing
- Vomiting with blood
- Bloody or black stool
- Shortness of breath
- Dizziness or light-headedness
- Pain radiating into your neck and shoulder

In addition, know that heartburn caused by simple acid reflux is normally worse *after* meals. If your heartburn worsens *before* meals, it may be a sign of an ulcer.

Overeating is the most common cause of heartburn. But it's not the only one. Some people get heartburn without overindulging. To squelch the fire, heed these tips from experts.

**Don't overdo it.** Stomach acids can be forced up into the esophagus when there's too much food in your belly. Fill your belly more, and you'll force up more acid. There can be many reasons for heartburn, but for the occasional sufferer, it's usually eating too much food too fast, says Samuel Klein, M.D.

**Feed that hamburger to the dog.** Greasy, fried, and fatty foods tend to sit in the stomach for a long time and foster surplus acid production. You can discourage future attacks if you avoid fatty meats and dairy products, says Larry I. Good, M.D.

**Think mild, for spice isn't always nice.** Chile peppers and their spicy cousins may seem like the most likely heartburn culprits, but they're not. Many people with heartburn can eat spicy foods without added pain, says Dr. Klein. Then again, some can't.

## Antacids Do Help

Over-the-counter digestive aids are generally effective and safe. One would hope so; Americans pay billions of dollars a year for these medications. The antacids that got the highest marks from our experts were many of the most common names—all those whose labels say they're made from a mixture of magnesium hydroxide and aluminum hydroxide. (One constipates and the other tends to produce diarrhea; combined, they counter each other's side effects.)

Although the mix may be relatively free of side effects, it still is not a good idea to stay on these antacids for more than a month or possibly two, says Francis S. Kleckner, M.D. They are so effective that they could mask a serious problem that requires a physician's care, he says. Our experts agree that liquid antacids, although not as convenient as tablets, are generally more effective.

**Be cautious about the Florida sunshine tree.** Acidic foods like oranges and lemons may seem like trouble, but the acid they contain is kid stuff compared to what your stomach produces, says Francis S. Kleckner, M.D. He suggests you let your tummy decide on these foods.

**Take an antacid.** "An over-the-counter antacid such as Maalox or Mylanta will generally bring fast relief from occasional heartburn," says Dr. Klein. These products help neutralize the acid in your stomach, while acid blockers like Pepcid AC, Zantac 75, and Tagamet can decrease the production of acid in the stomach for several hours. You can take these before a meal as well as after. (For more on antacids, see "Antacids Do Help.")

**In this case, milk doesn't do a body good.** Fats, proteins, and calcium in milk can stimulate the stomach to secrete acid. "Some people recommend milk for heartburn—but there's a problem with it," says Dr. Klein. "It feels good going down, but it stimulates acid secretion in the stomach."

**Leave the mints at the cash register.** Mints are one of several foods that tend to relax your lower esophageal sphincter, the little valve that keeps acid in your stomach—and the little lid that can often protect you even when you do overindulge.

Other foods that can relax your sphincter include beer, wine, other alcoholic beverages, and tomatoes.

**Go easy on the caffeine.** Caffeinated drinks such as coffee, tea, and cola may irritate an already inflamed esophagus. Caffeine also relaxes the sphincter.

**Say no to cocoa.** The number one food to avoid when you're experiencing heartburn is chocolate. The sweet confection deals those with heartburn a double whammy. It is nearly all fat, *and* it contains caffeine. (For chocolate addicts, however, here's good news. White chocolate, while just as fatty, has little caffeine.)

**Swear off fizzy drinks.** All those little bubbles can expand your stomach, producing the same effect on the sphincter as overeating, says Dr. Good.

**Clear the air.** "It doesn't matter whether it's yours or someone else's tobacco smoke—avoid it," says Dr. Kleckner. It will relax your sphincter and increase acid production.

**Check your waistline.** The stomach may be compared to a tube of toothpaste, says Dr. Kleckner. If you squeeze the tube in the middle, he says, something's going to come out of the top. A roll of fat around the gut squeezes the stomach much as a hand would squeeze a tube of toothpaste. But what you get is stomach acid.

**Loosen your belt.** Think again of the toothpaste analogy, says Dr. Kleckner. "Many people can get relief from heartburn simply by wearing suspenders instead of a belt."

**If you're lifting, bend at the knees.** If you bend at the stomach, you'll be compressing it, forcing acid upward. "Bend at the knees," says Dr. Kleckner. "It's not only a way to control acid, it's also better for your back."

**Check your medicine cabinet.** You may find the source of your grief lurking inside. A number of prescription drugs, including some antidepressants and sedatives, may aggravate heartburn. If you have heartburn and are on any prescription drug, review it with your physician, says Dr. Kleckner.

**Vow to eat dinner earlier tomorrow night.** "Never eat within $2\frac{1}{2}$ hours before bedtime," says Dr. Kleckner. A bulging stomach and gravity working together are a sure way to force stomach acid upward into the esophagus.

*Cures from the Kitchen*

An oft-touted remedy for heartburn is 1 teaspoon of apple cider vinegar in a half-glass of water sipped during a meal. "I've used it many times—it definitely works," says home-remedy expert Betty Shaver. It may sound bizarre to ingest an acid when you have an acid problem, admits Shaver, but there are good acids and bad acids.

# Herbal Heartburn Helpers

Walk into your health food store, and chances are you'll find a number of herbs reputed to fight heartburn. Herb researcher Daniel B. Mowrey, Ph.D., studied the evidence thoroughly and concluded that *some* herbal remedies do relieve and prevent heartburn.

**Ginger.** This, says Dr. Mowrey, is the most helpful. "I've seen it work often enough that I'm convinced," he says. "We're not sure how it works, but it seems to absorb the acid and have the secondary effect of calming the nerves." Take it in capsule form just after you eat. Start with two capsules and increase the dosage as needed. You know you've taken enough, says Dr. Mowrey, when you start to taste ginger in your throat.

**Bitters.** A class of herbs called bitters, used for many years in parts of Europe, is also helpful, Dr. Mowrey says. Examples of common bitters are gentian root and goldenseal. "I can vouch that they work," he says. Bitters can be taken in capsule form or as a liquid extract, just before you eat.

**Aromatics.** The aromatic herbs, such as catnip and fennel, are also reputed to be good for heartburn, but the research on these is sporadic, says Dr. Mowrey.

**Don't lie flat.** If you lie flat, you'll have gravity working against you. Stay upright and the acid in your stomach is more likely to stay in your stomach. "Water doesn't travel uphill, and acid doesn't either," says Dr. Kleckner.

**Be a block head.** When you finally do lie down, elevate the head of your bed 4 to 6 inches. You can do this by putting blocks under the legs of the bed or by slipping a wedge under the mattress at the head of the bed. (Extra pillows, however, cannot be expected to do the trick.) Keeping the bed on a slant will discourage the heartburn from returning.

**Take life a littler easier.** "Stress," says Dr. Klein, "may cause an increase in acid production in the stomach. Some good relaxation techniques may be of help in reducing your level of tension, allowing you to rebalance your unbalanced body chemistry."

## PANEL OF ADVISORS

**Larry I. Good, M.D.,** is a former member of the Long Island Gastrointestinal Disease Group in Merrick, New York. He also was an assistant professor of medicine at the State University of New York at Stony Brook.

**Francis S. Kleckner, M.D.,** is a gastroenterologist in Allentown, Pennsylvania.

**Samuel Klein, M.D.,** is a William H. Danforth professor of medicine and nutritional science and director of the Center for Human Nutrition at Washington University School of Medicine in St. Louis.

**Daniel B. Mowrey, Ph.D.,** of Lehi, Utah, is a psychologist who specializes in psychopharmacology and who has been researching the use of herbs in medicine for 15 years. He also is president of American Phytotherapy Research Laboratory in Provo, Utah, and the author of *Herbal Tonic Therapies*.

**Betty Shaver** is an herbalist and a lecturer on herbal and other home remedies who is based in Grahamsville, New York.

# HEAT EXHAUSTION
## 27 Tactics to Stave Off Trouble

Each summer, with everything from garden hoes to golf clubs in hand, the same people who are cautious enough to carry umbrellas when rain is predicted push themselves beyond safe limits in the sun.

The not-uncommon result: heat exhaustion, a condition in which an excessive loss of body fluid results in a rise in body temperature.

It's important to understand that no one is immune to heat exhaustion, not even the most finely conditioned athlete, says Richard Keller, M.D. That's because the hotter we get, the more we perspire, and if we sweat *too* much, we start to run low on water.

Heat exhaustion is caused by water depletion (dehydration) or in rare cases—rare because of Americans' typically high-salt diets—salt depletion. (We lose salt along with our sweat.)

Thirst is likely to be the first symptom, followed by loss of appetite, headache, pallor, dizziness, and a general flulike feeling that may include nausea and even vomiting. In more extreme cases, the heart may race and concentration may become more difficult.

Hopefully, you won't find yourself in that situation. Here's how to avoid it and, if necessary, how to cope with it.

**Get out of the sun.** This is as critical as it is obvious, especially for the person already experiencing heat exhaustion. Otherwise, body temperature could continue to rise, even if you're resting and drinking water, Dr. Keller

## WHEN TO CALL A DOCTOR

If it's not treated, heat exhaustion can progress to heatstroke, which can be deadly. Yet it is sometimes difficult to distinguish between heat exhaustion and heatstroke, says Richard Keller, M.D.

Of course, no one goes directly from feeling fine to the brink of death—no matter how hot it is, says Larry Kenney, Ph.D.

For this reason, a person who does not respond within 30 minutes to self-help measures for heat exhaustion should be taken to the doctor. It's important to get emergency care quickly, says Dr. Kenney, noting that complications such as shock and kidney shutdown could develop.

"If you have heat exhaustion, the worst you'll get is confused. If you have trouble walking or become unconscious, then you're getting into heatstroke," says Dr. Kenney.

Heatstroke is a major malfunction of the body's thermoregulatory system—internal temperature is allowed to rise dangerously high. Symptoms can be similar to those of heat exhaustion—dizziness and nausea, for example. In addition, the person may become very disoriented and even agitated. When the body quits regulating temperature, the heatstroke victim typically stops sweating—but not always.

People under 30 can sweat the whole way through, Dr. Keller says, "provided they're in pretty good shape."

Although fainting may or may not signal heatstroke, it warrants immediate medical care. "If they revive quickly—say, in 2 to 5 minutes—that's more likely heat exhaustion," says Dr. Keller, adding that seizure and coma are additional possibilities with heatstroke.

Unless heatstroke strikes in a hospital parking lot, you'll need to administer some fast first aid. Here are recommendations on how to treat heatstroke until you can get to a doctor.

**Cool with water.** "Splash the person with water instead of immersing him in cool water, if possible," Dr. Keller says. "The water will evaporate on the skin more quickly and have a cooling effect."

**Apply cool towels.** Again, this is a better choice than immersing the person in ice-cold water.

**Take advantage of technology.** If possible, move the person into an air-conditioned setting.

**Force fluids.** Water is best, provided the person is conscious, Dr. Keller says.

**Take charge.** Some of those afflicted let pride get in the way of treatment. Roofing, for example, can be intensely hot work. "The hot tar is 325°F when you're putting it down," says roofing safety director David Tanner. Add the sun's heat and the humidity, and, he says, "We've had people wait too long, become delirious, and just start running across the roof and almost fall off."

says. Even returning to the sun many hours later can cause a relapse in some cases.

**Drink water.** It's still the best beverage to turn to for hydration, says Dr. Keller. It should be taken a little at a time, not gulped down. "Ideally, you would have loaded up on water ahead of time—*before* going out into the sun," he adds.

**Eat more fruit and vegetables.** "They have a fairly high water content and good salt balance," Dr. Keller says.

**Drink diluted electrolyte beverages.** Gatorade, perhaps the best-known example, is widely used by professional sports teams. Football teams, for instance, often have twice-daily practices in July and August, and players who sweat heavily can lose a lot of potassium and sodium, says former New York Jets head trainer Bob Reese. "We have Gatorade and water available on the field at all times," he says.

**Avoid salt tablets.** Once routinely handed out to athletes and anyone else who wanted them, most doctors now consider these pills bad medicine. "They do the opposite of what they're supposed to do," says Larry Kenney, Ph.D. "The increased salt in the stomach keeps fluids there longer, which leaves less fluid available for necessary sweat production."

**Avoid alcohol.** Booze fast-forwards dehydration, says Danny Wheat, the head trainer for the Texas Rangers baseball club. The team often plays in 100°F-plus conditions in Arlington, Texas. "We stress to players that the night before a day game, they should limit their alcohol consumption," he says.

**Avoid caffeine.** Like alcohol, it speeds dehydration and can make you sweat more than normal, says Dr. Keller.

**Don't smoke.** Smoking constricts blood vessels, Dr. Keller says, and can impair your ability to acclimate to heat.

**Acclimate slowly.** "You can't work and live in air-conditioning all the time and then go out and be a weekend warrior," says Dr. Keller. "Starting early in the season, you should get some outdoor time every day and slowly build from there."

**Go slower.** Whatever you're doing outside, you should do it more slowly than usual when it's extremely hot, Dr. Keller suggests.

**Pour a cold one—on yourself.** Dousing your head and neck with cold water will help if it's hot and dry outside, says Dr. Kenney, because the water evaporates and cools you off. "In humid conditions," he says, "there's probably no benefit."

**Be your own fan.** Use a newspaper, a baseball cap—whatever you have—to keep yourself in a cool breeze.

**Cheat the sun.** You can't beat the sun, so do what you have to do outdoors early and late in the day. "On hot days, we start work at daylight," says roofing safety director David Tanner. "Then we knock off about 2 or 3 o'clock in the afternoon."

**Hit the scales.** Heat exhaustion doesn't necessarily develop in 1 day. You could be dehydrating gradually over several days. "During training camp, we check players' weight every day to make sure the water they sweat off in practice is getting put back," Reese says.

**Drink like a baby.** Pedialyte and other rehydrant formulas for infants are effective enough that the Texas Rangers give them to their players in extremely hot weather, Wheat says. The primary ingredients are sugar, sodium, and potassium.

Drinking 1 quart before a race or tennis match and 1 quart during or after the workout might not be a bad idea, says Dr. Keller.

**Give the meteorologist a little credit.** Granted, 2-inch snowfall predictions sometimes materialize as 10-inch snowfalls. But when it comes to summertime heat and humidity, the forecast is usually accurate. When they say it is going to be hot enough to fry an egg on Main Street, don't make that the day to begin painting your house.

**Wear a hat.** Choose a hat that shades your neck and is well-ventilated. A wide-brimmed hat with lots of tiny holes, for example, is a good choice. "The blood vessels in your head and neck are very close to the skin surface, so you tend to gain or lose heat there very quickly," says Dr. Kenney. "The top of the head is especially sensitive in people who are bald or balding."

**Don't bare your chest.** "You pick up more radiant heat exposure with your shirt off," says Lanny Nalder, Ph.D. "Once you start perspiring, a shirt can act like a cooling device when the wind goes through," he adds.

**Carry a spare.** If your shirt gets wet with perspiration, take it off and wash it as soon as possible. "The dried salt from your sweat impairs the 'breathing' quality of the shirt," Dr. Nalder says. Change it and wash it as soon as possible.

**Wear cotton/polyester blends.** They breathe better than shirts that are 100 percent cotton or 100 percent tightly woven nylon.

**Wear light colors.** They reflect the heat, says Dr. Nalder, while dark colors absorb it.

## PANEL OF ADVISORS

**Richard Keller, M.D.,** is an emergency room physician at St. Therese Hospital in Waukegan, Illinois.

**Larry Kenney, Ph.D.,** is a professor of physiology and kinesiology in the Noll Physiological Research Center at Pennsylvania State University in University Park.

**Lanny Nalder, Ph.D.,** is a professor in the department of health, physical education, and recreation and director of the Human Performance Research Center and the Wellness Center at Utah State University in Logan.

**Bob Reese** is the former head trainer for the New York Jets and past president of the Professional Football Athletic Trainers Society. He is now an associate professor at the College of Health Sciences in Roanoke, Virginia.

**David Tanner** is safety director and project manager for Tip Top Roofers in Atlanta.

**Danny Wheat** is the head trainer for the Texas Rangers baseball club in Arlington, Texas.

# HEMORRHOIDS
## 18 Tips to Find Relief

Hemorrhoids are among the most common of all health ailments, afflicting 8 out of 10 of us at one time or another. Even Napoleon had hemorrhoids. It is said the distracting pain of the emperor's hemorrhoids contributed to his defeat at Waterloo.

Hemorrhoids are swollen veins in or around the anus. They become more prevalent as people age but are also associated with pregnancy and childbirth, chronic constipation, and chronic diarrhea.

Much like varicose veins, hemorrhoids occur when normal blood vessels expand under pressure. Heredity makes some people more vulnerable to hemorrhoids, but they can also be caused by—and remedied by—such things as diet and toilet habits.

## WHEN TO CALL A DOCTOR

If you've never had hemorrhoids, but all of a sudden you experience discomfort, it may well be related to something else. If discomfort is accompanied by itching and you've recently returned from a trip abroad, for example, you might have parasites. You will need medical treatment to get rid of them.

Bleeding from the rectum always warrants a trip to the doctor, says Edmund Leff, M.D. "Hemorrhoids can never become cancer, but hemorrhoids can bleed and cancer can bleed."

At other times, an enlarged vein in your anus can clot, creating a big, blue, swollen, hard area that's very painful, says John O. Lawder, M.D. In most cases, your doctor can easily extract the clot.

Hemorrhoids that don't heal may require medical intervention to halt bloodflow to the tissue or to remove it. Options include laser and traditional surgery and sclerotherapy (in which a chemical solution is injected to shrink the vessel).

Here's what our experts suggest to relieve the pain and discomfort of this common problem.

**Strive for soft and easy bowel movements.** Straining on the toilet provides just the kind of pressure needed to engorge and swell the veins in your rectum. Hard stools then make matters worse by scraping the already troubled area. Solution? Drink lots of fluids, eat plenty of fiber, and refer often to the following remedies.

**Ease the passage of stools.** Once you've increased the fiber and fluids in your diet, your stool should become softer and pass with less effort. You may help your bowels move even more smoothly by lubricating your anus with a dab of petroleum jelly, says Edmund Leff, M.D. Using a cotton swab or your finger, apply the jelly about ½ inch into the rectum.

**Clean yourself tenderly.** Your responsibility to your hemorrhoids shouldn't end when you're through moving your bowels. It's extremely important to clean yourself properly and gently, says John O. Lawder, M.D. Toilet paper can be scratchy, and some types contain chemical irritants. Purchase only unscented white toilet paper, and dampen it under the faucet before each wipe.

**Use premoistened wipes.** The Kimberly-Clark Corporation has recently launched a product, Cottonelle Fresh Rollwipes, that offers water-moistened flushable toilet paper sheets on a roll. Preparation H Medicated Wipes, another alternative, are four times larger than medicated pads and contain aloe to soothe the area as you wipe. They're also safe to flush.

**Don't scratch.** Hemorrhoids can itch, and scratching can make them feel better. But *don't* give in to the urge to scratch. You can damage the walls of these delicate veins and make matters much worse for yourself, says Dr. Lawder.

**Don't lift heavy objects.** Heavy lifting and strenuous exercise can act much like straining on the toilet, says Dr. Leff. If you're prone to hemorrhoids, get a friend to help or hire someone to move that piano or dresser.

**Soak in the tub.** The sitz bath—sitting with your knees raised in 3 to 4 inches of warm water in a bathtub—is a remedy that still tops the list of most experts as a way to deal with hemorrhoids. The warm water helps kill the pain while increasing the flow of blood to the area, which can help shrink the swollen veins, says J. Byron Gathright Jr., M.D.

**Apply a hemorrhoid medication.** There are many hemorrhoid creams and suppositories on the market, and while they generally will *not* make your problem disappear (contrary to what the ads may say), most are designed as local painkillers and can relieve some of the discomfort, says Dr. Gathright.

**Choose a cream.** Choose a hemorrhoid cream over a suppository, says Dr. Leff. Suppositories are absolutely useless for external hemorrhoids. Even for internal hemorrhoids, they tend to float too far up the rectum to do much good, he says.

**Work wonders with witch hazel.** A dab of witch hazel applied to the rectum with a cotton ball is one of the very best remedies available for external hemorrhoids, especially if there's bleeding, says Marvin Schuster, M.D. Witch hazel causes the blood vessels to shrink and contract.

While anything cold, even water, can help kill the pain of hemorrhoids, icy cold witch hazel provides even more relief. Chill a bottle of witch hazel in an ice bucket or the refrigerator. Then take a cotton ball, soak it in the witch hazel, and apply it against your hemorrhoids until it's no longer cold, then repeat, suggests Dr. Schuster.

**Try stoneroot.** "I have one patient who has found that collinsonia is the only thing that will control his hemorrhoids," says Grady Deal, D.C., Ph.D. Collinsonia, also known as stoneroot, is an old-fashioned herbal remedy, popular in the last century, although it can still be found in some health food stores today.

Herbalists describe *Collinsonia canadensis* as an herb whose main use is to strengthen the structure and function of the veins. It is particularly good for the treatment of hemorrhoids, acting as an astringent that may help shrink the painful veins, says Dr. Deal.

Take two 375-milligram capsules twice a day with a full glass of water between meals for acute problems. Some people need to take a maintenance dose of two tablets daily indefinitely to control symptoms, says Dr. Deal. (But check with your doctor first.) "I keep them on hand all the time for hemorrhoid patients," he says.

**Watch your weight.** Because they have more pressure on the lower extremities, overweight people tend to have more problems with hemorrhoids, just as they do with varicose veins, explains Dr. Lawder.

**Control your salt intake.** Excess sodium can make your hemorrhoids worse. Salt retains fluids in the circulatory system that can cause veins in the anus and elsewhere to bulge, says Dr. Lawder.

**Avoid certain foods and drinks.** While certain foods won't make your hemorrhoids worse, they can contribute to your anal misery by creating further itching as they pass through the bowels. Watch out for excessive coffee, strong spices, beer, and cola, says Dr. Leff.

**Lie on your left side if you're pregnant.** Pregnant women are particularly prone to hemorrhoids, in part because the uterus sits directly on the blood vessels that drain the hemorrhoidal veins, says Lewis R. Townsend, M.D. A special hemorrhoid remedy if you are pregnant is to lie on your *left* side for about 20 minutes every 4 to 6 hours, he says. This helps decrease pressure on the main vein, draining the lower half of the body.

**Give it a little shove.** Sometimes the word *hemorrhoid* refers not to a swollen vein but to a downward displacement of the anal canal lining. If you have such a protruding hemorrhoid, try gently pushing it back into the anal canal, says Dr. Townsend. Hemorrhoids left hanging are prime candidates to develop into painful clots.

**Buy a special pillow.** Sitting on a doughnut-shaped cushion (available in drugstores and medical supply stores) can take pressure off painful hemorrhoids, says Dr. Townsend.

**Try the ClenZone.** This little appliance attaches to your toilet seat and squirts a thin stream of water into your rectum after every bowel movement. It cleanses you and serves as a soothing mini-sitz bath at the same time.

ClenZone is available directly from Hepp Industries, Inc., 687 Kildare Crescent, Seaford, NY 11783. It costs from $25 to $70.

## PANEL OF ADVISORS

**Grady Deal, D.C., Ph.D.,** is a nutritional chiropractor in Koloa, Kauai, Hawaii. He is also the founder and owner of Dr. Deal's Hawaiian Wellness Holiday health spa in Koloa.

**J. Byron Gathright Jr., M.D.,** is chairman emeritus of the department of colon and rectal surgery at the Ochsner Clinic Foundation and clinical professor of surgery at Tulane University, both in New Orleans. He is also past president of the American Society of Colon and Rectal Surgeons, and Secretary General of the International Society of University Colon and Rectal Surgeons.

**John O. Lawder, M.D.,** is a family practitioner specializing in nutrition and preventive medicine in Torrance, California.

**Edmund Leff, M.D.,** is a colon and rectal surgeon in Phoenix and Scottsdale, Arizona.

**Marvin Schuster, M.D.,** is director emeritus of the Marvin M. Schuster Center for Digestive and Motility Disorders at the Hopkins Bayview Medical Center, and professor emeritus of medicine and psychiatry at Johns Hopkins University School of Medicine, both in Baltimore.

**Lewis R. Townsend, M.D.,** has a private practice in Bethesda, Maryland. He is a clinical instructor of obstetrics and gynecology at Georgetown University Hospital and former director of the physicians' group at Columbia Hospital for Women Medical Center, both in Washington, D.C.

# HICCUPS
## 17 Home-Tested Cures

Pregnant women know a secret many of the rest of us don't. Before they're born, babies hiccup in the uterus. A pregnant woman can feel the little spasm and see her tummy move, too.

Most of us hiccupped before we were born and keep on doing it every now and then for the rest of our lives. Why? Nobody is really sure. Some scientists believe hiccupping is the last vestige of a primitive reflex that at one time served some useful purpose, now long forgotten. They have a better idea, though, about what causes hiccups—eating too fast and swallowing too much air.

Hiccups usually stop spontaneously after several seconds or minutes. Once in a while, though, bouts can last a very long time. Mull over this medical curiosity: Charles Osborne of Anthon, Iowa, started hiccupping in 1922 and hiccupped for the next 65 years. That's 430 million times!

Hiccup cures date to antiquity and number in the hundreds, perhaps thousands. The general goal of all hiccup cures is either to increase carbon dioxide levels in the blood or to disrupt or overwhelm the nerve impulses causing the hiccups. Read on. Maybe one of these treatments will be your sure cure.

**"Mac" McCallum's guaranteed gulp.** "I cure my hiccups by filling a glass of water, bending over forward, and drinking the water upside down," says Richard McCallum, M.D. "That always works, and I firmly recommend it for my normally healthy patients."

That cure came through for musician Mark Golin, who found himself beset with hiccups after a late-night gig in New York City. "A woman told me to bend over and drink the water from the opposite side of the glass," he says. "It worked then and has worked dozens of times since then."

**The Dreisbach deflator.** As a hard-driving researcher for a major northeastern publishing company, Christine Dreisbach Murray knows what it's like to work through lunch and sometimes suffer the consequences—a bad bout of hiccups. "I used to try holding my breath," she says, "but lately, I've been blowing air out of my body in a slow, steady stream." Simple as it sounds, that seems to work, she says.

**Betty Shaver's sensation swallower.** "When you're eating, just be quiet and eat," says herbal remedy expert Betty Shaver. "Then you won't get hiccups."

That's probably sage advice, but for those who are already afflicted, Shaver offers this remedy. "Hold your breath for as long as possible and swallow at the time you feel the hiccup sensation coming. Do that two or three times, then take a deep breath and repeat again. That should do it," she says.

That cure has worked wonders for one well-known author who used to get the hiccups when forced to read aloud before her elementary school classmates, and who has suffered since then when making public appearances. "I always needed something that would work quickly, because I wouldn't start hiccupping until the kid ahead of me got up to read," she says. "Swallowing is the only thing that got me through the *Dick and Jane* series."

**The half-minute hiccup helper.** Dawn Horvath can diagnose digestive disturbances with great dexterity. She's a researcher like Murray, a profession that seems to know no end of alimentary ailments.

Horvath's helper goes like this: "Fill a Dixie cup with water and place it on the counter, then press your index fingers in your ears. Bend over at the waist and pick up the cup with the pinky finger and thumb of each hand and, while holding your breath, drink the water down in one or two gulps."

**The tot tickler.** When you have a roomful of active kids running around giggling and laughing at the day-care center, you can bet some will end up with hiccups before the day is done.

"I tickle them while they hold their breath, and they try hard not to laugh," says child-care expert Ronnie Fern. "It works, too," says she. "I suppose it makes you gasp for breath and makes your diaphragm go back to doing what it's supposed to do."

**Pat's brown bagger.** We were going to leave out the old tip about breathing into a brown paper bag, figuring everybody probably knew it already and—worse yet—that it never worked very well anyway. But then we started hearing tales about Pat Leayman, a mail clerk for a major firm located in the industrial heartland. Seems she's cured large numbers of hiccupping mail workers (must be something in the stamps) using nothing more than that old brown paper bag!

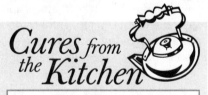

*Cures from the Kitchen*

"One cure I find effective is a teaspoon of sugar, swallowed dry," says André Dubois, M.D. "That quite often stops the hiccups in minutes. The sugar is probably acting in the mouth to modify the nervous impulses that would otherwise tell the muscles in the diaphragm to contract spasmodically."

# The Laundry List

The truth must be told. Doctors approach the occasional bout of hiccups exactly the same way the rest of us do—by running through a list of favorite treatments until they find one that works.

Thoughtfully, the *Journal of Clinical Gastroenterology* published a list of suggested hiccup cures to help those doctors whose personal lists were a little weak. Here are the journal's recommendations.

- Yank forcefully on the tongue.
- Lift the uvula (that little boxing bag at the back of your mouth) with a spoon.
- Tickle the roof of your mouth with a cotton swab at the point where the hard and soft palate meet.
- Chew and swallow dry bread.
- Suck a lemon wedge soaked with Angostura bitters.
- Compress the chest by pulling the knees up or leaning forward.
- Gargle with water.
- Hold your breath.

The journal didn't list these treatments, but you may want to give them a try.

- Suck on crushed ice.
- Place an ice bag on the diaphragm just below the rib cage.

"It's in the technique," Leayman says, sensing our skepticism. "You have to blow in and out exactly 10 times, and you have to do it really hard until you're red in the face. You also have to do it fast, and you have to form a good seal around your mouth with the bag so that no air gets in. If you follow those directions exactly," she says, "the bag will work every time."

## PANEL OF ADVISORS

**André Dubois, M.D.,** is a gastroenterologist in Bethesda, Maryland.
**Ronnie Fern** is director of the ACJC Day-Care Center in Easton, Pennsylvania.
**Richard McCallum, M.D.,** is a professor of medicine and chief of the gastroenterology and hepatology division at the University of Kansas Medical Center and the Kansas City Veterans Administration Medical Center in Kansas City, Kansas.
**Betty Shaver** is an herbalist and a lecturer on herbal and other home remedies who is based in Grahamsville, New York.

# HIGH BLOOD PRESSURE
## 19 Pressure-Lowering Strategies

High blood pressure has been called a "silent" disease because it causes no symptoms for years or even decades. In fact, more than a third of the approximately 50 million Americans with high blood pressure don't know they have it.

But even in the absence of symptoms, high blood pressure, also called hypertension, can damage blood vessels and greatly increase the risk for stroke, kidney disease, and heart disease. That's because your arteries can take only so much force. When blood rushes through them at high pressure, it causes the arteries to thicken and harden over time. This, in turn, puts extra strain on the heart and increases the risk of blood-blocking clots, says Howard Weitz, M.D.

Smoking, obesity, and a sedentary lifestyle all contribute to high blood pressure, but in the majority of cases doctors don't know for sure what causes it. Studies have clearly shown, however, that most people with high blood pressure

## WHEN TO CALL A DOCTOR

Your blood pressure readings ideally should be below 120/80 millimeters of mercury (mm Hg). If either of these numbers is elevated, it's time to get serious and make the necessary changes to bring the numbers down.

Lifestyle changes may lower blood pressure to a healthful range, but many people also require medications. The main classes of blood-pressure-lowering drugs include diuretics, which reduce fluid in the body; beta-blockers, which slow heart rate; and ACE inhibitors, which cause blood vessels to dilate.

The drugs are quite safe, but they can cause a variety of side effects, including dizziness or dehydration, says David M. Capuzzi, M.D., Ph.D. They can also cause blood pressure to drop too low in some cases.

Report side effects to your doctor right away, Dr. Capuzzi advises. With so many drugs available, your doctor probably won't have any trouble finding one that provides the benefits without the discomfort.

can control or even eliminate it with some basic lifestyle changes, says Nilo Cater, M.D.

**Know your numbers.** Because high blood pressure causes no symptoms at first, there's no way to know you have it without being tested. You can test it yourself at home with a blood pressure cuff, sold in drugstores.

Studies show that people who check their blood pressures at home several times a month may keep it under better control. It's also a good way to rule out "white-coat hypertension," in which blood pressure spikes in the doctor's office but is normal the rest of the time. A recent study found, however, that white-coat hypertension may actually be associated with increased cardiovascular risk.

"I usually ask people to bring their home monitoring devices into the office so that we can make sure they're accurate," says Dr. Weitz.

**Lose weight if you need to.** It's the most important thing you can do to manage high blood pressure, says Dr. Cater. If you're overweight, you're two to six times more likely to develop high blood pressure. The heavier you are, the worse your blood pressure is likely to be.

That's because the more you weigh, the more blood circulates through your arteries, causing an increase in pressure. As a result, both the heart and circulatory system are under increased strain to move the blood throughout the enlarged body.

You don't necessarily have to lose a lot of weight to improve your blood pressure readings. In fact, research suggests that losing as little as 5 to 10 percent of your weight may be enough to lower your blood pressure to a healthier range.

Despite the plethora of weight-loss plans around, the basic approach is pretty simple: Consume fewer calories than you burn by practicing portion control, reduce your consumption of high-fat (and high-calorie) foods, and exercise regularly.

**Get some exercise every day.** Regular exercise can lower blood pressure by 5 to 10 percent, says David M. Capuzzi, M.D., Ph.D. That may not sound like much, but it's often enough to keep high blood pressure from developing.

Research suggests that you'll get the most benefits by exercising 5 hours a week. Jogging, bicycling, and weight lifting are excellent exercises, but vigorous daily activities, such as walking or brisk gardening, can also make a difference.

**Give up cigarettes.** If you're a smoker, this is probably the last advice that you want to hear, but it makes a real difference. Every time you smoke, your blood pressure shoots upward, staying high for an hour or more. Put another way, even if you smoke only 10 cigarettes a day, your blood pressure may be constantly in the danger zone.

Smoking is probably the hardest habit to break. Some people succeed by going cold turkey, but you're more likely to be successful if you get some help by attending stop-smoking workshops, for example, or using nicotine patches or other medications to break tobacco's grip. (For more tips on how to beat smoking, see Addiction on page 7.)

**Learn about DASH.** It stands for Dietary Approaches to Stop Hypertension. Apart from the use of medication, it's one of the most effective ways to keep blood pressure in a healthful range. The diet includes:

- Eight to 10 daily servings of fruits and vegetables
- Seven to eight daily servings of whole grains
- Two to three daily servings of low-fat dairy foods
- Two or fewer servings of meat

People who follow the diet are often able to lower systolic pressure (the first reading in your blood pressure measurement) by more than 11 points and diastolic pressure (the second reading) by more than 5 points. Those are about the same improvements that some people get from taking medications.

"The DASH diet is a little difficult for people to follow, but it's ideal for the patient who is motivated to stick with it," says Dr. Weitz.

**Shake the salt.** There has been a lot of controversy about sodium's role in contributing to high blood pressure. Doctors have known for years that people who are "sodium-sensitive" have blood pressure spikes when they get too much salt in their diets. But what about the rest of us?

As it turns out, nearly everyone may benefit by eating less salt. Sodium attracts water, so too much dramatically increases your blood volume (much of which is water to begin with). This, in turn, raises blood pressure. The American Heart Association suggests that everyone should limit salt consumption to no more than 2,400 milligrams daily by using low-sodium or sodium-free processed foods, for example, and avoiding pickles, sauerkraut, or other salty foods.

**Add salt at the table, not in the kitchen.** Foods absorb a lot of salt when they cook, which reduces the intensity of the flavor. That means you have to keep sprinkling on the salt to get the taste you want. So add salt at the table to get the most flavor with the smallest sprinkle.

**Read food labels.** Sodium hides in some unexpected places. Even healthful, whole grain breakfast cereals may contain 100 milligrams (or more) of sodium per serving. Snack foods like potato chips are in a class by themselves: An 8-ounce bag of chips may contain 1,300 milligrams of sodium, more than 50 percent of the maximum daily limit recommended by the American Heart Association. Checking labels while keeping a running tally of your daily sodium intake is the best way to maintain healthful limits.

**Get enough potassium.** Think of potassium and sodium as being at opposite ends of a seesaw. As your levels of potassium increase, sodium levels decline, leading to a reduction in blood pressure. The Daily Value for potassium is 3,500 milligrams, but people who are using some diuretics—medications to control high blood pressure—may need a little more, explains Dr. Weitz. The richest sources of potassium are fresh foods of all kinds, especially fruits and vegetables.

**Get enough calcium and magnesium.** These minerals aren't a treatment for high blood pressure, but your blood pressure may rise if you don't get enough calcium and magnesium in your diet, says Kristine Napier, R.D.

Be sure to get 1,000 to 1,200 milligrams of calcium daily. Some of the best sources include low-fat or fat-free milk, fortified soy milk, and fortified orange juice.

For magnesium, eat plenty of leafy green vegetables, whole grains, and legumes. Lean meats and poultry also contain healthful amounts of magnesium. The Daily Value is 400 milligrams daily.

**Put fish on the menu.** It contains omega-3 fatty acids, which can help lower blood pressure, can reduce the risk of blood clots in the arteries, and have been shown to reduce death rates in people who have already had a heart attack, says Dr. Cater. All fish contain omega-3s, but the best sources are fatty fish, such as salmon, mackerel, and tuna. Canned sardines are also a good source of omega-3s.

**Season with garlic.** Evidence from numerous studies suggest that garlic can reduce blood pressure. Try to get the equivalent of about 1 gram of raw garlic per day.

**Supplement with coenzyme Q$_{10}$.** It improves energy supplies to heart muscle cells, helping them pump more efficiently with less effort. That, in

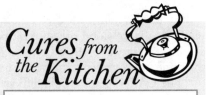

## Cures from the Kitchen

The omega-3 fatty acids in fish may lower blood pressure slightly and reduce the risk of blood clots in the arteries. But what if you don't like fish? Try flaxseed. It has a pleasant, nutty taste, and it's loaded with omega-3s along with cholesterol-lowering fiber.

You can mix a tablespoon or two of flax in a glass of water and slug it down once a day. A more flavorful option is to sprinkle the ground seeds on breakfast cereals or mix them into meat loaf, stews, or other cooked dishes.

When you shop for flax, get the ground variety—or buy whole seeds and grind them at home. Don't bother eating the whole seeds, because they'll pass through your digestive tract without being absorbed.

turn, helps lower blood pressure. Experts recommend taking about 100 milligrams per day.

**Try hawthorn.** This herb boasts a long tradition as a remedy for heart ailments. European and Chinese doctors use it to lower blood pressure. Take 400 to 600 milligrams daily.

**Drink moderately.** Small amounts of alcohol don't affect blood pressure and may even be good for the heart. Too much alcohol, on the other hand, causes blood pressure to rise. For men, two drinks daily are the upper limit; women should have no more than one drink each day.

"We don't advise people who don't drink to start," Dr. Weitz adds. The benefits of alcohol for cardio protection are modest at best, but the potential risks from alcohol are significant.

**Manage stress.** Emotional stress doesn't cause long-term increases in blood pressure, but it can cause the numbers to rise temporarily. Stress can also trigger heart attacks in those with underlying cardiovascular problems, says Dr. Weitz.

Allow yourself time to slow down and relax—with meditation, exercise, deep breathing, or other stress-reduction techniques. "Stress is hard for people to eliminate in real life," Dr. Weitz adds. "It often requires professional counseling or techniques such as biofeedback to get adequate results."

**Take snoring seriously.** Frequent snoring may be a symptom of sleep apnea, a condition in which breathing intermittently stops during sleep. "It can definitely raise blood pressure, and it can also bring about heart irregularities called arrhythmias," says Dr. Weitz.

Apart from snoring, symptoms of sleep apnea include morning headaches or feeling tired when you get up. "If we suspect sleep apnea, we'll usually refer people to a sleep laboratory for evaluation," he adds.

**Keep an eye on cholesterol.** High cholesterol doesn't cause high blood pressure, but it can make the arteries narrower, less flexible, and less likely to dilate during exercise or at other times when the heart needs more blood, says Dr. Weitz. Elevated cholesterol also results in fatty deposits, or plaque, on artery walls. Continued high blood pressure can cause the deposits to rupture, increasing the risk of dangerous clots. "Eighty percent or more of heart attacks are caused by the rupture of plaque," he says.

As part of your overall treatment plan for high blood pressure, you'll probably be advised to keep your total cholesterol under 200, but lower is better. Dietary changes, such as eating more fiber and reducing your consumption of saturated fat, can cause cholesterol to drop significantly. Getting regular exercise, losing weight, and, if necessary, taking medications are also important parts of long-term cholesterol control.

# HIGH CHOLESTEROL
## 37 Steps to Total Control

Your heart beats an average of 100,000 times a day. With every beat, it sends 2 to 3 ounces of blood whooshing through your vascular system—some 60,000 miles of arteries, veins, and capillaries.

The heart's an impressive organ, but its efforts won't do much good unless the vascular highway is free from obstructions. But for millions of Americans, buildups of cholesterol and other fatty substances in the arteries restrict the flow of blood and promote the development of blood clots. Over time, this can lead to heart attacks, strokes, and other vascular diseases.

Cholesterol itself isn't harmful. In fact, the body produces this waxy substance daily to manufacture cell membranes, bile acids, vitamin D, and a variety of sex hormones. Problems only occur when cholesterol levels in the blood rise to unhealthy levels.

We often talk about cholesterol as though it's a single substance, but there are two main types:

• Low-density lipoprotein (LDL) is the harmful form. High levels of LDL promote the development of a dense, fatty layer called plaque on artery walls. As the plaque layer gets thicker over the years, it's harder for blood to squeeze by. Plaque also promotes the development of blood clots that can impede or stop the flow of blood. It's best to keep your LDL level under 100.

## WHEN TO CALL A DOCTOR

Ideally, your levels of "good" HDL cholesterol should be above 40 (and preferably above 60), and your levels of "bad" LDL below 100. Your total cholesterol, which is the sum of HDL, LDL, and other blood fats, should be well below 200.

If your numbers aren't as good as they should be, your doctor may advise you to take cholesterol-lowering drugs. They are very effective but are usually recommended only when lifestyle changes aren't effective.

Your doctor will look at more than just cholesterol numbers when considering drugs, adds Nilo Cater, M.D. Other risk factors for heart disease, such as smoking or a family history of heart problems, will also determine whether or not you need medication.

- High-density lipoprotein (HDL) is *beneficial*. Its job is to remove excess LDL from the blood and carry it to the liver for disposal. Strive to keep this level *above* 40.

Aim to keep your total cholesterol level, which is the sum of HDL, LDL, and other blood fats, below 200.

Medications are sometimes required to bring cholesterol into a healthful range, but many people can control it by making simple changes in their diets and lifestyles.

**Cut way back on saturated fat.** Found in meats, butter, and a variety of packaged foods, saturated fat is converted by the liver into cholesterol. If your cholesterol is already hitting the danger zone, limit saturated fat to less than 8 percent of total calories, says Kristine Napier, R.D.

"Don't eat red meat more than once or possibly twice a week, and limit servings to about the size of a deck of cards," she advises.

Even if you make few other changes in your diet, cutting back on saturated fat could lower your total cholesterol as much as 20 points in 6 to 8 weeks, she says.

**Eat more fiber.** Found in plant foods, dietary fiber—especially the soluble fiber in oats, beans, barley, and asparagus—is essential for lowering cholesterol. Unfortunately, most Americans get only 12 to 14 grams of dietary fiber daily, a far cry from the 25 to 35 grams that doctors recommend.

Fiber lowers cholesterol in several ways, Napier explains. It absorbs water and swells in the stomach, increasing your feeling of fullness. In addition, soluble fiber dissolves and forms a gel in the intestine. The gel traps cholesterol molecules before they get into the blood.

"Everyone should have at least one source of soluble fiber daily," Napier says. More is better: Researchers have found that people who get 7 grams of soluble fiber daily have lower blood cholesterol levels, which may help reduce the risk of heart disease.

**Cook with olive oil.** It's the oil of choice throughout the Mediterranean, and the payoff is clear. People in Greece, Spain, and other Mediterranean countries are about half as likely as Americans to die of heart disease, even when their cholesterol levels are fairly high.

Olive oil–along with canola, sunflower, and other oils high in monounsaturated fats–lowers levels of harmful LDL without lowering HDL at the same time. "Olive oil, especially extra-virgin, is also rich in phytochemicals that help prevent cholesterol from sticking to artery walls," Napier says.

Olive oil isn't medicine, of course. It's still 100 percent fat, which means it can add a lot of excess calories to your diet. The idea is to use it in place of butter or other fats in the diet, not in addition to them.

**Make your meals meatless.** Most of the saturated fat in the American diet comes from meat, which is why anyone with high cholesterol should consider following a vegetarian diet, at least most days of the weeks. A mostly vegetarian diet not only can lower cholesterol levels, for some people it can also help to stabilize arterial deposits that have already formed, says David M. Capuzzi, M.D., Ph.D.

"If you get your dietary fat down to 12 to 15 percent of total calories, you can have dramatic reversals," Napier adds.

**Boost fiber with psyllium.** One tablespoon of this crushed seed, available in most drugstores, provides as much fiber as a serving of bran cereal. If you some-

## Do just 1 thing

Try a new margarine. Traditional margarine is made with hydrogenated fats, which can raise cholesterol as much as saturated fat does. Some new margarines (such as Benecol and Take Control), however, contain plant sterols, compounds that help prevent cholesterol from getting into the blood.

One large study found that people who used Benecol for 1 year had a drop in total cholesterol of 10 percent and a decrease in LDL of 14 percent, according to Nilo Cater, M.D.

"I definitely recommend these products," he says. "They're the single most effective dietary tool we have to lower cholesterol." Even people who are on medications can get an additional 15 percent reduction in LDL by having two servings (1 tablespoon counts as a serving) daily.

times find it difficult to get enough fiber-rich foods in your diet, you may want to take a tablespoon or two of psyllium daily. You can mix it in water and belt it down, for example, or sprinkle it on cereals, smoothies, or other foods.

"Psyllium is a good source of soluble fiber," says Nilo Cater, M.D. "Adding 3 grams of soluble fiber to the diet gives about a 5 percent reduction in LDL within a month or two."

**Fill up on oats.** This cereal grain has gotten a lot of attention for its cholesterol-lowering prowess for good reason: The soluble fiber in oatmeal and oat bran help prevent cholesterol from getting into the bloodstream.

Studies find that eating as little as 1 cup of cooked oat bran daily can lower cholesterol as much as 5 percent within a month or two, says Dr. Cater. But cooked oat bran is different from instant oatmeal. "One packet of instant oatmeal has about 1 gram of soluble fiber, so you'd have to eat three servings to get an appreciable effect," he notes.

**Put fish on the menu.** It contains omega-3 fatty acids, healthful fats that lower LDL and triglycerides—harmful blood fats that have been linked to heart disease—while raising HDL at the same time. Fatty fish such as salmon, mackerel, and tuna contain the most omega-3s, Napier says.

**Eat flax.** A nutty-tasting grain seed, flax is loaded with cholesterol-lowering omega-3s. It's also rich in soluble fiber and phytoestrogens, which help with cholesterol control, Napier says.

"Don't use flaxseed oil," she adds. "You'll be missing out on the fiber as well as some of the phytoestrogens." Also, the oil contains many more calories than the seeds, so using too much can lead to weight gain, and you can even raise your cholesterol levels as a result of the weight gain.

Health food stores and most supermarkets sell whole or ground flaxseed. If you buy the whole form, grind it at home; the whole seeds aren't broken down during digestion, Napier says.

**Follow the "rule of five."** Some breakfast cereals, especially the super-sugary kind, are fiber lightweights, but others provide a real fiber kick. Check the labels. Buy only cereals that provide at least 5 grams of fiber per serving. Fiber One, for example, packs 28 grams of fiber in just 1 cup, Napier says.

**Enjoy whole grains.** Forget "white" anything—white rice, white bread, or white flour. Most of the fiber has been stripped away during processing. Whole grains, on the other hand, are loaded with it. A slice of whole wheat bread, for example, has about 2 grams of fiber, three times more than a slice of white bread.

**Switch to brown rice.** It takes longer to cook than the white varieties, but it's higher in fiber and contains more rice oil, which is thought to have cholesterol-lowering effects, Napier says. You can also buy instant brown rice, which cooks faster.

**Eat more grapefruit.** It contains a type of fiber called pectin, which blocks the absorption of cholesterol and other fats into the blood. Red grapefruit is better than white because it's richer in the carotenoid called lycopene, an antioxidant that helps prevent LDL from sticking to artery walls.

**Snack on nuts.** Even though they're almost dripping with fat, studies find that people who eat nuts are less likely to develop heart disease. Most nuts are high in monounsaturated and polyunsaturated fats. Replacing saturated fat in the diet with these "good" fats can cause a significant drop in LDL, says Dr. Cater.

**Include milk in your diet.** While full-fat milk, cheese, and other dairy foods are extremely high in saturated fat, fat-free and low-fat dairy foods have negligible amounts. Plus, studies suggest that low-fat dairy foods can help high blood pressure, Napier says.

**Add mushrooms to recipes.** Studies show that shiitake mushrooms can lower cholesterol and triglyceride levels. Health food stores and many grocery stores often carry fresh shiitake mushrooms. Try sautéing them for tasty and healthful additions to soups, stews, sauces, omelets, and stir-fried meals.

**Crunch into an apple.** Apples are rich in the soluble fiber pectin. Experts have found that pectin mops up excess cholesterol in your intestine, like a sponge soaks up spills, before it can enter your blood and gunk up your arteries. Then the pectin is excreted, taking fat and cholesterol along with it.

**Eat vitamin C–rich foods.** This vitamin is an antioxidant that helps prevent cholesterol from sticking to artery walls and blocking the flow of blood. You can get a lot of vitamin C in your diet by eating plenty of fruits and vegetables, especially green and red peppers, spinach, tomatoes, and oranges or other citrus fruits.

Because it takes a lot of vitamin C–about 500 milligrams daily–to control cholesterol and reduce the risk of heart disease, it makes sense to take a supplement as part of a vitamin C–rich diet, Dr. Capuzzi says.

**Drink green tea.** It's rich in polyphenols, antioxidants that keep LDL from sticking to artery walls. Black tea contains some of the protective compounds, but green tea, which undergoes less processing, is a better source.

**Add soy to your diet.** It's a staple in Asian cuisine, which may be one reason heart disease is much less common in Asian countries than in the United States.

Soy foods such as tofu, tempeh, and soy milk contain chemical compounds called isoflavones, which appear to reduce the amount of cholesterol that the liver produces. People who eat about an ounce of soy protein daily can have drops in total cholesterol of about 10 percent.

"Soy is most effective in people with very high cholesterol levels of 240 or above," Dr. Cater adds. "It appears to be less helpful if your cholesterol is lower than that."

To incorporate more soy in your diet:

- Eat whole soybeans. They contain more of the beneficial compounds than processed soy foods. Soak the dried beans overnight, drain the water, and then cook them in a covered container for 2 to 3 hours. If this sounds like too much work, eat edamame (green soybeans), a favorite snack in Japan that is now available in Asian grocery stores in the United States.

- Add tofu to recipes. It has little flavor of its own, but it absorbs the flavors of other ingredients. Tofu is commonly added to stews, casseroles, or stir-fries in place of cheese or meat.

- Try tempeh. Along with miso, it's a fermented soybean product with a slightly smoky taste—and it's exceptionally high in isoflavones.

- Make a soy smoothie. A delicious way to get more soy in your diet is to blend 1 to 3 ounces of tofu, a variety of fresh fruits, and 1 cup of soy milk.

**Toast your health with wine.** Dozens of studies suggest that drinking moderate amounts of red wine can reduce the risk of heart attack—possibly by 30 to 50 percent, in some cases. Wine raises levels of HDL and helps prevent blood clots from forming in the arteries. It also contains antioxidant compounds that reduce cholesterol buildup in the arteries.

"Red wine tends to get most of the attention, but research suggests that any form of alcohol may help," says Dr. Cater.

More isn't better, however. The risks of consuming too much alcohol vastly outweigh the cholesterol-controlling benefits. Men are advised to have no more than two drinks daily; for women, one drink is the upper limit.

**Cook with garlic.** It's loaded with sulfur compounds that may lower blood pressure and cholesterol and reduce the tendency of platelets—cell-like structures in blood—to form clots. There's even some evidence that garlic may reverse existing cholesterol buildup. "Garlic will not have a dramatic impact on cholesterol buildup in the arteries, but it has some potential health benefits," agrees Dr. Capuzzi.

If the taste of garlic isn't for you, you can get the same benefits by taking enteric-coated garlic tablets. The coating allows the tablets to pass intact through the stomach to the small intestine, where they're absorbed into the blood.

**Add more onions to recipes.** They contain a powerful antioxidant called quercetin, which helps prevent LDL from accumulating in the arteries. In addition, the sulfur compounds in onions raise levels of beneficial HDL. Eating half of a raw onion a day may raise HDL as much as 30 percent.

All onions are helpful, but red and yellow onions contain the highest levels of other antioxidants called flavonoids.

**Shop for color.** The next time you're in the produce department at the supermarket, take a look at all the pretty colors: Fruits and vegetables with red, orange, and yellow hues are all rich in carotenoids, plant pigments that make cholesterol less likely to stick to artery walls, Napier says.

Carotenoid-rich foods include tomatoes, red peppers, sweet potatoes, and watermelon. Studies find those who eat the most fruits and vegetables—and get the most carotenoids—are less likely to develop heart disease than those who get smaller amounts.

**Ask your doctor about niacin.** Also known as vitamin $B_3$, niacin can raise levels of beneficial HDL by as much as 25 percent, while lowering LDL about 10 percent, says Dr. Cater.

Unfortunately, it takes high doses of niacin—anywhere from 1,000 to 3,000 milligrams daily—to have these effects. And side effects, including uncomfortable skin flushing, are common. "At the amounts needed to obtain the beneficial effects, niacin is a drug, not a vitamin," says Dr. Cater. "It should only be taken under the supervision of a physician."

**Sprinkle fenugreek on food.** In a human clinical trial involving 20 people between ages 50 and 65, researchers found that taking either 12.5 grams or 18 grams of fenugreek for 30 days resulted in a significant reduction in total cholesterol levels, specifically LDL. Try sprinkling some of the ground seeds on food,

## Cures from the Kitchen

When you're trying to lower cholesterol, beans are among the best foods you can eat. They're very high in soluble fiber, which "traps" cholesterol in the intestine and helps keep it out of the bloodstream.

All beans are high in fiber, but some varieties really stand out. Black beans, for example, have 7½ grams of fiber in a half-cup serving. Lima and kidney beans have about 6½ grams, and black-eyed peas contain about 5½ grams.

The drawback to beans, of course, is that they take forever to cook. Make life easy and use canned beans. They're just as good at lowering cholesterol as the dried kind.

shooting for 1 to 2 tablespoons of ground fenugreek seeds three or four times a day.

**Take good-for-you guggul.** Guggul is an herb closely related to myrrh. A study with humans showed that 100 milligrams of guggul taken daily can decrease total cholesterol by almost 12 percent, and LDL and triglycerides also declined by about the same percentage. The recommended standardized dose is 25 milligrams three times a day. When your lipid levels have normalized, experts suggest reducing the dose to 25 milligrams once a day.

**Pop a ginger pill.** Ginger gives you a double bonus of protection because it temporarily lowers elevated blood pressure and reduces LDL while raising HDL levels explains Tieraona Low Dog, M.D. She advises taking one 550-milligram capsule three times a day. Depending on what your lipid profile looks like after 8 weeks, then take more or less.

**Dig some dandelion.** Cholesterol, which is a building block for hormones, is produced in the liver. Dandelion is a bitter, and bitters help normalize liver and pancreatic function, which affects the way your body metabolizes fat, including cholesterol. Take a cup or two of dandelion root tea before meals advises herbalist Betzy Bancroft.

**Maintain a healthy weight.** If you're overweight, your metabolism undergoes changes that can cause cholesterol levels to rise. "Losing even 5 to 10 percent of your weight if you're overweight can lower LDL," says Dr. Cater. If you change the composition of your diet in order to lose weight—by eating less fat and more fiber, for example—LDL will drop even more.

**Get regular exercise.** Walking, swimming, jogging, and even lifting weights can raise beneficial HDL 10 to 15 percent, says Dr. Cater. And because people who exercise also may lose weight, it can cause a corresponding drop in LDL.

Any exercise is beneficial, but you'll get the most benefits if you do it regularly—say, for 20 to 30 minutes each day, 5 to 6 days a week.

**Try to quit smoking.** Smoking lowers levels of HDL and increases LDL. It also damages LDL molecules in the blood, making them more likely to stick to artery walls.

## PANEL OF ADVISORS

**Betzy Bancroft** is a professional member of the American Herbalists Guild and manager of Herbalist and Alchemist in Washington, New Jersey.

**David M. Capuzzi, M.D., Ph.D.,** is a professor of medicine, biochemistry, and molecular pharmacology and director of the Cardiovascular Disease Prevention Center at Thomas Jefferson University Hospital in Philadelphia.

**Nilo Cater, M.D.,** is an assistant professor of internal medicine and a nutrition scholar at the Center for Human Nutrition at the University of Texas Southwestern Medical Center at Dallas.

**Tieraona Low Dog, M.D.,** is a family physician in Albuquerque and a professional member of the American Herbalists Guild.

**Kristine Napier, R.D.,** is nutrition director of Nutrio.com, author of *Eat to Heal*, and coauthor of *Eat Away Diabetes*.

# HIVES
## 9 Hints to Stop the Itch

Hives are a common skin condition that trigger inflammation and itchy raised areas known as wheals. The itching is intense and often distracting.

They typically occur when you're exposed to certain foods, drugs, insect bites, plants, metals, or other allergens. This exposure causes special cells in your body to start releasing histamine, making blood vessels leak fluid into the deepest layers of your skin.

Yet allergic reactions aren't the only cause of hives. Emotional stress, cold

## WHEN TO CALL A DOCTOR

Hives can kill by blocking breathing passages. If you get hives in your mouth or throat, call your emergency number (911 in most areas) immediately. If you know that you're subject to this kind of reaction, you should be under a doctor's care and have a readily available supply of epinephrine. This life-threatening allergic reaction, called anaphylaxis, causes several symptoms, usually immediately or within 2 hours of exposure to the offending substance.

Symptoms of anaphylaxis include hives; a sense of uneasiness; agitation; tingling, itchy, and flushed skin; coughing; sneezing; and difficulty breathing as the windpipe swells and closes off. Your heart may malfunction and beat erratically. You may also go into shock.

People with chronic hives (longer than 6 weeks) or with severe acute hives should also see a doctor.

weather, even sunshine can trigger them. The wheals may disappear in minutes or hours, but usually within a couple of days. While you wait for them to disappear, follow these tips to relieve the itch and swelling.

**Send antihistamines to the rescue.** Over-the-counter antihistamines are about the best thing you can do without a prescription, says Leonard Grayson, M.D. Diphenhydramine (Benadryl) and chlorpheniramine (Chlor-Trimeton) are the most commonly used and are often found in cold and hay fever medications.

*Caution:* Most antihistamines make you drowsy.

**Cool down.** Applying cold compresses, sitting in cool baths, or rubbing an ice cube over the hives are the best, and only, topical treatment for hives, Dr. Grayson says. The cold shrinks the blood vessels and keeps them from opening, swelling, and allowing too much histamine to be released. "But it's only temporary," he says. "And if you get hives from cold weather or water, you're out of luck." Hot water only makes the itching worse.

**Use calamine lotion.** This astringent is famous for taking the itch out of poison ivy, but it may help temporarily soothe the itch of your hives as well. Since astringents reduce discharge, they may keep the blood vessels from leaking fluid and histamine. Other astringents that may help hives include witch hazel and zinc oxide.

---

## A Touch of the Natural

For those willing to try something different, here are a few alternatives.

**Take tea and see.** If you suspect emotions cause your hives and if you want to stay away from synthetic internal medication like antihistamines, try a nerve-calming herb tea, suggests herbologist Thomas Squier. He recommends peppermint or passionflower teas. Chamomile, valerian, and catnip are other common sedative herb teas.

**Make a poultice or paste.** Herbal manuals often list a poultice of crushed chickweed leaves as a remedy for itchy skin. Some people make a paste of water and cream of tartar and apply it to the hives, replacing it when the paste dries and crumbles.

**Put on pressure.** Natural medicine expert Michael Blate says that he's had success in getting rid of hives with acupressure. Deeply massage the point on your trapezius muscle (running between your neck and shoulder) located midway on the muscle and just an inch or so over the backside of the ridge. "If it doesn't hurt somewhat, you haven't found exactly the right point," he says.

**Try the alkaline answer.** "Anything that's alkaline usually helps relieve the itch," Dr. Grayson says. So try dabbing milk of magnesia on your hives. "It's thinner than calamine, so I think it works better," he says.

**Help with hydrocortisone.** If you have just a small number of small hives, a hydrocortisone cream like Cortaid applied directly on the hives may relieve the itching for a while, says Jerome Z. Litt, M.D.

**Remember that an ounce of prevention is worth a pound of hives.** "There are myriad causes of hives," says Dr. Litt. "You have to be a detective to find out what causes them." Some of the more common causes are medications, foods, cold, insect bites, plants, and emotions. Once you find out, of course, try to avoid exposure. If you know you're likely to get hives for whatever reason, he suggests, take an antihistamine beforehand. It may prevent them.

## PANEL OF ADVISORS

**Michael Blate** is founder and executive director of the G-Jo Institute of Columbus, North Carolina, a natural health organization that promotes acupressure and oriental traditional medicine.

**Leonard Grayson, M.D.,** is a skin allergy specialist and former clinical associate allergist and dermatologist at Southern Illinois University School of Medicine in Springfield.

**Jerome Z. Litt, M.D.,** is a dermatologist and assistant clinical professor of dermatology at Case Western Reserve University School of Medicine in Cleveland. He is the author of *Your Skin: From Acne to Zits.*

**Thomas Squier** is a retired former U.S. Army Special Forces instructor at the JFK Special Warfare Center and School, Survival-Evasion-Resistance-Escape/Terrorist Counteraction Department of Fort Bragg, North Carolina. He is a Cherokee herbologist and grandson of a medicine man. He also writes a newspaper column called "Living off the Land."

# HOSTILITY
## 11 Soothers for Seethers

Fits of rage and hostility are so common these days that colorful terms such as *going postal* and *smackdown* have sadly become part of our everyday language. Left unchecked, however, hostility is serious business. It can blot out the lucrative deal landed at work, sabotage your efforts as a parent, and destroy everyday good deeds.

---

### Why Are We So Mad?

The number of theories for why we're so hostile these days is as long as the list of things that set us off. But experts have found a few common reasons why we seem to be more hot-tempered today.

*We're overworked.* "The average adult is working more hours than ever before," says Karyn Buxman, R.N. With technological advances like pagers and cell phones, we're always on the clock. Those pressures build up over time and make us quite angry, she adds.

*We're more accepting of it.* In our fathers' day, a man was the voice of reason, staying ever calm, cool, and collected. Today, professional wrestlers are among our role models. We get the message that it's okay to snap at whoever ticks us off. "Unfor-tunately, in today's day and age, we are more *laissez-faire* about behavior," says Dr. Hauck. "We feel it's okay to blow up at our boss or call someone a nasty name on an airplane."

*We're wired that way.* Combine the reasons above with the fact that we've been genetically programmed to react decisively when faced with a crisis. It's a fight-or-flight survival mechanism that dates back to the days when cave dwellers roamed the earth, says Aaron R. Kipnis, Ph.D. But instead of burning off all that aggressive energy by battling a mammoth beast as our ancestors used to, today it often builds up and has nowhere to go. As a result, that charged energy sometimes gets taken out on your boss, the guy who cut you off, or your spouse.

People who think it's okay to let anger fly, rationalizing that it's good to get it out, are probably harming themselves more than they think, says Paul A. Hauck, Ph.D. "Inappropriately expressed or repressed anger can overshadow all the good things a person does," he says. "Anger can ruin you if you let it."

It doesn't take a degree in subatomic physics to know that explosive anger eventually takes its toll on a person. Numerous research studies have shown that angry people face heart disease in record numbers compared to their calmer counterparts. Uncontrolled anger has also been linked to other conditions, including white-blood-cell-count abnormalities, asthma, diabetes, and anorexia nervosa, as well as to everyday complaints such as backaches.

If the toll on your body isn't big enough for you, consider how it affects the quality of your everyday life. "Anger, if not expressed appropriately or if repressed, can be the dynamite that explodes an important relationship or gets you fired from a job," says Dr. Hauck.

No one is suggesting that you never get angry. How you handle that charged energy, though, is what separates hotheads from those who keep their cool.

## Anger Avoidance

The real secret to controlling your rage is to never let yourself get to the exploding point. Here's what our experts suggest to keep your anger from building up.

**Exercise at lunch.** Anger and tension tend to build up as the day progresses. By swimming laps or walking at lunch, you'll relieve some of the hostility and tension that have built up in the first half of the workday. "Find a form of exercise that you enjoy and that helps to relieve the everyday stresses, and you'll be less susceptible to letting rage get the best of you," says Aaron R. Kipnis, Ph.D.

**Take an extra 10.** Once a week, treat yourself to a 70-minute lunch break—without your beeper and cell phone—and don't be in a hurry to get back to the grind. Chances are you're working 50-plus hours a week, and that extra 600 seconds without any communiqués from your boss, coworkers, or spouse won't get you canned and will do you wonders, says anger-management expert John Lee.

**Break the chain.** Plan ahead to avoid a buildup of minor everyday things that could make you blow your top. For example, if you're taking an airplane trip, take a book or crossword puzzles with you, because chances are you'll have delays, says Lee.

**Brainstorm.** Make mental notes of things that have upset you in the past and think of other ways to respond in the future, says Marilyn J. Sorensen, Ph.D.

"If you don't put new behaviors or thinking into your repertoire, you will continue to act the same way," she says. Ask yourself if this is really the behavior and image you want to project. If not, think of other ways to see the situation and consider what you could do or say differently.

**Prepare for hecklers.** Stand-up comedians like Chris Rock have deep reservoirs of comebacks to deal with hecklers. You should, too, suggests Karyn Buxman, R.N. "We all work with certain people who push our buttons," she says. Think ahead and develop a humorous and *kind* response or two to keep them off balance. Humor is a great tool to diffuse tense situations.

## Anger Diffusion

Despite our best efforts, we all get angry sometimes. Here's how to keep your flash of fury from turning into an ugly incident.

**Call a time-out.** If you find yourself coming to a boil, remove yourself from the situation to clear your head, suggests Dr. Sorensen. "Call 'time-out' to let the other person know you are not going to continue the interaction at that time," she says. Tell a loved one or coworker that you're angry right now and suggest a later time to readdress the problem.

**Give time travel a try.** Take a page from Michael J. Fox in *Back to the Future* and transport yourself 10 months or 10 years into the future—without that

---

### Are You About to Blow?

The symptoms leading up to full-blown rage are easy to spot, according to Lynne McClure, Ph.D. Here are four signs that you might be about to erupt.

*Palpitations.* Your heart feels as if it were about to pound its way out of your chest, and your breathing becomes quite shallow.

*Overheating.* Your body temperature rises, and you start to sweat. "That's where the old saying, 'Boy, did he get hot under the collar' comes from," says Dr. McClure.

*Fixation.* You're consumed with whatever is making you angry. "If you're in a meeting with 14 people and find that you're completely riveted on that one person that made you angry 2 weeks ago, then you have a problem," she says.

*Overreacting.* You're letting other everyday things, such as the absence of toner in the office copier, set you off. "When little things get you enraged, that's often a sign that you have unresolved anger," says Dr. McClure.

souped-up DeLorean, of course. "Will what's making you angry right now really matter in 10 years, 10 months, or even 10 minutes?" asks Buxman. "For 99 out of 100 things, probably not."

Also, if you're about to do something impulsive, think about the future repercussions of your action.

**Keep your hands busy.** When anger strikes, do something constructive with your hands, legs, feet, face, and jaw—anything that will release the tension in your muscles and distract yourself. For instance, if you're at home, take a bath towel in both hands and twist it as tightly as you can, suggests Lee. As you twist it, let out sighs, moans, or grunts. After 10 to 15 minutes, imagine that the knots that used to be in you are now in the towel.

If rage visits you in the office, grab a toy. "To ease the potential anger-producing incidents at work, people should have toys or things to amuse them in their desk, whether that's wind-up toys or cushy balls," says Buxman.

**Divert your attention.** If, for example, the person in front of you in the "10 items or less" supermarket line has 36 items and you're Yosemite Sam–angry about it, Buxman recommends distracting yourself until the counting-challenged shopper has made it through the checkout line. Flip through a supermarket tabloid article, check out what's on TV tonight, or talk to the more rule-abiding person in line behind you.

**Don't drink alone.** When you're angry, a can—or 12—of beer may seem like your best friend. But drowning your anger with alcohol, especially alone, only makes the problem worse. It's when you're drunk that you're most likely to leave the boss a threatening voice mail. Instead, call your best friends and invite them out for a gripe session/happy hour. Sure, enjoy a few drinks, but use the time to vent your anger and get it out of your system. Before you know it, you'll be laughing and will have forgotten whatever had you steamed in the first place.

**Scream up a storm.** If you've had a bad day at work, Lee suggests pulling into the nearest parking lot and, with the windows rolled up, screaming as loud as you possibly can. Swear. Name names. If you're at home, take a pillow and holler into it. The pillow will muffle the noise so that the nosy neighbor can't hear you. How long should you scream? "As long as you have the energy to yell," says Lee. "It might seem simple, but you're releasing that anger right away."

## PANEL OF ADVISORS

**Karyn Buxman, R.N.,** is a public speaker who specializes in therapeutic humor and is the president of HUMORx, a company that helps people manage their stress and organizations improve their bottom line through humor, based in Hannibal, Missouri.

**Paul A. Hauck, Ph.D.,** is a psychologist in Moline, Illinois.

**Aaron R. Kipnis, Ph.D.,** is a psychotherapist in Santa Barbara, California, and the author of *Angry Young Men.*

**John Lee, M.A.,** is the founder and director of several mental health programs related to anger management and the author of *Facing the Fire.*

**Lynne McClure, Ph.D.,** is president and consultant of McClure Associates in Mesa, Arizona, and the author of *Anger and Conflict in the Workplace* and *Risky Business: Managing Employee Violence in the Workplace.*

**Marilyn J. Sorensen, Ph.D.,** is a clinical psychologist and the author of *Breaking the Chain of Low Self-Esteem* and *Low Self-Esteem: Misunderstood and Misdiagnosed.*

# HOT FLASHES
## 18 Ways to Put Out the Fire

Perhaps the most common complaints women have about menopause revolve around the dreaded hot flashes—waves of heat that start in the chest and spread to the neck and head, leaving them sweaty, hot, flushed, irritable, and uncomfortable.

According to Mary Jane Minkin, M.D., about 75 percent of women experience hot flashes. A single hot flash can last anywhere from 30 seconds to 30 minutes, but 2 to 3 minutes is the norm. Women typically experience them for 3 to 5 years.

As if hot flashes weren't bad enough, they turn into an even more annoying beast in the twilight hours. Nocturnal flashes, or night sweats, wake women at all hours of the night, soaking them in pools of sweat. Since night sweats disrupt sleep cycles, they may be even more difficult to deal with than daytime hot flashes. They can leave a woman fatigued, exhausted, and begging for one good night of sleep.

## WHEN TO CALL A DOCTOR

Hot flashes and night sweats are rarely serious enough to demand medical attention. Still, if you are just feeling lousy or haven't slept well in weeks, you shouldn't put up with them, says Mary Jane Minkin, M.D. "Your doctor can make it better."

Hot flashes and night sweats are the result of the drop in estrogen that women experience during perimenopause (the 2 to 8 years before menopause) and menopause, which actually occurs after 12 months with no periods. This estrogen deficiency, as well as other hormonal changes, interferes with the way your body regulates heat.

If the heat is too much to bear, the tips below can help you get a handle on both daytime and nighttime hot flashes.

**Banish binge drinking.** Dr. Minkin says that drinking a *glass* of wine a day is fine. If you're drinking a *bottle* a day, however, it might be a problem. Along with its other health risks, excessive alcohol is definitely a strong aggravator of hot flashes. Alcohol causes blood vessels to dilate. More blood rushes through, goes to the surface of the skin, and produces a hot flash.

## Do just 1 thing

Smash out cigarettes. Cigarettes have been clinically shown to bring on menopause 2 years earlier, but that's not the only reason to quit smoking, says Mary Jane Minkin, M.D. Smoking's indirect effect on blood vessels definitely brings on hot flashes, she says. If you're already getting frequent hot flashes, it's just going to make them worse. So add hot flashes to your list of 2,000 reasons to quit smoking already.

**Wean yourself off the bean.** Hot caffeinated beverages are another common hot flash–aggravator. "You can drink soda or hot herbal tea if you'd like," says Dr. Minkin. "It's not the heat or the caffeine alone that seem to cause hot flashes. But the combination of the two really seems to bring them on strong."

**Rely on exercise.** Not only does it give strength to your heart and bones, regular exercise also reduces the occurrence of hot flashes and night sweats. "I'm a big believer in exercise," says Dr. Minkin. Exercise reduces menopausal symptoms, helps you sleep, keeps bones strong, and maintains heart health. Exercise three to five times a week for 30 to 45 minutes at a time.

**Find a low-sweat form of exercise.** There's just one problem with recommending exercise for menopausal women. "When women have hormonal problems, the last thing they want to do is sweat," points out Larrian Gillespie, M.D. She recommends a low-sweat form of exercise such as swimming, yoga, or Pilates, an exercise system that improves flexibility and strength without building bulk.

**Know the truth about hormone replacement.** There's a myth that it's dangerous to go on and off hormone replacement therapy (HRT). "I don't know how it got started," says Dr. Minkin. The truth is, HRT is a very flexible thing. So if hot flashes and night sweats make both your days and nights miserable, Dr. Minkin recommends at least trying HRT for a couple of months. If you don't like it, you can always go off the medicine whenever you want. If you decide you want to go back on it again, you can do that, too.

**Consult your calendar.** "One thing I do encourage women to do if they're going to stop estrogen is to stop in a cool month," says Dr. Minkin. If you stop in the month of July, you'll discover that a 90°F summer afternoon is a really bad time to get hot flashes.

**Try some black cohosh.** "Black cohosh is mysterious," says Dr. Minkin. The herb is not a plantlike estrogen, like the phytoestrogens found in soy and flax, and nobody is really sure why it works so well. Still, Dr. Minkin admits, dozens of studies and her own patients have convinced her that black cohosh is a legitimate herb for relieving hot flashes. The most commonly available brand is Remifemin, which you can find in drugstores. Follow label directions.

**Discover red clover.** Another herb that might be effective against hot flashes is red clover. A natural phytoestrogen, this herb was proven useful in clinical studies. The most commonly available brand is Promensil. You should be able to find it at a drugstore near you. Follow label directions.

**Study your soy options.** Incorporating more soy foods into your diet may be quite helpful for overcoming hot flashes and other menopausal symptoms. The advantage of soy, which is bursting with phytoestrogens, is its wide availability. Your best bet is to shoot for one to two servings a day (the amounts found in a typical Asian diet). You're likely to find a wide array of soy foods at your grocery store, including edamame, tofu, and miso. You also may want to ask your doctor about soy-based forms of hormone replacement therapy.

**Eat other foods rich in phytoestrogens.** Soy products aren't the only foods that can give you a good dose of hot flash–relieving phytoestrogens. Other foods to incorporate into your daily diet include chickpeas, lentils, and almost any kind of bean.

**Try deep belly breathing.** In some women, belly breathing alone can help reduce the severity of a hot flash. To give it a try, lie on your back with your hands on your abdomen. Imagine that your abdomen is a balloon that you fill with air as you inhale and deflate as you exhale. Repeat this six to eight times a minute whenever you experience hot flashes.

**Depend on old-fashioned sleep aids.** If night sweats keep you up at night, try these time-tested tips from Dr. Minkin: drinking a warm glass of milk, taking a warm bath, or simply not focusing on the day's events.

**Rely on cotton.** If night sweats are a persistent problem, all-cotton sheets and pillowcases will "breathe" and wick moisture away from your skin. Avoid flannel, satin, or cotton/polyester blends, which trap wetness around your body. It may also help to keep a light cotton quilt at the foot of your bed. If you get the chills following a nocturnal flash, pull this over you for comfort. Other cottony items to have on hand while fighting night sweats include an all-cotton, short-sleeved, knee-length nightgown, all-cotton underwear, and a small cotton towel to wipe up the sweat. Avoid full-length nightgowns and other blends of underwear. They'll only trap heat and make you feel uncomfortable.

**Keep a fan next to your bed.** It can cool you down at night during those heat waves. Or install a ceiling fan over your bed.

**Imagine yourself naked.** Sometimes, the power of positive thinking can overcome all other forms of intervention. Take a few long, deep breaths and imagine yourself naked, rolling gently through cold mountain snow. If all else fails, it's worth a shot.

### PANEL OF ADVISORS

**Larrian Gillespie, M.D.,** is a retired assistant clinical professor of urology and urogynecology and president of Healthy Life Publications. She is the author of *The Menopause Diet* and *The Goddess Diet.*

**Mary Jane Minkin, M.D.,** is a clinical professor at Yale University School of Medicine and an obstetrician-gynecologist in New Haven, Connecticut. She is the coauthor of *What Every Woman Needs to Know about Menopause.*

*Cures from the Kitchen*

Steep yourself some sage tea. This common kitchen herb is often the herbalists' choice for reducing or eliminating night sweats. To make a cup of sage tea, place 4 heaping tablespoons of dried sage in 1 cup of hot water. Cover it tightly and steep for 4 hours. Then, when you need it, strain the concoction, reheat it, and drink it up.

# Impotence

## 14 Secrets for Success

Improved treatments for impotence are gradually shedding light on this once hushed-up diagnosis. In fact, it's come so out into the open that following prostate cancer surgery, Senator Bob Dole even starred in television commercials for Viagra, a drug for impotence, also called erectile dysfunction, or E.D.

Doctors define impotence as the consistent inability to sustain an erection sufficient for sexual intercourse.

It's more common than many people realize, affecting somewhere between 10 and 15 million American men, becoming more prevalent with age. For instance, about 5 percent of 40-year-old men experience impotence, but for 65-year-old men that number jumps to 15 to 25 percent.

And even more men have an occasional problem achieving an erection.

"If men are honest, every one of them will tell you they've experienced impotence at least one time in their lives," says Neil Baum, M.D. "Not every incident is a '10.' It can be devastating when it occurs," he says. "A man's whole concept of his masculinity may be undermined."

Until the early 1970s, experts thought underlying problems in the psyche caused most erection problems. Today, the medical community recognizes that most impotence is actually caused by a disease, an injury, or a medication with impotence-related side effects.

Here's what our experts advise to overcome impotence.

**Give yourself time.** "As a man gets older, it may take a longer period of genital stimulation to get an erection," says Dr. Baum. "For men ages 18 to 20, an erection may take a few seconds. In your thirties and forties, maybe a minute or two. But if a 60-year-old doesn't get an erection after a minute or two, that doesn't mean he's impotent. It just takes longer."

The time period between ejaculation and your next erection also tends to increase with age. In some men ages 60 to 70, it may take a whole day or longer to regain an erection. "It's a normal consequence of aging," says Dr. Baum.

## WHEN TO CALL A DOCTOR

Men of every age can be treated for impotence. When home remedies fail to help, a urologist can assess your problem and offer a wide array of therapies that may resolve the problem. Here are the main avenues of treatment identified by the National Kidney and Urologic Diseases Information Clearinghouse.

- Drug therapy, including testosterone replacement therapy and drugs that allow more bloodflow into the penis, such as Viagra
- Vacuum devices that draw blood into the penis and hold it there for an erection
- Surgically implanted devices that can be mechanically expanded when an erection is desired
- Surgery to correct bloodflow problems to the penis

**Consider your medication.** Prescription drugs might be at the root of the problem. Or it might be those over-the-counter antihistamines, diuretics, or sedatives you're using. Realize, of course, that not every individual reacts to medications the same way.

Drug-induced impotence is most common in men over 50, says Dr. Baum, with almost 100 drugs identified as potential causes of impotence. In fact, an *American Medical Journal* study of 188 men found that drugs were the problem 25 percent of the time.

If you suspect your medication, consult your doctor or pharmacist and ask about changing the dosage or switching to a different drug. Do not, however, attempt to do this on your own.

**Beware of recreational drugs.** Other troublemakers include cocaine, marijuana, opiates, heroin, morphine, amphetamines, and barbiturates.

**Go easy on the alcohol.** Shakespeare was right when he said in *MacBeth* that alcohol provokes desire but takes away the performance. That happens because alcohol is a nervous-system depressant. It inhibits your reflexes, creating a state that's the opposite of arousal, says Richard E. Berger, M.D. Even two drinks during cocktail hour can be a cause for concern, he says.

Over time, too much alcohol can cause hormonal imbalances.

"Chronic alcohol abuse can cause nerve and liver damage," says Dr. Baum. Liver damage results in an excessive amount of female hormones in men. Without the right proportion of testosterone to other hormones, you won't achieve normal erections.

**Know that what's good for the arteries is good for the penis.** The penis is a vascular organ, says Irwin Goldstein, M.D. The same things that clog your arteries—dietary cholesterol and saturated fat—also affect bloodflow to the penis. In fact, he says, all men over age 38 have some narrowing of the arteries to the penis.

So watch what you eat. "High cholesterol is probably one of the leading causes of impotence in this country," says Dr. Goldstein. "It appears to affect erectile tissue."

**Don't smoke.** Studies show that nicotine can be a blood vessel constrictor, says Dr. Baum.

University of California researchers summarized 20 years of scientific research about the connection between smoking and impotence. Forty percent of the 3,819 men with impotence studied over the years were current smokers, compared to just 28 percent of men in the general population.

Tobacco use is "an important risk factor" for impotence, they concluded.

**Feel good about your body.** Thinking about taking off a few pounds? Studying karate? Starting a weight-training program? Do it. The better a man feels about his body, the better he'll feel going into the event, says James Goldberg, Ph.D.

**Don't overdo exercise.** Excessive exercise stimulates the body's natural opiates, the endorphins. "We're not sure how they work, but they tend to lessen sensation," says Dr. Goldberg. Exercise is good for you, but you can get too much of a good thing.

**Wait out pain.** Your body also produces its own opiates when you're in pain, says Dr. Goldberg. These opiates can turn off any sexual stimuli. There's not much you can do, he says, except wait for a better time.

**Relax.** Being in a relaxed frame of mind is crucial to maintaining an erection. Here's why. Your nervous system operates in two modes. When the sympathetic nerve network is dominant, your body is literally "on alert." Adrenal hormones prepare you to fight or take flight. Nerves shuttle your blood away from your digestive system and penis and into your muscles.

You can turn on your sympathetic nervous system just by being too anxious, says Dr. Baum. For some men, the fear of failure is so overwhelming that it floods the body with norepinephrine, an adrenal hormone. That's the opposite of what you need to have an erection.

The key here is to relax and let your parasympathetic nervous system take over. Signals that travel along this network will direct the arteries and sinuses of the penis to expand and let more blood flow in.

**Avoid whole-body stimulants.** That means caffeine and certain questionable substances touted as potency enhancers. As discussed above, it's important to be relaxed during sex, says Dr. Goldberg. Stimulants tend to constrict the smooth muscle that must dilate before an erection occurs.

**Refocus your attention.** One way to relax is to focus with your partner on the more sensual aspects of intimacy. Play with and enjoy each other without worrying about an erection.

"The skin is the largest sexual organ in the body," says Dr. Goldberg, "not the penis."

**Plan ahead.** Decide in advance what you'll do if you don't get an erection, suggests Dr. Berger. If you're not so focused on the erection itself, it makes it easier for the erection to come back, he says.

**Talk to your partner.** Don't risk increasing the tension in the bedroom by maintaining a sullen silence. Together, play detective and figure out what's going on. Pressure at work? Strain over a child's illness? A touchy, unresolved issue?

"If you understand some of the things that can cause impotence, you can find a way to explain it without attributing it to something that's not there," says Dr. Berger. "And you should talk about what your alternatives are. Will you continue your lovemaking in a different way? Don't let the erection, or lack of it, interfere with your intimacy."

## PANEL OF ADVISORS

**Neil Baum, M.D.,** is an associate clinical professor of urology at Tulane University School of Medicine and a staff urologist with Touro Infirmary, both in New Orleans.

**Richard E. Berger, M.D.,** is a urologist and a professor at the University of Washington in Seattle and director of the Reproductive and Sexual Medicine Clinic at the university.

**James Goldberg, Ph.D.,** is research director of the Bari/Goldberg Clinic at Chula Vista, California.

**Irwin Goldstein, M.D.,** is a professor of urology at Boston University School of Medicine.

# INCONTINENCE
## 22 Tips to Gain Control

Urinary incontinence is a symptom, not a disease. But the consequences of involuntary loss of urine can be debilitating to a person's self-esteem, social life, and job.

That's why Robert Schlesinger, M.D., calls incontinence a "social disease."

"People will go to almost any extent to adjust their lives to it. We had one woman who didn't go out of her house for 3 years because she was so ashamed."

No one should have to be stigmatized by incontinence, says Katherine Jeter, Ed.D. "Nearly everybody can be made better or cured." That's saying something, when you consider that more than 13 million adult Americans are incontinent.

Two types of incontinence are stress and urge incontinence. If coughing, laughing, exercising, or sneezing cause you to leak small amounts of urine, you may have stress incontinence, which is the most common form in women and

## WHEN TO CALL A DOCTOR

"The vast majority of people with mild to moderate symptoms do not have to rush off to see a doctor. Give yourself 3 months to see if lifestyle measures work," says Abraham N. Morse, M.D.

Other symptoms—painful urination, for example, incontinence that accompanies painful intercourse, or urine that's cloudy or tinged with blood—are signs that it's time to call a doctor right away. Urinary tract infections or even tumors can cause the bladder to go into overdrive.

You should also call a doctor if you're having large "accidents" rather than small leaks. Or if accidents are accompanied by numbness or weakness in your arms or legs, vision changes, or a change in bowel habits. These symptoms may be a sign of nerve damage or other neurological problems, such as Parkinson's disease.

is treatable. Physical changes resulting from pregnancy, childbirth, and menopause are the common culprits behind stress incontinence.

Urge incontinence happens when you suddenly feel the need to urinate and then lose control of your bladder. It seems to strike for no apparent reason, and more women than men are affected. Inappropriate bladder contractions (otherwise known as an overactive bladder) are the most common underlying cause of urge incontinence and can develop when the muscles and nerves that control the bladder's "holding" ability are damaged. A variety of conditions can cause such damage, including urinary tract infections and vaginal childbirth.

In most cases, incontinence is a matter of degree. But it is not a normal part of aging, says Neil Resnick, M.D. "It's not inevitable, and it's not irreversible." Sometimes minimal effort can reduce, even prevent, the problem. Here are some ways to help yourself.

**Keep a bladder diary.** For a week, write down everything you ate, drank, when you went to the bathroom, and when you leaked urine, Dr. Jeter suggests. The diary will help you and your doctor track down the cause.

**Go easy on fluids.** Your bladder diary may reveal that you've been downing gallons of water a day, Dr. Jeter says. "Usually, it's because a person is on a diet that requires forcing liquids. If you drink a little less, your incontinence problem should ease up."

Take note of the timing, too. It's better to sip water throughout the day rather than pouring it down all at once. And it's especially important to stop drinking water within 3 to 4 hours of going to bed, especially if you get up several times during the night to go to the bathroom, adds Joseph Montella, M.D.

**But not too easy.** Cutting your fluid intake to below-normal levels without your doctor's approval can lead to dehydration, worsening urinary problems and possibly causing serious illness. Doctors usually advise people to drink eight glasses of water daily to prevent dehydration.

**Avoid alcohol.** Booze is a great stimulant for trotting to the bathroom.

**Avoid caffeine.** Caffeine is another well-known diuretic. Caffeine also irritates the bladder and stimulates muscle contractions, which can aggravate the symptoms of urge incontinence, explains Abraham N. Morse, M.D.

Caffeine is found in beverages, but also in foods such as chocolate and in medications such as Excedrin. Doctors advise limiting caffeine intake to no more than 200 milligrams daily, about the amount in 12 ounces of coffee. Your diary will help you notice whether you're getting too much.

Switching to decaffeinated coffee or to tea will help, but it may not eliminate the problem, Dr. Morse adds. Other substances in coffee and tea also act as bladder irritants.

# Do just 1 thing

Bladder drill training is one of the best treatments for certain types of incontinence. The idea is simple. Rather than going to the bathroom every time you get the urge to urinate, only go at specific times—every hour on the hour, for example, whether you feel the urge or not.

Do this for 5 to 7 days, then increase the interval between bathroom visits to 1½ hours, advises Abraham N. Morse, M.D. Do this for another 5 to 7 days, then increase the interval to 2 hours. Keep increasing the time intervals until you reach 4 hours.

Hold your urine as best you can between bathroom breaks. You might experience leaks, but that's okay. As long as you stick to the clock, you'll eventually gain more control.

This method can be highly effective, but no one knows why. "We don't know whether it truly retrains the bladder to function normally," says Neil Resnick, M.D., "or whether it trains the brain to cope with a persistent bladder dysfunction."

"Studies have shown that about 50 percent of people will have significant improvement with bladder training alone," adds Dr. Morse.

**Avoid grapefruit juice.** Grapefruit juice is a famous diuretic, which is why it formed the basis for a once-popular diet.

**Substitute cranberry juice.** Cranberry juice is key to bladder health because its acidity helps prevent urinary tract infections, a common problem to people who live with many forms of incontinence. Cranberry juice also helps deodorize the urinary tract, making accidents a little less noticeable.

**Drink "flat" water.** The carbon dioxide bubbles in fizzy water and soft drinks make the urine more acidic, which can trigger the urge to urinate, says Dr. Morse.

**Stay loose.** Constipation can contribute to incontinence. So eat a high-fiber diet, and be sure to drink adequate amounts of fluid. One incontinence clinic's prescription is daily helpings of popcorn!

**Don't smoke.** Nicotine and other chemicals in tobacco smoke can irritate the bladder, says Dr. Montella. "People who smoke may have chronic irritation that can lead to an overactive bladder," he explains.

Also, if you have stress incontinence, coughing can trigger leaking.

**Lose excess weight.** Foundation president Cheryle Gartley says that letters from patients seen at the Simon Foundation for Continence in Wilmette, Illinois, show people who lose even a few pounds can reduce incidents of incontinence.

**Try "double voiding."** When you urinate, stay on the toilet until you feel your bladder is empty. Then, stand up and sit down again, lean forward slightly at the knees, and try again.

**Know when you should go.** It's a good idea to empty your bladder on a regular basis, Dr. Jeter says. For example, don't sit at the dinner table and hold it until dinner's over. Holding too long may lead to bladder infection and an overstretched bladder. Also, if you have a too-full bladder and a weak sphincter muscle, she says, you're likely to leak when you cough, sneeze, or laugh. Your best bet is to empty your bladder before and after meals, and at bedtime.

**Do special exercises.** Kegel exercises were developed in the late 1940s by Arnold Kegel, M.D., to help women with stress incontinence during and after pregnancy. The experts say that these exercises reduce and may even prevent some forms of incontinence in both sexes and at all ages. Here are the guidelines from the National Association for Continence.

1. Without tensing the muscles of your legs, buttocks, or abdomen, imagine that you're trying to hold back a bowel movement by tightening the ring of muscles (the sphincter) around the anus. This exercise identifies the back part of the pelvic muscles.

2. When you're urinating, try to stop the flow, and then restart it. This identifies the front part of the pelvic muscles. (For women: Imagine you're trying to grip a slipping tampon.)

3. You're now ready for the complete exercise. Working from back to front, tighten the muscles while counting to four slowly, then release. Do this for 2 minutes, at least three times a day—that's at least 100 repetitions.

**Anticipate accidents.** If you know you're going to sneeze, cough, lift, or bounce up and down, squeeze that sphincter ahead of time to ward off an accident.

**Don't panic if you have no warning.** If you have urge incontinence, you have almost no warning of the need to go. Don't panic. Instead, at first notice, relax. The same muscles you use to clench your buttocks can also be used to short-circuit those "gotta go" sensations. Clench the muscles as tightly as you can, and hold the tension for a few seconds. Doing this several times in a row often makes the urge to urinate disappear. "It's like biting your lip when you have to sneeze," says Dr. Morse.

When the urge sensation passes, walk slowly, without panic, to the nearest restroom.

**Quiet your mind.** Another strategy for sudden urges is to "breathe deeply, calm yourself down, and have confidence that you're not going to make a mess," says Dr. Morse. If you can calm yourself for 30 to 60 seconds, there's a good chance the urge will go away, he explains.

"The idea is to get control over your bladder, rather than having a panic situation," adds Dr. Montella. "Wait until you're calm, then go to the bathroom."

**Be ready for emergencies.** If incontinence at night is a problem, keep a bedpan or commode within reach of your bed.

**Compensate for your age.** As you age, it takes longer to get places—including the bathroom. So make sure you always know where the bathroom is, and position yourself as close as possible to it, says Dr. Jeter.

**Buy special supplies.** There are several brands of absorbent underpants, pads, and shields. The products absorb 50 to 500 times their weight in water, neutralize odor, and congeal fluid to prevent leakage. The kind you need depends on your individual anatomy and the kind and degree of incontinence you have. It's understandable if you're embarrassed to buy them. Find an understanding pharmacist and ask to have your purchase waiting for you when you arrive, or purchase them online and have them delivered to your door.

**Reduce the tension in your life.** "Whenever you're anxious or depressed, your body sensations are magnified in a negative way," says Dr. Morse. "If you're anxious to begin with, feeling as though you have to rush to the bathroom is one more thing that can put you over the edge."

Take a hint from your bladder and unwind. Give yourself an hour each day to do something that's just for you, like taking a long walk, watching some television, or going to a movie or museum.

## PANEL OF ADVISORS

**Cheryle Gartley** is president of the Simon Foundation for Continence in Wilmette, Illinois.

**Katherine Jeter, Ed.D.,** is founder of the National Association for Continence in Spartanburg, South Carolina.

**Joseph Montella, M.D.,** is director of urogynecology at Jefferson Medical College of Thomas Jefferson University in Philadelphia.

**Abraham N. Morse, M.D.,** is an assistant professor of urogynecology at the University of Massachusetts Medical School in Worcester.

**Neil Resnick, M.D.,** is a professor of medicine and chief of the division of geriatric medicine at the University of Pittsburgh Medical Center.

**Robert Schlesinger, M.D.,** is a urologist at Faulkner Hospital in Jamaica Plain, Massachusetts.

# INFERTILITY

## 19 Ways to Get a Baby on Board

Few experiences can compare to the joy of bringing a child into the world. And virtually nothing is as distressing as trying to make a baby—and failing.

Infertility is the inability to conceive a child within 1 year. A variety of factors contribute to infertility, including genetics, health conditions, and lifestyle choices. And while infertility may be traced to a single cause in either you or your partner, it can also be caused by a combination of factors, from infection to stress to medications.

If you and your partner have been unable to get pregnant, you're far from alone. Overall, 2.1 million married couples face infertility. Of these couples, the problem occurs in a man's reproductive system 30 to 50 percent of the time and in a woman's reproductive system—which has more tasks to perform in the baby-making process—50 to 70 percent of the time.

But take heart, especially if you're an older mommy wanna-be. While you and your partner will want to see a doctor to determine the exact cause of your infertility, there's a lot that you can do on your own to increase your odds of conceiving a child. Try one or all of these expert-recommended tips.

## Do just 1 thing

Kick those butts. "No question about it—smoking is a major factor in infertility," says John Jarrett, M.D. "If both partners smoke, their chances of successful conception drop as much as 50 percent."

In men, the heavy metals in cigarette smoke get inside the head of the sperm and poison the mechanism by which the sperm penetrates the egg, says Dr. Jarrett. In women, the heavy metals prevent cell division from occurring, which leads to a miscarriage.

Women over 35 who are planning to have children have another urgent reason to quit. Smoking makes you infertile by bringing on menopause an average of 2 years earlier.

WHEN TO CALL A DOCTOR

If you're under age 35, and you and your partner have not been able to conceive during a year of unprotected sex, see your gynecologist. If you're age 35 or older, see your doctor if you haven't conceived after 6 months.

## Remedies for Women

**Plan ahead, if you can.** Unfair as it is, it's a biological fact: A woman's age dramatically impacts her fertility, says Robert Stillman, M.D. Population studies indicate that more than 90 percent of women under the age of 24 are able to conceive successfully. That figure drops sharply with age; by the time women are between the ages of 35 and 44, the odds are a little better than 1 in 3.

That's *not* to say that if you're in your twenties or early thirties, you should have children if you're not emotionally or financially prepared, says Dr. Stillman. But knowing up front that your odds of conceiving dwindle with age can help you make an informed decision about when to get pregnant.

**Practice think-ahead birth control.** If you're over 35, it may be better to avoid two birth-control methods: Depo-Provera ("the Shot") and Norplant, advises Dr. Stillman. Both can linger in a woman's body long after she stops taking them—sometimes, up to several years. If you prefer a hormonal method of birth control (rather than, say, condoms or diaphragms), use the Pill, recommends Dr. Stillman. "When you're ready to conceive, there will be less chance of a long delay."

If you're under 35, Depo-Provera and Norplant are probably quite safe, says Dr. Stillman. "There will be enough time for them to leave your system, even at the end of the spectrum."

**Get to your "fertility weight."** Twelve percent of all infertility cases stem from weighing too much or too little. If you're overweight, losing just 5 to 10 percent of your weight may dramatically improve your chances of ovulating and conceiving. If you're drastically underweight, try your best to gain. "Women biologically need a certain amount of body fat to carry and bear a child," says Dr. Stillman.

**Keep up with your workouts.** It's a myth that women should stop working out while they're trying to conceive, says John Jarrett, M.D. In fact, regular exercise can help you cope with the emotional stress that you might be feeling as you try to get pregnant.

**Time your ovulation.** Women typically ovulate—release an egg from an ovary—10 to 14 days before they menstruate. To find out when you ovulate, buy an ovulation detection kit, recommends Linda C. Giudice, M.D. These kits, which you can buy over the counter, measure your levels of urinary luteinizing hormone (LH), a hormone that stimulates egg maturation and release. Use the test between 8:00 A.M. and 10:00 A.M., when LH typically surges, she says.

**Get a jump on your hormones.** The ovulation detection test typically reads positive 24 hours *before* you actually ovulate. When you get that positive result, have intercourse that night (or day), the next day, or both, says Dr. Giudice.

**Or throw timing out the window.** If a woman is on a reliable 28-day cycle, she ovulates around day 14, says Dr. Jarrett. "So having sex on days 10, 12, 14, 16, and 18 will pretty much cover your bases."

**Lie still.** Lying still for 5 to 10 minutes after intercourse may improve your chances of conceiving, because it helps keep your partner's semen where it needs to be, says Dr. Stillman. (It's not necessary to do something drastic to keep semen inside you, he adds. So forget about hanging upside down in gravity boots.)

**Say *sayonara* to soy foods.** Women who are trying to conceive should avoid soy foods, such as tofu and soy milk, advises Dr. Stillman. "They contain plant estrogens, called phytoestrogens, that compete with a woman's natural estrogen, and they can throw off a woman's ovulation cycle," he says. "We've seen women who have stopped ovulating completely."

**Choose vitex.** Also known as chasteberry, vitex stimulates the pituitary gland to increase the production of LH, explains Serafina Corsello, M.D. This results in higher levels of progesterone during the second phase of a woman's menstrual cycle, called the luteal phase. Progesterone is important for fertility because it helps develop a thick, blood-rich uterine lining into which a fertilized egg can implant. Many women between ages 30 and 45 have a drop-off in progesterone, which leads to shortened cycles and the inability to plant an egg. You should use vitex for several months before attempting to become pregnant. A standard dose is 40 drops of standardized extract once a day, or one 650-milligram capsule up to three times a day.

**Try false unicorn root.** While it hasn't yet been researched scientifically, this herb is considered *the* fertility herb by many herbalists. It's thought to contain compounds called steroidal saponins that herbalists suspect may be responsible for its normalizing effect on female hormones. Use 5 to 15 drops of the tincture (available in health food stores) for 3 to 6 months.

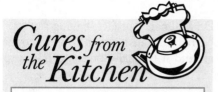

## Cures from the Kitchen

Daddy wanna-bes should consider filling their plates with fresh fruits and vegetables. The nutrients they contain may help "grow" healthy sperm.

Here's why. A preliminary study conducted at the Cleveland Clinic Urological Institute's Center for Advanced Research in Human Reproduction and Fertility suggests that abnormally high levels of free radicals may cause infertility in some men. Free radicals are "crippled" oxygen molecules that are generated naturally by our body processes. They damage healthy cells—and, possibly, sperm.

"Sperm require small amounts of free radicals to fertilize an egg," says study author Ashok Agarwal, Ph.D. "But too many free radicals can damage the sperm's cell membrane and DNA, compromising the sperm's ability to fertilize."

The researchers theorize that antioxidant vitamins, such as beta-carotene, vitamin C, and vitamin E, may benefit the sperm of men under high oxidative stress—for example, smokers and avid exercisers—because these vitamins may help neutralize free radicals.

## Remedies for Men

**Stay out of hot tubs.** Hot tubs can be detrimental to a man's fertility because the intense heat can kill the sperm in his testes, says Dr. Stillman. Steam rooms are fine, however.

**Say bye-bye to briefs.** It really is true: It's better to wear loose, baggy underwear that allows your testicles to "breathe," says Dr. Giudice. "Briefs raise the temperature of a man's testicles, which can kill sperm or can decrease the ability of sperm to fertilize an egg."

**Try Proxceed.** Men with low sperm count may want to try this dietary supplement, specifically designed to optimize sperm quantity and quality. It contains L-carnitine and acetyl-L-carnitine, which play a role in the process of sperm development, maturation, and maintenance. "Some urologists and infertility folks recommend that men with low sperm counts try it," says Dr. Giudice. "There may be something to it." Proxceed is available online, directly from the manufacturer.

## Remedies for Men and Women

**Break out the condoms.** If you're not currently in a monogamous relationship but want to have children someday, use a condom—every time. Sexually transmitted diseases such as chlamydia and gonorrhea, which often cause no symptoms, can cause infertility in both men and women.

**Don't overdo the deed.** Having sex until you're ready to drop will *not* increase your chances of conceiving, says Dr. Stillman. "In fact, having sex four or five times a day is counterproductive." That's because a man's sperm count drops dramatically right after ejaculation, and it typically takes 48 hours to reach pre-ejaculation levels.

**Drink lightly or not at all.** Research shows that women who consume as few as five drinks a week may hinder conception. Men who consume large amounts of alcohol can impair their fertility as well. A heavy drinker may end up with a damaged liver. Estrogen levels rise in men with liver damage, which can often cause impaired sperm production.

## PANEL OF ADVISORS

**Ashok Agarwal, Ph.D.,** is director of the andrology laboratory and sperm bank at the Cleveland Clinic Foundation in Ohio.

**Serafina Corsello, M.D.,** is medical director of the Corsello Center for Complementary-Alternative Medicine in New York City. She is the author of *The Ageless Woman.*

**Linda C. Giudice, M.D., Ph.D.,** is director of the division of reproductive endocrinology and fertility at Stanford University.

**John Jarrett, M.D.,** is a reproductive endocrinologist in Indianapolis.

**Robert Stillman, M.D.,** is a clinical professor in the department of obstetrics and gynecology at Georgetown University School of Medicine in Washington, D.C., and medical director at the Shady Grove Fertility Reproductive Science Center in Rockville, Maryland.

# INGROWN HAIR
## 10 Ways to Get a Clean Shave

An ingrown hair lives up to its name, for instead of growing outward, it grows back into the skin. When the tip of the hair punctures the skin, it can cause inflammation and pain. Naturally curly hairs, especially beard hairs in African-American men, are commonly ingrown.

If inflammation is also a problem, many experts recommend letting the hair grow if feasible. When hairs are longer, they don't twist around and puncture the skin.

Dermatologists say that tweezers are the only way to get rid of an ingrown hair, but there are other methods to make sure ingrown hairs don't return. Follow these tips to ease your discomfort.

**Send tweezers to the rescue.** If you can see an ingrown hair beneath the skin, apply a warm, damp compress for a couple of minutes to soften the skin, advises Rodney Basler, M.D. Then sterilize a needle or tweezers and pluck the hair. Follow with an antiseptic such as hydrogen peroxide or rubbing alcohol.

**Bring the hair to the surface.** If you can't see the ingrown hair, don't go fishing for it, Dr. Basler warns, "because it might not be an ingrown hair at all." Instead, treat it with a warm compress until you can see a hair lurking there. Then use a sterilized needle or tweezers, followed by an antiseptic.

**Think about growing a beard.** "The curlier your hair is, the more likely you are to get ingrown hairs," says Dr. Basler. If it's a real problem, seriously consider growing a beard.

**Soften your whiskers.** If there's no way you can have a beard, properly preparing your whiskers for shaving helps prevent ingrown hairs. Wash your face thoroughly with soap and water for 2 minutes, recommends Jerome Z. Litt, M.D. That softens the hair. Rinse well, apply shaving cream or gel, and leave it on for 2 minutes to further soften the hair.

**Hide behind your shadow.** Reconcile yourself to having a continual five o'clock shadow, Dr. Basler says. Don't shave close. The best way to do this, he says, is to use an electric razor.

**Don't double up.** Double-track razors are double trouble. The first blade cuts and sharpens the hair; the second blade cuts below the skin level, Dr. Litt says. The result: The sharpened hair curls around and slips back into the skin. Instead, use a single-track razor and settle for a shave that isn't as close.

**Train your whiskers.** Does your beard grow in several directions? Dr. Litt advises you to train it to grow out straight. Do this by shaving in two directions: down on the face, and up on the neck (to prevent neck nicks). Don't shave in all kinds of different directions or back and forth. "You won't get as great a shave at first," he says, "but if you keep shaving down on the face and up on the neck, your beard should start growing out straight in a matter of months."

**Try the aftershave special.** Put a damp towel on your face for a few minutes after shaving, Dr. Basler says. "It softens the whiskers so they're less able to repenetrate the skin." Use a creamy aftershave lotion, not the typical alcohol-loaded aftershave splash. "It's soothing and keeps the hair moisturized," he says.

**Fight infection.** If a whisker burrows inside your skin despite your best efforts, you can cut down on the amount of bacteria it carries with it. A 10 percent benzoyl peroxide solution has some antibiotic effect, Dr. Basler says, and probably will help if used as an aftershave. Typical aftershaves contain lots of alcohol and may also help decrease the bacterial load.

**Ladies, shave down instead of up.** "Women typically shave their legs from ankle to knee," Dr. Litt says. This is against the grain and can cause ingrown hairs. Instead, shave down, from knee to ankle.

## PANEL OF ADVISORS

**Rodney Basler, M.D.,** is a dermatologist and assistant professor of internal medicine at the University of Nebraska College of Medicine in Lincoln.

**Jerome Z. Litt, M.D.,** is a dermatologist and assistant clinical professor of dermatology at Case Western Reserve University School of Medicine in Cleveland. He is the author of *Your Skin: From Acne to Zits.*

# INGROWN NAILS
## 7 Feet-Treating Methods

Few things drive a man or woman to distraction more than an ingrown nail. The pain can bedevil even the most placid people. How can a minor problem hurt so much?

Ingrown nails typically start when a nail—usually on the big toe—grows or is pushed into the soft, tender tissue alongside it. People whose toenails are somewhat convex are more susceptible, but anyone can fall victim. The result: red, painful, tender toes.

Although the long-term goal is to prevent future ingrown nails, the immediate aim of most folks is to soothe the pain. Here's how to accomplish both.

**Try an over-the-counter product.** There are a variety of nonprescription products that may soften the nail and the skin around it, thus relieving pain,

### WHEN TO CALL A DOCTOR

If your toe becomes infected, you should definitely see a physician, says Suzanne M. Levine, D.P.M. Signs to look for include swelling, redness, and pain or warmth when touched. Pus-filled blisters may also form. To reduce inflammation until your appointment, periodically soak your foot in an iodine solution, then apply an antibiotic cream.

"If you let an ingrown nail become seriously infected," she cautions, "you can end up in big trouble. Several patients have come to me only after their toes became red and swollen with pus. If your circulation is poor, you run the risk of gangrene."

Sometimes a bloody growth, called proud flesh, builds up on the side of the nail. This inflamed soft tissue can become quite sensitive when it extends into the nail groove. Doctors may cut away a small portion of the ingrown nail during a minor operation and prescribe antibiotics to fight infection.

says podiatrist Suzanne M. Levine, D.P.M. Dr. Scholl's Ingrown Toenail Relief Strips and Outgro Solution are two that may help. Make sure you follow directions to the letter. *Don't* use them if you have diabetes or impaired circulation.

**Get a wisp of relief.** Your mission is to help that embedded toenail grow out over the skin folds at its side. Start by soaking your foot in warm water to soften the nail, says Frederick Hass, M.D. Dry carefully, then gently insert a *wisp* (not a wad) of sterile cotton beneath the burrowing edge of the nail. The cotton will slightly lift the nail so that it can grow past the tissue it is digging into. Apply an antiseptic as a safeguard against infection. Change the cotton insert daily until the nail has grown past the trouble spot.

**Remember: V is *not* for victory.** Whatever you do, don't fall for that old wives' tale about cutting a V-shaped wedge out of the center of the nail, warns Glenn Copeland, D.P.M. "People think that an ingrown nail is too big and that if you take a wedge from the middle, the sides will grow toward the center and away from the ingrown edge. That's utter nonsense. All nails grow from back to front only."

**Let your toes breathe.** Simply put, ill-fitting footwear can cause an ingrown nail, especially if your nails tend to curve. That's why you should avoid pointed or tight shoes that press on toenails, says Dr. Levine. Opt instead for sandals, where appropriate, or wide-toed shoes. If necessary, she says, modify offending shoes by cutting out the portion that presses on your toe. That may seem a little drastic, but a badly ingrown nail will put you in a drastic mood. Likewise, stay away from tight socks and panty hose.

**Cut nails with precision.** Never cut your nails too short, says Dr. Hass. Soften them first in warm water to reduce possible splitting, then cut straight across with a substantial, sharp, straight-edged clipper. Never cut a nail in an oval shape so that the leading edge curves down into the skin at the sides. Always

## Protect Those Toes from Accidents

While ingrown nails come mostly from improper cutting, they can also result from any number of accidents, says Frederick Hass, M.D. Stubbing your toe is one cause. Dropping a heavy object on your foot is another.

"I'd recommend stout, comfortable shoes for housework," he says. "If you constantly handle heavy objects such as machinery and crates at work, I'd definitely advise work shoes with steel toeboxes. They can protect your toes in all but the most serious accidents."

leave the outside edges parallel to the skin. And don't trim the nail any deeper than the tip of the toe; you want it long enough to protect the toe from pressure and friction.

**Fix mistakes properly.** If you accidentally cut or break a nail too short, carefully smooth it with an emery board or nail file at the edges so that no sharp points are left to penetrate the skin, says Dr. Hass. "Don't be tempted to use scissors, no matter how small they are. There is simply not enough space for you to work them properly, and they often leave a sharp edge."

## PANEL OF ADVISORS

**Glenn Copeland, D.P.M.,** is a podiatrist at the Women's College Hospital in Toronto. He is also consulting podiatrist for the Canadian Back Institute and a podiatrist for the Toronto Blue Jays baseball team.

**Frederick Hass, M.D.,** is a general practitioner in San Rafael, California. He is on the staff of Marin General Hospital in Greenbrae.

**Suzanne M. Levine, D.P.M., P.C.,** is a podiatrist and a podiatric attending physician at New York–Presbyterian Hospital. She is the author of *Your Feet Don't Have to Hurt.*

# INSOMNIA
## 22 Steps to a Good Night's Sleep

Insomnia ranks right behind the common cold, stomach disorders, and headaches as the reasons people seek a doctor's help. In a Gallup poll of more than 1,000 adults, one-third complained that they woke in the middle of the night and couldn't fall back to sleep.

At one time, doctors might have automatically prescribed a pill or two to ease you into dreamland, but that isn't always the case today. Researchers and doctors are learning more about sleep each year, broadening their knowledge of how to deal with its related problems.

Indeed, there are quite a few commonsense approaches that you can use to try to correct the problem yourself. It may take just one therapy; it may take a combination. In any case, the key to success is discipline. As Michael Stevenson, Ph.D., says, "Sleep is a natural physiological phenomenon, but it's also a learned behavior."

## WHEN TO CALL A DOCTOR

Serious sleeping troubles sometimes can result in what experts call chronic insomnia, which could have profound underpinnings, such as psychiatric disturbance, breathing problems, or unexplained leg movements during the middle of the night. Experts agree that if you can't easily fall asleep or stay asleep throughout the night for a month or so, it may be time to consult an expert.

According to the American Sleep Disorders Association, first explain your problems to your personal physician. If your doctor can't offer any advice, have her recommend a sleep-disorders specialist.

**Set a rigid sleep schedule 7 days a week.** Sleep medicine experts insist on people trying to be as regular with their habits as possible, says Merrill M. Mitler, Ph.D.

The key is to get enough sleep so that you can make it through your day without drowsiness. To achieve that goal, try to get to bed at the same time each night, which will help set your system's circadian rhythm, the so-called body clock that regulates most internal functions. Just as important is arising at the same time each morning.

Set a sleeping time of, say, 1:00 to 6:00 A.M. If you're sleeping soundly through that 5-hour period, add 15 minutes each week until you find yourself waking in the middle of the night. Work on getting through that waking period before adding another 15 minutes. You'll know when you reach the point where you've had enough sleep—you'll wake up refreshed, energetic, and ready to take on the day.

If you wake up during the night and can't get back to sleep in 15 minutes, don't fight it, says Dr. Mitler. Stay in bed and listen to the radio until you're drowsy again.

Again, be sure to wake up at the appointed hour in the morning; don't sleep in, trying to make up for "lost" sleep. That goes for the weekends as well. Don't sleep late on Saturday and Sunday mornings. If you do, you may have trouble falling asleep Sunday night, which can leave you feeling washed out on Monday morning.

**Don't waste your time in bed.** As you grow older, your body needs less sleep. Most newborn babies sleep up to 18 hours a day. By the time they're 10 years old, their need usually drops to 9 or 10 hours.

Experts agree that there is no "normal" amount of sleep for an adult. The average is 7 to 8 hours, but some people operate well on as few as 5 hours, while others need up to 10 hours. The key is to become what experts call an efficient sleeper.

Go to bed only when you're sleepy, advises Edward Stepanski, Ph.D. If you can't fall asleep in 15 minutes or so, get up and do something pleasantly monotonous. Read a magazine article, not a book that may engross you. Knit, watch television, or do a puzzle. Don't play computer games that excite you or perform goal-oriented tasks such as the laundry or housework.

When you feel drowsy, go back to bed. If you can't fall asleep, repeat the procedure until you can. But remember: Always wake up at the same time in the morning.

**Set aside some "quiet time" before bed.** "Some people are so busy that when they lie down to go to sleep, it's the first time all day that they've had to think about what happened that day," says psychiatrist David Neubauer, M.D.

An hour or two before going to bed, sit down for at least 10 minutes or so. Reflect on the day's activities and try to put them into some perspective. Review your stresses and strains, as well as your problems. Try to work out solutions. Plan tomorrow's activities.

This exercise will help clear your mind of the annoyances and problems that might keep you awake once you pull up the covers. With all that mental detritus out of the way, you'll be able to fill your mind with pleasant thoughts and images as you try to drift off to sleep. If, for some reason, cold reality begins to seep into your conscience, shut it out by saying, "Oh, I've already dealt with that, and I know what I'm going to do about it."

**Don't turn your bed into an office or a den.** "If you want to go to bed, you should be prepared to sleep," says Magdi Soliman, Ph.D. "If there's something else to do, you won't be able to concentrate on sleep."

Don't watch TV, talk on the phone, argue with your spouse, read, eat, or perform mundane tasks in bed. Use your bedroom only for sleep and sex.

**Avoid stimulants after twilight.** Coffee, colas, and even chocolate contain caffeine, the powerful stimulant that can keep you up, so try not to consume them past 4:00 P.M., says Dr. Mitler. Don't smoke either; nicotine is also a stimulant.

**Say no to a nightcap.** Avoid alcohol at dinner and throughout the rest of the evening, suggests Dr. Stevenson. And don't fix a so-called nightcap to relax you before bed. Alcohol depresses the central nervous system, but it also disrupts sleep. In a few hours, usually during the middle of the night, its effects wear off, your body slides into withdrawal, and you'll wake up.

**Question your medication.** Certain medications, such as asthma sprays, can disrupt sleep. If you take prescription medication routinely, ask your doctor about the side effects. If she suspects that the drug could be interfering with your sleep, she may be able to substitute another medication or adjust the time of day you take it.

**Examine your work schedule.** Research has shown that people who work on "swing" shifts—irregular schedules that frequently alternate from day to night—have problems sleeping, says Mortimer Mamelak, M.D. The stress of an up-and-down schedule may create jet lag–like tiredness all the time, and sleep mechanisms can break down altogether. The solution: Try to get a steady shift, even if it's at night.

**Eat a light snack before bedtime.** Bread and fruit will do nicely an hour or two before you hit the hay, says Sonia Ancoli-Israel, Ph.D. So will a glass of warm milk. Avoid sugary snacks that can excite your system or heavy meals that can stress your body.

Use common sense. If you're older, don't drink a lot of fluids before bed, or bathroom duty might call in the middle of the night.

**Create a comfortable sleep setting.** "Insomnia can often be caused by stress," says Dr. Stevenson. "You get into bed, and you're nervous and anxious,

## Light Up Your Life

Researchers at the National Institute of Mental Health (NIMH) found that bright lights in the morning could help chronically poor sleepers set their circadian rhythms, or "body clocks," on a more regular pattern.

According to Jean R. Joseph-Vanderpool, M.D., who conducted sleep research there for many years, many people find they just can't get started in the morning.

That's why when his research subjects woke up, say, around 8:00 A.M., they were placed in front of high-intensity, full-spectrum fluorescent lights for 2 hours—strong light that resembles what you might encounter on a summer morning in Washington, D.C. Those lights, in turn, told the body it's morning and time to get moving. Then, in the evening, they would wear dark glasses so that their bodies would know it was time to begin to wind down.

After several weeks of the therapy, Dr. Joseph-Vanderpool's patients reported more alertness in the morning and better sleep at night.

At home, he says, you can accomplish the same effect by walking around the neighborhood, sitting in the sun, or doing some yardwork as soon as you arise. During the winter, consult your doctor about the best type of artificial light to use.

and the nervous system is aroused, and that impairs your ability to sleep. Soon, the bedroom becomes associated with sleeplessness, and that triggers a phobic response."

You can change that by making the bedroom as comfortable a setting as possible. Redecorate with your favorite colors. Soundproof the room and hang dark curtains to keep out the light.

Buy a comfortable bed. It doesn't matter whether it's a coiled-spring mattress, a waterbed, a vibrating bed, or a mat on the floor. If it feels good, use it. Wear loose-fitting sleep clothes. Make sure the bedroom's temperature is just right—not too hot, not too cold. Be sure there's no clock within view that can distract you throughout the night.

**Turn off your mind.** Keep yourself from rehashing a stressful day of worries by focusing your thoughts on something peaceful and nonthreatening, says Dr. Stevenson. Play some soft, soothing music as you drift off or some environmental noise, such as the sound of a waterfall, waves crashing on a beach, or the sound of rain in a jungle. The only rule: Be sure it's not intrusive and distracting.

**Use mechanical aids.** Earplugs can help block out unwanted noise, especially if you live on a busy street or near an airport, says Dr. Ancoli-Israel. Eyeshades screen out unwanted light. An electric blanket warms you, especially if you're a person who always seems to be on the brink of a chill.

**Learn and practice relaxation techniques.** The harder you try to sleep, the greater the chances you'll end up gnashing your teeth all night rather than stacking some Zzzs. That's why it's important to relax once you're in bed.

"The one problem with insomnia is that people often concentrate too much on their sleep, and they press too hard," Dr. Stevenson says. "The key to successfully falling asleep is to reduce your focus and avoid working yourself into a frenzy."

Biofeedback exercises, deep breathing, muscle stretches, or yoga may help. Special audiotapes can teach you how to progressively relax your muscles.

Here are two techniques that doctors have found particularly successful.

- Slow down your breathing and imagine the air moving slowly in and out of your body while you breathe from your diaphragm. Practice this during the day so that it's easy to do before you go to bed.

- Program yourself to turn off unpleasant thoughts as they creep into your mind. To do that, think about enjoyable experiences you've had. Reminisce about good times, fantasize, or play some mental games. Try counting sheep or counting backward from 1,000 by 7s.

# The Herbal Approach

Help for insomnia may be as close as the herbal aisle of your grocery store. Here are a few herbs to try.

**Valerian.** This is the best-studied herbal sleep aid. Research shows that extracts of the root not only help you fall asleep faster but also improve sleep quality. Try taking this herb 30 to 45 minutes before bedtime. The typical dosage is one 150- to 300-milligram capsule standardized to 0.8 percent valeric acid.

**Kava kava.** When insomnia results from anxiety, this herb is particularly effective. Studies suggest that kava kava promotes sleep by acting upon the brain's emotion centers and by relaxing muscles. Taking one or two 400- to 500-milligram capsules an hour before bed should help you get the sleep you need.

**Chamomile.** A bright, daisylike flower, chamomile has an age-old reputation for calming nerves and gently aiding sleep. Drinking one or two cups of tea before bed will help soothe you into sleep.

**Take a warm bath.** One theory suggests that normal body temperatures play off the body's circadian rhythm. Those temperatures are low during sleep and at their highest point during the day.

Along those lines, it's thought that the body begins to get drowsy as temperature drops. Therefore, a warm bath taken 4 to 5 hours before bedtime raises that temperature. Then, as it begins to fall, you'll feel more tired, which makes it easier to fall asleep.

**Take a hike.** Get some exercise late in the afternoon or early in the evening, suggest Drs. Neubauer and Soliman. It shouldn't be too strenuous—a walk around the block is just fine. Not only will it fatigue your muscles, but it will also raise your body temperature and may help induce sleepiness as a warm bath would. Exercise also may help trigger the deep, nourishing sleep that your body craves most for replenishment.

**Try sex before bedtime.** For many, it's a pleasurable and mentally and physically relaxing way to let loose before settling down to sleep. Indeed, some researchers have found that hormonal mechanisms triggered during sexual activity help enhance sleep.

But again, it depends on the person, according to James K. Walsh, Ph.D. "If sex causes anxiety and creates problems, it's not such a good idea. But if you find it enjoyable, it can do a lot for you."

# PANEL OF ADVISORS

# IRRITABLE BOWEL SYNDROME
## 20 Coping Suggestions

Many people with irritable bowel syndrome, or IBS, develop a sixth sense about public restrooms. They know where to find one in a hurry, and they're accustomed to leaving a table of friends at dinner or a sale at Bloomingdale's to dash to the bathroom.

Doctors aren't sure what causes IBS, but many believe it's a muscle contraction or "motility" disturbance. The walls of the intestines are lined with layers of muscles that contract and relax as they move food from the stomach through the intestinal tract. In people who don't have IBS, the muscles contract and relax in regular rhythm. In people with IBS, the contractions are stronger—and they last longer.

Another theory blames an overgrowth of intestinal bacteria, says Mark Pimentel, M.D. In one study, doctors at Cedars-Sinai Medical Center in Los Angeles found that 78 percent of the 202 IBS patients they studied have a condition known as "small intestine bacterial overgrowth," in which the bacteria that normally live in the colon somehow find their way into the relatively sterile small intestine. The small intestine responds with an increase in gas and bloating after meals, as well as noticeable changes in the usual bowel habits. There is some controversy about this theory, however.

The upshot of coping with IBS means identifying the food, drinks, or stressful events that trigger alternating bouts of diarrhea, constipation, and abdominal pain. Sometimes, people with IBS get all three at the same time. A sense of bloating or fullness and mucus in the stool are other complaints.

Some doctors think that IBS may be second only to the common cold as America's most widespread medical complaint. Yet there's plenty of good news: For one, IBS does not appear to raise your risk for colorectal cancer. And IBS doesn't trigger changes in the bowel tissue or cause inflammation. After a diagnosis of IBS, these tips can ease symptoms and discomfort.

**Take the news in stride.** "There's a very good connection between stress and an irritable bowel," says Douglas A. Drossman, M.D. What you don't want to do is get stressed *because* you have an irritable bowel and thereby create a vicious

## WHEN TO CALL A DOCTOR

Like clockwork, you've always gone once a day. Gradually, you pass stools only every 3 days. Or vice versa. Or you have alternating constipation and diarrhea. These changes, or any other changes in bowel movements, especially when accompanied by abdominal pain that seems aggravated in stressful situations and relieved by passing stools, are the cardinal signs of irritable bowel syndrome.

Other symptoms may indicate a more serious condition. See your doctor if you have:

- Blood in your stool
- Unexplained weight loss
- Diarrhea that causes you to wake up at night
- Constipation, diarrhea, abdominal pain, or any combination of the three so severe that you can't work for several days or engage in social activities

cycle. Especially during flare-ups of abdominal pain, it's important to take a deep breath. "Think about what's happening. Recognize that it's happened before and it will pass. Know that you're *not* going to die—because people don't die from an irritable bowel," he says.

**Become a more relaxed person.** Anything you can do to help yourself unwind should help to alleviate your symptoms, says Dr. Drossman. You may benefit from relaxation techniques, such as meditation, self-hypnosis, or biofeedback. If the stress in your life is particularly problematic, consider psychological counseling. The key is to find what works for *you*.

**Keep a stress diary.** People with an irritable bowel have an intestinal system that overreacts to food, stress, and hormonal changes. "Think of your irritable bowel as a built-in barometer, and use it to help you determine what things in your life are most stressful," says Dr. Drossman. If, for instance, you have stomach pain every time you talk to your boss, see it as a sign that you need to work on that relationship (perhaps by talking it over with your boss, a friend, a family member, or a therapist). Simply keep a record of your symptoms for a week or two, taking note of what was happening just before their onset to see if any patterns emerge.

**Log in your food and beverage intake, too.** Certain foods and beverages, just like stress, can activate an irritable bowel, so it's also helpful to record in your diary the foods and beverages that give you the most trouble, says Dr. Drossman.

**Add fiber to your diet.** Many people with IBS do much better simply by adding fiber to their diets, says James B. Rhodes, M.D. Fiber tends to be most effective with people who tend toward constipation and small, hard stools, but it may also help you if you're experiencing diarrhea. The best fiber to add to your diet is the insoluble type—found in bran, whole grains, fruit, and vegetables.

**Send psyllium seed to the rescue.** An easy way to increase your fiber intake is with crushed psyllium seed, says Dr. Drossman. It's a natural laxative sold in drugstores, supermarkets, and health food stores. Unlike chemical laxatives often found on the same shelves, psyllium-based laxatives such as Metamucil or Konsyl are nonaddictive and generally safe, even when taken over long periods.

**Drink lots of fluid.** To keep your bowels moving smoothly, you need not only fiber but also fluids. You'll need more on August days when you play tennis than on December days that you spend at the movies, but in general, you should drink between six and eight glasses of fluid a day, says Dr. Rhodes.

---

## Visualize Yourself Pain-Free

It's normal to panic during an attack of abdominal pain. But ironically, stress makes the pain worse by tensing the bowel.

How can you break this nasty cycle?

With visualization, says Donna Copeland, Ph.D. It's a very effective tool for dealing with pain and anxiety, she says. Learning visualization techniques with a professional is probably the best route. But there's nothing wrong with trying a few on your own.

Dr. Copeland suggests the following: If you feel pain, stop what you're doing, find a comfortable place to sit or lie down, close your eyes, and—instead of focusing on your pain—see yourself:

- Diving expertly into the warm ocean surf off a beautiful, white-sanded tropical island beach

- Standing atop a tall, snow-crested mountain, breathing the cool air, and listening to the crunch of snow under your feet

- Sitting in a large wooden hot tub, chatting idly with several of your closest friends

- Walking through a lush garden in a far-off, exotic land

**Reconsider dairy products.** One fluid you may be better off without is milk. "A large number of people who say they have IBS are really lactose intolerant," says William J. Snape, M.D. It means that your body has difficulty absorbing lactose, an enzyme found in milk. Your doctor can test you for lactose intolerance, or you can give up dairy products for a couple of days and see how you do. In either case, you may find that this one dietary change can clear up all your problems. (For more information on lactose intolerance, see page 366.)

**Cut out the fat.** Here's one more good reason to eat a low-fat diet. "Fat is a major stimulus to colonic contractions," says Dr. Snape. In other words, it can worsen your IBS. A good place to begin to cut the fat out of your diet is by eliminating heavy sauces, fried foods, and salad oils, he says.

**Pass on the gas.** Some people with IBS are particularly sensitive to gas-inducing foods, says Dr. Rhodes. If you fall into this group, you may find relief by avoiding such flatulence champs as cooked dried beans, cabbage, Brussels sprouts, broccoli, cauliflower, and onions.

**Go easy on the bran.** If you're adding fiber such as bran to your diet, add it slowly to give your body time to adjust. Too much fiber, too fast, can produce gas, says Dr. Rhodes.

**Beware of spicy foods.** Some people with IBS are sensitive to foods laden with peppers and other spices, says Dr. Rhodes. Try eating a lot of spicy foods for 1 week and a lot of bland foods the next week, and note if your condition changes, he suggests.

**Don't brew trouble with coffee.** Coffee is a major cause of woe among people with IBS, says Dr. Snape. To some extent, the culprit may be caffeine, but it may also be the resins in the coffee bean itself. You may get some relief if you switch to decaffeinated. If you don't, try cutting down on all coffee.

**Reconsider alcohol.** Alcoholic beverages can exacerbate your problems, but it's probably not the alcohol itself, says Dr. Snape. Rather, it's the complex carbohydrates in beer and the tannins in red wine that probably cause the most grief. People with IBS should avoid these two drinks, he says.

**Put out that cigarette.** "A large number of people experience IBS problems with smoking," says Dr. Snape. The most probable culprit is the nicotine, so if you're trying to quit with the help of nicotine gum, you may not see any difference in your tummy problems.

**Spit out the gum.** Nicotine gum is not the only kind of gum that can give you troubles. Gums and candies artificially sweetened with sorbitol are not easily digested and can worsen your IBS, says Dr. Drossman. While the amount of sorbitol found in one stick of gum or one hard candy isn't likely to affect you greatly, if you gobble up 10 or more pieces a day, it's time to cut back.

**Eat regular meals.** It's not only *what* you eat, but *how* you eat that can vex an irritable bowel, says Dr. Snape. Digesting a lot of food eaten all at once over-stimulates the digestive system. That is why it's much better to eat frequent smaller meals than infrequent larger ones.

**Go for a jog.** "Good body tone, good bowel tone," says Dr. Rhodes. Exercise strengthens the entire body, including the bowel. It helps relieve stress, and it releases endorphins that help you control pain. All in all, regular exercise will more than likely calm your irritable bowel. Be careful, however, not to overdo it. Too much exercise can lead to diarrhea.

**Call a hot-water bottle to the rescue.** If you experience abdominal pain, the best thing to do is to sit or lie down, take a deep breath, and try to relax. Some people also find that putting a hot-water bottle or a heating pad on their tummy helps, says Dr. Snape.

## PANEL OF ADVISORS

**Donna Copeland, Ph.D.,** is a professor of pediatrics (psychology) and chief of the behavioral medicine section at the University of Texas M. D. Anderson Cancer Center in Houston. She is also a clinical psychologist and past president of the American Psychological Association's Division of Psychological Hypnosis.

**Douglas A. Drossman, M.D.,** is a professor of medicine and psychiatry with the division of digestive diseases and codirector of the UNC Center for Functional Gastrointestinal and Motility Disorders at the University of North Carolina at Chapel Hill School of Medicine. He is a gastroenterologist with psychiatric training.

**Nancy Norton** is founder of the International Foundation for Functional Gastrointestinal Disorders in Milwaukee.

**Mark Pimentel, M.D.,** is assistant director of the gastrointestinal motility program at Cedars-Sinai Medical Center in Los Angeles, and lead author of a 2000 study in the *American Journal of Gastroenterology* on bacterial overgrowth and irritable bowel syndrome.

**James B. Rhodes, M.D.,** was a professor of medicine with the division of gastroenterology at the University of Kansas Medical Center in Kansas City.

**William J. Snape Jr., M.D.,** is a clinical professor of medicine at University of California, Irvine; medical director of clinical motility laboratory at California Pacific Medical Center in San Francisco; and director at the Bowel Disease and Motility Center at Long Beach Memorial Medical Center in Long Beach.

# Jet Lag
## 21 Hints for Arriving Alert

Want to induce your own jet lag without a trip to Europe? Try this: In the spring, set the clock ahead 3 hours—instead of 1 hour—for daylight saving time.

The endless summer night might be fun, but the end result would be jet lag, because adjusting your inner body clock isn't as easy as changing the time of the clock on the wall.

Yet when you fly across several time zones, you ask your body to adjust to a new time and a new place. It takes awhile for the internal clock to reset itself to the new day or night cycle. That's why you get jet lag. And the more time zones you cross, the more you suffer.

No matter which way you're going, each time zone crossed requires about 1 day of adjustment, says Charles Ehret, Ph.D.

The previously mentioned inner body clock, says Dr. Ehret, is really a whole set of clocks controlled by a master clock. "Every cell in the body is a clock," he explains, "and they're all brought together by a special pacemaker in the brain."

Normally your body clock operates on cycles approximately 24 to 25 hours long. But rapid time changes disrupt all that. The result is jet lag—fatigue, lethargy, inability to sleep, trouble concentrating and making decisions, irritability, perhaps even diarrhea and a lack of appetite.

Though you can't make time stand still, there's a lot you *can* do to take some of the zap out of jet lag.

**Live on a schedule.** Weeks, or at least days, before you leave, maintain a sensible schedule. "People who have no order in their lives—who stay up late to watch a movie and start doing their laundry at 2:00 A.M.—have more trouble with jet lag," says Dr. Ehret. Make sure your circadian rhythms, also called body clock cycles, are in sync.

**Get enough sleep.** Shortchange yourself on sleep before your trip, Dr. Ehret says, and you can count on making jet lag worse. "Give yourself about 15 extra minutes of sleep each of the last few nights before you travel."

# Fight Jet Lag with Feast and Fast

The now-famous anti–jet lag diet developed by Charles Ehret, Ph.D., grew out of extensive animal research at the Argonne National Laboratory. In actuality, it is more than a diet. Daylight, social cues, sleeping patterns, and mental and physical exercise all play a role in making the diet work, Dr. Ehret says.

But the core of the plan involves a 4-day sequence of feast-fast/feast-fast prior to the day of arrival. For these purposes, feast means to eat as much as you want, and fast means to eat lightly.

Here is a sample menu for a fast day.

*Breakfast:* Two eggs, any style, and one-half piece of lightly buttered toast—214 calories.

*Lunch:* One chicken breast, skin removed; 1 cup of bouillon; ½ cup of low-fat cottage cheese—245 calories.

*Supper:* One small bowl of pasta, lightly buttered with margarine; one piece of bread, lightly buttered; 1 cup of cooked vegetables (broccoli, string beans, summer squash, or carrots); one alcoholic beverage (optional)—355 calories.

Caffeine is also a major part of the plan. Experiments with laboratory animals, Dr. Ehret says, have shown that caffeine can be used to reset body clocks.

Now let's examine some additional aspects of Dr. Ehret's plan as applied to a westward flight with a 3-hour time change—for example, a trip from New York to San Francisco in which you arrive in San Francisco at 8:30 A.M. local time.

**Change your caffeine habits.** Three days before the flight, stop consuming caffeine, except from 3:00 to 4:30 P.M. One day before the flight, caffeine is allowed only between 7:00 and 8:00 A.M. On the day of the flight, drink two to three cups of black coffee. But do this no later than 11:30 A.M. and have no more caffeine the rest of the day.

**Set your watch to the new destination time.** Start acclimating yourself to the time change; stay mentally active in the half-hour immediately preceding breakfast time at your destination.

**Pass up breakfast with the passengers.** Arrange to have breakfast at the breakfast time of your destination. In this situation, it would be soon before landing.

**Eat a hearty lunch with the natives.** You may arrive in San Francisco in the morning, but put off eating until lunchtime. But it's also a feast day, so enjoy.

**Fly by day, arrive at night.** "The best plan is to arrive at your destination in midevening, get something light to eat, and go to bed by 11:00 P.M. destination time," says Timothy Monk, Ph.D.

This scenario, Dr. Monk says, gives your body optimal opportunity to adjust to the change in time zones.

**Drink plenty of fluids during the flight.** Airplane cabins are notoriously dry, Dr. Monk says, and fluids help combat the dehydration that induces fatigue. Dehydration obviously won't help you beat jet lag.

**Avoid alcohol.** Alcohol is a diuretic and further dehydrates you. Ask for juice or water instead.

**Pretend you're not on a plane.** Flight attendant Jonie Nolan does this when she's not working and just traveling as a passenger. "I get a pillow and shut my eyes, but I don't go to sleep, and I pretend I'm not on the flight," she says. "I daydream, thinking pleasant, positive thoughts or just making plans for what I'm going to do next week." This helps her reduce stress before asking her body to suddenly shift 2 to 3 hours.

She says that she hasn't tried this on really long flights but finds it effective for trips where she crosses a couple of time zones.

**Do as the Romans do.** When you arrive, start adapting to your new environment as quickly as possible. "Get involved—notice the new street names and the language of the people," says Dr. Ehret. "This helps you adjust."

**Socialize.** This is especially important if your body craves sleep but it's only midafternoon at your destination. "When we're socializing, our bodies assume it's daytime because human beings are, by nature, daytime creatures," says Marijo Readey, Ph.D.

**Don't nap.** Or if you do, limit the nap to 1 hour. Napping, Dr. Monk says, just delays your adjustment to the new time zone.

**Soak up some sunshine.** Get out in the sun at your destination as much as possible, says Dr. Monk. This exposure helps keep your biological clock in the stimulated and awake state during daylight hours at your destination.

When light strikes the eye, neurotransmitters are released that send an immediate signal to specific regions of the brain, Dr. Ehret explains. In turn, these brain regions signal the rest of the body that your awake-and-active phase is about to begin.

**Make a date with the sun.** Some experts feel that the time of day you get out in the sunshine is also important. Light earlier in the day appears to shift

# How Three Famous Globe-Trotters Tried to Cope

If you need a personal strategy for beating jet lag, check out tips from famous globe-trotters Henry Kissinger, Dwight D. Eisenhower, and Lyndon Johnson.

In his book *Overcoming Jet Lag*, Charles Ehret, Ph.D., described each method, noting that while none is very reliable, they're also not harmful either.

**Take the diplomatic route.** Several days before the flight, go to bed 1 hour earlier and get up 1 hour later. This was former Secretary of State Henry Kissinger's routine. The problem with this plan, Dr. Ehret says, is the rigidity it demands. Kissinger couldn't always follow it consistently, and most people would probably have the same problem. There's also no proof, Dr. Ehret adds, that this approach measurably reduces jet lag.

**Arrive extra early.** Former President Eisenhower tried to arrive several days ahead of time before meeting with foreign leaders. The problem with Eisenhower's plan, Dr. Ehret says, is that often he didn't arrive early enough to compensate for the one-time-zone-crossed-equals-one-day-of-adjustment rule.

**Live by your home clock.** After arriving at a new destination, former President Lyndon Johnson insisted on maintaining his old schedule—eating and sleeping at his usual time. He even arranged meetings at hours that were convenient by Washington, D.C., time but not so convenient for the foreigners with whom he was meeting.

Perhaps you can get away with this if you're the president of the United States, Dr. Ehret says, but for the average traveler, it may be hard to get dinner reservations for 2:00 A.M.—even in Paris.

the body's clock to an earlier hour, while light later in the day seems to shift the body's clock to a later hour, according to Al Lewy, M.D., Ph.D.

So if you've traveled east, Dr. Lewy suggests getting outside light in the morning. And if you've traveled west, he recommends getting outside light in the afternoon. This only works, however, if you're crossing six or fewer time zones.

**Exercise.** Exercise, especially outdoors, gets your body pumped up, helps alertness, and gets you out in the sunlight.

A study at the University of Toronto also suggests that exercise reduces the number of days that jet lag affects you. Researchers exposed golden hamsters (nocturnal animals with stable activity rhythms) to artificial light and advanced the onset of darkness 8 hours, simulating the conditions of a long flight east.

After darkness, one group of hamsters exercised on a running wheel. The other group mostly slept. While the nonrunning hamsters took 5.4 days to adjust and to resume normal nocturnal activity, the running hamsters adjusted in just 1.6 days.

**Think before you react.** Put off all important decision-making for 24 hours or at least until you feel well-rested, advises Dr. Ehret. You won't do your clearest thinking after a long trip.

In business, he says, "People have made bad deals and later identified jet lag as the reason."

**Reverse the process.** If possible, use these tips to prepare for your return flight home, too. Jet lag is a two-way sky.

## PANEL OF ADVISORS

**Charles Ehret, Ph.D.,** is a pioneer in the field of chronobiology, the study of time's effect on plants, animals, and people. He is a retired senior scientist from the Argonne National Laboratory, a unit of the U.S. Department of Energy.

**Al Lewy, M.D., Ph.D.,** is a psychiatrist at Oregon Health Sciences University School of Medicine in Portland. He has done studies on the effects of sunlight on the human body clock.

**Timothy Monk, Ph.D.,** is a professor of psychiatry and director of the human chronobiology research program at the University of Pittsburgh School of Medicine.

**Jonie Nolan** has been a flight attendant for Trans World Airlines, now American Airlines, since 1981. She is based in St. Louis.

**Marijo Readey, Ph.D.,** was formerly a researcher at the Argonne National Laboratory, a unit of the U.S. Department of Energy.

# KNEE PAIN
## 23 Ways to Handle the Hurt

The knee is the strongest of the 187 joints in the human body, absorbing a force equivalent to $4\frac{1}{2}$ times your body weight just when you walk down the stairs. Yet despite its power, the knee is also the joint that typically causes the most suffering.

As Americans have become more active, sports-related knee injuries have become more common. But you don't have to be an athlete to experience knee pain. Automobile accidents commonly involve knee injuries. So do falls. Some knee pain stems from overuse or age-related wear and tear on the joint. The most common cause of knee pain is osteoarthritis, a degenerative wearing down of the cartilage cushions in the joint, causing bones to scrape painfully against each other.

In large measure because of osteoarthritis, which is much more common in people over age 45, knee pain tends to be a particular problem for older Americans. One study reported that 18 percent of men and 24 percent of women over 60 experienced knee pain on most days. The oldest Americans had the highest

## WHEN TO CALL A DOCTOR

Abrupt twisting motions (like in basketball or skiing) or an impact to the side of the knee (perhaps from a car accident or football tackle) may cause an injury to the cruciate ligament or the medial or lateral collateral ligaments of the knee. These injuries may or may not involve pain when they occur, but you may hear a buckle sound or "pop." Tendinitis and ruptured tendons may occur with overuse, or when you attempt to break a fall.

These injuries may be followed by swelling, tenderness, radiating pain, and perhaps some discoloration and loss of motion.

They should be iced, and they require medical care as soon as possible.

rates of knee pain, with 24 percent of men and 30 percent of women ages 85 to 90 having pain in their knees.

Part of the problem is design, or rather the inability of knee design to change whenever human beings place new demands on it. "The knee, without question, is ill-suited for the jobs we ask it to do," says James M. Fox, M.D. It wasn't designed for football, soccer, automobile accidents, carpentering, plumbing, or squatting and kneeling all day long.

If your knees ache because of overuse or abuse, here are a few things you can do to make amends.

**Take a load off.** Body weight is a major contributor to knee problems, says Dr. Fox. For every pound you weigh, that's multiplied by about six in terms of the stress placed across the knee area. If you're 10 pounds overweight, that's an extra 60 pounds your knee has to carry around. As Dr. Fox observes, "You don't put a Mack truck on Volkswagen tires."

**Don't bother with braces.** Knee braces can be purchased at just about any sporting goods store, but the experts say to leave them on the shelf. Some braces are truly meant to be preventive, but these are typically very complex, custom-designed, and cost from $300 to $1,000. "The wraps or braces you buy off the shelf at a sporting goods store shouldn't be used for anything more than to remind you that you have a bad knee," says Dr. Fox.

Some of them can do more harm than good, by pushing your kneecap into the joint, says trainer Marjorie Albohm.

**Go homeopathic.** Traumeel tablets and creams containing chamomile, echinacea, belladonna, calendula, and arnica are said to relieve knee pain. Dissolve the tablets under the tongue every few hours, or apply the cream directly to the knee. Be careful not to rub the cream onto broken skin, however.

**Reach for a nonprescription medication.** Ibuprofen is the over-the-counter painkiller of choice recommended by our experts. It reduces inflammation and provides pain relief without causing as many stomach problems as aspirin. Acetaminophen is a fine painkiller and causes fewer stomach problems, but it does little to reduce inflammation.

Studies have also shown ibuprofen can significantly improve joint mobility in people with acute knee ligament damage.

**Ask for a prescription.** A newer class of anti-inflammatory pain relievers, COX-2 inhibitors, offers the same benefits as ibuprofen while being even easier on the stomach. Many doctors now recommend celecoxib (Celebrex) or rofecoxib (Vioxx) for people with severe pain and a history of gastrointestinal problems.

**Try an alternative.** Glucosamine and chondroitin have been gaining in popularity in the treatment of osteoarthritis. Although controlled studies of these compounds have produced mixed results, they do appear to have a significant impact on pain. So far, their effect seems to be slightly less robust than nonsteroidal anti-inflammatory drugs such as ibuprofen, and their full effect is not seen for 4 to 6 weeks. Larger trials are underway.

**Take your vitamins.** Certain vitamins can help rebuild cartilage and tendons and reduce joint pain. Some experts recommend vitamin A (5,000 IU per day), vitamin $B_6$ (50 milligrams per day), vitamin C (1,000 milligrams, two times per day), vitamin E (400 IU per day), and niacin (35 milligrams of niacinamide per day).

**Try the rub that soothes.** Some menthol lotions produce heat, which can relieve symptoms and make you feel more comfortable, says Dr. Fox. By covering the knee in plastic after applying the lotion, you can make the liniment even hotter. Be careful that you don't burn your skin or cause irritation.

**Find a spicy cure.** Over-the-counter creams that contain capsaicin, an extract from chile peppers, may tone down knee pain. The creams, such as Zostrix and Capzasin-P, may be irritating to the skin, so try a small test spot for a few days before applying it to your entire knee, and don't apply it to broken skin.

**Target knee swelling.** Three natural substances may help to reduce inflammation within a sore joint. Fifty to 100 milligrams of grape seed extract a day is a safe dose to take indefinitely. Or try taking 1,000 milligrams of bromelain, a pineapple extract, or 500 milligrams of curcumin, a compound from the spice turmeric, three times a day for up to a month. If swelling persists after that, see your health care provider.

**Strengthen with exercise.** The only things holding the knee together are the muscles and the ligaments, says Dr. Fox. Building up the muscles is critical, because the muscles are the real supporting structures. If they don't have their power or endurance, you're going to be in trouble with your knees.

Stronger muscles provide you with a stronger joint, one that's better able to withstand the considerable strain that even walking or stairclimbing places on the knees. The goal of these exercises is to strengthen your quadriceps, the muscles in front of your legs, and your hamstring muscles, in the back of your thighs. These two muscles must be in balance, says Dr. Fox. If just one or the other is developed, it causes stress on the knee joint.

The following exercises are not hard to do, and they hurt a lot less than aching knees.

***Isometric knee builder.*** Sit on the floor with your sore knee straight out in front of you. Place a rolled towel under the small of the knee, then tighten the muscles in your leg without moving the knee. Hold that contraction and work up to where you can keep the muscles taut for at least 30 seconds, then relax. Repeat this tightening and relaxing process up to 25 times.

***Sitting leg lifts.*** Sit with your back against a wall and place a pillow in the small of your back. (Sitting against a wall ensures that the leg muscles do the lifting. This type of leg lift won't aggravate back pain.) Once you're in that position, do the isometric contraction described above for a count of five, then raise your leg a few inches and hold it to a count of five, then lower it and relax for a count of five. Work up to doing three sets of 10 lifts each, always using the five-count for pacing.

***Hamstring helper.*** Lie on your stomach with your chin to the floor. With an ankle weight (or a sock filled with coins and draped over your ankle) and your knee bent, slowly lift the lower leg 6 to 12 inches off the floor, then slowly lower it back down, stopping before you touch the floor. Repeat the movement again, always working slowly and steadily through each repetition. Work up to three sets of as many of these as you can comfortably do (largely determined by the amount of weight you use).

A word of caution: If an exercise causes increasing discomfort or pain, stop, Dr. Fox advises. You have to listen to your body. Don't work through the pain.

**Try to modify.** Athletes with chronic knee problems have to modify their levels of training or daily activity, says Albohm. "But that doesn't mean turning into a couch potato." If you like racquetball and you have a chronic knee condition that racquetball gradually made worse, you're probably going to have to get away from that, she says.

Options? Try swimming, biking, or rowing, all activities that are beneficial to health without placing great strain on the knees. The key phrase is "non-weight-bearing" activity. In fact, by helping to strengthen thigh muscles, non-weight-bearing exercises such as biking and rowing can give you better knees without sacrificing aerobic capacity or caloric burn.

Whatever you do, don't give up a healthy lifestyle because of knee pain. No one should have to stop being active, Albohm says. Simply avoid anything that causes pain in that knee.

**Change to a softer running surface.** A lot of runners' pain is caused by tendinitis that results from poor training habits, says Dr. Fox. These are not significant mechanical problems, he says, and they can often be minimized by a change in running surface.

For starters, run on grass before asphalt and asphalt before concrete. Concrete is the hardest surface of all and should be avoided as much as possible. Don't make a habit of jogging on sidewalks. Try to find a golf course to run on once the golfers have left.

"When you run a mile, your foot is striking the ground between 600 and 800 times," Dr. Fox adds.

**Try RICE.** Following any activity that causes knee pain, Albohm says, immediately rest the area and apply ice, compression, and elevation for 20 to 30 minutes. That advice is commonly called RICE, short for rest, ice, compression, and elevation.

"Don't underestimate the power of ice," says Albohm. Ice is a tremendous anti-inflammatory and will really help the condition.

Keep your icing routine simple, she says. When you return from working out, just prop the leg up, wrap an elastic bandage around it, and apply an ice pack for 20 to 30 minutes. That should always be your first try at relieving pain.

**Use heat with caution.** When there is *no* swelling present, using a heating pad before an activity may let you exercise with less pain. But, Albohm cautions, if there's any swelling, don't use heat. Also, don't use heat *after* an activity, she says. We're assuming the area is becoming irritated by activity, and heat is only going to increase any irritation that's there.

**Update your shoes.** If your shoes can't absorb the shock anymore, says Gary M. Gordon, D.P.M., that shock has to go someplace. So it goes through your foot, up your shin, and into your knee. Sometimes it keeps on going, up to your hip and back as well.

"I tell runners that if they run 25 miles a week or more, they need new shoes every 2 to 3 months," Dr. Gordon says. If they run less than that, they need new shoes every 4 to 6 months. Aerobic dancers and basketball and tennis players who work out twice each week can probably get by with new shoes every 4 to 6 months. But if they exercise four times or more each week, they also need new shoes every 2 months. Most people don't want to hear that. (Except maybe the shoe salespeople.)

**Exercise in water.** The buoyancy of water makes it the perfect place to gently exercise a sore knee joint. Try your regular knee exercises underwater. Swimming and water walking will keep you in shape without putting stress on your knees.

**Get into low gear.** Many experts like bike riding, either stationary or freewheel, as an alternative to the knee strain and pain that can be caused by running. But biking is a great way to stay in shape and take a load off your knees only if you do it with caution. Cyclists can also damage their knees, typically by thinking that the harder it is to pedal, the more exercise you get. Harder pedaling puts more strain on the knees. In general, a lower gear, which makes it easier to pedal, is a better gear, Albohm says.

**Find the trigger point for pain.** There's a trigger point on the inside of the thigh that contributes to "weak knee syndrome," says masseur Rich Phaigh. That trigger point is responsible for a lot of generalized pain on the inside of the knee, too.

To get rid of that pain, move your hand straight up from the kneecap along the front of the thigh for about 3 inches, then move it inward for another 2 to 4 inches. With the tip of your thumb, press in firmly and hold until you feel the muscle release its tension. That can be anywhere from 30 to 90 seconds, Phaigh says. Then release.

**First and finally, stretch.** Many of fitness consultant Lisa Dobloug's clients are older and have special needs when it comes to protecting their knees. Her emphasis is on the quality—not quantity—of exercise and the importance of stretching.

It's very important to warm up and cool down properly, she says. Take about 10 minutes and do very light stretching before you begin exercising. Maybe go through the motions of whatever exercise you'll be participating in without really extending it. Then do a little aerobics—jogging in place or walking around. After you're done working out, you should stretch for flexibility and to counteract the pounding that the exercise put your knees through.

Here's one stretch that Dobloug likes for postworkout stiffness. Lie down on your back and pull your knees into your chest, then start to straighten one leg, she says. Act like you're trying to press your heel toward the ceiling. Hold the stretch for a count of 10 while breathing slowly, then relax. Repeat with the other leg.

## PANEL OF ADVISORS

**Marjorie Albohm** is a certified athletic trainer at Ortho Indy in Indianapolis. She served on the medical staffs for the 1980 Winter and 1996 Summer Olympics and the 1987 Pan American Games.

**Lisa Dobloug** is a fitness and spa consultant in Washington, D.C. She is president of Saga Fitness. Many of her clients are older people who wish to remain active and who appreciate her sound advice about warming up, stretching, and cooling down.

**James M. Fox, M.D.,** specializes in arthroscopic and reconstructive knee surgery at the Southern California Orthopedic Institute in Van Nuys, California. He is the author of *Save Your Knees* and was a member of the medical staff for the 1984 Summer Olympics.

**Gary M. Gordon, D.P.M.,** has a sports medicine practice in Glenside, Pennsylvania, where he specializes in podiatric medicine and foot surgery.

**Rich Phaigh** is codirector of the American Institute of Sports Massage in New York City and the owner of a therapeutic massage clinic in Eugene, Oregon. He has taught more than 250 classes in advanced therapeutic technique in the United States and abroad. Phaigh has worked on the likes of running stars Alberto Salazar and Joan Samuelson.

# LACTOSE INTOLERANCE
## 14 Soothing Ideas

Even though low-fat dairy products are considered by most to be healthy foods, not everyone can digest them with ease. In fact, an estimated 30 million to 50 million Americans are lactose intolerant, which means they face a host of digestive problems whenever they eat dairy foods. Just how many dairy foods a lactose-intolerant person can eat without causing symptoms varies from person to person.

Lactose intolerance occurs when the small intestine doesn't produce enough lact*ase*, an enzyme required for the digestion of lact*ose*, the natural sugar found in dairy products. Although it can be annoying, lactose intolerance is not a serious medical problem.

Most people develop some degree of lactose intolerance by the time they're 20, according to Seymour Sabesin, M.D. But you can have your ice cream and eat it, too. Here's how.

**Take the tolerance test.** Since everyone's degree of tolerance is different, find out how much of a good thing you can have before you stop enjoying it, says Theodore Bayless, M.D. The obvious thing to do is decrease the amount of milk and dairy products you eat until your symptoms go away.

Even a few sips of milk can bother some people, he says. About 30 percent of lactose-intolerant people will get symptoms only after a quart, and maybe 30 to 40 percent from a glass.

**Don't forget your calcium.** "Milk products are a major source of calcium," Dr. Bayless cautions. "Most people should get the calcium equivalent of two glasses of milk daily." If milk is your main source of calcium and you cut back on it, then you should supplement your diet with substitutes like Tums, or sardines with bones, spinach, or broccoli, he says. Calcium-fortified juices and cereals, calcium supplements, and lactase enzymes, pills, or lactase-treated milk can also help you maintain a healthy calcium intake level.

**Never drink milk alone.** "Some people find that their symptoms disappear if they consume their dairy products with meals," Dr. Bayless says.

**Inoculate yourself.** It may be worth trying to take just a small amount of milk products each day, gradually increasing the dose to build up your tolerance, Dr. Bayless suggests. Back off if your symptoms reappear.

**Eat yogurt.** The fermentation process that produces yogurt depends on organisms that also produce lactase, the enzyme in short supply in lactose-intolerant people, says Naresh Jain, M.D. The bacteria themselves also probably break down the lactose in the milk. About 70 to 80 percent of otherwise healthy lactose-intolerant people should be able to tolerate yogurt quite well.

Dr. Sabesin notes that yogurt has only about 75 percent of the lactose content of an equal amount of milk. That difference, he says, may be all you need to be able to tolerate lactose. About 4 to 6 ounces a day is about all you need to keep gas away.

Here are some other tips on yogurt.

*Choose regular over frozen.* Yogurt is made from pasteurized milk. But sometimes manufacturers repasteurize the yogurt before they freeze it. "This would kill the beneficial organisms that produce lactose," says Dr. Jain. So try to find yogurt that has not been repasteurized. Look for the National Yogurt Association's Live and Active Cultures (LAC) seal on the label to be sure that the product you purchase meets the association's minimum standard of 10 million organisms per gram.

*Choose fat-free.* "Fat slows gastric emptying," Dr. Jain says. Yogurt with fat in it sits in the stomach for a longer time. This means stomach acid may have more of a chance to kill the beneficial organisms. Since lactose digestion takes place in the small intestine, you want your organisms to get there as soon as possible, even if your stomach acid doesn't kill them. Although this is still only a theory, Dr. Jain says, it's probably best to stick with fat-free yogurt.

*Eat it every day.* "We gave study subjects yogurt on a regular basis every day," Dr. Jain says, "and we demonstrated improvements in their digestion."

**Add your own lactase.** Several companies make lactase enzyme and add it to milk. Or you can buy it in liquid form and add it yourself. Lactaid, resulting from research done by Dr. Bayless and David Paige, M.D., at Johns Hopkins University Hospital in Baltimore, are tablets you can take when you eat lactose-containing foods. Also, a few drops of lactase liquid in a quart of milk renders the milk flatulence-free with a slightly sweeter taste.

"The only problem is whether you add enough lactase," Dr. Sabesin says. "Each person has a different degree of lactose intolerance, so it's a matter of trial and error." The tablets and drops are available over the counter in drugstores. Supermarkets nationwide carry tummy-ready Lactaid milk.

**Try buttermilk.** "Buttermilk should be pretty much tolerable," Dr. Jain says. That's because it contains less lactose per 1-cup serving than whole, fat-free, and all varieties of milk in between. Despite its name, buttermilk also has less fat and less cholesterol than even 2 percent milk.

**Say "cheese."** "Cheese has less lactose in it than milk," Dr. Jain says. Hard cheeses are the best, Dr. Bayless says, because they are most fermented.

"Swiss cheese and extra-sharp Cheddar cheese contain only a trace amount of lactose and are thus less likely to produce digestive upset," says Dr. Sabesin.

**Know that acidophilus milk doesn't help.** Although acidophilus organisms are highly beneficial for digestion, they colonize the *large* intestine, notes Jeffrey Biller, M.D. Lactose digestion occurs in the *small* intestine, so acidophilus just passes by the lactose.

**Beware of fillers.** Lactose is a very common filler in many kinds of medication and nutritional supplements. "In some pills and for some people," Dr. Jain warns, there's enough lactose to cause the symptoms of lactose intolerance. Read labels carefully. Ask your pharmacist if your medication has a lactose filler.

**Call a hotline.** Lactaid has a toll-free phone line for questions about lactose intolerance. The phone number is (800) LACTAID.

## PANEL OF ADVISORS

**Theodore Bayless, M.D.,** is the clinical director of the Meyerhoff Digestive Disease Center at the Johns Hopkins University Hospital in Baltimore.

**Jeffrey Biller, M.D.,** is a gastroenterologist at the Center for Pediatric Gastroenterology and Nutrition in Boston.

**Naresh Jain, M.D.,** is a gastroenterologist in Niagara Falls, New York.

**Seymour Sabesin, M.D.,** is a gastroenterologist and director of the section of digestive diseases at Rush–Presbyterian–St. Luke's Medical Center in Chicago.

# LARYNGITIS
## 15 Hoarseless Hints

For those who love to talk or sing, laryngitis can be a real, er, pain in the neck. Think of an opera singer sidelined on opening night because all she can coax out of her mouth is a croak. Ponder the politician who can't filibuster to stall debate on the Senate floor.

Most of us don't depend on our voices nearly as much as folks at the Metropolitan Opera or lawmakers in Washington, D.C., but laryngitis can be troubling nevertheless. The most noticeable symptoms are the loss of voice or hoarseness. The throat may also be raw or tickle, and those with laryngitis often feel an urge to clear their throats.

The common cold and other viral infections of the upper airways are the most common causes of laryngitis. Laryngitis may also accompany the flu, bronchitis, pneumonia, measles, whooping cough, or any infection of the upper airways. As any opera singer will tell you, excessive use of the voice, exposure to tobacco smoke, even allergic reactions, can bring it on, too.

What's the physical cause of all those bad vibrations? For you to sound like you, the air you exhale through your larynx—that voice box commonly known as your Adam's apple—has to vibrate through your vocal cords in just the right way. When the cords are scarred or swollen, they don't create the right shaped "container" for that air. That allows breath to escape.

Even a slight change in the vocal cords can render a person's voice unrecognizable. The vocal cords contain a central muscle bundle, various layers of connective tissue, and a skinlike covering called the mucosa. "An alteration in any one of these layers can disrupt the optimal vibration through the tissue," says Scott Kessler, M.D.

If your timbre is now as deep and croaky as Lauren Bacall's, follow our experts' tips to recover your true voice.

**Don't talk.** No matter what triggered the laryngitis, the most important thing you can do for your voice is to give it a rest, says Laurence Levine, M.D., D.D.S. Try to go a day or two without talking.

## WHEN TO CALL A DOCTOR

If your voice loss is accompanied by pain so severe that you have trouble swallowing your own saliva, see a physician immediately, says George T. Simpson II, M.D. Swelling in the upper part of your larynx may be blocking your airway.

You should also contact your physician if you find yourself coughing up blood, hear noises in your throat when you breathe, or find that continued voice rest does nothing to alleviate your hoarseness. When laryngitis persists, it may signal the presence of a throat tumor. In any case, consult your doctor if your voice doesn't return to normal within 3 to 5 days.

**Don't even whisper.** If you have to communicate, pass notes. "Whispering causes you to bang your vocal cords together as strongly as if you were shouting," explains George T. Simpson II, M.D.

**Don't take aspirin.** If you've lost your voice because you were yelling too loudly, you've probably ruptured a capillary, says Dr. Levine. So stay away from aspirin. Aspirin increases clotting time, which can impede the healing process.

**Use a cold-air humidifier.** The mucosa that blanket your vocal cords need to be kept moist. When they're not, mucus can become sticky and adherent, a virtual flypaper for irritants. Fight back with a cold-air humidifier, says Dr. Kessler.

**Steam it away.** Steaming can also restore moisture. Robert Feder, M.D., a doctor and singing coach, suggests hanging your head over a steaming bowl of water for 5 minutes twice a day. To avoid burns, keep the bowl on a steady surface and your face about an arm's length away from the water.

**Drink plenty of fluids.** Dr. Simpson favors 8 to 10 glasses a day, preferably water. Dr. Feder recommends juice and tea with honey or lemon.

**Don't use ice.** Warm fluids are best, says Dr. Feder. Cold drinks can just aggravate the problem.

**Breathe through your nose.** "Breathing through your nose is a natural humidifier," says Dr. Kessler. "People who have a deviated nasal septum breathe through the mouth while asleep. That exposes the voice to dry and cold air. Evaluating how you breathe is critical to understanding the nature of hoarseness."

**Nix the cigarettes.** Smoking is a prime cause of throat dryness, says Dr. Kessler.

**Choose your cough drops wisely.** Avoid mint and mentholated products, says Dr. Feder. They can temporarily paralyze your throat muscles and slow down the recovery process. Stick to honey- or fruit-flavored soft cough drops instead.

**Beware of airplane air.** Talking on an airplane can sabotage your voice. That's because the pressurized air inside the cabin is so dry. To keep your cords moist, breathe through your nose, says Dr. Kessler. Chew gum or suck on lozenges so that you'll have no choice but to keep your mouth closed.

**Check your medication.** Certain prescription drugs can be very drying, our experts say. Check with your doctor if you're uncertain. Likely culprits include blood pressure and thyroid medications and antihistamines.

**Don't strain, amplify.** If your job requires you to raise your voice to be heard, use mechanical means to make yourself louder. "Often, we don't make enough use of amplification systems to protect voice function," says Dr. Levine.

**Respect your voice.** If you have a presentation to do and you find yourself hoarse, it's better to cancel than risk doing long-term damage to your voice, says Dr. Kessler.

**Consider voice training.** If you find yourself speaking a lot, consider getting some voice training. In a nontrained voice, the muscles that suspend the larynx strain against each other, says Dr. Levine. Training the voice can get those muscles to work together as a team.

## PANEL OF ADVISORS

**Robert Feder, M.D.,** is an otolaryngologist in the Los Angeles area. He is the physician on-call for the Music Center, the Performing Arts Center of Los Angeles County. He is also a former professor of drama and a former professor of otolaryngology at UCLA.

**Scott Kessler, M.D.,** is a New York City otolaryngologist specializing in performing-arts medicine. He is the physician for many of the performers at the Metropolitan Opera and the City Opera, as well as for cast members of Broadway plays and cabarets. He is also on the staffs of Mount Sinai and Beth Israel Hospitals in New York City.

**Laurence Levine, M.D., D.D.S.,** is an associate clinical professor of otolaryngology at Washington University School of Medicine in St. Louis and an otolaryngologist in Creve Coeur and St. Charles, Missouri.

**George T. Simpson II, M.D.,** was chairman of the department of otolaryngology at Boston University School of Medicine, University Hospital, and Boston City Hospital. He was also an attending physician at Children's Hospital Medical Center and the Veterans Administration Hospital and a member of the scientific advisory committee for the Voice Foundation.

# LEG PAIN
## 6 Tips to Ease the Pain

A variety of problems can lead to aching legs, including back problems, infections, and nerve damage. Overuse or injury also can cause leg pain. Most commonly, leg pain stems from trouble with the arteries or veins, such as varicose veins, phlebitis, or intermittent claudication.

Fortunately, simple home remedies can help relieve most leg pain. Here's some advice about curbing leg pain associated with intermittent claudication. (For more information on phlebitis and varicose veins, see pages 457 and 601.)

Intermittent claudication, a chronic pain experienced in the calf when walking, is estimated to afflict 3 to 10 percent of the entire American population, with significantly higher rates among people age 70 and older. Though a painful and serious condition in its own right, intermittent claudication is really the *symptom* of a larger, more serious problem—peripheral vascular disease.

Just as plaque-clogged blood vessels in the heart lead to angina (chest pains), intermittent claudication signals the onset of restricted bloodflow in the "periphery," that is, the area farthermost from the heart—the arms and legs.

"We're talking about the symptom phase of arterial disease," says Jess R. Young, M.D. "If you get arterial disease in the heart, you get angina and heart attacks. If you get it in the head circulation, you get strokes. Intermittent claudication is the same process, but in the legs and arms."

For that reason, intermittent claudication should not be taken lightly. If you've been diagnosed as having this condition, you should continue seeing your doctor to regularly monitor the underlying disease resulting in the pain you now feel in your legs. The pain, after all, is only a symptom. The real disease is a killer. In fact, patients with intermittent claudication have a life expectancy 10 years less than people of the same age who don't have this symptom.

On the upside, there are a number of things that you can do at home to rid

## WHEN TO CALL A DOCTOR

Leg pain is a symptom of many conditions, some very serious. If your pain is severe, worsens rapidly, or lasts for more than a week, see your doctor as soon as possible.

Chronic foot problems that get infected are a leading cause of amputation in people who have intermittent claudication. If you have a cut, scrape, blister, or other foot problem that develops the redness, swelling, heat, and pain of infection, seek immediate medical help.

yourself of claudication's pain and help slow the progression of peripheral vascular disease.

**Stop smoking.** "The number one thing on everyone's list with this affliction should be to stop smoking," says Dr. Young. About 75 to 90 percent of all people with intermittent claudication are smokers.

Stopping smoking is so important, in fact, that our experts say you must quit before any other remedy listed below will work. Is it worth it? Consider the following: Cigarette smoking increases the damage the disease can do by substituting carbon monoxide for oxygen in the already oxygen-starved muscles of your legs. Nicotine also causes constriction of the arteries, which further restricts bloodflow, possibly damaging the arteries themselves and leading to blood clots. In extreme cases, these clots can result in gangrene and may require amputation of a limb.

**Start walking.** "Next to stopping smoking, exercise is most important," says Dr. Young. The type of exercise he's talking about, and the type our experts overwhelmingly recommend, is the simplest of all—walking.

"Get out every day for at least an hour of walking exercise," says Dr. Young. "You can break that up any way you want, but you have to bring on the discomfort of intermittent claudication to have the walking do any good." Walk until you bring on the pain, he says, but don't stop at the first sign of pain. "Wait until it gets moderately severe. Then stop and rest a minute or two until it goes away, then start up walking again." Repeat that pain/walk cycle as often as you can during your 60 minutes of daily walking.

Be warned, however, that improvement won't happen overnight. "It will be 2 to 3 months, minimum, before you see results," says Dr. Young. So don't get discouraged.

A study at the Claude D. Petter Older Americans Independence Center at the University of Maryland showed just how much walking can improve the lives of patients with intermittent claudication. Patients who participated in a 6-month exercise program increased the distance they could walk without pain by 134 percent. The bloodflow in their calves increased 30 percent. Perhaps most important, the changes weren't just in the gym. The 28 patients studied also increased their everyday activity level by 38 percent. The benefit of exercise was highly significant when the active group was compared to a control group of patients who didn't change any of their habits for the study.

**Exercise rain or shine.** "Walking is the best *singular* exercise," says Robert Ginsburg, M.D., "but bicycling on a stationary bike can also help if it works the calves." In fact, any indoor exercise that works the calves enough to bring on the pain of claudication can help. Some exercises to try include toe raises, stair-climbing, running in place, jumping rope, and dancing (get your doctor's okay before trying these more strenuous exercises).

**Take a load off.** Obesity can be a major problem for those with claudication, not only because of the strain it places on circulation but also because of the damage it inflicts on the feet.

"You're traumatizing tissue in the feet that just doesn't have a good enough blood supply to take that abuse," notes Dr. Young.

**Avoid heating pads.** Because of the restricted bloodflow in the legs, people who have intermittent claudication often experience cold feet, too. But regardless of how cold your feet may be, never warm them with a heating pad or a hot-water bottle. Because bloodflow is restricted, the heat can't be dissipated and could actually burn your feet. Try loose wool stockings to warm your feet instead.

**Know your blood pressure and cholesterol level.** "If you have intermittent claudication, you should also be checked for high blood pressure and high cholesterol," says Dr. Young. "These are important risk factors that tend to markedly increase the severity of the underlying disease, and it's very important to keep both of those conditions tightly controlled."

## PANEL OF ADVISORS

**Robert Ginsburg, M.D.,** is the former director of the Center for Interventional Vascular Therapy at Stanford University Hospital.

**Jess R. Young, M.D.,** is the former chairman of the department of vascular medicine at the Cleveland Clinic Foundation in Ohio.

# MARINE BITES AND STINGS
## 15 Soothing Strategies

Where unsuspecting swimmers swim, dangerous creatures lurk. Forget the relatively rare sharks. Jellyfish, sea urchins, stingrays, spiny fish, coral, and even microscopic parasites are far more likely to make a day at the beach feel like, well, no day at the beach.

Jellyfish are the most common culprits of ocean vacations gone awry. Their flowing, translucent tentacles are covered with stinging capsules called nematocysts. When a tentacle brushes up against your skin, the nematocysts are ejected, piercing the skin and injecting stinging venom. The result: a burning, throbbing, itching sensation, which can feel as minor as a paper cut or more like a bee sting.

Unfortunately, jellyfish aren't the only stinging fish in the sea. Stingrays, scorpion fish, and even catfish all have venomous spines. Sea urchins, though not usually venomous, have protruding spines that can pierce barefoot beach-goers.

All this might make fresh water swimming seem less hazardous. Not necessarily. A dip in a lake could impart an annoying itch. That would be swimmer's itch—a condition caused by larval flatworms that burrow into the skin and die. Each one leaves a bump, called a papule, that can be even itchier than a mosquito bite, says Harvey Blankespoor, Ph.D. Although it can occur in marine waters, where it's known as clam digger's itch, it is more often reported in lakes and ponds in the northern tier of the United States.

To prevent these painful encounters, avoid swimming in infested waters, especially after stormy weather, and be careful not to step on beached creatures that might appear to be dead. Choose a beach with trained lifeguards, who are likely to be familiar with the species you may encounter.

Here's how to soothe yourself if sea creatures attack.

## Jellyfish Stings

**Pour on the vinegar.** Ordinary vinegar may be your best defense against nematocytes left behind by many, but not all, jellyfish. "The weak acid is useful to stop them from firing," says Joseph Burnett, M.D. Pour vinegar di-

## WHEN TO CALL A DOCTOR

Jellyfish stings are usually mild, although two species found in the South Pacific, the Portuguese man-of-war and the box jellyfish, are more painful than others. Any time a jellyfish sting causes severe pain that is not alleviated by over-the-counter medications, get to a doctor, recommends Joseph W. Burnett, M.D. Also, any sting on the eye could injure the cornea and merits a trip to the emergency room. One phone number to keep handy is the National Marine and Freshwater Envenomation Hotline. The toll-free hotline can be reached at (888) 232-8635.

An allergic reaction to a jellyfish sting is rare but not unheard of, and it requires an immediate call to the doctor. Symptoms include:

- Difficulty breathing
- Swelling around the mouth
- Swelling of the limb where the sting occurred
- Shortness of breath
- Wheezing
- Chest pain
- Dizziness
- Nausea
- Stomach cramps

Infections that result from marine injuries, indicated by pain, redness, swelling, or discharge, should also be addressed by a doctor, who will clean the injury and prescribe antibiotics.

rectly over the affected area for about 30 seconds, he suggests. Once you've neutralized the nematocysts, you can safely pick off the tentacles. If you don't have any vinegar with you, ask a lifeguard. Some of them keep a bottle in their first-aid kits.

While vinegar is recommended for most jellyfish stings, there is one exception: It may actually worsen the already furious pain of a Portuguese man-of-war, prevalent in the waters of Hawaii and the South Pacific. Man-of-wars are easy to identify by their iridescent blue gas-filled floats, which makes their bodies easy to avoid, but their long tentacles can extend more than 40 feet in the water. If you think you've been stung by a man-of-war, don't apply vinegar or anything else, just remove the remaining nematocysts and seek immediate medical attention, particularly if you are in severe pain.

If you haven't neutralized them, avoid removing any tentacles adhering to the skin with your bare fingers—you could get another sting. "Pick off the big pieces with a gloved hand, tweezers, or scrape them off with the edge of a shell, a sand shovel, or the dull side of a knife blade," says Jeffrey N. Bernstein, M.D.

**Slather on a slurry.** Don't have vinegar? Coat the sting with a mixture of 50 percent baking soda and 50 percent salt water. This treatment will prevent additional venom from being released. As with vinegar, this tip is not recommended for Portuguese man-of-war stings.

*Caution:* Don't use *fresh* water if you haven't inactivated the nematocysts with vinegar or baking soda. Fresh water may stimulate the release of more venom.

**Rinse it with salt water.** If you don't have anything to neutralize the stingers, flush the area with ocean water. "Salt water is handy and safe," observes Craig Thomas, M.D. Avoid other old wives' remedies like alcohol, ammonia, urine, and bleach. They may be harmful, causing the nematocysts to discharge more venom.

**Charge it!** One common method for removing the desensitized nematocysts is to cover the sting with shaving cream to help draw them out and then scrape them off with a credit card, says Dr. Bernstein. Don't have a can of shaving cream in your beach bag? Ask a lifeguard. Some keep it in their first-aid kits. Do this only after you've treated the area with vinegar or baking soda, since pressure will otherwise trigger more stinging.

**Heat it up.** Dr. Bernstein and his colleagues conducted a study to determine whether heat or ice worked better to relieve the pain of jellyfish stings. In the test, 9 people were treated with ice packs. Just over half reported pain relief within an hour. Of the 18 people treated by immersing the stung area in hot water, almost all felt no pain an hour later. "Water should be hot to the touch, but obviously not so hot that you burn yourself," explains Dr. Bernstein. After the jellyfish nematocysts have been scraped off, immerse the sting in hot water until you feel no pain when you remove it. If hot water is unavailable, apply a heating pad to the area instead. No studies have supported using heat to treat man-of-war stings, however.

**Put it on ice.** While heat may be more effective, ice is often handier at the beach. After scraping off the nematocysts, place an ice pack or a bag of ice directly on the sting for some pain relief, says Dr. Bernstein. Keep it on until the pain subsides.

**Head to the drugstore.** For the pain of a jellyfish sting, take aspirin, acetaminophen, or ibuprofen, says Dr. Burnett.

"Topical preparations don't work in the initial treatment phase. They don't penetrate deeply enough to ease the pain. An over-the-counter hydrocortisone cream or a topical antihistamine may be helpful if symptoms persist beyond 24 hours. Consult a physician if symptoms last more than a few days," Dr. Bernstein advises.

## Other Water Woes

**Care for sea urchin injuries.** A stroll along coastal waters could prove painful if you step on a hidden sea urchin. These creatures have sharp, brittle spines that penetrate the skin, then break off. Surprisingly, small pieces embedded in the skin may be best with no treatment at all. "Big, loosely penetrated spines can be plucked off, but otherwise they have to be dug and cut out, which does more harm than good," says Dr. Thomas. The spines will either work themselves out or dissolve within 3 weeks. It's rare for infection to occur, but watch for signs of redness and swelling.

**Treat venomous fish stings.** Stingrays hide just beneath the sand. Surprise one, and you're likely to discover that the end of its tail contains a powerful stinger. Stingray stings are immediately painful, just like a bee sting, says Dr. Thomas. To relieve pain, remove the stinger and any poison tissue remaining on your skin by rinsing with salt or fresh water. Then, pull out any embedded parts with a tweezers. Immerse the wound in hot water, about the temperature of bathwater. Soak for 30 to 90 minutes.

Other fish, like catfish or scorpion fish, have venomous spines that cause a painful reaction if they scrape skin. Again, immersion in hot water will bring relief. "We recommend hot water for most marine venoms because the heat disables the venom's proteins," says Dr. Bernstein.

**Quell coral pain.** Coral can give snorkelers or waders a nasty scrape. "These cuts are a combination of a sting, from the nematocysts in the coral, and a dirty cut. Therefore, they get infected often," says Dr. Thomas. Clean the wound thoroughly, removing any fragments of coral in the skin with a tweezers. Then, scrub the area with gauze soaked in clean, fresh water, and coat with an antiseptic such as Bactine. Fresh water, in treating coral cuts, is unlikely to trigger nematocysts and is essential for cleaning the wound.

**Soothe sea lice.** Not really lice at all, sea lice are jellyfish larvae, sometimes encountered in warm ocean waters. Often, they get trapped inside a swimmer's bathing suit or under a T-shirt. Once they sit there for a while, they start stinging. "It causes an almost allergic reaction," says Dr. Bernstein. "You'll get an itchy irritation in the area around the waistband or under the bathing suit." First, shower to remove any larvae that might still be on your skin. Then, treat the itch with an over-the-counter antihistamine, like Benadryl, or a hydrocortisone cream.

**Squelch swimmer's itch.** Swimmer's itch, which is really a by-product of an encounter with a waterborne parasite, can affect every part of the body that's in contact with the water, leaving a small, round, itchy bump wherever the parasite has entered. It shows up within 15 minutes of contact with the parasite and lasts for 1 to 2 weeks. Here are a few recommended remedies for soothing that itch.

***Try over-the-counter treatments.*** Swimmer's itch that covers the entire body or is intensely irritating could require a doctor-prescribed antihistamine, warns Dr. Blankespoor. Less-severe cases can be treated with topical anti-itch formulas, such as cortisone creams. Or look for a nonprescription cream or ointment containing benzocaine, such as Boil-Ease, to relieve itching.

***Don't drip dry.*** Toweling off the moment you step out of the lake won't always protect you against swimmer's itch. But some species of the parasite only enter as the water dries on the skin, so it's a good idea to dry yourself immediately after a swim.

## PANEL OF ADVISORS

**Jeffrey N. Bernstein, M.D.,** is medical director of the Florida Poison Information Center in Miami and the National Marine and Freshwater Envenomation Hotline.

**Harvey Blankespoor, Ph.D.,** is a biology professor at Hope College in Holland, Michigan, who studies swimmer's itch.

**Joseph W. Burnett, M.D.,** is a professor and chairman of dermatology at University of Maryland in Baltimore, and president of the International Consortium for Jellyfish Stings.

**Craig Thomas, M.D.,** is the president of Hawaii Emergency Physicians Associated and the coauthor of *All Stings Considered.*

# MEMORY PROBLEMS
## 21 Ways to Forget Less

Spend some time with the older adults in your life, and you'll probably start hearing jokes about getting senile—usually because someone forgot an appointment or can't remember a word that's right on the tip of her tongue.

Despite the occasional humorous comments about memory loss, one of the greatest fears people have is losing their memory or mental abilities over time. It's worth remembering that there's a huge difference between occasional "senior moments" and conditions such as dementia or Alzheimer's disease, which are caused by underlying disease.

High blood pressure, for example, can contribute to declines in memory. So can depression, fatigue, high cholesterol, stroke, side effects from medications, and a variety of nutritional deficiencies. It's essential to see a doctor if your memory is suddenly worse than it used to be, or if it seems to be going downhill over time.

## WHEN TO CALL A DOCTOR

Because memory declines can be caused by many physical problems, such as depression, thyroid disorders, nutritional deficiencies, or even urinary tract infections, it's important to see a doctor as soon as you notice any changes, says Cynthia R. Green, Ph.D.

Ask yourself if your memory has gotten significantly worse in the last 6 months, suggests Dr. Green. "Are the changes seriously affecting your ability to function? Are your friends or family concerned? The answers to these questions will give you a sense of the seriousness of the changes," she says.

Another thing to consider is whether you're taking a new medication, Dr. Green says. Many drugs, including antihistamines and medications for heartburn, anxiety, and high blood pressure, have memory impairment as a side effect. In many cases, switching to a new drug or changing the dose may be all that's needed to reverse the problem.

# Do just 1 thing

Pay attention. If you find that your memory isn't as good as you'd like it to be, make a special effort to focus your attention on the things you want to remember.

"The number one reason we forget things is that we weren't paying attention in the first place," says Cynthia R. Green, Ph.D.

One way the brain sorts information is by routing it to short-term or long-term memory. Long-term memories tend to stay with us, while short-term memories tend to be fleeting. If you don't focus your attention on remembering new things, they'll never make the transition into long-term memory.

"My favorite technique for remembering names is repetition, in which I say the name back to the person," says Dr. Green.

You can use the same technique for anything. When you put the car keys down, for example, simply repeat to yourself where you're putting them. When you meet someone new, repeat the name in your mind a few times. Making the effort to remember things will help ensure that you do.

Occasional forgetfulness is rarely a sign of disease, however. Nor is it something you necessarily have to live with. With a combination of mental exercises and lifestyle changes, there's a good chance that you can improve your memory and keep it strong for years to come.

**Give your mind a workout.** The brain is like any other part of the body. The more it's exercised and challenged, the stronger it gets over time, says Gunnar Gouras, M.D.

People who are mentally active form additional neural connections, Dr. Gouras explains. In other words, they have a larger "reserve" of brain circuits, so they're more likely to stay mentally sharp. A study of 678 nuns, for example, found that those with the most education and language abilities were less likely to develop Alzheimer's later in life.

So keep your mind busy. Do crossword puzzles. Read challenging books. Play Scrabble or go to the movies. Virtually any activity that keeps the mind active could help reduce the risk of age-related memory declines.

**Put information into chunks.** It's easy to forget—or fail to learn—information that comes in large chunks. It's much easier to remember things when you break them down into smaller chunks, says Cynthia R. Green, Ph.D.

Phone numbers are a good example. They're customarily divided into three units—the area code, the first three numbers, and the final four numbers. They're fairly easy to remember because they're broken into small, manageable pieces of information.

You can use this same technique to manage all kinds of information. When you shop, for example, divide the shopping list into logical pieces: produce, freezer, and dairy foods.

**Form mental pictures.** It's easier to remember things when you have a visual image in your mind to go along with them. Suppose you've just been introduced to someone named Bill at a party. Repeat the name a few times in your mind, and also form a mental picture of a $1 bill. The combination of mental repetition and a visual image will help you remember his name in the future.

**Make mental connections.** When you were in school, you probably learned to spell "principal" by thinking of the word "pal." It was a way to link new information with something you already knew. It's a quick and easy way of giving information meaning, says Dr. Green.

"I was at a conference and I met a woman named Regina," says Dr. Green. "As soon as she said her name, I connected it to a friend of mine who's also named Regina, which made the name easier to remember."

You can form connections with almost anything. Suppose the number on your gym locker is 23. Link it to something that you already know, like the expression "23 skidoo." The connection doesn't have to make literal sense. In fact, it might be more memorable if it doesn't make sense, Dr. Green explains.

**Try the storytelling technique.** Another way to remember names or other information is to weave them into little mental stories, says Dr. Green. If you meet someone named Frank Hill, for example, you might think something like, "Frankly, he's getting over the hill."

**Write it down.** Appointment books, calendars, and notepads are invaluable memory aids. Apart from the fact that you can write things down and look them up later, the act of writing can make them easier to remember, says Dr. Green.

**Create "forget-me-not" spots.** Some things are always getting lost or forgotten—car keys and reading glasses, for example. One of the best memory aids is simply to put these and other commonly lost items in the same places all the time.

The minute you walk in the door, put your keys on a table by the door, Dr. Green suggests. Keep your reading glasses next to the couch or bed. As long as you're consistent, you'll never have to worry about losing these or other items again.

**Prioritize sleep.** "My wife says women don't have time to sleep," says Allan Hobson, M.D. "But the brain needs sleep to perform adequately. When you're asleep, it works on information you've gathered." Shoot for at least 8 hours a night. "Of course, some people can get by on less, but 8 hours is needed on average, and some people may need 10 hours. If you're experiencing poor cognitive function, take a good look at how much sleep you're getting, and sleep more if needed," Dr. Hobson suggests.

**Take a multivitamin.** The B vitamins, especially vitamin $B_{12}$, play a key role in memory and mental functions. "As people get older, it becomes harder to absorb B vitamins from the diet," says Dr. Green. "A vitamin $B_{12}$ deficiency can cause significant memory loss."

She recommends a multivitamin that provides 100 percent of the Daily Value for vitamins $B_6$ and $B_{12}$ and folic acid. Supplements in gel, liquid, or powder forms may be better absorbed than solid supplements, she adds.

**Get extra vitamin E.** It's an antioxidant nutrient that helps block the harmful effects of free radicals, unstable oxygen molecules in the blood. It can reduce buildups of cholesterol and other fatty substances in blood vessels in the brain, and it also appears to reduce inflammation. "A large study suggests that antioxidants can slow the progression of Alzheimer's disease," Dr. Gouras says.

Vitamin E is mainly found in nuts, wheat germ, and cooking oils, so it's difficult to get enough in your diet without taking supplements. The optimal dose has not been established, but 400 to 1,000 IU vitamin E daily is probably sufficient, says Dr. Gouras.

**Give ginkgo a try.** Researchers at the Medical Research Centre at the University of Surrey in Guildford, England, found that people ages 50 to 59 who took 120 milligrams of ginkgo three times daily had improvements in memory, concentration, and alertness. An herb, ginkgo appears to improve circulation and helps brain cells get all the nutrients that they need to stay healthy.

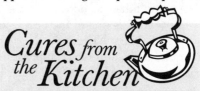

## Cures from the Kitchen

A leading theory of memory loss is that unstable oxygen molecules in the body, called free radicals, damage cells and blood vessels in the brain. You can't rid yourself of free radicals, but you can curtail some of their harmful effects by eating fruits and vegetables.

"Fruits and vegetables contain vitamins and antioxidants that fast food doesn't, and they're probably protective against some age-related diseases of the brain," says Gunnar Gouras, M.D.

The next time you're pushing a shopping cart through the produce aisle, focus on fruits and vegetables with the most brilliant hues—they're the ones with the highest concentration of antioxidants, adds Cynthia R. Green, Ph.D.

**Consider Siberian ginseng.** Feeling stressed and forgetful? Some experts recommend Siberian ginseng. Ginseng may aid memory by supporting the function of the adrenal gland, thereby helping with stress management. Try taking 100 to 200 milligrams a day.

**Rely on rosemary.** "When my daughter was studying for her college chemistry final, I told her to dab some essential oil of rosemary in her hair," recalls herbalist Brigitte Mars. "She also dabbed on the oil just before taking the test. Smelling the scent during the test reminded her of the material she'd studied, so she was able to remember what she'd learned." You could also place 1 to 3 drops of essential oil of rosemary on a cotton ball or tissue, tuck it in your sleeve, and inhale as needed for the same effect.

"Rosemary is one of the best essential oils to aid memory and reduce anxiety," adds Mars. Never take the oil by mouth, however, as many essential oils are quite toxic, and never apply it undiluted to the skin, because the essential oils are concentrated and will cause irritation.

**Exercise regularly.** Walking, biking, and other forms of exercise are among the best ways to increase bloodflow throughout the body, including in the brain. "Regular aerobic exercise also protects us from other illnesses such as stroke, diabetes, and high blood pressure, which contribute to memory problems," says Dr. Green.

**Keep stress at manageable levels.** People who are frequently tense or anxious tend to have high levels of cortisol and other stress hormones. Over time, elevated levels of these hormones can affect the hippocampus, the part of the brain that controls memory, says Dr. Green.

Stress and anxiety also affect memory indirectly, she adds. If you're tense all the time, you're more likely to have sleep problems—and the resulting fatigue can make it harder to remember things.

"You can't avoid stress entirely, but you can balance it with activities that help you relax," says Dr. Green. "It might be taking the time to do some coloring with your kids. Take a bath or have a massage. Anything that shifts your attention away from what's stressing you can be helpful."

**Keep cholesterol low.** Laboratory studies have shown that mice given a high-cholesterol diet are more likely to develop Alzheimer's disease at an earlier age than animals who get less cholesterol, says Dr. Gouras. In addition, current research suggests that adults who take statins—prescription medications that lower cholesterol—have a significantly lower risk of developing Alzheimer's disease.

More research is needed to conclusively show that lowering cholesterol—either with drugs or with dietary changes—will protect against Alzheimer's disease or memory loss, Dr. Gouras adds. But because lowering cholesterol has so many other benefits, such as reducing the risk of stroke or heart disease, it's worth the extra effort.

**Drink more water.** About 85 percent of the brain consists of water. People who don't drink enough can get dehydrated, which leads to fatigue and makes it harder to remember things. Try to drink at least eight 8-ounce glasses of water daily.

**Get some extra protection.** Over-the-counter analgesics such as aspirin, ibuprofen, and naproxen (such as Aleve) are known as nonsteroidal anti-inflammatory drugs, or NSAIDs. They're very effective for pain relief, and there's some evidence they also protect the brain. Studies have shown that people who take these drugs regularly are 45 to 50 percent less likely to develop Alzheimer's disease than those who don't take them, says Dr. Gouras.

**Don't give in to depression.** It makes it hard to concentrate, and it also causes people to feel tired and sluggish. Among elderly adults, in fact, depression is often mistaken for Alzheimer's disease or other forms of dementia, says Dr. Gouras.

"Depression can be caused by Alzheimer's disease, and it has been found that older patients who get depressed have a higher risk of developing Alzheimer's disease," says Dr. Gouras.

## PANEL OF ADVISORS

**Gunnar Gouras, M.D.,** is an assistant professor of neurology and neuroscience at the Joan and Sanford I. Weill Medical College of Cornell University and an Alzheimer's researcher at Fisher Center for Alzheimer's Research at Rockefeller University, both in New York City.

**Cynthia R. Green, Ph.D.,** is an assistant clinical professor of psychiatry at Mount Sinai School of Medicine of New York University in New York City. She is also president of Memory Arts, a consulting firm that provides memory fitness training to corporate executives, and the author of *Total Memory Workout.*

**Allan Hobson, M.D.,** is a professor of psychiatry at Harvard Medical School and director of the Neurophysiology and Sleep Laboratory at Massachusetts Mental Health Center in Boston.

**Brigitte Mars,** is an herbalist and teacher at the Rocky Mountain Center for Botanical Studies in Boulder, Colorado. She is also a professional member of the American Herbalists Guild.

# MENOPAUSE
## 18 Ways to Embrace the Change

Menopause is not a disease—though the way this natural process is portrayed in the press, you might think otherwise.

Don't believe the hype. Menopause does not have to be a horrendous life-altering change. Many women cruise through menopause with minimal symptoms, and many of the symptoms women do endure can often be controlled naturally.

Doctors commonly define menopause as the 366th or 367th day after a woman's last period (think 1 year and 1 day). This event can occur in a woman's forties or her sixties, but most commonly, the change takes place when a woman is in her early fifties.

The symptoms of menopause vary widely from woman to woman. They may not affect a woman at all, or they may hit like a blizzard in Buffalo. As women age, their estrogen levels drop, which triggers menopausal symptoms and also increases their risk of cardiovascular disease and osteoporosis. The most common symptoms are weight gain, vaginal changes (including dryness and loss of elasticity), sleep disturbances, emotional changes, and hot flashes.

Sound bad? It doesn't have to be. Eat right, exercise, and talk to your doctor about the possibility of hormone replacement therapy (HRT), other medications, or herbal remedies. They all can help smooth your transition, enabling you to enjoy the benefits of menopause: no more PMS, no more periods, and no more pregnancy worries.

### WHEN TO CALL A DOCTOR

Mary Jane Minkin, M.D., has a few rules for when you should see your doctor about menopause-related symptoms. First, she recommends an annual exam no matter what. Also, if you have irregular spotting or strange bleeding for any reason, see your doctor, she says. Finally, if menopause leaves you feeling unwell in general, see your doctor.

# Do just 1 thing

Exercise regularly. When it comes to enjoying a relaxing, comfortable menopause, regular exercise offers you the total package. "Exercise reduces menopausal symptoms, helps you sleep, helps your bones, and helps your heart," says Mary Jane Minkin, M.D.

Saying you're going to exercise is fine, but, as Larrian Gillespie, M.D., points out, most women only stick with it for about 6 weeks. That's why you have to find a variety of activities you truly enjoy.

Many problems women face as they grow older can be attributed to a loss of flexibility. To counteract this problem, Dr. Gillespie recommends a type of exercise called Pilates (pronounced "puh-LAH-teez") that focuses on flexibility and strength for the whole body without building bulky muscles.

Another issue women face as they begin an exercise program is a fear of sweat. "When women are overweight and have hormonal problems, they typically don't like to sweat," says Dr. Gillespie. Again, Pilates is a good, low-sweat alternative, as are swimming and yoga.

**Stamp out the butts.** Your chances of developing heart disease and osteoporosis jump during menopause. Smoking makes those odds rise even higher. That's not the only reason to quit. "Smokers have a 2-year-earlier menopause on average than non-smokers," says Mary Jane Minkin, M.D. Quitting smoking at an early age is critical both for your reproductive health and for a healthy transition into menopause. Granted, if you quit at 48, it won't stop early menopause, but if you're 22 or 23, it might help, she says.

**Refrain from binge drinking.** Too much booze is another no-no for both your bone and heart health as you transition into menopause. "Drinking a glass of wine a day is fine," says Dr. Minkin. But drinking a bottle a day is definitely not good for either your heart or your bones. Plus, she adds, alcohol brings on hot flashes, one of menopause's greatest discomforts.

**Bone up on calcium.** You can get a healthy dose of 1,000 milligrams a day of calcium from dairy products. "The reality, however, is that most women don't drink a lot of milk and eat a lot of cheese because they're legitimately worried about saturated fat and calories," says Dr. Minkin. To ensure adequate calcium intake, Dr. Minkin recommends taking 1,000 milligrams of supplemental calcium a day.

**Don't forget vitamin D.** This is the other nutrient that Dr. Minkin pinpoints as crucial to good menopausal health. The best way to get a daily dose of 400 IU of vitamin D is with a good multivitamin.

**Know the truth about HRT.** A persistent myth exists that it's dangerous to go on and off HRT. "It's not," says Dr. Minkin. In fact, she adds, women should feel free to experiment with HRT until they find the combination that works best for them—or decide they don't need it at all. "At no point do you have to make the decision, 'I'm going to do HRT for the rest of my life,' or 'I'm not going to do HRT for the rest of my life,'" she says. "If somebody wants to try it for a couple of months, that's fine. If somebody doesn't want to try it right now but maybe wants to give it a shot in a couple of months, that's fine, too."

Dr. Minkin also addresses the other major concern surrounding HRT—the risk of breast cancer. "Taking estrogen for 2 months will not give you breast cancer," she says. Taking HRT for more than 10 years might cause a slightly high risk, but even that's debatable. And HRT consistently turns up as one of the best remedies for one of the most troublesome symptoms of menopause: hot flashes, says Dr. Minkin.

**Know the truth about your diet.** "Women metabolize foods differently than men," says Larrian Gillespie, M.D. "Where men use carbohydrates for energy, women use carbohydrates to store as fat so we're able to procreate in the face of starvation." Plus, she notes, alterations in estrogen levels make these diet differences even more pronounced as we grow older. Read the tips below to fight menopause-related weight gain.

*Eat five or six smaller meals throughout the day.* To counteract the weight gain typical of menopausal women, Dr. Gillespie recommends eating five or six smaller meals interspersed throughout the day rather than three large meals. "These meals should each be around 250 to 300 calories," she adds.

*Focus on "good" carbohydrates.* To fight the foods that lead to weight gain, Dr. Gillespie recommends that menopausal (and premenopausal) women make diet decisions based on the glycemic index, a chart that ranks foods by their affect on your blood sugar. The higher a food's glycemic ranking, the more it boosts your blood sugar. She suggests focusing on foods with a low glycemic ranking, including beans, peanuts, most fruits, and sweet potatoes. Foods with a high glycemic ranking include bagels, corn chips, potatoes, and pretzels.

**Try a lubricant.** Another typical complaint of menopause is decreased sexual desire, sometimes caused by low estrogen-induced physical changes in the vagina. "If the lack of interest in sex is caused by physical discomfort, there are a number of over-the-counter lubricants you can try. You can also ask your doctor about estrogen creams, tablets, or rings," says Dr. Minkin. "If there are emotional issues involved, however, the couple really needs to focus on matters in their relationship."

**Try old-fashioned sleep aids.** If sleep is a problem, Dr. Minkin advises some of the old tricks your grandmother might have taught you. "Drinking a warm glass of milk, taking a warm bath, or not focusing on the day's events can all help you sleep more restfully," she says.

**Share your troubles with friends.** Much of the stress of menopause for women is due to other life changes that may be occurring at the same time. "Kids are finishing college and moving back home, parents are aging and developing health problems, and husbands are going through their second childhoods. These are all issues I hear from my patients," says Dr. Minkin. Friendships can help you overcome these emotional land mines. "Volunteer your time for a charitable organization, or join a menopause support group," she says. "These are great ways to meet friends, share life's stresses, or just get together and share experiences."

**Give your partner a book.** You might have menopause totally licked from your end. But your partner may be totally oblivious to the changes going on in your body and doesn't understand why things get tough for you from time to time. "Have your partner read up on it to understand the changes your body is going through and then hopefully react with patience and encouragement, says Dr. Minkin. Plus, your partner might even be able to help you get active about it and offer things you can do to make it better.

For more tips on the biggest bugaboo of menopause, see Hot Flashes on page 321.

**Buy black cohosh.** "This is my favorite herb to use for menopausal symptoms. It really does make a big difference," says Connie Catellani, M.D. Studies in menopausal women show that black cohosh alleviates symptoms of hot flashes, night sweats, vaginal dryness, sleep disturbances, nervousness, irritability, and depression. Research focusing on a standardized black cohosh extract called Remifemin has found it performs on a par with estrogen replacement treatment.

Scientists have yet to determine precisely how black cohosh works, but apparently it helps balance estrogen levels, Dr. Catellani says. Some doc-

*Cures from the Kitchen*

As a natural phytoestrogen, soy has proven useful for helping women overcome the symptoms of menopause in numerous studies. You can choose from a variety of soy food products readily available at your grocery store. Mary Jane Minkin, M.D., recommends 45 to 60 milligrams of isoflavones per day. One-half cup of tofu or a glass of soy milk each day are good sources of isoflavones.

tors say it shouldn't be used continually for more than 6 months since its long-term effects have not been studied. But there have been no reported adverse effects from its long-term use, and Dr. Catellani says, "Some women I treat have used it for 3 or 4 years with no problems."

To prevent menopausal symptoms, take one or two 40-milligram capsules or tablets of extract (standardized to 2.5 percent triterpene glycosides) twice a day. The dosage for standardized extract is ½ to 1 teaspoon (60 to 120 drops) twice a day, says Dr. Catellani. If you are currently taking HRT and would like to switch to black cohosh, talk to a health care practitioner. You may need guidance to make the transition. Otherwise, you'll have a flare-up of menopausal symptoms.

**Get milk thistle.** If you've been taking synthetic hormones and having symptoms related to excess hormone levels—such as breast tenderness, headaches, or bloating—it may mean that your liver isn't "clearing" the breakdown products of these drugs well, says Serafina Corsello, M.D. To help it out, she recommends milk thistle, or silymarin, an herb that protects the liver against harmful substances and even helps repair and regenerate injured liver cells. Milk thistle is best taken as a standardized extract.

The usual dose for milk thistle is 420 milligrams, divided into two to three doses a day for 6 to 8 weeks, then a reduction to 280 milligrams daily, Dr. Corsello says.

**Seek out St. John's wort.** Hormone-related depression, if experienced earlier in life, may return during menopause, Dr. Catellani says. St. John's wort, long recognized for its ability to fight "melancholy," has been shown to be as effective as some prescription antidepressants for mild to moderate depression. "It's less likely than prescription antidepressants to cause side effects, such as fatigue, loss of sexual interest, or dry mouth," she explains.

The dosage used in most clinical trials was 300 milligrams in capsule form, three times a day, of an extract containing 0.3 percent hypericin, one of the active ingredients in St. John's wort. And you may need to use it regularly for 2 to 3 weeks before you see an effect. If symptoms persist, seek immediate help from a qualified mental health professional.

**Consider kava.** Kava is emerging as the herb of choice for women who want to mellow out when life puts them on edge. In one study, women who took 100 milligrams of kava extract three times a day for 8 weeks reported less than half the anxiety and depression that women taking blank look-alike pills reported. Kava has few side effects compared with prescription anti-anxiety drugs, is not addictive, and in therapeutic doses does not affect concentration or alertness.

The standard dose is 70 milligrams of standardized kava extract, two to three times a day. "It does work, and it does have a sedating effect, so I might recommend it for short-term situational anxiety," Dr. Catellani says. "But personally, I prefer that women look at and change the things that are causing them anxiety, rather than just take a pill, whether it's herbal or not."

## PANEL OF ADVISORS

**Connie Catellani, M.D.,** is a physician in Skokie, Illinois.

**Serafina Corsello, M.D.,** is medical director of the Corsello Center for Complementary-Alternative Medicine in New York City. She is the author of *The Ageless Woman*.

**Larrian Gillespie, M.D.,** is a retired assistant clinical professor of urology and urogynecology and president of Healthy Life Publications. She is the author of *The Menopause Diet* and *The Goddess Diet*.

**Mary Jane Minkin, M.D.,** is a clinical professor at Yale University School of Medicine and an obstetrician-gynecologist in New Haven, Connecticut. She is the coauthor of *What Every Woman Needs to Know about Menopause*.

# MORNING SICKNESS
## 12 Ways to Counteract Queasiness

In her wisdom, perhaps Mother Nature came up with morning sickness to prepare women for even greater challenges in their journeys to motherhood. Then again, perhaps morning sickness is simply the body's way of adapting to rising estrogen levels. Whatever its origins, more and more doctors take it seriously these days.

Take Yvonne Thornton, M.D. She used to make light of her patients' complaints, she says, until she learned better. "What's a little nausea? I thought," she recalls. "And then I became pregnant. I was camped out by the toilet every 5 minutes!"

Morning sickness is really a misnomer for the vomiting and nausea that strike many pregnant women. It usually affects women in the first 3 months after conception, but sometimes it continues throughout the pregnancy. Some women find that nausea hits at any time of the day or night. Others report

## WHEN TO CALL A DOCTOR

Consult your physician about your morning sickness if:

- You notice you've lost a pound or two. Normally, weight gain during pregnancy continues even if you can't keep all your meals down.
- You feel dehydrated or are not urinating.
- You find that you can't keep anything down—no water, no juice, nothing—over a period of 4 to 6 hours.

At its most severe, morning sickness can spiral into a condition doctors call hyperemesis gravidarum. Left untreated, it can disturb the essential electrolyte balance in your body, cause pulse irregularities, and, in its severest form, damage the kidneys and liver. It also endangers your unborn child. The ketones that result when your body breaks down fat already stored in the body can cause neurological damage in the baby.

Women with hyperemesis gravidarum are usually hospitalized overnight and treated with an intravenous solution of glucose, water, and vitamins, as well as some medications.

feeling worse in the evening, after a long day at work. Some say that certain smells trigger it.

Typically, morning sickness begins around week 6 of pregnancy—about the same time the placenta begins serious production of human chorionic gonadotropin (HCG), a pregnancy hormone. In most women, symptoms peak during week 8 or 9 and wane after week 13.

The good news is that morning sickness seems to be a sign that the pregnancy is going well. A National Institute of Child Health and Human Development study of 9,098 pregnant women found that those who vomited during their first trimester were less likely to miscarry or deliver prematurely.

With that good news in mind, try these remedies so that you can say, "I've lost that queasy feeling."

**Experiment.** What worked for your sister, your best friend, or the woman down the street may not do it for you. "There are as many remedies as there are women," says certified nurse-midwife Deborah Gowen. You may need to try a couple of strategies before you find one right for you.

**Eat the way your baby eats.** The child growing inside you nourishes itself by raiding your bloodstream for glucose 24 hours a day. If you don't take care how you replenish the supply, your blood sugar levels can drop sharply.

Your best tactic, says nurse-midwife Tekoa King, is to switch the way you eat to the way the baby eats, a little bit at a time. Put glucose into your system quickly and easily by eating simple sugars, such as fruit sugars, that are already half broken down. Grapes and orange juice are excellent choices.

**Avoid fried, fatty foods.** That grilled cheeseburger with onion rings may have looked great to you last week, but you might not want to chance it now.

"Anything fried often seems to make pregnant women more nauseated," says King. The body takes longer to digest such foods, she says, which means they sit in the stomach longer.

**Carry raw almonds with you.** Snacking on them fulfills the requirement of small, frequent meals. They contain some fat, some protein, and are high in calcium and potassium. They're portable, too, and tastier than crackers, notes Gowen.

---

# Massage to the Rescue

The next time your mate expresses sympathy about your morning sickness, tell him he can do something to help—acupressure massage.

Daily allover massage is ideal as a preventive strategy, says Wataru Ohashi, an ohashiatsu teacher.

But if your partner won't go for that, show him the instructions for this quickie technique. It can help in a pinch.

Have the woman recline on her right side and sit behind her, supporting her back with your left leg. Slip your left arm under hers and grasp her left shoulder.

With your right hand, massage her entire neck three times. Then place your palm against the base of her skull and stretch her head away from her shoulders.

Next, use your thumb to press down her back in the grooves between the left shoulder blade and spine and then around the perimeter of her shoulder blade out toward her side. Keep the pressure on for 5 to 7 seconds per point. If you find a sore spot, gently give it extra attention. Slip your thumb as far under her shoulder blade as is comfortable for her.

Begin with gentle pressure and let your partner tell you if she wants more pressure. Always use your body weight, not your muscle power. "The feeling is totally different," says Ohashi.

"If you stimulate the external, you can eliminate the internal discomfort," says Ohashi. The trigger points you use in this exercise affect the stomach and the hormonal system, he adds.

**Keep nibbles on your night table.** If almonds don't appeal to you, or if nausea strikes in the morning, keep soda crackers by your bed. Moving around on an empty stomach can make you feel worse, says King. So eat something to bring your blood sugar up before you get out of bed in the morning, or in the middle of the night.

**Nibble to keep away heartburn, too.** "You should always have something in your stomach, even if it's just a cracker," advises Gregory Radio, M.D. "The stomach naturally makes more acids during pregnancy. Those acids need something to work against."

**Sip ginger ale.** Remember how your mom used to give you ginger ale to settle an upset stomach? Dr. Thornton is a ginger ale fan, too.

**If you're taking prenatal vitamins, check with your doctor.** In some instances, they can make you sick to your stomach, says Gowen. Your doctor or midwife may be able to switch you to a different brand or chewable vitamin that won't upset your stomach.

**Trust your body's wisdom.** "Eat whatever appeals to you, as long as you're not eating junk," says Gowen. "Avoid caffeine, artificial sweeteners, all drugs. But if all you crave is pasta, then eat it. It really does work when women listen to their bodies."

**Keep calm.** If you continue to put on weight, and dehydration isn't a problem for you, you're probably doing just fine.

"Women don't tend to lose beyond what their body stores can handle," says King. "I think we just don't know the magic of what goes on inside the mother. My belief is that you can really be fairly ill with morning sickness, yet you can continue nourishing your baby very well."

## Cures from the Kitchen

Although the kitchen may be the last room a nauseated, pregnant woman wants to visit, she'll find several helpful beverages there. Gregory Radio, M.D., recommends drinking small amounts of clear fluids frequently. Clear broth, fruit juice, and herbal teas such as ginger, raspberry leaf, and chamomile fill the bill. Ginger tea is especially known as a superior remedy for morning sickness. Researchers don't know how ginger calms nausea and stops vomiting, but they know that it does. "I don't mean to endorse a product," he says, but Gatorade is usually superb because it can help maintain your electrolytes—substances that regulate the body's electrochemical balance.

## PANEL OF ADVISORS

**Deborah Gowen,** a certified nurse-midwife, works for Women-Care in Arlington, Massachusetts.

**Tekoa King,** a nurse-midwife, has been delivering babies for more than a decade and has taught nurse practitioners at the University of California, San Francisco. She is affiliated with the Bay Area Midwifery Service.

**Wataru Ohashi** is an internationally known teacher of ohashiatsu and founder of the Ohashi Institute, a nonprofit organization in New York City.

**Gregory Radio, M.D.,** is a practicing obstetrician-gynecologist and chairman of primary care and the department of obstetrics and gynecology at Lehigh Valley Hospital in Allentown, Pennsylvania.

**Yvonne S. Thornton, M.D.,** is a maternal fetal medicine specialist and associate clinical professor of obstetrics and gynecology at Columbia University College of Physicians and Surgeons in New York City. She is also director of the Perinatal Center at St. Luke's Hospital, also in New York City.

# MOTION SICKNESS
## 24 Quick-Action Cures

The French call seasickness *mal de mer*, and even the most seasoned sailors can suffer from it. In the air, it's airsickness. On land, it's carsickness. And then there's amusement-park-ride sickness. At least one visitor a day turns green on Disney World's Space Mountain or Big Thunder Mountain roller coaster. Regardless of what you call it, it's all the same thing: that queasy, uneasy feeling collectively known as motion sickness.

"Motion sickness results when the brain receives wrong information about the environment," explains Rafael Tarnopolsky, M.D. To help keep our bodies in balance, our sensory systems continually collect information about our surroundings and send it to our inner ears, where, like computers, they organize the information before sending it on to the brain.

When our balance system notes a discrepancy between what our inner ears sense and what our eyes sense, motion sickness can take hold, says Horst Konrad, M.D. Not everyone gets it, but the signals are pretty clear when it does occur. Dizziness. Sweating. Pale skin and feelings of nausea. If things don't improve, you throw up.

Once you feel the symptoms coming on, motion sickness can be very difficult to stop, especially if you've reached your particular point of no return—usually once nausea sets in. But the following remedies can help nurse the symptoms, perhaps even cutting them short. Better yet, they may keep them from starting in the first place next time you're bobbing and rolling, rolling and bobbing along on a choppy sea's waves.

**Think about motion wellness.** "Motion sickness is partly psychological," says Dr. Konrad. "If you think you're going to throw up, you're probably going to." Instead, turn your thoughts to something wonderful.

**Leave nursing the sick to someone else.** It's a common occurrence. You're on a fishing boat. Everything's going along fine until someone gets sick. You watch in sympathy, maybe even offer a comforting shoulder. Before long, you're the next body down. Then another hits the deck. It's the domino theory in action. As cruel as it may sound, do your best to ignore others who are sick, says Dr. Konrad. Otherwise, you're liable to end up in the same proverbial boat.

**Get your nose out of the joint.** Bad odors such as engine fumes, the dead fish on ice in the back of the boat, or the airline food passing by on the flight attendant's cart can contribute to nausea, says Dr. Konrad. Aim your nose elsewhere.

**Butt out.** If you're a smoker, you may think that lighting up can calm you, deterring motion sickness. Wrong. Cigarette smoke contributes to impending nausea, says Dr. Konrad. If you're a nonsmoker, hightail it to the nonsmoking section of the plane, train, or bus when you feel queasiness coming on.

**Travel at night.** Your chances of getting sick diminish when you travel at night because you can't see the motion as well as you can during daylight, says Roderic W. Gillilan, O.D.

**Don't get friendly with unfriendly food.** If certain foods don't like you when you're standing still, they're going to like you even less when you're moving. As tempting as plentiful meals may be during your travels, don't overindulge, advises Robert Salada, M.D.

**Go ahead, get fresh.** Deter nausea with a breath of fresh air, suggests Dr. Salada. In a car, open a window. On a boat, stand out on deck and take in the sea breeze. On an airplane, turn on the overhead vent.

**Think before you drink.** "Too much alcohol can interfere with the way the brain handles information about the environment, setting off motion sickness symptoms," says Dr. Konrad. What's more, alcohol can dissolve into the fluids on your

# Cures from the Kitchen

Folk remedies for motion sickness have probably been around since before the first buggy ride. Here are some that are worth trying.

**Gingerroot.** Although the remedy is tried and true, ginger recently passed scientific scrutiny when an experiment showed that two powdered gingerroot capsules were more effective than a dose of Dramamine in preventing motion sickness. Ginger works, researchers theorize, by absorbing acids in your gastrointestinal tract.

**Olives and lemons.** Motion sickness causes you to produce excess saliva, which can make you nauseated, some doctors say. Olives, on the other hand, produce chemicals called tannins, which make your mouth dry. Hence, the theory goes, eating a couple of olives at the first hint of nausea can help diminish it, as can sucking on a mouth-puckering lemon.

**Soda crackers.** They won't stop salivation, but dry soda crackers may help absorb the excess fluid when it reaches your stomach. Their "secret ingredients" are bicarbonate of soda and cream of tartar.

inner ear, which can send your head spinning, he says. Drink in moderation, if at all, during plane and ship travel.

**Get enough sleep.** "Your chance of getting motion sickness increases with fatigue," says Dr. Gillilan. So be sure to get your usual quota of sleep before taking off on a trip. If you're a passenger in a car or plane, catching a few Zzzs while en route can help, too, if only to temporarily ward off potentially sickening stimuli.

**Sit still!** Your brain is already confused enough without your creating extra motion. Keep your head especially still.

**Get up front and out ahead.** In a car, move up to the front seat and focus on the road ahead or the horizon, says Dr. Tarnopolsky. This brings signals from your body and your eyes into balance.

**Better yet, get into the driver's seat.** When you're behind the wheel, you're sensibly looking straight ahead, says Dr. Gillilan, and you have the added advantage of anticipating any quick changes in motion.

**Get caught up on your reading some other time.** Don't read while you're riding in a car or on a rough plane or boat trip, says Dr. Tarnopolsky. The movement of the vehicle you're in makes the printed matter on the page move, which can lead to terrible dizziness.

If you must read, there are ways to do it without getting sick, says Dr. Gillilan. Among them:

- Slouch down in the seat and hold the reading material close to eye level. "It's not the reading itself that makes you sick," he says, "but the angle at which you're doing it. When you look down while traveling in a car, the visible motion from the side windows strikes the eyes at an unusual angle, and that triggers the symptoms. This method brings your eyes into the same position as if you were looking down the road."

- Hold your hands next to your temples to block out the action or turn your back to the window nearest you.

**Find the center of most resistance.** On a ship, get a cabin midship, where the least amount of rolling and bouncing occurs, advises Dr. Tarnopolsky. On a little boat, you may find no such escape, although a forward cabin may be smoother than aft.

**Wear acupressure wristbands.** Sold in many marine and travel shops, these lightweight wristbands have a plastic button that is supposed to be worn over what Eastern doctors call the Nei-Kuan acupressure point inside each wrist. Pressing the button for a few minutes protects you against nausea.

**Set your sights on something stationary.** It'll help get your sensory system back in balance. Standing in a bobbing boat and watching the horizon, however, may make you sick because the horizon will bob along with you. Instead, turn your sights to a stationary point in the sky or to the land in the distance.

**Take a preventive pill.** If motion sickness is as inevitable as snow in January, consider taking an over-the-counter medication like Dramamine or Bonine. Taken a few hours in advance, it can prevent symptoms from occurring in the first place, says Dr. Salada. One or two tablets last for up to 24 hours. But be sure to take the medication in advance, because it isn't effective once the symptoms start.

**Remember, time heals all wounds.** This includes motion sickness. You may feel like you're going to die—in fact, it may sound like a blessing—but motion sickness doesn't kill. Your body will eventually adjust to the environment in a ship or boat—although it might take a few days—and will stop reacting.

So be patient. Things will get better.

## PANEL OF ADVISORS

**Patricia Cowings, Ph.D.,** is director of the Psychophysiological Research Laboratory at NASA's Ames Research Center in Moffett Field, California.

**Roderic W. Gillilan, O.D.,** is a retired optometrist in Eugene, Oregon, where he still specializes in the treatment of motion sickness.

# A Space-Age Cure That Goes to Extremes

". . . four, three, two, one—liftoff!" With an earth-shaking roar, white-hot jets propel Spacelab 3 and its four-member crew into the stratosphere, where it turns its back on a world still tremulously shivering. But the folks in ground control aren't the only ones shaken up by the blast. A mere 7 minutes into the flight, one of the crew members has his first "vomiting episode," an incident that is rerun numerous times during the mission.

Being motion sick in space is a serious problem for astronauts. "At any one time, the whole crew could be incapacitated," says Patricia Cowings, Ph.D. "Potentially, it could be disastrous. Throwing up while wearing a helmet could be fatal." And there's no easy solution, since motion sickness medications can have dangerous side effects.

But new horizons are opening up, thanks to a biofeedback training program. For the past 25 years, Dr. Cowings and her colleagues have been making people sick in order to help astronauts feel better.

"Essentially, our routine involves bringing a person up to our lab and making him throw up," says Dr. Cowings, known to her colleagues as the "Baroness of Barf." A devious device aids this process: a chair that rotates while moving volunteers' heads at various angles, a process that throws off the inner ear's sense of balance in a few minutes. "It works on virtually everyone," she says.

While rotating, the subject is monitored for physiological responses such as heart rate, breathing rate, sweating, and muscle contractions. "No two people have exactly the same response," Dr. Cowings explains. "Motion sickness is actually a kind of fingerprint that's unique to each person." The fingerprint clearly drawn, each person can then be taught to control his unique responses through a combination of deep relaxation and exercise of muscles—muscles we don't realize we can exercise, like those in blood vessels.

If you can learn to successfully control your early responses, you may prevent more violent ones from coming up. The success rate is so great that Dr. Cowings and her colleagues patented the technique. "About 60 percent can completely eliminate their symptoms when we retest them in the chair. Another 25 percent can significantly decrease their responses. And the training remains effective for up to 3 years," she says.

The results are promising enough, says Dr. Cowings, that an actual cure for motion sickness is on the horizon.

**Horst Konrad, M.D.,** is former chairman of the Committee on Equilibrium of the American Academy of Otolaryngology/Head and Neck Surgery, and professor and chairman of the division of otolaryngology at Southern Illinois University School of Medicine in Springfield.

**Robert Salada, M.D.,** is an assistant professor of medicine at Case Western Reserve University School of Medicine in Cleveland. He is also director of the Travelers Health Care Center of the University Hospitals of Cleveland, a first-of-its-kind service that provides health information and immunizations to travelers and immigrants.

**Rafael Tarnopolsky, M.D.,** is a former professor of otolaryngology at the University of Osteopathic Medicine and Health Sciences in Des Moines, Iowa, who now lives in Pittsburgh.

# MUSCLE PAIN
## 40 Ways to Relief

Pain can strike any of the more than 600 muscles in your body, heralding itself as a strain, soreness, or a cramp.

In all three cases, overuse is to blame: doing too much, too soon, too often, says Ted Percy, M.D.

If you've already overdone it, don't worry. Here are a host of things that you can do to ease muscle pain.

**Take it easy.** "Every time you exercise, your muscles are injured," says Gabe Mirkin, M.D. "It takes 48 hours for muscles to heal from exercise. Soreness means damage, and you should stop exercising when you feel sore."

Of course, you don't have to be running a race or playing a hard tennis match to injure your muscles. Working in the yard, walking around the zoo all day, sitting in a position that you're unaccustomed to or that's awkward, or even just sitting in the same position for a long time, can cause muscle problems.

How much rest you should give your muscles depends on the severity of the injury and the situation, says Allan Levy, M.D.

A cramp may require only minutes of rest, a severe strain may need days or weeks. But sometimes you might not have the luxury of resting the muscle as long as needed. If you're out hiking and strain a muscle, for example, at least

## WHEN TO CALL A DOCTOR

Most of the time, the pain of a sudden muscle cramp, strain, or even extreme soreness is a lot more serious than the injury. But not always.

Cramping, for example, could be the result of a nerve injury, says Allan Levy, M.D. Or, in rare cases, it could be the result of phlebitis—inflammation of a vein. Phlebitis can become serious if a deep vein is involved, but is typically not serious when the inflammation is located in a superficial vein. (For more information, see Phlebitis on page 457.)

A strain may not even be what it seems. "This is very rare," Dr. Levy says, "but I had a patient who thought he had badly strained a thigh muscle on a stationary bike. It never improved, and we finally did surgery. He had a huge malignant tumor in the muscle."

The point here isn't to scare you, but to remind you that muscle problems that take on abnormal characteristics and linger *may* be more serious. Consult your doctor.

rest for a couple of hours, then carefully stretch the muscle before trying to continue, Dr. Levy advises.

**Put yourself on ice.** It's still the first line of defense against swelling and should be used immediately after injury, says Carol Folkerts, a former orthopedic coordinator of physical therapy. She recommends using an ice pack or wrapping ice in a towel or plastic bag and applying it for 20 minutes at a time throughout the day.

Keep the ice off the affected area for at least as long as you keep it on. "The ice constricts your blood vessels, and it's not good to constrict your blood vessels too long," Folkerts says. "You could kill the viable tissue in that area." People with heart disease, diabetes, and vascular diseases are especially vulnerable, and they should use ice with caution and only with the consent of their doctors.

**Wrap it up.** An elastic bandage will keep the swelling down. Just be careful not to wrap too tightly, Dr. Levy cautions, or you could cause swelling below the injured area. Compression may stop cramping, too, but Dr. Levy warns that's a rather painful approach.

**Put your feet up.** That is the advice if you've injured your foot or lower leg. Specifically, raise the injured body part higher than your heart to prevent blood from pooling and causing swelling, says former New York Jets head trainer Bob Reese.

**Follow up with heat.** After starting the ice, you may switch to heat for acute soreness or strain, Folkerts says. Typically, people like heat better; it's more relaxing. The heat dilates blood vessels and promotes healing.

Just remember not to switch from ice to heat too soon, or the injured area may swell. You don't have to switch over to heat at all unless you want to, Folkerts says. "You can stay with ice."

**Use heat-penetrating rubs carefully.** There isn't complete agreement among our experts on this point. "All the heat-penetrating rubs are valuable because they keep the temperature of the affected area up," says Dr. Levy.

But athletic trainers, for the most part, are less enthusiastic about these popular over-the-counter analgesics. "They can irritate the skin," says sports medicine expert Mike McCormick. "These rubs give a false sense of security—they warm, but it's surface warmth. They don't get the muscles warm."

## Stretch to Strengthen

Give muscles the attention they need, and they tend to do their jobs quietly. Ignore them, and they'll scream for attention by cramping or becoming strained when moved the wrong way.

When that happens, you may be able to quiet them again with some simple stretching. But if you want them to remain quiet, you probably will have to make stretching a regular part of your life.

Here are a few suggestions from doctors, athletic trainers, and physical therapists to help you keep your attention on work and play, not on muscle pain.

**Toe the towel.** To stretch and strengthen ankle muscles, sit on the floor and loop a towel around the ball of your foot while holding the ends of the towel in your hands. Alternately point your toes up and down while pulling ends of the towel toward your face and keeping your legs straight. Repeat several times with both feet.

**Toe the towel again.** Only this time don't move your toes. Lean back with the towel looped around your foot until you feel the stretch in the calf muscle. Hold for 15 seconds and repeat several times.

**Use the steps.** To stretch your calves, stand on the bottom step of a staircase and hold the railing for balance. Move one foot back so that the ball of the foot is at the edge of the step and your heel hangs off the back. Then, with both knees slightly bent, drop your heel below the step and feel a stretch in the back of your lower leg. Hold for 30 seconds, then switch legs.

**Get into bed.** Actually, sit with one leg stretched out on the bed and hang the other leg over the side. Then lean forward until you feel the

**Look for arnica on the ingredient list.** Old-time folk remedies for sore muscles contained arnica, a yellow-orange flower found in Europe and North America. Arnica-containing lotions are available at many health food stores and some supermarkets. Be careful to test a small patch of skin before applying it liberally, though: Some people are allergic to a chemical in the flower.

**Use an anti-inflammatory drug.** Take aspirin, ibuprofen—any of the over-the-counter nonsteroidal drugs, says Dr. Percy. They'll help reduce pain.

**S-t-r-e-t-c-h.** For cramps and spasms, if you gradually stretch the muscle out, you'll get the muscle to relax, says Dr. Levy.

Stretching exercises can take care of your soreness as it exists now, as well as prevent soreness in the future, McCormick adds.

Stretching is important because muscles injured during exercise shorten

stretch in your hamstring (the back of the thigh) and hold for 10 to 15 seconds. Repeat several times, then switch positions and stretch the other hamstring.

**Stand on one leg.** To stretch your quadriceps (the front of the thigh) muscles, stand on one leg and hold your opposite foot so that the ankle is touching your buttocks and your knee points toward the floor. Hold for 10 seconds. Repeat five times with each leg.

**Reverse the conventional situp.** For a safer way to strengthen abdominal muscles, lie back with your arms at your sides or your fingers on your stomach. Then bend your knees and raise them above your chest. Lower your legs slowly while concentrating on your abdominal muscles. Repeat 5 to 10 times.

**Reach back.** For a good shoulder stretch, place one arm, with elbow bent, behind your head, and using the opposite hand, gently pull your elbow behind your head.

**Reach around.** Another good shoulder stretch is to hold one arm, with elbow bent, across your midriff and use the opposite hand to gently pull the arm across the front of your body.

**Stretch your wrists.** Make a fist, then span or spread your fingers as far as possible. Relax. Repeat three or four times.

**Stretch your forearms.** Hold your arms straight out in front of your body with your palms facing down. Bend your hands up, so that your palms face away from you. Hold that stretch for 5 seconds. Then bend your hands down, so that your palms are facing toward you. Hold that stretch for 5 seconds. Repeat three or four times.

during the healing process, Dr. Mirkin explains. And unless the muscles are then lengthened, they will remain tight and thus are more likely to be injured or torn. (For instructions on stretching exercises, see "Stretch to Strengthen" on page 402.)

**Give your muscles a massage.** Rub gently, and, as with exercise, stop if it hurts, Dr. Levy says. You also may want to warm the sore area before massaging it.

**Wear warm clothing.** If you're exercising in cold weather and feel yourself getting stiff and a little sore, warm up by adding more clothes. You may be able to halt muscle problems right there.

In cold weather, Reese uses running tights under players' uniforms to retain the heat. "The players like the compressive feeling it gives them, and the tights support the muscles a little bit," he says.

**Change positions.** Whether you're bent over a keyboard typing or bent over a bicycle pedaling, your wrists and forearms are vulnerable to cramping and soreness, says Scott Donkin, D.C. But there's one important difference between cyclists and office workers—when cyclists buy bikes, there's usually a salesperson there to make sure they select the bike that best fits them. Yet office workers, who have fingers and hands of all different sizes, typically use the same office equipment. With the selection of ergonomic accessories out there for desk jockeys, all it takes is a little research and testing to find a setup that puts you in a comfortable, ergonomically correct position.

"The wrist and hands should be used in what is known as the neutral position," according to Dr. Donkin. "In this position, the wrist is bent neither forward, backward, inward, nor outward."

If you have long hands and fingers, you can reduce the strain by adjusting the keyboard to a more horizontal position (flat with the work surface) as long as it does not put your arms or shoulders in a strained position.

For those who have short hands and fingers, a higher incline on the keyboard, typewriter, or calculator will make the keys easier to reach.

**Repeat the activity that made you sore.** It sounds counterintuitive, but it helps. "Do the activity again the very next day," Reese says, "but with much less intensity. It will help work out some of the soreness."

**Follow a hard-easy/hard-easy workout pattern.** This is advisable because of the 48 hours needed for muscles to recover, says Dr. Mirkin. "All serious athletes train that way."

**Branch out.** This is perhaps an even better idea than the hard-easy routine, Dr. Mirkin says. If you're a walker experiencing sore lower leg muscles, mix in some swimming or bicycling (which works the upper legs) so that you can continue exercising while healing.

**Lose weight.** If sore muscles and muscle strains have become a chronic problem, the extra weight you're asking them to move may be at least partially to blame.

**Be realistic.** If running always makes you hurt, for example, then you may have to find another exercise. "Running is one of the most dangerous sports for injuries," Dr. Mirkin says.

---

# Banish Nighttime Leg Cramps

Few things hurt worse than a charley horse—the searing pain of a calf muscle cramp that can wake you from the dead of sleep.

What happened? Basically, your calf muscle got stuck. Leg muscles contract when you turn or stretch during sleep. When a muscle stays contracted, a sudden cramp can result.

Here's how to stop night cramps and, hopefully, head off a recurrence later in the night.

**Lean into the wall.** Stand 3 to 5 feet away from a wall, keeping your heels flat and your legs straight. Lean into the wall in front of you as you support yourself with your hands. Hold for 10 seconds and repeat several times.

**Massage the cramp.** Massage the calf by rubbing upward from the ankle toward your heart, advises Carol Folkerts, a former orthopedic coordinator of physical therapy. If night cramps are a constant problem, you may want to do this before you even try to sleep, she adds.

**Loosen the covers.** The pressure of heavy blankets on your legs could be partly to blame, says Folkerts.

**Wear roomy PJs.** Snug-fitting pajamas will only exacerbate nighttime leg cramps if you're prone to them.

**Use an electric blanket.** The electric blanket on your bed can do more than keep you warm all over on cold winter nights; it can also keep your calf muscles warm and pain-free, says Folkerts.

**Sleep on your side.** Sleeping on your stomach with your legs straight out and your calves flexed invites cramping, says Scott Donkin, D.C. "Try sleeping on your side with your knees bent upward and a pillow between them."

**Consider more calcium.** "A calcium deficiency can make the muscles trigger-happy; the contractions in the muscles are stronger," Dr. Donkin says. The Daily Value for calcium is 1,000 milligrams a day (1,200 if you're over age 50).

**Slow down instead of stopping suddenly.** After hard exercise or physical work, the bloodstream is loaded with lactic acid, which collects in the bloodstream when there is a lack of oxygen, explains Dr. Mirkin. When the acid reaches high levels, it disrupts normal chemical reactions of the muscles and can make your muscles hurt.

"The most effective way to clear the bloodstream is to continue exercising at a slow, relaxed pace," Dr. Mirkin advises. While this may lessen immediate soreness, it won't protect you from soreness the next day. That soreness, he says, is caused by torn muscle fiber.

**Change your shoes.** If you're wearing the wrong kind of shoes or wearing shoes that don't fit well, that could explain the foot, leg, and even back pains you feel while exercising, says McCormick.

**Be patient.** The more serious the injury—a severely pulled hamstring, for example—the more of this virtue you will need to ensure a relapse-free recovery.

**Loosen your clothing.** If you feel a leg cramp approaching, you may want to shed tights or any other snug clothing to give your muscles a little more room.

**Stand up.** It's simple, and perhaps all it takes to stop a cramp in the leg or foot, Dr. Levy says.

**Drink up.** Dehydration is often a big contributor to cramping, says McCormick. "We overstress the need to force liquids, especially before, during, and after physical activity. And for good reason."

## PANEL OF ADVISORS

**Scott Donkin, D.C.,** is a partner in the Chiropractic Associates in Lincoln, Nebraska. He is also an industrial consultant, providing tips on exercise to reduce stress for workstation users, and the author of *Sitting on the Job*.

**Carol Folkerts** is formerly an orthopedic coordinator of physical therapy at the University of Maryland Hospital in Baltimore.

**Allan Levy, M.D.,** has a private practice in sports medicine in Woodcliff Lake and is a team physician for the New York Giants football team.

**Mike McCormick** is a partner with AthletiCo Sports Medicine and Physical Therapy Center in LaGrange Park, Illinois.

**Gabe Mirkin, M.D.,** is an associate clinical professor of pediatrics at Georgetown University School of Medicine in Washington, D.C., and in practice at Mirkin Medical Consultants in Kensington, Maryland. He is the author of several sports medicine books, including *Women and Exercise*, and a syndicated newspaper columnist and radio broadcaster.

**Ted Percy, M.D.,** is an associate professor emeritus of orthopedic surgery and sports medicine and head of the sports medicine section at the Arizona Health Sciences Center at the University of Arizona College of Medicine in Tucson.

**Bob Reese** is the former head trainer for the New York Jets and past president of the Professional Football Athletic Trainers Society. He is now an associate professor at the College of Health Sciences in Roanoke, Virginia.

# NAIL BRITTLENESS
## 14 Strengthening Secrets

Paul Kechijian, M.D., compares a person's nails to a brick wall, with the material between the nail cells the mortar that binds the bricks together, and the cells that make up the nails the bricks.

Over time, your nails—like a brick wall—can become damaged and brittle. The main causes of brittle nails are aging, followed by frequent hand washing and drying, and exposure to household cleaning products, he says. All of these lead to diminished moisture in the hands. Exposure to nail cosmetics can also play a role.

Brittle nails come in two varieties: hard and soft, notes C. Ralph Daniel III, M.D.

Hard and brittle nails are caused by dehydration—too *little* moisture in and around nails. On the other hand, soft and brittle nails happen when there's too *much* moisture in and around nails. One type isn't more common than the other, according to Dr. Daniel. "I see about a 50-50 split between the two types," he says. "But both are treatable."

In the case of hard and brittle nails, you're battling Father Time. Your nails naturally get harder and more brittle as you age because they lose some of their natural moisture. If you don't replace that lost moisture, they may crack.

## WHEN TO CALL A DOCTOR

Paul Kechijian, M.D., suggests seeing a dermatologist if you've been applying a moisturizer for 2 weeks and are still experiencing brittle nails, or if your nails hurt or affect the everyday function of your hands.

Soft and brittle nails occur from constant immersion in water, leaving nails waterlogged. The water causes the nails to expand and then shrink, over time becoming brittle.

Here's what to do.

**Reach for hand cream.** Apply a moisturizing hand cream to your hands and nails after each washing and drying. The hand cream traps moisture, keeping your hands and nails from drying out, says Dr. Kechijian.

Because your nails, like an accordion, expand when they absorb water and then contract when the water evaporates, products that attract and bind moisture to your nails, morning and night, are most effective. Over-the-counter creams with 5 percent lactic acid, such as Lac-Hydrin Five, fit this description. "You might also try any glycolic acid preparation (Total Skin Care Glycolic Gel is one) or any good moisturizer available at your drugstore. Ask your pharmacist to recommend one, or try a few until you find one you like," Dr. Kechijian notes.

**Shop around.** Over-the-counter moisturizers are sold in many different scents and textures. Dee Anna Glaser, M.D., suggests finding your favorite aroma and feel. The reason? You're more apt to use a product you enjoy.

Dr. Glaser also encourages people with brittle nails to place small tubes of moisturizer wherever they'll need them so that they can apply it after every washing of their hands. For example, stash tubes by all the sinks at home as well as in your glove compartment and desk drawer at work.

**Avoid alcohol.** Some perfumed hand lotions contain alcohol. Avoid these types if your nails are brittle. The alcohol only makes your brittle nails worse because of the drying effect of the alcohol, says Dr. Daniel.

**Keep nails short and sweet.** Longer nails are more subject to trauma and are more likely to crack or get caught on something and tear. Dr. Kechijian also proposes cutting your nails after showering, when they're softer and less likely to break.

## Cures from the Kitchen

Rub oil or thick hand cream into your nails while applying your hand moisturizer for better results, says Audrey Kunin, M.D. You can use expensive store-bought creams or look in your kitchen for vegetable oil or shortening.

Dee Anna Glaser, M.D., recommends this extra-soothing nighttime treatment. Before you go to bed, apply vegetable oil to your hands, then put on vinyl gloves or wrap your hands in plastic wrap to keep the oil off bedspreads and pillowcases. The gloves or plastic wrap forces the oil to penetrate your skin, preventing your hands from getting too dry.

**Eat a well-balanced diet.** Brittle nails can be the result of something you are—or aren't—eating, says Dr. Glaser. "Eating a well-balanced diet and taking a daily multivitamin/mineral supplement to get your recommended daily allowance of vitamins and minerals are important. Any trendy diet in which only a few foods are eaten, or where certain groups of foods are excluded, can produce nail problems," she adds.

**Double glove.** If washing dishes is on your daily "to do" list, Dr. Kechijian suggests investing in several pairs of cotton gloves to use under your rubber dishwashing gloves. The vinyl exterior of the dishwashing gloves keeps the water and cleaning products off your nails, while the cotton gloves absorb sweat so that your nails and hands don't get soggy inside the glove. He recommends gloves from the George Glove Company. For more information, call their toll-free number at (800) 631-4292. Their products are also available on the Internet.

**Dish off some chores.** While agreeing wholeheartedly that people with brittle nails should wear gloves while doing household chores, Audrey Kunin, M.D., has an even better way to limit your water exposure: Get someone else to wash the dishes.

**Go with acetate, not acetone.** Use nail polish removers that contain acetate. "Acetone nail polish removers are stronger, but they can take much-needed moisture out of your nails and make them brittle," says Dr. Daniel.

**Add some calcium.** A lack of calcium in the diet is another cause of brittle nails, says Dr. Kunin. Calcium supplements can work wonders for strengthening nails. If you don't get three servings of milk, cheese, or yogurt every day, take a 500-milligram calcium supplement daily if you are under age 50, or 1,000 milligrams of calcium if you are over age 50.

**Give soy a try.** Boni Elewski, M.D., says that just 5 grams of soy protein a day helps toughen up brittle nails. Try tofu, tempeh, soy milk, or frozen edamame, all available in most grocery stores. For example, each 8-ounce serving of soy milk provides 6 grams of soy protein and is cholesterol-free.

**Horse around with biotin.** Years ago, Swiss researchers proved that the B vitamin biotin increased the toughness of horses' hooves, says Dr. Daniel. Today, doctors recommend the vitamin for toughening human nails.

"Biotin doesn't work in every case, but I've found it to be effective in anywhere from one-third to one-half of the cases I've seen," says Dr. Daniel.

Cauliflower is a rich source of biotin, as are legumes such as peanuts and lentils; however, you'd have to eat a lot of them to get enough biotin. Instead, Dr. Daniel suggests that if you have brittle nails, take 300 micrograms of biotin

## No Thumbs-Up for Nail Strengtheners

The corner drugstore is often the first stop for people with brittle nails. They turn to nail strengtheners in the hope of transforming their brittle nails into unbreakable ones. Our experts say that these nail strengtheners aren't all that they're cracked up to be.

Nail strengtheners purportedly contain an ingredient that binds to damaged nails to make them thicker. But you can't change the quality of the nail simply by applying something to the surface, says Paul Kechijian, M.D. Instead of fixing the problem of brittle nails, he says, they merely camouflage the brittleness.

---

four to six times a day with food. This dosage should increase your nail thickness within 6 months.

**Manage your meds.** Some common drugs, such as diuretics, can cause dehydration and could worsen a preexisting case of brittle nails. Check with your doctor if you think your medications are contributing to your brittle nails.

## PANEL OF ADVISORS

**C. Ralph Daniel III, M.D.,** is a clinical professor of dermatology at the University of Mississippi Medical Center in Jackson.

**Boni Elewski, M.D.,** is a professor of dermatology at the University of Alabama at Birmingham.

**Dee Anna Glaser, M.D.,** is an associate professor of dermatology at St. Louis University School of Medicine.

**Paul Kechijian, M.D.,** is an associate clinical professor of dermatology and chief of the nail section at the New York University Medical Center in Great Neck.

**Audrey Kunin, M.D.,** is a cosmetic dermatologist from Kansas City, Missouri, and the founder of the dermatology educational Web site DERMAdoctor.com.

# NAIL DISCOLORATION
## 7 Nail Remedies

You can learn a lot about yourself simply by looking at your nails.

"Nail discoloration can be caused by a variety of conditions, such as reactions to medications (blue discoloration), bacterial infection (green/black), fungal infection (yellow), or even melanoma (black or brown discoloration)," says Audrey Kunin, M.D. Smoking can stain nails a very unattractive brown, while the wrong nail polish can leave them tinged an unnatural orange-yellow.

According to Coyle S. Connolly, D.O., the most common cause of discolored nails is a condition called onychomycosis. This nail fungus occurs when organisms known as dermatophytes move in under your nails. According to the National Onychomycosis Society, 11 million new cases are diagnosed each year.

Why so common? Toenails and fingernails and surrounding skin are prone to everyday wear and tear, which invite dirt, germs, and infection-causing fungi to take up residence there.

The first sign of a fungal infection is a change in color. The nail often becomes yellow to brown, and then it gets thicker and may develop a bad odor. Debris may collect beneath the nail, and a white area on the nail edge may form as the nail begins to lift from the nail bed. The infection can spread to other nails and even the skin. Toenails are affected more frequently than fingernails. This whole process often happens more frequently with age, says Dr. Connolly.

Here's how to keep this from happening to you.

**Keep clean.** Because fungi are everywhere, including the skin, they can be present months before they find opportunities to strike and before signs of infection appear. By following proper hygiene and regularly inspecting your feet and toes, you can reduce your chances of the problem, or even stop the chain of events once it starts, says Paul Kechijian, M.D.

"Clean, dry feet resist disease. A strict regimen of washing the feet with antibacterial soap and water every night before bedtime, and remembering to dry thoroughly, is the best way to prevent an infection," says Dr. Kechijian. This habit helps rid the feet of excess bacteria from shoes and gives them a full night of cleanliness before they are back into shoes.

## WHEN TO CALL A DOCTOR

According to Coyle S. Connolly, D.O., onychomycosis is not a problem to be ignored. "In fact, if left untreated, it can spread to other nails and make everyday activities, such as walking or writing, painful and difficult," he says.

See your doctor if:

- You notice unexplained changes in the color of your nail.
- Your nails look abnormally thick.
- Your nails are painful or tender.
- You have swelling on the skin surrounding the nail.
- You have a nail that appears to have separated from the nail bed.

"If it's a fungus, it's best to catch it in its earlier stages. If the discoloration is a symptom of something more serious, early detection is even more important," Dr. Connolly says.

Treating nail fungus can take some time—up to 6 months—so be patient. Follow the advice of your doctor and, most important, stick with the prescribed treatment regimen. The end result—healthy, clear nails—is well worth it.

Also, discolored nails might signal a more serious condition, such as heart disease, anemia, infection, or illness. See your doctor as soon as possible if you experience nail discoloration in conjunction with other symptoms, such as malaise.

**Snip nails short.** "Longer nails can get caught on things or rub against tighter shoes, which can cause the nail to lift from its bed," says Dr. Connolly. "That opening can invite fungus inside." Clip toenails straight across so that the nail doesn't extend beyond the nail bed, he suggests.

**Keep them cool.** Use a quality foot powder—talcum, not cornstarch—and wear shoes that fit well and are made of materials that breathe, says C. Ralph Daniel III, M.D. The reason? "Sweating makes matters worse, since it creates a warm, moist environment—perfect for spreading nail fungus," he says. The fungus digests the nail keratin, the protein that makes up the nail, causing the discoloration, which ranges from white to yellow and less often green to black.

**Wash your hands.** Fungal infection can spread from your feet to your hands. So wash your hands after inspecting your feet, says Dr. Connolly. Also, smooth away dead skin by gently scrubbing away with soap and water, because fungus often attaches itself to dead, dry skin and moves on to other areas. "Watch for any rash or nail involvement of any new rash," he advises.

**Watch those nail products.** Ordinarily, any moisture that collects underneath the surface of the nail passes through the porous structure of the nail and evaporates. Acrylic nails applied to the top of the nail may impede that, however. The water trapped below can become stagnant and unhealthy, ideal conditions for fungi and similar organisms to thrive, says Dr. Daniel.

Also, the pigments in some polishes can eventually turn nails an unflattering yellowish orange color. Cosmetology school director Rita Johnson says that the quality and the color of the product are usually the biggest factors.

Her colleague, Barbara Bealer, agrees. "Professional brands are often thicker, so they require fewer coats and usually don't stain as much as less-expensive polishes." In terms of color, red nail polish is the most likely to stain, followed by brown shades.

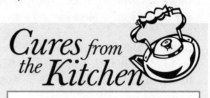

## Cures from the Kitchen

Superficial staining of the nail responds fairly well to swabbing clean, dry nails with a half-water, half-fresh-lemon-juice solution. Allow the nails to dry and repeat two or three times, says author Joni Keim Loughran. Moisturize afterward because lemon juice can dry out your nails and skin, she says. Skip a day or two and then repeat the process until the discoloration is gone.

One simple remedy is to vary your color choices—alternating lighter shades of nail polish with your reds and browns from time to time, suggests Bealer.

**Bring on the bleach.** Bleaching nails at home is relatively simple if you use this simple recipe, suggests Bealer: "Combine 10 parts water with 1 part chlorine bleach. Soak cotton balls or pads in this solution and use them to rub the stains. Repeat if needed, then wash your hands as usual." If stains are persistent, check the undersides of your nails. "Use a nail brush or toothbrush to make sure they are clean," she suggests.

Or, try using hydrogen peroxide every few days for 3 weeks to get your nails back to their normal color. Johnson suggests mixing 1 tablespoon of hydrogen peroxide with 3 tablespoons of baking soda. Apply to nails (underneath and over tops) with a cotton swab. Leave on for 3 to 5 minutes then rinse with warm water and apply hand lotion.

Johnson says that there are also over-the-counter nail bleaches, available at beauty supply stores, that will do the trick. Just follow the manufacturer's directions and warnings when using these products. You should see an improvement in 2 to 3 weeks, she notes.

# NAIL RIDGES
## 6 Ridge Reducers

Palm readers might be on to something after all. The only trouble is they could be looking at the wrong side of your hands. For it's not your palms, but your fingernails, that can predict your future health.

The ridges that appear in your nails, either vertically or horizontally, can indicate several serious medical conditions, says Dee Anna Glaser, M.D.

Vertical, or longitudinal, ridges, which run from the base of the nail to the tip, are most typical. They are usually normal and are related to aging or genetics. "Anyone over age 50 can expect to see more ridging in their nails as they age," says Paul Kechijian, M.D.

Severe ridging and cracking or sudden onset of vertical ridges serve as an alert to see a doctor, since they could be a sign of poor general health, poor nutrient absorption, or iron deficiency, says Dr. Glaser. They may also indicate rheumatoid arthritis or a circulatory or kidney disorder.

Horizontal, or transverse, ridges, which run from left to right, may occur as a result of severe psychological or physical stress, such as from infection or disease, says Dr. Glaser. Often called Beau's lines, they can occur after illness or trauma to the nail and with malnutrition. They can also be the result of habitually picking at or chewing your nail and cuticle, a nervous tic in some people. On the toenails, horizontal ridges may be related to sports injury and are common in soccer and tennis players.

Hormonal changes, genetics, and the way your body uses calcium are all factors that contribute to the rise of nail ridges. Nail ridges don't always signal a larger problem, though. "Remember, vertical ridges are like gray hair. You can expect to see more of them as you grow older," Dr. Kechijian reiterates. "They don't happen to everyone, but they are part of aging for many people." Nail ridging can cause the nails to become more susceptible to damage, but for the most part they're just a cosmetic problem. Here are some ways to reduce the ridges.

**Buff 'em.** Gently buff your nails with a buffing block to minimize the ridges, suggests Dr. Glaser.

Be gentle. Don't completely buff out the nail ridges, since severe buffing can weaken the nail plate, notes Dr. Kechijian.

---

# The ABC's of Nail Care

Because many nail disorders result from poor nail care, developing good nail habits today will help keep them healthy. Remember the following tips.

**Keep them short.** Shorter nails are less likely to crack or get caught on something and tear, says Paul Kechijian, M.D. He also suggests cutting your nails after bathing, when they're softer and less likely to break.

**Stay on the straight and narrow.** Nails should be cut straight across and rounded slightly at the tip for maximum strength, says C. Ralph Daniel III, M.D.

**Avoid biting your fingernails.** Your five-finger feeding frenzy worsens the condition of your nails, says Coyle S. Connolly, D.O.

**Eat a well-balanced diet.** Ridged nails can be the result of something lacking in your diet, says Dr. Glaser. "When people come into my office with severe nail changes, I immediately ask for their dietary history to make sure that they aren't on some fad diet keeping them from getting their recommended daily allowance of vitamins and minerals," she says. "If they're not eating a well-balanced diet, then a proper diet and a vitamin supplement might help the health of their nails."

**Don't overdo it with the emery board.** "Filing your nails is actually sanding your nails," says Dr. Kechijian. "If you oversand them, it will thin the nail and cause damage, which invites infection. So avoid overdoing it."

## PANEL OF ADVISORS

**Coyle S. Connolly, D.O.,** is an assistant clinical professor at the Philadelphia College of Osteopathic Medicine and a dermatologist practicing in Linwood, New Jersey.

**C. Ralph Daniel III, M.D.,** is a clinical professor of dermatology at the University of Mississippi Medical Center in Jackson.

**Dee Anna Glaser, M.D.,** is an associate professor of dermatology at St. Louis University School of Medicine.

**Paul Kechijian, M.D.,** is an associate clinical professor of dermatology and chief of the nail section at the New York University Medical Center in Great Neck.

# NAUSEA AND VOMITING
## 14 Stomach-Soothing Solutions

The world is full of things that make our stomachs turn. Depending on the situation, everything from eating egg salad to giving blood to reading credit card bills can make you clutch your belly in agony.

And what happens when that twisting, turning tummy becomes too much to bear? You guessed it—you vomit. Below are tips to help you keep nausea in check before the dreaded "V word" occurs. If it's too late, and you've already lost your lunch, there are tips to nurse your stomach—and the rest of you—back to good health.

## WHEN TO CALL A DOCTOR

"There are at least 25 different diseases that could cause chronic nausea," says Kenneth Koch, M.D. If your nausea just doesn't go away in a day or two, it's a good idea to see your doctor.

Vomiting, on the other hand, can be a sign of something serious. "If it's profuse, persistent, or bloody, seek help," advises Stephen Bezruchka, M.D. Also see a doctor if you've gone 24 hours without being able to keep any food down and nothing seems to help, Dr. Koch says.

"If your thirst is severe and you notice you're not urinating very much—and especially if you're also getting light-headed when you stand up, which are signs of dehydration—see a doctor," he adds. "If you know it's the flu, or you've just eaten something a little strange, you might try to go a bit longer."

Nausea can also be a sign of a heart attack. In which case, get to a hospital right away.

**Sip on syrup.** If you're not *that* nauseated, cola syrup seems to work really well, says Robert Warren, Pharm.D. The noncarbonated syrup has concentrated carbohydrates that may help settle the stomach. In fact, he says, any soft drink liquid concentrate or even plain sugar syrup (put ½ cup white sugar and ¼ cup of water in a saucepan, heat over medium heat stirring occasionally until it forms a clear liquid, and let cool) may help. Take 1 to 2 tablespoons for adults, at room temperature, as needed.

Emetrol is an over-the-counter product that works much the same way as cola syrup, except it doesn't contain caffeine, Dr. Warren says. It is more expensive than cola syrup, though. An alternative for people with diabetes is Bonine, a chewable motion-sickness tablet with no sugar.

**Choose clear liquids.** Even if you're craving food, stick with clear liquids like tea and juice, says nausea researcher Kenneth Koch, M.D. Drink the liquids warm or at room temperature, not cold, to avoid further shock to your stomach. Drink no more than 1 to 2 ounces at a time. One excellent choice might be peppermint tea. Mint has a very relaxing effect on your stomach.

**Make it flat.** "My mom used to give me 7 UP," Dr. Warren says. Other moms give cola or ginger ale.

Since our experts advise against cold beverages and carbonated ones, do as Stephen Bezruchka, M.D., suggests. Let carbonated drinks stand until flat and lukewarm. To hurry the process, pour the drink back and forth from one glass to another until it flattens out.

**Eat carbs first.** If you need something to eat, and your nausea isn't too bad, eat light carbohydrates in small amounts—toast or crackers, for instance, Dr. Koch says. As your stomach starts to settle, graduate to light protein, like chicken breast or fish. Fatty foods are the last thing to add to your diet. If your problem is not nausea but vomiting, start with Jell-O. Then follow the progression mentioned above to introduce other foods back into your diet.

**Get out of the pink.** The stomach soother Pepto-Bismol—as well as Mylanta and Maalox—is for disease-provoked stomach upsets, not for a queasy stomach. If your nausea is caused by inflammation or irritation, however, Dr. Koch says they're reasonable to start with. But none of our experts wholeheartedly recommend them. As Samuel Klein, M.D., notes, none is specifically designed for nausea. You should probably avoid these products altogether if you're already vomiting. By then, it's usually too late.

"Take them only if the vomiting is related to too much stomach acid. For instance, if you have a stomach ulcer or if something you ate is causing irritation," Dr. Klein says.

## Do just 1 thing

Try ginger. Daniel B. Mowrey, Ph.D., swears by it. "It will definitely take care of nausea," he says. Take capsules of the powdered root; the amount depends on how nauseated you are. "You know you've had enough when you burp and taste ginger," he says. Just be sure to avoid the fresh stuff. Fresh ginger is too strong for most people with nausea. Ginger ale or gingersnaps may work if your symptoms are very mild.

You could try taking ginger 30 minutes before you partake in an activity that you know will cause nausea (like going on a cruise). Take two 500-milligram capsules of dried ginger or drink an equivalent amount of ginger tea.

**Find relief in the meadow.** Meadowsweet, a pleasant-tasting wildflower, can be quite effective in reducing nausea, says Dr. Lois Johnson, M.D. To make a soothing cup of meadowsweet tea, mix 1 tablespoon of dried herb per cup of boiling water, and steep for 5 to 10 minutes before straining out the herb. Then sip on the concoction slowly. Rosemary is another ideal herb to add to the mixture.

**End it all.** One of the most effective ways to stop nausea is to allow yourself to vomit, Dr. Koch says. At the very least, you'll have a temporary respite from that queasy feeling. He doesn't recommend *making* yourself vomit, however.

## Press Your Luck

The Chinese have known for centuries that acupuncture is an effective, painless, drugless medication for nausea. And its cousin, acupressure, a needleless form of acupuncture, can also help. "The idea is to use it before you start vomiting," says acupuncturist Joseph M. Helms, M.D.

Apply pressure to the webbing between your thumb and index finger on either hand. Use firm, deep pressure and a rapid massaging movement for several minutes, he says.

Using the same kind of motion and pressure, Dr. Helms says, rub with your thumb or thumbnail on the top of your foot between the tendons of the second and third toes. With any luck, your nausea will pass after a few minutes.

**Replace important fluids and nutrients.** "The ultimate goals for someone who's got a lot of vomiting are to not get dehydrated and to not lose weight," Dr. Koch says. You lose a lot of fluid in vomiting, so the best thing you can do is drink water, tea, and weak juices to replace them. Gatorade, Pedialyte, or juices like apple and cranberry also help replace nutrients flushed out while vomiting.

**Sip—don't slurp.** Sipping your fluids in tiny swallows lets your irritated stomach adjust, Dr. Koch says. Sip no more than 1 to 2 ounces at a time. In addition, sipping small amounts enables you to determine how much fluid you can handle at one time.

**Use the color code.** If your urine is deep yellow, you're not getting enough fluid. The paler it gets, the better you're doing to prevent dehydration.

**Bathe yourself with herbs.** While ill, you might unintentionally vomit the herbs you took to feel better. A solution is an herbal bath to let herbs soak through your pores instead. Mix 1 tablespoon of fresh or powdered ginger with a quart of hot water, and

### Cures from the Kitchen

As long as you don't have diabetes, Hawaiian Punch may be a great remedy to try for nausea or an upset stomach. The refreshing red liquid has fructose, the same active ingredient as in the nausea reliever cola syrup. Plus, Hawaiian Punch is caffeine-free and just a quick convenience-store run away. As with other liquids used to relieve nausea, make sure you sip small amounts of Hawaiian Punch slowly.

let it cool. Then soak your hands or feet in the soothing bath until the vomiting subsides. If you have the flu, ginger also helps to open up the pores of your skin, allowing you to sweat until you break the fever.

## PANEL OF ADVISORS

**Stephen Bezruchka, M.D.,** is an emergency physician at Virginia Mason Hospital and Group Health Hospital in Seattle and an affiliate associate professor in the School of Public Health and Community Medicine at the University of Washington in Seattle.

**Joseph M. Helms, M.D.,** is a medical acupuncturist in Berkeley, California, and a clinical instructor at the UCLA School of Medicine in Los Angeles. He is the author of *Acupuncture Energetics.*

**Lois Johnson, M.D.,** is a physician in Sebastopol, California and a professional member of the American Herbalists Guild.

**Samuel Klein, M.D.,** is a William H. Danforth professor of medicine and nutritional science and director of the Center for Human Nutrition at Washington University School of Medicine in St. Louis.

**Kenneth Koch, M.D.,** is a gastroenterologist at the Milton S. Hershey Medical Center of the Pennsylvania State University in Hershey.

**Daniel B. Mowrey, Ph.D.,** of Lehi, Utah, is a psychologist who specializes in psychopharmacology and who has been researching the use of herbs in medicine for 15 years. He also is president of American Phytotherapy Research Laboratory in Provo, Utah, and the author of *Herbal Tonic Therapies.*

**Robert Warren, Pharm.D.,** is a pharmacist at United Pharmacy in Dinuba, California.

# NECK PAIN
## 27 Ways to Get the Kinks Out

When undue strain isn't placed on your neck, its seven vertebrae and 32 muscles do a pretty good job of holding up your 10- to 12-pound head. Still, that's a heavy load sitting on a relatively small structure, leaving your neck vulnerable to a variety of stresses that can result in acute or chronic pain.

A major cause of neck pain is holding your head in an awkward position for a long time, says former physical therapist Joanne Griffin.

Naturally, some people—because of their occupations—are more at risk than others. Hairstylists, for example, work in a bent-over position all day long, notes Robert Kunkel, M.D.

Regardless of your job or lifestyle, neck pain can be eased by applying a few time-tested methods, replacing bad habits with good ones, and giving your neck regular exercise. Help is on the way.

**Use ice.** Ice helps reduce swelling, so it's a good choice when stiffness settles in, Griffin says. If your neck has been slightly injured, apply an ice pack, wrapped in a thin cloth to protect your skin, for 15 minutes. Repeat every few hours as needed.

### WHEN TO CALL A DOCTOR

Severe or lasting neck pain may require a doctor's care. If, for example, you've been in an auto accident and have severe neck pain afterward, you may have whiplash and should see a doctor, advises Mitchell A. Price, D.C.

As a general rule, persistent neck pain warrants professional medical evaluation. "It's extremely remote, but it's possible that neck pain could be a signal that there's a tumor on the spine," says former physical therapist Joanne Griffin.

**Use heat.** After ice has reduced any inflammation, heat is a wonderful soother. Try a heating pad or a hot shower.

**Press on the painful spot.** Relieve muscle tension by applying moderate pressure to the area for 3 minutes. Don't press as hard as you can, but use your fingertips to exert steady, constant pressure on the affected point. At the end of 3 minutes, your pain should improve dramatically.

**Take a pain reliever.** Over-the-counter anti-inflammatories such as aspirin or ibuprofen will help reduce pain and inflammation. Follow label instructions.

**Try a homeopathic solution.** Traumeel, a product made from arnica, calendula, and belladonna, may help relieve muscle and joint pain according to some natural healing experts. Dissolve a Traumeel tablet under your tongue every couple of hours or apply it in cream form. Both are available at health food stores and drugstores.

**Turn to herbs.** Turmeric and ginger help reduce production of leukotrienes, substances that can trigger inflammation. Take 1 to 2 grams of each herb a day until your pain is relieved advises Mark Gostine, M.D.

**Add flaxseed oil to your juice.** Flaxseed contains alpha linolenic acid, a substance similar to the omega-3 fatty acids found in fish that can prevent joint swelling. Take 2 teaspoons a day, recommends Dr. Gostine. Refrigerate your flaxseed oil, since it spoils quickly.

**Give glucosamine a try.** Evidence suggests that this natural sugar may help repair joints. Dr. Gostine recommends taking 1,500 milligrams a day to ease neck pain, but be patient; it can take several weeks before you feel an effect.

**Take your vitamins.** Antioxidant vitamins such as vitamins C and E, taken on a regular basis, can help to prevent the painful deterioration of joints in your neck and elsewhere in your body. Take 1,000 milligrams of vitamin C and 400 IU of vitamin E daily.

**Sit in a firm chair.** Like the song says, the backbone is connected to the neck bone. Sitting in a chair without good back support can make neck problems worse and even cause new ones, says Mitchell A. Price, D.C.

**Support your lower back.** Roll up a towel and place it against the small of your back when sitting. It will better align your spine and provide additional support, says Griffin.

## Exercise Away Neck Pain

Even your neck muscles need to be stretched and strengthened. Here are some exercises to combat stiffness and prevent problems in the future. Do each exercise five times twice a day. Do the first three exercises for 2 weeks before starting the rest.

- Slowly tilt your head forward as far as possible. Then move your head backward as far as possible.

- Tilt your head toward one of your shoulders, while keeping your shoulder stationary. Straighten, then tilt toward the other shoulder.

- Slowly turn your head from side to side as far as possible.

- Place your hand on one side of your head while you push toward it with your head. Hold for 5 seconds, then relax. Repeat three times. Then do the same exercise on the other side.

- Do basically the same exercise as above, only provide slight resistance to the front of your head while you push your head forward. Then provide slight resistance to the back of your head while you push your head backward.

- Hold light weights—say, 3 to 5 pounds—in your hands while shrugging your shoulders. Keep your arms straight.

**Take a break.** Just as the feet need rest from constant standing, the neck needs a rest from constant sitting, says Griffin. Periodically stand up and walk around.

**Keep your chin up.** Keep your head level but pull your chin in as if you were making a double chin, says Griffin. Also, avoid lowering your head all the time when working at a desk or reading, she advises. This helps prevent stressing the muscles in the back of the neck.

**See eye to screen.** If you stare at a computer monitor all day, position it at eye level. If you force yourself to look up or down hour after hour, your neck may spasm, says Dr. Price.

**Get a telephone headset.** Holding the telephone in the crook of your neck and shoulder so that you can talk and write at the same time puts your neck in an awkward position—an invitation to stiffness and pain.

**Sleep on a firm mattress.** A lot of neck problems begin, and worsen, with poor sleeping habits that put the spine out of alignment. Having a firm mattress is important, Dr. Price says.

**Toss your pillow aside.** "A lot of people with neck pain feel better sleeping flat—without a pillow," Dr. Kunkel says.

**Get a cervical pillow.** These pillows, which cost as little as $20, give the neck proper support, Dr. Price says.

**Don't sleep on your stomach.** This is bad not only for your back but also for your neck, says Dr. Price. Instead, sleep in the fetal position—on your side with your knees up toward your chest.

**Wrap up.** When it's cold and damp outside, cover your neck well. The weather can aggravate neck stiffness and pain, Dr. Kunkel says.

**Relax.** Just being tense can tighten the muscles in your neck and put you in pain. If you're under a lot of pressure or feel tense a lot, meditation or progressive relaxation can help. Also, audiotapes are available to teach you how to relax.

## PANEL OF ADVISORS

**Mark Gostine, M.D.,** is president of Michigan Pain Consultants, based in Grand Rapids.

**Joanne Griffin** was formerly a senior physical therapist and inpatient headache treatment therapist in the New England Center for Headache at Greenwich Hospital in Connecticut.

**Robert Kunkel, M.D.,** is a consultant in the department of neurology at the Cleveland Clinic Headache Center in Ohio. He also is president of the National Headache Foundation.

**Mitchell A. Price, D.C.,** is a chiropractor in Reading, Pennsylvania.

# NIGHT BLINDNESS
## 11 Ways to Deal with the Dark

Call it the deer-caught-in-the-headlights phenomenon. It's that frightening time of day or night when there's been an extreme change in light, drastically reducing visibility. Night blindness affects everyone to some degree, because it usually takes a moment for the retina to adjust to changes in light, explains Alan Laties, M.D.

But for some people, night blindness is more than momentary.

"Nearsighted people can at times be slower to adapt to the dark," says Dr. Laties. Other people simply *can't* see in the dark. These people have a rare condition called congenital stationary night blindness.

Unfortunately, doctors don't have a bag of ready-to-issue cures for night blindness. But if you don't see well at night and your doctor has ruled out an eye disorder, our experts offer the following practical advice for driving safely at night, when night blindness poses the biggest problem.

**Drive safely at night.** On a clear day from the driver's seat, you can usually see 1,200 to 1,500 feet down a straight road, says Quinn Brackett, Ph.D. But at night with only your headlights as your guide, you can see only 300 to 400 feet. So it's important to give yourself every advantage.

## WHEN TO CALL A DOCTOR

If you're having problems with night vision, you should have your eyes examined by an ophthalmologist, advises Alan Laties, M.D. It's the best way to protect your vision.

Occasionally, night blindness can be an early symptom of a progressive eye disease. One example is retinitis pigmentosa (RP), which affects an estimated 100,000 people in the United States, according to Jill C. Hennessey, M.S.

**Take off the shades.** Don't wear sunglasses at night or even at dusk, no matter how stylish. They will further reduce light coming into your eyes, says Dr. Brackett.

**Get a pair of night glasses.** Millions of people take advantage of glasses to improve their vision. Glasses can improve night myopia, which is defective night vision, especially of distant objects, says Creig Hoyt, M.D.

Pilots will tell you that they have more trouble seeing runways at night. To combat this problem, at night they often wear glasses with stronger prescriptions, Dr. Hoyt says. What works for a pilot trying to land a plane on a narrow strip of pavement ought to help you keep your car on the driveway and out of the front yard.

Consider wearing a stronger prescription at night or getting glasses for night driving, even if you currently don't wear glasses during the day, Dr. Hoyt says.

**Keep your headlights clean.** Dirty headlights really reduce visibility and will only make an already bad problem worse, says safety researcher Charles Zegeer.

**Plan ahead.** Careful route planning can make night driving easier and safer. When possible, says Dr. Brackett, select roads that are divided or have very little traffic.

**Slow down.** That way, you give yourself more time to react to any unexpected hazards. Increase your regular following distance by 3 to 4 seconds to allow extra stopping time.

**Expect the unexpected.** The roads don't belong just to cars, but to walkers, runners, cyclists, and wayward deer as well. It's your responsibility to watch for others sharing the road.

**Respect the rain and fog.** These two conditions make night driving especially dangerous, Zegeer says. He recommends keeping your headlights on low beam in fog for better visibility.

**Don't take chances.** If fog or travel conditions become too bad, says Zegeer, pull off at a rest area, service station, or parking lot. Stay off the shoulder of the road.

**Look to the right.** "Look at the roadway's edge to the right to help you avoid the glare of oncoming headlights," Dr. Brackett suggests.

**Leave the driving till tomorrow.** If night blindness while driving is really a problem, drive only during the day. Even good lighting conditions at night, such as those in a big city, can be troublesome to someone with night blindness.

# NOSEBLEED
## 15 Hints to Stop the Flow

Whether it's a boxer in the ring, a kid who took a ball to the nose, or an office worker who collided with a door, nosebleeds are always alarming and often painful.

Vast amounts of blood circulate through capillaries in the nose, so bleeding can be copious when blood vessels break. Nosebleeds can also occur when your mucous membranes become irritated by a cold or winter's dry indoor heat. People with high blood pressure or atherosclerosis (hardening of the arteries) are especially vulnerable to nosebleeds, as are those taking certain medications, such as anticoagulants, anti-inflammatories, and aspirin. Nose blowing, nose picking, excessive sneezing, allergies, and foreign objects in the nose can also prompt it to bleed.

Whatever the cause, you can do many things to stop most nosebleeds. Here's what the experts say.

**Blow the clot out.** Before you try to stop your nosebleed, give your nose one good, vigorous blow says Alvin Katz, M.D. That should remove any clots that are keeping the blood vessel open. A clot acts like a "wedge in the door," he explains. Blood vessels have elastic fibers. If you can get the clot out, you can get the elastic fibers to contract around that tiny opening.

## WHEN TO CALL A DOCTOR

Nosebleeds can be serious. Head for the ER if:

- You've applied pressure for 10 to 15 minutes, but your nose still bleeds.
- Your nosebleed results from a head injury. This may indicate other skull or facial injuries. Bleeding that appears thin and watery could indicate the presence of cerebral fluid.
- You have been diagnosed with atherosclerosis or high blood pressure, and your nose has bled for more than 10 minutes.
- You find yourself bleeding from the *back* of the nose.

Nosebleeds can be fatal if they go on long enough. In rare instances, continuous bleeding may indicate the presence of a growth.

Finally, if your nosebleeds become more frequent and don't seem to be associated with a cold or an irritation of the mucous membranes, schedule an appointment with your physician.

**Pinch the fleshy part of your nose.** As soon as you've blown your nose, use your thumb and forefinger to squeeze shut the soft part of the nose. Apply continuous pressure for 5 to 7 minutes. If the bleeding doesn't stop, pinch again for another 5 to 7 minutes. The bleeding should stop by the time you're through.

**Sit up straight.** If you lie down or put your head back, you'll just swallow blood, says Dr. Katz.

**Apply ice.** "Sometimes an ice pack can help quite a bit," says Christine Haycock, M.D. The cold encourages the blood vessels to narrow and reduces bleeding.

**Don't pick.** It takes 7 to 10 days to completely heal the rupture in the blood vessel that caused your nose to bleed. Bleeding stops after the clot forms, but the clot becomes a scab as healing continues. If you pick your nose during the next week and knock the scab off, you'll give yourself another nosebleed, says Jerald Principato, M.D.

**Apply an antibiotic/steroid ointment.** Applying a bit of ointment inside your nose two or three times a day will destroy any staph bacteria, says Gilbert Levitt, M.D. This stops the itching and prevents the crusting of mucus that might tempt you to pick.

**Take iron.** If you're prone to nosebleeds, consider taking a multivitamin with iron to help your body rapidly replace the blood supply, says Dr. Levitt. Iron is a vital component of hemoglobin, a key substance in red blood cells. But unless blood tests show you're anemic, you only need to get the Daily Value of 18 milligrams a day.

**Watch your aspirin intake.** Aspirin can interfere with clotting. If you're prone to nosebleeds, don't take unnecessary aspirin.

**Watch your salicylate intake, too.** John A. Henderson, M.D., advises his patients to avoid foods high in salicylates, an aspirin-like substance found in coffee, tea, most fruits, and some vegetables. Foods on that list include almonds, apples, apricots, bell peppers, berries, cherries, cloves, cucumbers, currants, grapes, mint, peaches, pickles, plums, raisins, tangelos, tomatoes, and wintergreen.

**Control your blood pressure.** People with high blood pressure are prone to nosebleeds. So follow your doctor's advice carefully and stick to a low-fat, low-cholesterol diet, says Dr. Levitt. If you have high blood pressure and a blood vessel breaks, better that it should break outside the cranial cavity than inside, which would cause a stroke. In these situations, nosebleeds are like a built-in pop-off valve.

**Get your fair share of vitamin C.** Vitamin C is necessary for the formation of collagen, a substance essential to the health of body tissue, says Dr. Henderson. The collagen in the tissues of your upper respiratory tract helps mucus stick where it's supposed to, creating a moist, protective lining for your sinuses and nose. Make sure you're getting the recommended Daily Value of 60 milligrams a day.

**Humidify the air.** When you breathe, that same moist lining in your nose works to make sure that the air that reaches your lungs is well-humidified. So it follows that when your surroundings are dry, your nose has to work harder. A cold-mist humidifier, operating when the air is dry, helps moisturize airways and tissue linings.

Dr. Katz recommends that you fill the humidifier with distilled water to protect yourself from impurities in tap water. Also, be sure to clean the unit properly, according to the manufacturer's instructions, at least once a week.

**Be careful in choosing oral contraceptives.** Estrogen influences blood supply and mucous production. Anything that changes the estrogen balance in your body—including menstruation—can make you more prone to nosebleeds. Certain oral contraceptives also alter the balance. If nosebleeds are a problem

## The Ringside Remedy

In a professional boxing match, trainers have exactly 1 minute between rounds to stop a nosebleed.

Angelo Dundee, a Florida-based trainer to 15 world champion boxers, including Muhammad Ali and Sugar Ray Leonard, has his technique down pat.

"I take a piece of cotton and make a wick out of it. I dip it into Adrenaline 1:1000 and screw it into the nasal passage. Then I put pressure on that side of the nose," Dundee says.

"If you've got bleeding on both sides, I screw a cotton wick into each nostril and tell the kid, 'Breathe from your mouth and give the blood a shot to congeal.' Then I'll take a gauze pad and squeeze hard on the dead meat right in the middle of the nose. You know, the place where the nostrils meet down at the bottom of the nose? You can press as hard as you want. It won't hurt. That seems to stop it."

Adrenaline 1:1000 is available by prescription only. Its primary ingredient is an epinephrine-like substance, which is also a component of several over-the-counter nasal products, such as Afrin and Neo-Synephrine.

and estrogen hormone is a suspect, discuss this with your doctor when you choose your birth control pill.

**Don't smoke.** Along with the 2,001 other bad things it does to the body, smoking really dries out the nasal cavity, says Mark Baldree, M.D. It can make you more prone to nosebleeds.

## PANEL OF ADVISORS

**Mark Baldree, M.D.,** is an otolaryngologist in Phoenix. He is a staff member in the division of otolaryngology in the department of surgery at Good Samaritan Hospital in Phoenix.

**Angelo Dundee,** of Weston, Florida, is a boxing trainer who has been a trainer for 15 World Heavyweight boxing champions, including Muhammad Ali and Sugar Ray Leonard.

**Christine Haycock, M.D.,** is a professor of clinical surgery at the University of Medicine and Dentistry of New Jersey/New Jersey Medical School in Newark. She maintains a private practice in Newark.

**John A. Henderson, M.D.,** is an assistant clinical professor of surgery at the University of California, San Diego, School of Medicine and an otolaryngologist and allergist in San Diego.

**Alvin Katz, M.D.,** is an otolaryngologist and surgeon director of the Manhattan Eye, Ear, Nose, and Throat Hospital in New York City. He is past president of the American Rhinologic Society.

**Gilbert Levitt, M.D.,** is a retired otolaryngologist and former clinical instructor of otolaryngology at the University of Washington School of Medicine in Seattle.

**Jerold Principato, M.D.,** is an associate clinical professor of otolaryngology in the department of surgery at George Washington University School of Medicine and Health Sciences in Washington, D.C. He is also an instructor at the American Academy of Otolaryngology and an otolaryngologist in Bethesda, Maryland.

# Oily Hair
## 16 Neutralizing Solutions

Blondes may have more fun, but they also have more oily hair. And those with silky, baby-fine hair tend to have the worst problems with oiliness.

The reason is that those with finer hair have more hair per square inch of scalp. At the base of each hair shaft are sebaceous glands, which produce sebum, the fatty "oil" in oily hair. The more hair, the more oil glands. And the more oil glands, the more oil.

Blondes with fine hair have as many as 140,000 oil glands on their scalps, according to hair-care specialist Philip Kingsley. Compare that with redheads, who average 80,000 to 90,000 hairs per head. They rarely have oily hair, he says. Brunettes typically fall somewhere in the middle.

The texture of your hair also makes a difference, says Thomas Goodman Jr., M.D. Oil wicks onto fine, straight hair very easily. Wiry hair doesn't seem to get as oily.

Intense heat and humidity can also accelerate oil production. So can hormonal changes. For instance, androgen, a male hormone, can activate the sebaceous glands. Stress boosts bloodstream levels of androgen in women as well as in men.

Because they have more androgen than women, men tend to have oilier hair. Another reason is that men tend to have finer hair than women, says Kingsley. Men average 311 hairs per square centimeter of scalp, compared with 278 for the average woman. "That's a significant 10 to 15 percent difference," he says.

Since you're stuck with the *type* of hair Mother Nature gave you (if not the color), here's what our experts advise.

**Shampoo frequently.** The most important thing you can do to combat an excessively oily scalp is to shampoo once a day, particularly if you live in a city. When summer heat and humidity stimulate your scalp's oil glands, shampooing twice a day may be advisable, says Lowell Goldsmith, M.D.

"The sebaceous glands are producing oil continuously," he says. The goal is to shampoo often enough to keep up with the secretion and remove it.

**Choose a see-through shampoo.** "Clear, see-through shampoos tend to have less goo in them," says Dr. Goodman. They clean away oil better, without leaving a residue behind.

**Give yourself a scalp massage.** This should be done right before the shampoo, never between shampoos, says Kingsley. That little bit of extra oil expressed during a scalp massage would make your hair feel even more oily.

**Double bubble.** Excessively oily hair may need to be shampooed twice, says Dr. Goldsmith. "For people with especially oily hair or scalps, I suggest a double shampoo, leaving the shampoo on the scalp for 5 minutes each time. This won't harm the hair or scalp," he says.

**Get out of condition.** If you have oily hair that tends to flatten out as the day goes on, the last thing you want to do is coat it with more oil. Try going without a conditioner, suggests Dr. Goodman.

**Just aim for the ends.** If you find you do need a conditioner, look for a product that contains the least amount of oil or one that is largely oil-free. Then, just condition the ends instead of the roots.

## Cures from the Kitchen

Your mother told you never brush your hair near food, but that doesn't mean the kitchen can't provide some home remedies for oily hair. Try these hair-care pro tips.

**Try an apple cider vinegar rinse.** Put a teaspoon of apple cider vinegar in a pint of water and use as your final rinse. This solution removes soap residue that can weigh down oily hair. And don't worry about smelling like a salad; the vinegar's aroma subsides quickly.

**Freshen up with lemon.** Squeeze the juice of two lemons into a quart of the best water you can find, says hairstylist David Daines. Distilled water is a great choice.

**Switch to beer.** "Mousse dries the hair too much and clogs the pores," says Daines. He favors fresh beer as a setting lotion for oily hair. Store it in a closed plastic container in your shower; otherwise, it will keep for only a couple of days.

**Test for oil after shampooing.** "Each amount of shampoo can only take away so much oil," says Dr. Goldsmith. "So don't skimp on the shampoo." Test yourself. After you shampoo and dry your hair, does it still feel oily? If it does, you haven't cleaned it well enough.

**Apply astringent.** You can help slow oil secretion by applying a homemade astringent directly to your scalp. Kingsley suggests applying a mixture of equal parts witch hazel and mouthwash, with cotton pads, to the scalp only. The witch hazel acts as an astringent, and the mouthwash has antiseptic properties, he says. If your scalp is very oily, use this before each shampoo.

**Dry hair in the opposite direction from which it grows.** Left on its own, oily hair tends to be limp and lank. To coax more fullness into it, be creative with your blow-drying technique, says Kingsley. Use a brush to lift the hair up at the roots, or bend forward at the waist and gently brush your hair up over the top of your head.

**Don't overbrush.** "People with oily hair have to be extra careful not to be overly vigorous with brushing," says Dr. Goldsmith. Brushing from the roots carries oil from your scalp to the ends of your hair.

**Get the right cut.** Beat the straight, matted-down hair blues by asking your stylist to cut body into your hair. "I cut from underneath, to help make the style stand up," says hairstylist David Daines. Layers are the key. If you wear your hair long and one length, the weight pulls it down, causing it to lie flat on your head.

**Learn to relax.** As described above, when you're under stress, your body produces more androgens. And androgens help boost oil production. Kingsley's advice? Relax. Experiment with different relaxation techniques, such as meditation, tai chi, and yoga, and practice the one that works best for you.

**Consider your birth control pill.** Birth control pills have a decided effect on a woman's hormone balance. That, in turn, affects oil production. Dr. Goodman suggests that you discuss excessively oily hair with your doctor when you choose an oral contraceptive.

## PANEL OF ADVISORS

**David Daines** is a professional hairstylist at Salon in New York City.

**Lowell Goldsmith, M.D.,** is a professor of dermatology and chairman of the department of dermatology at the University of Rochester School of Medicine and Dentistry in New York. He specializes in hair disorders.

**Thomas Goodman Jr., M.D.,** is a dermatologist and former assistant professor of dermatology at the University of Tennessee Health Science Center in Memphis. He is the author of *Smart Face*.

**Philip Kingsley** is a trained trichologist (hair-care specialist) who maintains salons in New York City and London. He's also the hair columnist for the style section of *The Times* of London and the author of *Hair: An Owner's Handbook*.

# OILY SKIN
## 7 Restoratives for a Shine-Free Face

Nobody's dying from oily skin, so researchers aren't exactly racing to find a cure. Sad to say, the most state-of-the-art advice experts have to offer is to keep your skin clean. No magic here.

Oily skin has many more *causes* than solutions, unfortunately. Heredity plays a big part. So do hormones. For instance, pregnant women sometimes notice an increase in skin oil as hormonal activity changes. Women taking certain types of birth control pills often do as well. Stress can cause the oil glands to kick into overdrive. The wrong cosmetics can easily aggravate an otherwise mild case of oily skin. Some of these causes are within your ability to control, but others you'll have to learn to live with.

Look on the bright side. Skin experts believe that there are some advantages to having oily skin. In the long run, they say that oily skin tends to age better and wrinkle less than dry or normal skin. Meanwhile, here are some tips for a cleaner, drier face.

**Make mine mud.** "Clay masks or mud masks are worthwhile," says Howard Donsky, M.D. Masks cleanse the skin of surface greasiness and tone the skin—for a while anyway. Realize, however, that their effects are only temporary.

Generally, the darker brown the clay or mud, the more oil it can absorb. White or rose-colored clays, though, are gentler and work best on sensitive skin.

**Splash on the hot suds.** "Hot water is a good solvent," says Hillard H. Pearlstein, M.D. For that reason, he recommends washing oily skin with very warm water and plenty of soap. This combination dissolves skin oil better than cold water and soap. "That includes the grit and grime you're trying to get rid of on your skin," he says.

**Seek out drying soaps.** "Given the state of the art in oily skin treatment, all you can really do is degrease the skin," Dr. Pearlstein says. Do that repeatedly with drying soaps and astringents.

Finding a drying soap is not a problem. (Finding one that *won't* dry the skin is actually more of a challenge.) Many dermatologists favor Ivory for oily skin, along with more specialized degreasing soaps such as Cuticura Mildly Medicated Soap, Clearasil soap, and Neutrogena Oily Skin Formula.

But there's really no reason to spend lots of money, says Kenneth Neldner, M.D. "Some people feel that soaps like Safeguard and Dial are fairly drying, and these should do the trick." The key is to use lots of soap and really scrub that skin, he says.

**Follow with astringents.** Astringents with acetone and alcohol are your best bet, says Dr. Neldner. Acetone is a great fat and grease solvent, and most astringents have a bit of acetone in them. If you use it regularly, you can surely remove oil from the skin.

Although most astringents contain alcohol, look for a brand that also contains acetones such as Seba-Nil, says Dr. Neldner.

For an effective, inexpensive astringent, you can use ordinary rubbing alcohol. For something still inexpensive but milder, try witch hazel, which contains some alcohol and also works well.

Nonalcohol astringents contain mostly water and are not as effective as those

---

## Forget the Food Connection

Although some magazines and skin-care books recommend special diets for reducing oily skin problems (usually by cutting out fried and fatty foods), our experts dismiss such things as pure fantasy and wasted effort.

"There's no relationship between diet and oily skin," says Hillard H. Pearlstein, M.D. "The condition is genetically determined, and you either have it or you don't. You can't turn off the oil glands with diet—all you can do is mop up."

Kenneth Neldner, M.D., agrees. "I don't think diet has any effect. If it does, there's nothing about it that's known to the medical community. I mean, if you have dry skin, there's nothing you can eat that will make your skin oily, so there's no reason to think it would work the opposite way for oily skin."

with alcohol and acetone, but they may help if you have sensitive skin. Worth noting: Dermatologists say that rather than washing your face several times a day, which can leave it too dry and irritated, you're better off carrying astringent pads with you and using them to cleanse the face.

**Select cosmetics with care.** "Cosmetics come in two major categories: oil-based and water-based. If you have oily skin, use only a water-based product," says Dr. Neldner.

Many cosmetics are specially formulated for oily skin. They are made to soak up and cover oiliness so that the skin doesn't look as greasy. But no cosmetic has any magical ingredient to slow or stop oil production.

**Take a powder.** Baby powder, that is. For additional shine-free protection, some women find that simple products such as Johnson's Baby Powder make a superb face powder when fluffed lightly over makeup. Another handy way to blot the shine is to use rice paper facial tissues. They're coated with a light layer of cornstarch and are easy to stow in your purse for midafternoon touch-ups.

## PANEL OF ADVISORS

**Howard Donsky, M.D.,** is a clinical instructor of dermatology at the University of Rochester and a dermatologist at the Dermatology and Cosmetic Center of Rochester in New York.

**Kenneth Neldner, M.D.,** is a professor emeritus in the department of dermatology at the Texas Tech University School of Medicine in Lubbock.

**Hillard H. Pearlstein, M.D.,** is an assistant clinical professor of dermatology at the Mount Sinai School of Medicine of New York University in New York City.

# OSTEOARTHRITIS
## 28 Ways to End the Ache

While there are no medical records to confirm when the first case of arthritis occurred, researchers have found evidence of the painful joint condition in fossilized remains of 85 million-year-old dinosaurs. Now *that's* a disease that's stood the test of time.

The most recent statistics show that arthritis afflicts more than 33 million Americans. It's actually an umbrella term for more than 100 different conditions, however. The most common type of arthritis, osteoarthritis, typically affects the fingers, knees, ankles, feet, hips, neck, and spine, causing stiffness and pain.

Osteoarthritis is usually considered just a natural sign of aging, the result of normal wear and tear on your joints. Some of the factors that influence it, like heredity, are out of your control. Others, including numerous lifestyle decisions, however, can help prevent and relieve the painful symptoms.

Here are the best remedies that our experts have to offer.

**Eat for the long haul.** Rather than focus on individual nutrients until your head starts to spin, Justus Fiechtner, M.D., recommends looking at the big picture as your best dietary approach. "Keeping your weight under control is the best thing you can do to prevent osteoarthritis," he says. "Eating a well-balanced diet is the best way to get there."

### WHEN TO CALL A DOCTOR

If arthritis pain is persistent or if you have 5 to 10 minutes or more of significant morning stiffness on any given morning, see your doctor, advises Ted Fields, M.D. Also see your doctor if you have loss of motion or swelling in a joint or if the pain stops you from activities that are important to you.

Talk to your doctor if acetaminophen or another over-the-counter pain reliever doesn't help with the pain, says Justus Fiechtner, M.D.

437

The Arthritis Foundation's suggestions for a proper diet are simple: Strive for balance and eat plenty of vegetables, fruits, and grains; take in only moderate amounts of sugar, salt, and alcohol; and limit your consumption of fat and cholesterol. The foundation also advises taking a multivitamin/mineral supplement to ensure that you get your daily requirements of necessary vitamins and minerals, especially calcium.

**Focus on fiber.** Eating high-fiber foods is important for preventing and minimizing osteoarthritis for two reasons, notes Neal Barnard, M.D. One, fiber fills you up on fewer calories, so you're less likely to overeat and gain weight. Two, fiber is the great garbage collector for your internal organs. It picks up inflammatory toxins and hormones that aggravate arthritis and carries them out, reducing your chances of experiencing osteoarthritis pain.

## Do just 1 thing

Get to your ideal weight. "Being overweight is like carrying around heavy luggage," says Neal Barnard, M.D. "It hurts the knees, hips—literally every joint in the body." It's not just the extra weight that causes arthritis problems in obese people, he says. Extra body fat causes hormonal changes and builds up levels of estrogen, and research suggests higher levels of estrogen lead to a higher risk of osteoarthritis. "The basic rule of thumb is that every extra 10 pounds increases the risk of osteoarthritis in the knees 30 percent," he says.

**Drink lots of water.** "Hydration helps prevent arthritis," says Michael Loes, M.D. Your joints need to be moist to move smoothly, just like a well-oiled machine. Dr. Loes recommends drinking 72 to 96 ounces of water every day to prevent osteoarthritis pain. If you drink lots of coffee or other caffeinated beverages, which act as diuretics and flush water out of your body, quaff even more water.

**Exercise aerobically.** Whether it's walking, riding a stationary bike, or swimming, daily aerobic exercise can help reduce stiffness and pain, preserving or improving the health of your bones and joints. If you're just getting started, Dr. Barnard recommends a half-hour walk three times a week.

**Work in some weight, or resistance, training.** Just as aerobic exercise is important, a weekly weight-training regimen is key to building strength in your muscles, bones, and joints. If your muscles aren't strong, joints tend to slip out of alignment, causing more pain for you. If you have osteoarthritis, talk to a physical therapist before beginning a weight regimen.

**Stretch.** The third critical aspect of your workout routine, stretching is important for maintaining the strength and agility of your joints. Start with gentle range-of-motion exercises. These include simply rotating your arms, legs, and trunk slowly in as full a range of motion as possible without pain. Dr. Loes recommends a Theraband stretcher, a small piece of elastic that offers resistance as you stretch various body parts. Similar products are available online and in sporting goods stores.

**Start slowly and gently.** Overexertion can make osteoarthritis pain worse. "If your exercise causes pain that lasts for more than ½ hour after you are finished, you probably did too much. Cut back and work up to an increased amount," says Dr. Loes.

If you're unsure of your limitations, rely on the trusted guidance of your doctor, who can diagnose your physical limitations, and your physical therapist, who can create a routine to keep you sufficiently challenged within those limits.

**Exercise after a hot shower.** The hot water loosens you up, says Ted Fields, M.D., so you're less likely to experience pain while exercising.

**Buy good shoes.** Walking is a great aerobic exercise to reduce your arthritis pain. If you plan on becoming a regular walker, however, Dr. Loes recommends investing in a good pair of walking shoes. Try to get comfortable, lightweight shoes that are made of breathable material, are wide enough to accommodate the ball of your foot, and have good arch support and a padded heel. He prefers Asics because of their silicone soles.

**Exercise on a soft, flat surface.** This minimizes the odds that you'll take jarring, hurtful steps that could irritate your arthritis. A smooth, grassy field or a vulcanized rubber running track, like the one at your local high school, are excellent choices.

**Make friends with water.** "In retirement communities, it's not the golfers who are the healthiest," says Dr. Loes, "it's the swimmers." Swimming tops all our experts' lists of low-impact, aerobic exercises for arthritis. Dr. Loes recommends the backstroke and sidestroke to condition the paraspinal muscles, which are the tiny nerve-rich muscles surrounding the spine. Strengthening these muscles will help ease back pain and improve mobility. Water aerobics also helps relieve and reduce arthritis pain.

If you don't have a pool at your disposal, Dr. Fiechtner says that simply stretching your arms and joints in a warm bath or shower can help, too.

**Buy a home bubbler or spa kit.** Hot tubs are a great place to do your stretching, says Dr. Fiechtner. "You can even buy bubblers and spas to put in your own bathtub if you don't have access to a hot tub," he says.

**Use Epsom salts.** Added to bathwater, these magnesium sulfate crystals provide extra-soothing comfort for arthritis pain because they help draw out carbon—one of the waste products of your body—through your skin.

**Stand up straight.** Bad posture puts a lot of pressure on your joints, causing wear and tear on your bones and cartilage—just as poor alignment in your car causes tires to wear unevenly. It also can cause a lot of extra pain for people with arthritis, says Alan Lichtbroun, M.D. So stand up straight now; it could save your knees and hips in the long run.

**Get hot or cold.** If you feel arthritis pain flaring, Dr. Fields recommends heat or ice to quell the burning. Use ice for sudden flare-ups, chronic pain, or when your joints are inflamed. And reserve the heat treatment—like a hot bath, heating pad, or a hot pack wrapped in a towel—for when you feel sore and achy.

**Rely on acetaminophen.** Safe and effective, taking acetaminophen on a daily basis is the standard recommendation for minor arthritis pain. "Tylenol is the mainstay of operation," says Dr. Fiechtner. "It doesn't work for everybody, obviously, but it seems to work well if you don't take too much of it."

"The problem with taking many over-the-counter pain relievers every day is that they increase your risk of developing stomach ulcers," says Dr. Fiechtner. He recommends acetaminophen because unlike aspirin, ibuprofen, and naproxen (Aleve), which can all cause ulcers, acetaminophen is not associated with stomach problems.

**Make friends with SAM-e.** Used as a treatment for depression in Europe, SAM-e (S-adenosylmethionine) also helps arthritis, explains Sol Grazi, M.D. "SAM-e gets into the joint and serves as a building block to make the substances a joint needs." In addition to regenerating cartilage, SAM-e also reduces inflammation. To take advantage of SAM-e's benefits, take 200 to 800 milligrams daily until your joint pain lessens, Dr. Grazi recommends.

**Try MSM.** A sulfur-containing compound found in trace amounts in food, MSM (methylsulfonylmethane) is not as well-researched as other joint remedies. It does seem to relieve arthritis pain and inflammation by increasing the effectiveness of cortisol, the body's own natural inflammation fighter, explains Stanley Jacob, M.D. He recommends taking 1,000 milligrams twice a day with food for the first 2 to 3 days. Then each week, add an additional 1,000 milligrams to your daily intake until the pain subsides. A typical dose of MSM ranges from 2,000 to 8,000 milligrams a day.

**Love your joints with ginger.** Some studies indicate that this amazing root blocks inflammation as well as anti-inflammatory drugs do (and without side effects). Steep a few slivers of fresh ginger in a tea ball in 1 cup of freshly boiled water for 10 minutes. Let it cool to sipping temperature and drink up.

**Try glucosamine and chondroitin sulfate.** With all the buzz surrounding these two supplements, you might think they're *the* definitive cure for arthritis. But the jury is still out on that decision, with some of our experts a bit skeptical over the stellar study results of these supplements. Still, the literature seems to indicate that the combination works, says Dr. Fiechtner.

Dr. Fiechtner recommends 500 milligrams of a standardized glucosamine/chondroitin sulfate supplement three times a day. (Take it four times a day if you weigh more than 200 pounds or if you currently have joint pain.) Allow at least 3 weeks to see results.

**Take a daily C supplement.** Try a daily dose of vitamin C to preserve the health of your collagen and connective tissue. Take at least 100 milligrams a day.

**Add in vitamin E.** Vitamin E furthers the work of vitamin C in preserving joint health and relieving osteoarthritis pain. Take 400 to 600 IU each day.

**Mix in magnesium.** In addition to these other nutrients, Dr. Loes recommends 60 milligrams of magnesium a day. "Aside from just helping bones, magnesium helps to ward off cramps and improves sleep," he says.

**Don't forget vitamin D.** Vitamin D tops Dr. Fields's list of useful vitamins for arthritis. He recommends a multivitamin that provides at least 400 IU of vitamin D. Low levels of this vitamin can lead directly to osteoarthritis.

**Get your omega-3s.** The anti-inflammatory effects of omega-3 fatty acids seem to play a role in reducing arthritis pain, explains Dr. Barnard. Add flaxseeds or flax oil to your diet. Try to get 2 teaspoons every day for a healthy dose of omega-3s.

**Mix them with omega-6s.** "The most recent research seems to indicate that combining omega-3s with an omega-6 fat like borage oil, black currant oil, or evening primrose oil makes it even more effective," says Dr. Barnard. Try to get 1.4 grams of gamma linolenic acid (GLA), the most helpful omega-6.

**Find a capsaicin cream.** Capsaicin, the active constituent of hot peppers, is available over the counter in a topical cream. (The most commonly available brand is Zostrix.) Smearing capsaicin cream over your joints inhibits your nerve cells' ability to transmit pain impulses, effectively wiping out arthritis pain. You can find capsaicin cream over the counter at virtually every drugstore in the United States.

## PANEL OF ADVISORS

# OSTEOPOROSIS
## 20 Ways to Preserve Bone Strength

The word *osteoporosis* means "porous bones." Comparing two sets of x-rays—one from someone with healthy bones and the other from someone with osteoporosis—makes it immediately clear why the name is appropriate.

The healthy bones appear on x-rays as a lot of white shapes because the x-rays bounce right off the bone and are not captured on film. In someone with osteoporosis, however, you'd see a lot of dark shadows because the bones are so porous that x-rays pass right through them.

In the United States, about 8 million women and 2 million men have osteoporosis. Millions more have low bone density. Weak bones break easy—so easily, in fact, that even the mildest stresses, such as coughing, bending over to tie your shoes, or lifting a sack of groceries, can cause fractures.

The scary thing about osteoporosis is that it's a "silent" disease. It develops over decades without causing pain or other symptoms. You won't even suspect there's a problem until one day you fracture a bone performing a mundane task. Once osteoporosis has progressed this far, it can't be reversed, says Melba Iris Ovalle, M.D.

## WHEN TO CALL A DOCTOR

All people age 65 or older should have a bone-density test to determine if they're at risk for osteoporosis—or if they already have it, says Robert R. Recker, M.D.

Those with one or more risk factors for osteoporosis—such as a family history of the disease, a history of alcohol or tobacco use, the use of bone-weakening medications (such as steroids or antiseizure drugs), or early menopause—should get the test as early as age 50, Dr. Recker adds.

Your doctor will probably advise you to have a test called DEXA, which measures bone density of the hip and spine. If the density is lower than it should be, your doctor may advise you to take estrogen or other medications to prevent further bone loss and add bone density.

The good news is that bone is constantly regenerated—new cells are created while older cells are taken away. There are many ways to enhance this process and restore bone while also reducing the rate at which bone is removed, including prescription medication. Whether you have osteoporosis already or you want to be sure you never get it, here are some bone-banking strategies to keep your skeleton strong.

**Eat a calcium-rich diet.** Think of calcium as the cement that makes bones strong. Even though bones are loaded with calcium, cells called osteoclasts constantly break down bone and "steal" calcium for use in other parts of the body. If you don't get enough calcium in your diet, your bones will give up the calcium for other functions in your body.

Your peak bone-building years end at age 30. After that, bones can get perilously weak, especially after menopause, when declines in estrogen levels cause women's bones to lose calcium at an accelerated rate. Get a bone-density test at the first signs of menopause. Men also go through a similar process as women with a decline in their testosterone levels, almost like a menopause, although not as dramatic. Therefore, men are also susceptible for bone loss, and screenings should begin at 50 to 60 years of age, says Dr. Ovalle.

If you're 30 years or younger, you should get 1,200 milligrams of calcium daily. From ages 30 to 50, you need 1,200 to 1,500 milligrams daily, and after age 50, you need 1,500 to 2,000 milligrams of calcium each day.

"Your body only absorbs about 30 percent of the calcium you ingest," says Dr. Ovalle. "You have to overshoot in order to actually get the calcium that your body needs. Of course, follow your doctor's recommendations for the appropriate amount of calcium needed for your age and medical situation."

Calcium is among the easiest nutrients to get in your diet, especially if you eat dairy foods, says Robert R. Recker, M.D. A glass of low-fat milk, for example, has about 300 milligrams of calcium. Yogurt and cheese also provide ample amounts. Three to four servings daily of low-fat milk or other dairy foods will provide all or most of the calcium that your bones need to be healthy.

**Choose fortified foods.** If you don't enjoy the taste of dairy foods, or if you find you have trouble digesting them, there are plenty of dairy-free calcium sources to choose from. "If you don't eat dairy, the best thing is to eat a lot of fortified foods," says Dr. Recker.

Many fortified juices and breakfast cereals contain as much calcium as a glass of milk, says Dr. Ovalle. Some breads and snack bars are also fortified with calcium.

**Load up on produce.** Salad greens, broccoli, Brussels sprouts, and other fruits and vegetables provide healthful amounts of calcium. "With green vegetables, fortified foods, and perhaps daily supplements, you can get all the calcium that you need," Dr. Ovalle says.

**Eat soy foods.** Some brands of soy foods are calcium-fortified, but that's not the only reason that soy protects the bones. Soy contains phytoestrogens, chemical compounds that act like a weaker form of the bone-protecting estrogen that women can incorporate in their diet.

"Most brands of soy milk have just as much calcium per serving as regular milk. Preliminary studies suggest the phytoestrogens in soy help increase bone density," says Dr. Ovalle.

**Supplement your diet.** The average American does not consume enough calcium every day to prevent osteoporosis. Even women who eat healthy diets may fall short on calcium because so little of this mineral is absorbed. It makes sense to make up the difference with supplements, Dr. Ovalle says.

Because your body can absorb only 500 to 600 milligrams of calcium at a time efficiently, it's a good idea to take one supplement in the morning and another in the evening, says Dr. Recker. Look for supplements containing 500 milligrams of calcium, and take them two or three times daily. Another, less expensive option is to buy a big bottle of Tums, a calcium-based antacid. If you're getting your calcium from an antacid, choose tablets that are aluminum-free. Aluminum can hinder the body's ability to get enough calcium into the bones.

**Take supplements with meals.** Calcium is absorbed most efficiently in an acidic environment, Dr. Ovalle explains. "You should take supplements with food because that's when gastric acidity rises."

**Consider citrate supplements.** All calcium supplements are equally effective, but those that contain calcium carbonate may cause stomach bloating. Supplements with calcium citrate are easier on the stomach, says Dr. Ovalle.

Also, calcium citrate supplements don't require a high-acid environment for good absorption. They're a good choice for people with ulcers or heartburn, who may be taking medications that reduce the production of stomach acid.

**Get enough vitamin D.** This nutrient is vital for bone health because it helps transport calcium from the blood into your skeleton. Fortified milk and cereals are fortified with vitamin D. It's also found in most multivitamins. "Older people don't absorb vitamin D as well as they did when they were younger, so supplementation makes sense," says Dr. Ovalle.

People 50 years and under are advised to get 400 IU vitamin D daily. After age 50, bump it up to 800 IU, Dr. Ovalle advises. Always check first with your doctor to see if this is appropriate for you to do.

**Enjoy the sun.** Millions of people avoid the sun to protect their skin, but they may be harming their bones. Every time sunshine strikes your skin, your body produces bone-protecting vitamin D. Assuming you don't use sunscreen, 20 minutes of sun exposure gives you about 200 IU vitamin D, says Dr. Ovalle. Sunscreen blocks out vitamin D production almost completely.

If you tend to avoid the sun, or if you live in a climate with a lot of overcast days, it's especially important to take a multivitamin/mineral supplement and to eat foods fortified with vitamin D.

**Make soup.** Here's an easy and unique way to get more calcium in your diet. Make a homemade stock for soup from bones. Add a little vinegar when preparing the stock. The vinegar dissolves the calcium out of the bones. One pint of this soup offers as much calcium as about a quart of milk.

**Eat less salt.** Americans get tremendous amounts of dietary sodium, and our bones may be paying the price. Salt depletes the body's calcium stores in two ways. It reduces the amount that's absorbed from foods or supplements, and it increases the amount that's excreted. "The greater your intake of sodium, the greater the loss of calcium," says Dr. Recker.

The upper limit for sodium is 2,400 milligrams daily, but less is better. It's okay to sprinkle a little salt on your food, but try to avoid processed and packaged foods, which tend to be very high in sodium. Better yet, check food labels at the grocery store, and only stock up on foods that are low-sodium or sodium-free.

**Drink alcohol in moderation.** For men, that means no more than two drinks daily; for women, one drink is the upper limit. Excessive alcohol con-

**What the Doctor Does ...**

Melba Iris Ovalle, M.D., has dedicated much of her professional career to preventing and treating osteoporosis. Her dedication doesn't stop at the office. She spends a lot of time making sure that her bones—and the bones of her husband and children—are as strong and healthy as possible.

"I keep a few light weights by the nightstand, and I lift them every morning to strengthen my upper body," she says. She also walks her three dogs every morning, which helps strengthen bones in her legs and hips.

"I make sure that everyone in the family gets enough calcium," says Dr. Ovalle. "For breakfast, we have cereal, milk, and juice. During the day, I also try to have at least one serving of dairy—yogurt, a cheese stick, or a glass of milk."

Everyone in the family takes calcium supplements, Dr. Ovalle adds, and regular exercise is always on the agenda. "Exercise and a calcium-rich diet are essential," she says. "Most people could prevent osteoporosis just by doing those simple things."

sumption decreases bone formation and reduces your body's ability to absorb calcium.

Alcohol can hurt in yet another way. People who drink heavily tend to have poor diets, which results in lower calcium intake and a greater risk of osteoporosis and fractures.

**Drink fewer soft drinks.** They contain phosphorus, a mineral that binds to calcium and reduces its ability to get into bones, says Dr. Ovalle. Another problem with soft drinks is that they often take the place of calcium-rich milk in the diet, she adds.

**If you smoke, try to quit.** On top of all the other health benefits of not smoking, here's another one: Lifelong smokers are 10 to 20 times more likely to develop osteoporosis than nonsmokers, says Dr. Recker.

**Get plenty of exercise.** It slows the rate of bone loss and can lead to an increase in bone density. Virtually any type of exercise is helpful, but the best for bone health are weight-bearing exercises, such as walking, in which you move your body against gravity, and resistance exercises, such as lifting weights, says Dr. Recker.

Exercise has other benefits as well. Because it improves muscle tone, coordination, and balance, it can dramatically reduce the risk of falls, the leading cause of fractures in the elderly, says Dr. Ovalle.

You don't have to be a hard-core athlete to build stronger bones with exercise. You don't even have to join a gym. Any activity that gets you on your feet and moving against gravity for 30 minutes four or five times a week adds significant amounts of bone to your skeleton. Add a 15-minute weight-lifting session, and your bones get even stronger.

"Start with 30 minutes three times a week, then gradually work up to five times a week," says Dr. Ovalle. "It isn't necessary to do the exercise all at once. You can spread it out—by getting 15 minutes in the morning, for example, and another 15 minutes later in the day."

What exercises are best for bones? Here are some of your options.

- Walking is a weight-bearing exercise that increases stress on bones in the legs and hips. The stress stimulates bone-building cells to create new bone, which is why women who walk regularly have greater bone density and get fewer fractures than those who are sedentary. "I've seen increases in bone density of 1 to 2 percent when people exercise along with calcium/vitamin D regimens," says Dr. Ovalle.

- Running, dancing, aerobics, and other high-impact activities are even better for bone growth than walking. If you already have osteoporosis, ask your doctor if your bones are strong enough for high-impact exercises.

- Flexing your wrists—by holding a soup can in each hand and bending your wrist toward your forearm, for example—strengthens wrist bones and reduces the risk of fractures or other injuries.

- Household activities can strengthen the bones just as much as "formal" workouts, as long as you do them vigorously. Yard work is a good choice because it involves a lot of pushing and pulling. Even cleaning the house—sweeping, vacuuming, and walking up and down stairs—helps keep bones strong.

## PANEL OF ADVISORS

**Melba Iris Ovalle, M.D.,** is medical director of the Osteoporosis Center of Evanston Northwestern Healthcare in Highland Park, Illinois.

**Robert R. Recker, M.D.,** is director of the Osteoporosis Research Center at Creighton University School of Medicine in Omaha, Nebraska.

# PET PROBLEMS
## 31 Treatments for Cats and Dogs

Anyone who has ever brought home a cuddly puppy or a rambunctious kitten knows the joy of pet ownership. And their numbers are rising. The American Pet Products Manufacturers Association found in 2001 that there were 68 million pet dogs and 73 million pet cats in the United States.

Unfortunately, loyalty and playfulness aren't the only things pets bring into the home. Along with the fun may come a variety of unpleasant surprises: putrid skunk odor and pesky fleas, to name a few. The good news is that a host of old-fashioned home remedies and safe new products can protect you and your pet from common pet problems. Here's what the experts recommend.

### Skunk Stink Solutions

Skunks are nocturnal, so chances are your pet's encounter with one of the brazen, odoriferous black-and-white critters will occur at night, when pet stores and dog-grooming parlors are closed. Even though there are a variety of commercial products that make skunk odor disappear, there are also several homemade remedies that you can use right away. For best results, try them outside (if weather permits). Also, make sure to first carefully rinse your pet's eyes with water; the skunk probably sprayed Fido's eyes for investigating something he shouldn't have. And don't let any of the remedies get into his eyes while you're washing him.

**Try a chemist's solution.** Chemist Paul Krebaum of Lisle, Illinois, first happened upon a skunk-odor cure when trying to rid his laboratory of the lingering odor of thiols: natural, bad-smelling compounds that resulted from his professional experiments. Since skunk spray also produces thiols, he tried the same solution when his neighbor's cat was sprayed, and it worked.

Krebaum's formula was published in *Chemical and Engineering News* and has since become a favorite of veterinarians and dog groomers.

Here's how to make it. Mix 1 quart of 3 percent hydrogen peroxide (the kind you find at the drugstore) with ¼ cup of baking soda and 1 teaspoon of liquid soap. If your pet is large, you can add a quart of room-temperature water.

## WHEN TO CALL A VETERINARIAN

Even though most pet owners can tell when their furry companions aren't feeling well, they can't actually tell you what's wrong. It can be difficult to distinguish between a serious illness and an innocuous ailment, since many of the symptoms can be the same.

   This medical alert guide, with advice from Amy Marder, V.M.D., tells you when a symptom is serious enough to warrant a vet's emergency care. *These symptoms could mean that your pet's life is literally on the line. Call your veterinarian immediately for advice.*

- Blood in the stool, bleeding from mouth and rectum, or vomiting and bloody diarrhea can be a sign of many things, including internal hemorrhage from poisoning.

- Copious diarrhea that comes on every half-hour or hour, with no eating or drinking in between, can cause shock.

- Difficulty in breathing, especially with blue gums, can be a sign of heart failure.

- Abdominal swelling with attempts to vomit, especially in the deep-chested dog breeds, is a symptom of bloat, "a serious emergency," Dr. Marder says, often requiring immediate surgery.

- Frequent drinking and urination, accompanied by depression, vomiting, diarrhea, and discharge of reddish mucus, 6 to 8 weeks after heat in an unspayed, intact (virgin) female dog or cat are signs of pyometra, which is a very common and very deadly uterine infection. It comes on slowly over months or years and is also marked by irregular heat periods.

- Difficulty in giving birth is an emergency. Some strain is involved in a normal birth, but if there's continuous labor without results, it could be life-threatening.

- Seizures should be reported to a vet immediately. The cause could be poisoning. Don't try to restrain the animal during convulsions.

- Itching, pain, loss of appetite, lethargy, fever, swollen joints, and/or lameness can be indicators of a tickborne disease in your pet. Prompt diagnosis and treatment with antibiotics can save your pet, so see a veterinarian as soon as possible if you notice these signs. If you live in an area where your dog comes into contact with fleas, you may want to ask your veterinarian about the Lyme vaccine for dogs. There is no vaccine for cats yet.

"Use a sponge or cloth to really work the solution into the animal's fur, especially in spots where he got sprayed," says Krebaum. Let your nose be your guide. Once the smell is gone, rinse thoroughly with room-temperature to slightly warm water.

Krebaum warns pet owners not to bottle and store the mixture. The oxygen it produces can be *explosive* if it is put in a closed container. In the open air, it's perfectly safe for you and your pet.

**Use douche on your pet's fur.** A commercial vinegar-and-water douche, such as Massengill or Summer's Eve, comes in handy at the oddest moments. The vinegar is helpful for covering up skunk odor, says veterinary technician Mary Ann Scalaro. Use rubber gloves to protect yourself from the skunk odor. Pour the douche over your pet's fur, and rub it in. Sponge it on your pet's face. Don't let the animal get wet again, because water washes out the vinegar and the smell will return.

You'll have to repeat the treatment at least once, so you'll probably need several bottles, says Scalaro.

**Reach for a juicy solution.** Tomato juice works about as well as vinegar because of its high acidity, Scalaro says. Bathe your animal in tomato juice, working the juice thoroughly through the fur. Rinse well. Repeat, if necessary, until the odor is reduced. Its drawbacks are that it's red (meaning your white cat or dog may get a dye job), and it's messy and sticky. Also, you'll need a lot of it. Still, it's better than skunk odor.

**Be prepared.** If your pet attracts skunks like, well, like a dog attracts fleas, make sure you have one or more of the commercial products created specifically for this problem on hand. Most contain enzymes and bacterial cultures that break down the substance in skunk spray responsible for the odor. They include Skunk-Off and Stinkeroo Too. "Skunk-Off works surprisingly well," says Deborah Patt, V.M.D., "and it won't hurt clothing or furniture."

A nonenzyme product is SkunkKleen by G. G. Bean, Inc. Unlike products with enzymes, it has no odor of its own and doesn't create one when it meets up with skunk smell, and it has a much longer shelf life, say its manufacturers. It's also nontoxic and safe to use, they say. Still another product is All-Purpose Elimin-Odor from Pfizer Animal Health. These products should work immediately, although they often require repeat applications. They are available at pet stores.

# Freedom from Fleas

Fleas are as prolific as they are resilient. Consider the facts. In 9 months, the time it takes to make one human baby, two fleas can generate *millions* of descendants. Adult fleas live 1 to 2 months on pets, they can survive the most frigid winters, and immature fleas can go 6 to 12 months without eating. But they're more than a simple nuisance: Fleas can cause anemia in pets and transmit disease and parasites.

Unfortunately, some products traditionally used to fight fleas are pretty unpleasant, too. The Humane Society of the United States has issued warnings about flea and tick products containing certain chemicals, called organophosphate insecticides and carbamates, based on a troubling report by the Natural Resources Defense Council (NRDC). The report asserted that these insecticides can be especially harmful to children and pets, but even adults are at risk.

Fortunately, safe and effective alternatives to organophosphate insecticides abound.

**Attack internally.** Add garlic and brewer's yeast to your pet's daily diet. Both ingredients are said to make a flea's tastebuds curl in disgust. Some pet owners swear by this, despite the lack of scientific proof.

Sprinkle a tablespoon of brewer's yeast on your pet's food each day. Dogs over 50 pounds can have up to 2 teaspoons of garlic a day. Give smaller dogs $\frac{1}{4}$ to $\frac{1}{2}$ teaspoon a day. Cats should have only $\frac{1}{8}$ teaspoon or less garlic each day for not more than 2 weeks.

**Use a natural flea fighter.** Treat your pet with natural products. At the first sign of fleas, bathe your pet with a shampoo or dip that contains d-limonene, says entomologist Fred Hink, Ph.D. This chemical is from the peel of ripe oranges and other citrus fruits. It's also used in soaps and perfumes. The FDA has even approved it for use in food products.

The shampoo is sold under the name Pet Stop. A pump spray is also available, but the shampoo or dip is easier to use, he says.

**Give an herb bath.** At the first sign of fleas, bathe your pet with a natural pet shampoo that contains flea-repellent herbs. Shampoos such as Cloud Nine and All The Best, which contain pennyroyal, eucalyptus, or certain other herbal oils, boost the bathwater's flea-killing power. Or if you're using the d-limonene shampoo, add a few drops of one of these oils to the bathwater for extra potency. Don't use the oils without diluting, since they may burn the skin. A badly flea-infested dog needs a bath about every 2 weeks; a cat, about once a month.

**Groom your pets.** Remove fleas by combing your pets regularly with special flea combs and bathe them with a pesticide-free pet shampoo. These simple steps can often be effective alternatives to powerful pesticides, says the Humane Society.

**Forget electronic warfare.** Those high-tech, expensive flea collars that produce ultrasound get a lot of attention, but "they don't work," Dr. Hink says.

"They have no effect on adult fleas. Fleas and other insects, as far as we know, simply have no receptors for those wavelengths."

**Read labels carefully.** On the advice of the Humane Society, do your best to avoid flea-killing products that contain organophosphate insecticides such as chlorpyrifos, dichlorvos, phosmet, naled, tetrachlorvinphos, diazinon, and malathion. Products with carbamates, listed as carbaryl or propoxur on labels, should also be avoided.

These chemicals lead to a buildup of acetylcholine, the body's messenger chemical, interfering with the normal functioning of the nervous system. Experts calculate that a child's exposure to an organophosphate insecticide on the day of a pet's treatment may exceed safe levels.

Small children and cats are most vulnerable to toxic effects of these pesticides, not only because of their body size but also because of their behavior. Small children crawl and play on the ground and put objects in their mouths. Your pets, especially cats, may also be at risk because they groom themselves extensively, ingesting pesticides as they lick their fur. Do not use these products on very young, pregnant, elderly, or sick pets unless directed by your veterinarian.

Some of the products containing these potentially harmful pesticides are being phased out, but many more are still finding their way onto store shelves.

**Don't use dog products on cats.** Follow the label directions carefully for any flea or tick product. A product that may be safe for dogs can kill a cat, says Marvin Samuelson, D.V.M.

**Be cautious with powders.** Flea powders you shake on the pet's fur *can* be helpful but are frequently misused, Dr. Samuelson says. The problem is in the labeling, which says to sprinkle or dust the animal. "Sprinkle" means a pinch to one person and half the can to another. If you prefer this type of flea product, talk with your vet about how much you should use based on your pet's size and needs.

**Call on Avon.** Avon's bath oil, Skin-So-Soft, has been shown to be an effective flea repellent. University of Florida researchers sponge-dipped flea-ridden dogs with a solution of 1.5 ounces of Skin-So-Soft to 1 gallon of water. A day later, flea counts had dropped 40 percent. "Fleas have a keen sense of smell," the researchers reported, speculating they don't like Skin-So-Soft's woodland fragrance.

**Consider new topical products.** Newer topical insecticides for pets were created to be less toxic to humans and animals than the old organophosphate chemicals or carbamate-based products. These include imidacloprid (Advantage) and fipronil (Frontline).

**Be clean, clean, clean.** Here's the first technique you can do for your home, not just for your pet. "In summer, wash the pet's bedding in hot, soapy water once a week and dry it in a hot dryer," says Richard Pitcairn, D.V.M., Ph.D. "Also, vacuum your rugs every 2 to 3 days. Ninety percent of fleas are found where the animal sleeps." If you're battling an infestation, make sure to throw away the vacuum cleaner bag after each use so that the flea eggs don't hatch and start the problem again.

**Use natural powders.** They contain flea-repelling herbs such as rosemary, rue, wormwood, pennyroyal, eucalyptus, or citronella, and sometimes tobacco powder. Sprinkle the powder on your carpets. You can also dust the powder in all the nooks and crannies that you can't reach by vacuuming. You can buy these powders at stores that carry natural pet products or from online suppliers. Two brands are Royal Herbal and Natural Animal. Follow manufacturer's instructions carefully. Some herbs, such as pennyroyal and tobacco powder, can be toxic in large amounts.

**Stunt their growth.** The least toxic method to flea prevention is an insect-growth regulator. One such product contains methoprene, which has the brand name Precor. "This inhibits development of the flea larvae by blocking the pupa stage," Dr. Samuelson says. "It doesn't kill existing fleas, but it stops their reproduction. It's not toxic to warm-blooded animals." Methoprene is deactivated by sunlight, so it's only good in the house, where most fleas live anyway, and in the car, where you and your pet have surely deposited them. Treat your home, especially your pet's bedding, twice a year.

Other insect-growth regulators that kill future generations of fleas include a pyriproxyfen, which is found under the name Nylar, and lufenuron. All are recommended as much safer than traditional pesticides by the National Resources Defense Council and the Humane Society of the United States, and they are found in products both for use on the pet and for household control. One product that contains Nylar and can be used for indoor cleaning is EctoKyl. Lufenuron is an ingredient in an oral pill for pets called Program.

## Tick Talk

Ticks suck blood from warm-blooded creatures. They can spread Rocky Mountain spotted fever, Lyme disease, and ehrlichiosis. The good news is that they're easier to control than fleas.

**Groom them away.** After your dog comes in from the fields or woods, go over him with a fine-toothed flea comb, says Dr. Pitcairn. This helps catch ticks that haven't attached themselves yet. Concentrate on the neck and head and in and around the ears. Ticks love to burrow there because they are warm and protected.

**Pull them out.** Clean your hands, the area around the site of the bite, and a pair of tweezers with disinfectant. Use your fingers if you wear latex gloves. Grab the tick as close to your pet's skin as possible, then pull gradually and slightly twist. If you pull slowly, you will get the head out, too. But if you don't, it's not a major concern. Leaving the head embedded may cause a minor inflammation, but it clears up rapidly, Dr. Pitcairn says. Be sure to wash your hands thoroughly after removing a tick.

## Stop Itching

You might call them hot spots, or summer eczema, but when your pet is literally mutilating himself trying to relieve itching, you need to do something about it.

"There is no such disease as summer eczema in dogs," says Donna Angarano, D.V.M. Most of the time in dogs, you're seeing flea allergy at work. It's not the flea *bite* but the flea *saliva* that's driving your pet mad. Just one flea is enough. A vet should diagnose this condition because other allergies, parasites, and illnesses can also cause "summer eczema."

**Kill the fleas.** If you know it's a flea allergy, see above. You have to go after the fleas. The allergy often worsens with age, says Dr. Angarano.

"You can't cure the allergy," adds Dr. Samuelson, "but you can remove the cause. Some studies link flea allergy to a boom-or-bust cycle. Owners let fleas get out of control, then kill them all, then lose control again." So don't let fleas run rampant in the first place.

**Treat the wound.** Clip the hair off around the hot spot, clean it with warm water, and apply an astringent to dry it out. Dr. Angarano recommends Domeboro astringent, available over the counter. Following label directions, mix the two packets of Domeboro with water. Soak a clean, dry cloth with the solution, then apply the solution once or twice a day until the area stops oozing and is healing.

**Ease the sting.** A product containing aloe vera may help soothe and dry. "Powders and ointments often make it worse," Dr. Angarano says.

**Keep it clean.** An open wound like a hot spot is a natural for a bacterial infection, so monitor it and keep it clean.

## Tame Unwelcome Mats

Laura Martin knows mats. She raises Old English sheepdogs at her Jen-Kris Kennels in North Barrington, Illinois. Here are her tips for smooth, matless fur.

**Cut vertically.** "Most people cut mats horizontally, parallel with the skin," Martin says. "Of course, that leaves a big hole. You should cut a mat vertically, moving out away from the skin from the base of the mat. That way you cut the matted hair lying horizontally, but leave the hair that's still vertical. You'll be breaking big mats into smaller ones, and you'll have nowhere near as big a hole when you're done. Use sharp-edged but blunt-tipped scissors."

**Use your fingers.** When you get down to the smaller mats, pull them apart with your fingers, Martin says. Then comb or brush them out with a metal-toothed comb or a wire pin brush.

**Loosen mats with spray.** Protein-lanolin sprays, such as Soft'n Silky and Pro-Groom, can help. Spray the product on the mat. Let it sit 10 minutes, and then cut the mat, Martin says. It will cut the procedure's time in half.

**Don't forget the paws.** If your pet gets a mat between his paws, cut the mat horizontally and remove the whole clump.

## Sticker Solutions

Most of the time, prickly stickers that get caught in your pet's fur are just an annoyance. They're a hassle to remove, and if you leave them in, they can mat fur. But sometimes they're more dangerous. Foxtails, for instance, can literally burrow their way into ears and through skin and body openings, causing severe infections, Dr. Pitcairn says. That's why removing stickers is essential.

**Comb or brush them out.** Use a metal comb with wide teeth to pull stickers out of fur before matting begins. Hold the comb against the skin to make the grooming easier.

**Use your fingers.** If there are only a few stickers or if they are in the ears or between the toes, use your fingers to pull them out. (If this job is bothersome, just think, at least they're not ticks!) If the sticker is too deep in the ear for you to see, however, don't try to remove it. You may push it right through the eardrum, Dr. Pitcairn warns. Instead, put some vegetable or mineral oil in the ear to soften the sticker and take your pet to the veterinarian as soon as possible.

## Evict Ear Mites

Pets with ear mites scratch their ears incessantly. If you look down the ear canal, you'll see dark debris, like coffee grounds. Once a dog or cat gets ear mites, they unfortunately seem prone to the problem for life.

Although prescription medication is a common method of attack, Dr. Pitcairn recommends these natural remedies.

**Try the herb mite helper.** Mix ½ ounce of almond oil and 400 IU of vitamin E in a dropper bottle, Dr. Pitcairn says. Once a day for 3 days, put a warmed dropperful or two in each ear and massage the ear well. Let your pet shake her head. Then clean out the opening with cotton swabs (don't stick the swab into the ear canal). The oily mixture smothers the mites and helps healing. Refrigerate the mixture between uses.

**Send yellow dock to the rescue.** After 3 days of almond oil treatments, let your pet's ears rest for 3 more days. Then try this approach to inhibit or kill the mites. Add 1 pint of boiling water to 1 slightly rounded teaspoon of the herb yellow dock. Cover tightly and steep for 30 minutes. Strain and let cool slightly, so the liquid is warm but not hot. Once a day for 3 days, put a warmed dropperful or two in each ear and massage the ear well. Let your pet shake her head. Then clean out the opening with cotton swabs (don't stick the swab into the ear canal). Refrigerate the mixture between uses. Let your pet's ears rest for 10 days. Then do one more 3-day yellow dock treatment as outlined above.

## PANEL OF ADVISORS

**Donna Angarano, D.V.M.,** is an associate dean and professor of dermatology at the College of Veterinary Medicine at Auburn University in Alabama.

**Fred Hink, Ph.D.,** is a professor emeritus in the department of entomology at Ohio State University in Columbus.

**Paul Krebaum** is a chemist and independent consultant in Lisle, Illinois.

**Amy Marder, V.M.D.,** is an assistant clinical professor of medicine at Tufts University School of Veterinary Medicine in Medford, Massachusetts and a veterinary behavior consultant at the New England Veterinary Behavior Associates in Lexington, Massachusetts. Dr. Marder heads the behavioral department at the Animal Rescue League of Boston. She is also former vice president of behavioral medicine at the American Society for the Prevention of Cruelty to Animals (ASPCA) and past president of the American Veterinary Society of Animal Behavior.

**Laura Martin** is a breeder of Old English sheepdogs in North Barrington, Illinois. She has been breeding and showing dogs for 20 years.

**Deborah Patt, V.M.D.,** runs a small-animal clinic, the Patt Veterinary Hospital, in Gilbertsville, Pennsylvania.

**Richard Pitcairn, D.V.M., Ph.D.,** of the Animal Natural Health Center in Eugene, Oregon, is the author of *Dr. Pitcairn's Complete Guide to Natural Health for Dogs and Cats.*

**Marvin Samuelson, D.V.M.,** is a veterinary dermatologist with Animal Dermatology and Allergy Associates in Topeka, Kansas. He is a past director of the Veterinary Teaching Hospital at Texas A&M University in College Station.

**Mary Ann Scalaro** is a former veterinary technician at the Hollis Veterinary Hospital in Hollis, New Hampshire.

# PHLEBITIS

## 13 Remedies to Keep It at Bay

If blood flowing through the veins is a peaceful river, then phlebitis is the body's equivalent of the Hoover Dam.

Those who have experienced phlebitis know it as much more: a painful, frightening affliction that can claim a victim's life without warning via a blood clot lodged in the veins of the lungs.

Phlebitis just means inflammation of the veins. It is more correctly known as thrombophlebitis. "Thrombo-" is for the blood clot that is its trademark and primary danger. Two basic types of phlebitis exist: deep vein thrombophlebitis, or DVT for short, which is the more dangerous condition, and superficial phlebitis, the more common, less serious condition that we will deal with here. Both are caused by long periods of inactivity, such as a long car trip or a lengthy bed rest. Your genes might also put you at a greater risk for developing this condition.

"Deep vein thrombophlebitis is something we're always on guard against," says Michael D. Dake, M.D., "because those people can develop a moving blood clot that would have direct access to the lungs if it broke loose and traveled through the system. DVT usually requires hospitalization and treatment with anticoagulants. The blockages that occur in superficial phlebitis, however, tend not to break loose."

### WHEN TO CALL A DOCTOR

Even the most innocent phlebitis can be the sign of a more serious ailment. Swelling or tenderness around a reddened area on your leg is something you should at least ask your physician about. If you have a history of commonly developing superficial phlebitis or varicose veins, you might also be at risk for deep vein thrombophlebitis. Finally, see your doctor if you feel any prolonged pain or swelling in your calf or thigh, and the pain is coming primarily from the back of the calf.

While it sounds disturbing, you probably don't have to stress over the tender, ropy veins of superficial phlebitis you may feel just below your skin's surface. Here are some home remedies that may help complement your doctor's care.

**Get off the Pill.** "If you've had a history of phlebitis or blood clots, you definitely shouldn't use oral contraceptives," says Jess R. Young, M.D. The incidence of deep vein thrombophlebitis in oral contraceptive users is estimated three to four times higher than in nonusers. Such a relatively high rate of deep vein clotting also puts the person with superficial phlebitis at a high risk for recurrence.

**Give it rest and warmth.** Treat superficial phlebitis by elevating the leg and applying warm, moist heat, says Dr. Dake. While it is not necessary to remain in bed, resting with the leg elevated 6 to 12 inches above the heart seems to speed healing. The inflammation of superficial phlebitis usually disappears in a week to 10 days, though it may take 3 to 6 weeks to completely subside.

## Cures from the Kitchen

High-fiber foods are important to your vein health for one simple reason—they keep you regular. If you're constipated, you tend to push too much and too frequently when you have a bowel movement, which puts extra pressure on the valves of your legs. Try to get around 30 grams of fiber a day from foods like bran cereals, oatmeal, and beans. And remember to drink extra water. Without water, adding fiber can make your constipation worse.

**Get some exercise.** "Exercise—primarily walking—tends to keep the veins emptied," says Robert Ginsburg, M.D. Keeping your legs moving when they feel fine will help improve your circulation, so it's a good way to prevent a recurrence of phlebitis. "The veins are a low-pressure system, and if the valves that keep blood from flowing backward in the legs aren't working properly, such as in varicose veins, the only way you're going to prevent blood from pooling is by walking."

**Walk when you have to ride.** Planning a long trip by car? If you've had phlebitis in the past, then make sure your wheels aren't the only things in motion. The main thing is to stop frequently and exercise, says Dr. Dake. "Don't just stop one time during the day and walk a mile, but rather, stop four or five times and walk shorter distances." Exercise prevents your circulation from becoming sluggish as a result of sitting motionless for long periods of time.

**Beware the friendly skies.** The scientific literature is littered with reports of people stricken with deep vein thrombophlebitis following long airplane flights. Nobody seems to be quite sure why this happens, although cabin pressure, lack of motion, and alcohol intake are possible culprits. The condition is so common that it's now known as economy class syndrome, because it rarely seems to strike those passengers seated in roomy, first-class seats.

"Long plane rides or car trips, or really any long period of inactivity, can increase the risk of thrombosis," says Dr. Young. But on airplanes you tend to be confined to your seat more than when traveling by car. So if you have phlebitis, get out of your seat and walk up and down the aisle every 30 minutes after taking off.

To help maintain good relations with your neighbors, he says, "It might be good to request an aisle seat."

**Know your risks.** Once you've had phlebitis, you're at increased risk of getting it again. Long periods of bed rest make you especially vulnerable. While you might not be able to prevent prolonged bed rest following an injury or serious illness, certain types of risks, such as elective surgery, can be avoided if you're prone to clotting disorders. Consult your doctor for specific risk factors, but keep in mind that getting up and around can help reduce the risks of developing phlebitis after surgery.

**Put your feet up when you're laid up.** "If you've had phlebitis and you're going to be bedridden for any length of time," says Dr. Young, "elevate the foot of the bed several inches to increase bloodflow through the veins." He also suggests that you exercise your legs as much as you can while in bed.

Try this exercise once an hour: Flex your feet, lifting your toes while keeping your heels down, as though you're pumping a piano pedal. Repeat for a minute or two.

**Wear support stockings for relief.** These stockings, available in drugstores and department stores, impede the blood's tendency to pool in the small blood vessels closest to the skin. While there's no documented evidence showing that support stockings do any good in *preventing* phlebitis, they do seem to relieve pain and make some people feel better. The best advice? Wear support stockings if you're prone to swollen legs and ankles or varicose veins.

**Investigate aspirin.** Some studies suggest that the blood-thinning properties of aspirin may help reduce phlebitis by preventing rapid clot formation in those prone to the disease. These studies advise that you take aspirin before prolonged periods of bed rest, travel, or surgery, all of which tend to make circulation sluggish and increase the possibility of clotting.

While such a simple recommendation sounds enticing, some doctors hedge on its effectiveness. "I'm not sure aspirin will be that protective against clotting," says Dr. Dake. Even if you do opt for aspirin, this is a *medical* treatment—see your doctor first.

**Try horse chestnut.** Available in tincture or capsules, this herb can really improve stressed veins by helping to strengthen and repair blood vessels that have lost their elasticity, says Mindy Green, director of education at the Herbal Research Foundation. Take 300 milligrams twice a day to relieve symptoms.

**Add vitamin E.** Another natural remedy to try is vitamin E for its mild blood-thinning action. Take doses of 400 to 800 IU daily.

**Add another reason to quit.** If you smoke and experience recurring cases of phlebitis, you should quit, says Dr. Young. "You could have a case of Buerger's disease that just hasn't moved to the arteries yet." Buerger's disease is characterized by severe pain and blood clots, usually in the legs. It is directly related to smoking, and the only cure is to give up all forms of tobacco. "Occasionally, Buerger's will start out as phlebitis," he explains. It's possible that Buerger's could be misdiagnosed as phlebitis, in which case continued smoking would be *very* hazardous to your health.

## PANEL OF ADVISORS

**Michael D. Dake, M.D.,** is an associate professor of radiology and chief of the division of cardiovascular and interventional radiology at Stanford University Medical Center.

**Robert Ginsburg, M.D.,** is the former director of the Center for Interventional Vascular Therapy at Stanford University Hospital.

**Mindy Green** is the director of education at the Herbal Research Foundation in Boulder, Colorado.

**Jess R. Young, M.D.,** is the former chairman of the department of vascular medicine at the Cleveland Clinic Foundation in Ohio.

# PHOBIAS AND FEARS
## 12 Coping Measures

"There are as many different kinds of phobias as there are different kinds of people," says phobia expert and psychologist Jerilyn Ross.

In the classic sense, a phobia is "an irrational, involuntary, inappropriate fear reaction that generally leads to an avoidance of common everyday places, objects, or situations," says Ross.

In the real sense, though, a phobia is the fear of fear itself. "A phobia is a fear of one's own impulses," says Ross. "It's a fear of having a panic attack, feeling trapped, and losing control."

Phobias are classified into three types: simple or specific phobias, social phobias, and agoraphobia. People with specific phobias experience a dread of certain objects, places, or situations. People with social phobias avoid public situations, like parties, because they're afraid they'll do something to embarrass themselves. Agoraphobics are victims of a complex phenomenon based on a fear of being in public places without a familiar person or an escape plan.

The onset of a phobia is generally unprovoked and rapid. "Usually, people who develop phobias do so in areas in which they had no previous fear," says Ross.

Increasing evidence suggests that phobias are caused by a combination of psychological and biological factors. First, they tend to run in families, sug-

## WHEN TO CALL A DOCTOR

If your phobia interferes with your life, seek professional help. Who you seek out is as crucial as seeking help itself. "It's important that you get help from someone who understands phobias," says phobia expert and psychologist Jerilyn Ross. "Many phobics end up going from doctor to doctor and hospital to hospital, so find a professional who specializes in phobias and anxiety-related disorders."

gesting some genetic basis. So if one of your parents had a phobia, you may be predisposed to one, but not necessarily the same one. More often than not, phobias strike people who have a history of separation anxiety and perfectionism.

People with phobias always recognize that their fear is inappropriate to the situation, says Ross. For example, if you're flying on an airplane during a thunderstorm, feeling fearful is a normal reaction. If, however, your boss tells you you'll have to take a business trip in a few weeks and you immediately start worrying about having a panic attack on the plane, that's inappropriate to the situation.

## Blame It on Your Ears

Just when you think that your phobia may be all in your mind, along comes Harold Levinson, M.D., who says it's not in your mind at all. It's in your inner ear.

Dr. Levinson has specialized in inner ear–determined disorders since successfully treating his dyslexic and attention-deficit hyperactivity disorder (ADHD) patients with inner ear–enhancing medications. "Not only did the learning, attention, and balance/coordination/ rhythmic symptoms improve, but so did their phobia problems," he says.

It was his unique background as both a psychiatrist and a neurologist that led him to this conclusion. "A significant number of my dyslexic and ADHD patients with inner ear problems also had phobias identical to the patients I was treating in my psychiatric practice. Psychotherapy neither explained nor helped phobic symptoms, however, whereas these medications often helped dramatically and rapidly."

After 35 years of research on more than 35,000 patients, Dr.

Levinson believes that 90 percent of all phobic behavior is a result of an underlying malfunction within the inner ear system and its supercomputer, the cerebellum.

"The sensory and motor mechanisms controlled by the inner ear are not functioning correctly," he explains. For example, balance is controlled in the inner ear. If it is not working correctly and your balance is off, you might be afraid of heights or falling or tripping. Similarly, if your eye and hand coordination is impaired, you won't be able to read and write correctly.

Dr. Levinson acknowledges that his was a minority point of view 30 years ago. But thousands of success stories are nothing to snicker at, and current independent research is substantiating his original concepts. Dr. Levinson is convinced that a trip to an ear specialist is at least worth a try for those who have phobias and related learning, concentration, and balance/coordination, and rhythmic disturbances.

Sound like something you've experienced? If so, here's some rational advice for irrational behavior from those who deal with the problem every day.

**Reverse your thinking.** In a phobic situation, negative thoughts and scary images trigger the physical symptoms of fear, explains Manual D. Zane, M.D. You should allow the fear to come, but try to shift from the negative thoughts—"That dog will bite me"—to something realistically positive like—"The dog is tightly leashed and can't get away."

**Come face-to-face with fear.** Avoiding your fear prevents you from overcoming it, says Dr. Zane. Instead, desired control can be achieved through a process called exposure treatment, in which you expose yourself to the object of your fears little by little. Gradually, you'll learn that what you imagine and expect to happen does not actually occur. Such graduated exposure also helps you get used to the object of your fear, he says.

For example, say your phobia is spiders. In exposure treatment training, you start to face your fear—usually in the presence of another person—by looking at pictures of spiders. When you learn to handle this, you may move on to looking at a dead spider, then a live spider, and you may even progress to holding one in your hand. Each time you may still feel some fear, but you learn that the awful things you dread don't actually occur.

**Pat yourself on the back.** Functioning successfully with a level of fear is a big achievement, says Dr. Zane. Dealing with it successfully is much more plausible and realistic than trying to completely erase your fear. Each encounter that you overcome in your exposure treatment training should be considered a personal victory, thus helping build your self-confidence.

**Play mind games.** "When you feel your fear taking hold, do manageable things like counting backward by 3s from 1,000, reading a book, talking aloud, or taking deep breaths," says Dr. Zane. "When you are involved with doing something manageable in the present, you reduce your involvement with fear-generating thoughts and images. Your body quiets down, and you maintain control."

**Measure your fear.** Label your fear on a scale of zero to 10, suggests Dr. Zane. You'll find that the severity of your fear is not constant, that it goes up and down. Write down thoughts or activities that make it increase and decrease. Knowing what triggers, increases, and decreases the fear may help you learn to control it.

**Look over the rainbow.** Use thoughts, fantasies, and activities that make you feel good to shift yourself away from frightening thoughts, suggests Dr. Zane. For example, think more about the high probabilities of a safe flight and the

# How to Fight a Panic Attack

"I felt like I was standing in the middle of a six-lane highway with cars coming at me from either side." That's how 26-year-old Tanis describes how it felt whenever she tried to leave her home. Tanis has the most common of all phobias, agoraphobia, a fear of being away from a safe person or place.

Just the thought of venturing outside of her Virginia home brought on a paralyzing panic attack. "One moment you feel fine, then the next moment you feel like you are about to die," she says. "Physically, my heart started beating faster, I got nauseated, and I felt shaky and as though I was about to faint." For Tanis, these were the signs of a full-blown phobia.

She did manage to leave her house for therapy, though, and that did the trick. Now she ventures out all the time, trying to help those still stuck inside. Here are some of the tactics Tanis learned in therapy that helped set her free.

**Recognize the attack.** "If a panic attack comes on, recognize it for what it is," she says. "You've had them before, so you know you're not going to die. You've gotten through it before and you can do it again. Acceptance is the key."

**Be sensitive to yourself.** People with phobias are usually perfectionists and are hard on themselves, but you shouldn't be, says Tanis. When you are going through the exposure treatment, be easy on yourself. Give yourself credit because you went through the exposure, even if it brought on an attack.

**Go slowly.** Start out slowly, but do some exposure treatment every day. Set goals for yourself, such as an 8-week goal and a 16-week goal. Once you start dealing with your phobia over and over again, it really does become conditioned. "As impossible as that may sound to a phobic, you can do things like a normal person again."

pleasures of lying on the beach in Hawaii instead of focusing on and reacting to only the unlikely dangers of the flight.

**Beware of the effects of caffeine.** "People who have repeated panic attacks may be very sensitive to caffeine," says David H. Barlow, Ph.D. "Caffeine recreates some of the symptoms they have during panic attacks, but this doesn't mean they should avoid it, since avoidance may only perpetuate the panic cycle."

As the stewardess comes walking down the aisle with the drink cart, remember that caffeine isn't limited to coffee. It's also in tea; certain soft drinks, such as colas; and chocolate.

**Burn that adrenaline.** "With panic attacks, you have an excess of adrenaline in the body, and when you move, you burn it up," says Christopher McCullough, Ph.D. Don't try to sit still and relax. You need to move to burn up the adrenaline, so walk around or exercise during the attack.

**Play muscle games.** If you can't move around, the next best thing to do is to tighten and relax various muscles in your body. "Tighten the large muscles of your thigh, then do a quick release," suggests Dr. McCullough. Then go on to the other muscles in your body. "This kind of rhythmic tensing and releasing will also burn up the adrenaline," he says.

## PANEL OF ADVISORS

**David H. Barlow, Ph.D.,** is a professor and director of the Center for Anxiety and Related Disorders at Boston University.

**Harold Levinson, M.D.,** is a psychiatrist and neurologist in Great Neck, New York. He discovered that an inner ear dysfunction was responsible for dyslexia and related learning, concentration, and phobic or anxiety disorders. He is coauthor of *Phobia Free.*

**Christopher McCullough, Ph.D.,** has a practice in San Francisco. He is the founder and former director of the San Francisco Anxiety and Phobia Recovery Center. He is coauthor of *Managing Your Anxiety* and author of *Always at Ease* and *Nobody's Victim.*

**Jerilyn Ross, M.A., L.I.C.S.W.,** is president and chief executive officer of the Anxiety Disorder Association of America, director of the Ross Center for Anxiety and Related Disorders in Washington, D.C., and coauthor of *Triumph over Fear.*

**Manuel D. Zane, M.D.,** is founder and former director of the Phobia Clinic at White Plains Hospital Medical Center in New York.

# Pizza Burn
## 6 Cooling Treatments

It's commonly called "pizza burn" or "pizza palate," but the nasty mouth burns from digging into too-hot food could just as easily be called "baked potato burns," "lasagna burns," or "coffee burns." Pizza just gets the bad rap.

Because the tissue on the roof of your mouth is only millimeters thick, any super-hot food or liquid can burn there and cause swelling and irritation. The most common culprit is, of course, pizza.

"It's a common problem, but it still can be quite painful," says Van B. Haywood, D.M.D. "Like a skinned knee, it's going to take some time to heal, whether you treat it or not."

Here are some wise things to do the next time you singe the roof of your mouth.

**Apply some ice.** Putting an ice cube in your mouth right away brings down the temperature, eases the pain of the burn, and helps control the swelling, says Kimberly Harms, D.D.S., much like plunging your hands into cold water after burning them. Just pop a piece of ice into your mouth and suck.

**Reach for some Häagen-Dazs.** We know, this remedy is going to be pretty tough to take! If keeping an ice cube in your mouth is too irritating, then a few

### WHEN TO CALL A DOCTOR

A pizza burn will completely heal on its own in a week to 10 days. But, if you have a lesion, bump, or scratch, painful or not, that does not disappear within 2 weeks, then it's time to see your dentist, because you could have a much more serious problem.

"Sometimes what we think is discomfort caused by pizza burn can be a cancerous lesion," says Van B. Haywood, D.M.D. The discomfort of both can feel the same in the beginning, but will last much longer with a lesion.

scoops of ice cream can help put out the fire on the roof of your mouth, says Dr. Haywood. Not in the mood for butter pecan? Try a milkshake instead.

**Gargle with salt water.** Rinsing your mouth with a warm salt-water rinse—½ teaspoon of table salt mixed in an 8-ounce glass of warm water—cleanses the area and helps heal the burn, says John J. Caimi, D.M.D.

**March to the nearest drugstore.** Apply an over-the-counter topical anesthetic such as Orabase (other brands are just as effective) directly to the burn to help protect the wound, soothe the pain, and speed the healing process, suggests Dr. Harms.

**Avoid crunchy and hot foods.** Change your eating habits for a few days, suggests Dr. Haywood. "You'll want to stay away from Tabasco sauce and limit your intake of spicy foods for a few days after suffering a pizza burn," he says. "Those types of foods will aggravate the burn and cause you more pain."

Also avoid crunchy foods with sharp edges like potato chips and pretzels, which can aggravate the lesion, says Dr. Caimi. And, maybe you should strike pizza from your dietary list for a week or so. Sticking with a bland diet while the thermal irritation heals is a must.

"Most people will eat bland and soft foods for a couple days after this happens—without even thinking about it," says Dr. Haywood.

**Learn from your burn.** Next time, take more care when you order pizza, slurp drive-thru hot coffee, or munch on just-microwaved food. The latter is important since microwaved foods often cook unevenly, so the outside and inside may have different temperatures—and potentially cause pizza palate.

"There's usually a lesson in the mistake," says Dr. Haywood. "Let the pizza or other hot food cool for a minute or so before you take your first bite."

## PANEL OF ADVISORS

**John J. Caimi, D.M.D.,** is a dentist in Ridgway, Pennsylvania. He has been in practice for more than 23 years.

**Kimberly Harms, D.D.S.,** is a dentist in Farmington, Minnesota, and a consumer advisor for the American Dental Association.

**Van B. Haywood, D.M.D.,** is a professor at the Medical College of the Georgia School of Dentistry in Augusta.

# POISON PLANT RASHES
## 18 Itch Relievers

Question: What's the most common allergy in the country?

The answer, surprisingly enough, is poison ivy, oak, and sumac allergy. About 85 percent of people are susceptible to becoming allergic to this trio. Though it may take a day to develop, the symptoms are unmistakable. The red rash and unceasing itchiness can make a case of poison plant rash positively unbearable. The irony is that most people don't even know that these symptoms signify an allergy.

---

## Urushiol Oil: Evil and Persistent

Urushiol oil, the active ingredient in poison ivy, poison oak, and poison sumac, is one of the most potent external toxins we know, says William L. Epstein, M.D. "The amount needed to cause a rash in very sensitive people is measured in nanograms, and it could take as little as 1 nanogram. But most sensitive people will react in the 100-nanogram range." Consider that a nanogram is a mere *billionth* of a gram; that means it would take less than ¼ *ounce* of urushiol to cause a rash in every person on earth. Five hundred people could itch from the amount covering the head of a pin.

James A. Duke, Ph.D., whose interest in "this evil plant" was sparked by "an early application of poison oak as a substitute for toilet paper," says that its well-known itch is not the only problem; its long life can fool you, too. Specimens of poison ivy several centuries old have caused dermatitis in sensitive people, says Dr. Duke.

"When the Japanese restored the gold leaf on the golden Temple in Kyoto, they painted urushiol lacquer on it to preserve and maintain the gold," Dr. Epstein says. "The main message for tourists there is, 'Don't try to steal the gold.'" You'll be caught red-handed. Literally.

## WHEN TO CALL A DOCTOR

About 15 percent of the 120 million Americans who are allergic to poison plants are so highly sensitive that they break out in a rash and begin to swell in 4 to 12 hours instead of the normal 24 to 48. Their eyes may swell shut and blisters may erupt on their skin.

"This is one of the few true emergencies in dermatology," says William L. Epstein, M.D. "Get to a hospital as soon as possible. A shot of corticosteroids will bring the swelling down."

The nagging itch and telltale red rash are caused by the toxin urushiol oil, found in poison ivy, poison oak, and poison sumac. Some people are more sensitive to it than others. A few lucky people are not sensitive to it at all—they can literally roll in the stuff and not get a reaction. But our experts don't advise it. Sensitivity to urushiol can develop at any time.

If you've been messing around in a poison patch, you'll soon know whether you're immune or not. But as ugly as the rash looks, it's the itch that'll do you in. Here's what you can do about it.

**Know your enemy.** Ideally, avoid getting a poison plant rash in the first place. You can try to avoid poison ivy, poison oak, and poison sumac simply by steering clear—if you know what it looks like.

Poison ivy plants have clusters of three shiny leaves, the source of the saying "Leaves of three, let it be." It can grow as a vine or as a shrub, but it always has hair on its trunk. Poison ivy is found throughout most of the country.

Poison oak can be a high-climbing vine or a shrub. Its notched leaves look like those of the common white oak tree. Its berries grow in clusters and are green in summer and off-white in winter. Poison oak grows mostly in the western and southeastern states.

Poison sumac stems each have 7 to 13 leaflets. Poison sumac grows as a tall shrub, sporting green berries in summer that turn yellow-white in winter. It can be found in the northern part of the country and sometimes in the Deep South, too.

Even in winter, when there are no leaves, the poison lurks in roots and stems, waiting to pounce. So you must be on guard for these poison plants all year around.

**Block that ivy.** If you know you're going to be around poison ivy, like when you're about to clear it out of your yard, prepare yourself first. IvyBlock is a lotion that actually prevents urushiol from penetrating your skin. The lotion also leaves a slightly visible film on the skin so that you can see exactly where you're protected. IvyBlock and similar products are available at drugstores.

**Wash up.** If, despite your best efforts, you've been exposed, pour rubbing alcohol over your skin immediately. The alcohol removes the urushiol oil from your skin, says William L. Epstein, M.D. Don't use a washcloth, however, to apply the alcohol, because it just picks up the urushiol oil and spreads it around.

However, if you steer clear of poisonous plants and are confident you've not been exposed, it's a good idea to avoid using alcohol-based skin cleansers *during* your hike or picnic because alcohol will remove the layer of oil your skin creates to protect itself, and any exposure you might get later in the day would be worse.

**Rinse well.** "Water inactivates urushiol," Dr. Epstein says. Soap is unnecessary. But after being exposed, you must douse yourself *immediately* with water from your hose or canteen or the next stream. "The best possible treatment is alcohol followed by water," he says. Again, don't use a washcloth.

**Use what you have.** If you don't have rubbing alcohol at your disposal, opt for several premoistened towelettes (like baby wipes) if you have them. If you have a cooler handy, rub ice on the affected area.

**Wash everything.** That means everything that may have come in contact with the poisonous plant: your clothes, your dog, your backpack. One patient who drove home after handling poison oak kept picking it up for weeks from the steering wheel of his car, says Dr. Epstein.

**Pop a pill.** A few hours to a few days after exposure to the poisonous plants, the rash develops, along with

## Do just 1 thing

Use calamine lotion. The time-honored mainstay in poison treatment is calamine lotion, a popular skin protectant with a cooling, soothing action that distracts your skin from the itching sensation, says Robert Rietschel, M.D.

With poison ivy, poison oak, and poison sumac, the blood vessels develop gaps that leak fluid through the skin, causing blistering and oozing, he explains. "When you cool the skin, the vessels constrict and don't leak as much," he says.

Most calamine lotions contain only about 5 percent calamine, which is actually a form of crystallized zinc. As the lotion dries on your skin, it leaves a powdery residue that absorbs the oozing, develops a crust, and keeps your skin from sticking to your clothes, Dr. Rietschel notes. He suggests applying calamine lotion three or four times a day. To keep your rash from getting too dry and making the itch even worse, stop using calamine when the oozing stops, he says.

its maddening itch. Oral antihistamines are high on Robert Rietschel, M.D.'s, list of poison plant rash remedies. There are two over-the-counter brands to choose from: Chlor-Trimeton, which contains the active ingredient chlorpheniramine maleate, and Benadryl, which contains the active ingredient diphenhydramine hydrochloride. "You even could take your hay fever medicine if it happens to be an antihistamine," he adds.

**Try other drying agents.** "Although not as popular and soothing as calamine, there are other skin soothers that can be just as effective. Some of them, however, often have a lot of alcohol and tend to sting," Dr. Rietschel warns. Use them as you would calamine—that is, until the oozing stops. Otherwise you can get the rash too dry, and it will crack and cause more itching. Zinc oxide, witch hazel, baking soda, and Burow's solution (aluminum acetate), which is sold under brands like Domeboro, all work well.

**Cover with a compress.** Put a cotton cloth soaked in cool water over the rash and let a fan blow over it, Dr. Rietschel advises. The cooling and evaporating effect works the same as calamine lotion, although there's no residue to soak up the oozing.

**Irritate it to distraction.** "Counterirritants like menthol and phenol confuse the nerve endings in the skin and provide a cooling sensation," Dr. Rietschel says. "But they can sting and sometimes aren't sufficient to give you the relief you need." Menthol and phenol are available in anti-itch creams.

**Counterattack with cortisone.** Over-the-counter cortisone creams are too weak and "are absolutely worthless in knocking out a significant rash," Dr. Rietschel says. "But they can relieve minimal itching." Start using them about 2 weeks into the rash, when it's healing, scaling, and itching.

**Try an oatmeal onslaught.** Colloidal oatmeal dries up oozing blisters. Aveeno is the most popular commercial preparation for skin care and

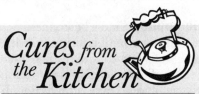

## Cures from the Kitchen

If you don't have an Aveeno oatmeal product readily at your disposal, regular oatmeal can work just as well. Make some soupy oatmeal and allow it to cool. Then scoop the mixture into an old sock and strain out the liquid. You can use this sock as a compress to apply to the rash for 10 minutes every 2 hours.

If you don't want to use your good socks, just strain the oatmeal mixture and smear the liquid over your rash five times a day. Do this until the symptoms subside.

comes with easy-to-follow instructions. Apply it with a cloth to the blisters, or use it in the bath.

**Find relief with jewels.** The most popular herbal treatment is jewelweed, also known as impatiens or touch-me-not. You slit the stem and put the juice on the rash. James A. Duke, Ph.D., says he uses jewelweed to stop the rash from developing. "I ball up the whole plant and make sort of a washrag out of it and wipe the poison sap off," he says. Jewelweed is fairly easy to find in the wild, if you know what to look for. The orange species blooms from June through September in moist, shaded areas. You may have difficulty finding jewelweed in health food stores. To order a 4-ounce bottle of the lotion, send a letter to Rainbow's End Herbals, 514 Gidsville Road, Amherst, VA 24521, or find the product online. Slather it on skin to soothe the itching.

**Try some other herbs.** Herbalists recommend washing the infected area with a grindelia tincture to soothe itching. Also, an echinacea wash helps fight inflammation in the blistered, irritated skin. Mix 1 part echinacea tincture with 3 parts water and then rinse the infected areas with the mixture several times a day.

**Get muddy.** Find a bentonite clay "mud pack" at a health food store, and mix it with water until it forms a thick goo. Spread it over the infected skin to dry up blisters and control the itch, then remove it when it wears off or gets itchy.

For added relief, add $\frac{1}{4}$ to $\frac{1}{2}$ teaspoon of powdered Oregon grape root to the clay poultice to fight off infection. If the rash feels hot, add a drop of lavender essential oil to produce a cooling effect.

**Don't get burned.** Don't try to rid your yard of urushiol by burning plants—urushiol takes to the air in a fire. You can inhale droplets of the oil and come down with serious lung infections, fever, and a body-wide rash.

## PANEL OF ADVISORS

**James A. Duke, Ph.D.,** teaches herbal healing at the Tai Sophia Institute in Columbia, Maryland. He is a retired economic botanist for the Agricultural Research Service of the USDA.

**William L. Epstein, M.D.,** is a professor emeritus of dermatology at the University of California, San Francisco, School of Medicine.

**Robert Rietschel, M.D.,** is a staff dermatologist at the Ochsner Clinic in New Orleans and clinical professor of dermatology at the Louisiana State University School of Medicine and Tulane University Medical Center in New Orleans.

**Varro E. Tyler, Ph.D.,** was a professor of pharmacognosy at Purdue University in West Lafayette, Indiana, and the author of *The Honest Herbal*. He also served as a *Prevention* magazine advisor.

# PREMENSTRUAL SYNDROME
## 29 Ways to Treat the Symptoms

Think of it as biological warfare, its battles played out on the fields of a woman's body and mind. Once a month, about 2 weeks before she begins to menstruate, the opposing armies—estrogen and progesterone—begin to amass. These female hormones, which regulate the menstrual cycle and affect a woman's central nervous system, normally work in tandem. It's only when one tries to outdo the other that trouble looms.

Some women escape the conflict altogether, their hormones striking a peaceful balance before a single sword is drawn. Others are less fortunate. For one woman, estrogen levels may soar, leaving her feeling anxious and irritable. In another, progesterone predominates, dragging her into depression and fatigue.

The battles can rage for days. You may feel bloated and gain weight, have a headache, backache, acne, allergies, or terrible breast tenderness. You may crave ice cream and potato chips. Your mood may shift without reason, swinging from euphoria to depression. Then, suddenly, the troops clear out and peace of mind returns—just as your period begins.

Premenstrual syndrome, or PMS, is believed to affect to varying degrees between one-third and one-half of all American women between the ages of 20 and 50, says Susan Lark, M.D.

## WHEN TO CALL A DOCTOR

The symptoms of premenstrual syndrome rarely call for medical intervention, but drastic circumstances demand drastic measures. If you've tried almost everything here and nothing seems to help, see your doctor about a prescription medication. In addition, if the symptoms of PMS are seriously affecting your health and other daily activities, see your doctor as soon as possible. Oral contraceptives and antidepressants may be appropriate treatment methods if nothing else can reduce your PMS symptoms.

Certain factors, such as bearing several children or being married, seem to increase the risk of PMS, says Guy Abraham, M.D., who has conducted extensive investigation into the disorder. (PMS is a major cause of divorce, he notes.)

The problem may have a genetic basis, says Edward Portman, M.D.

Not all women with PMS have the same symptoms and the same intensity of discomfort, says Dr. Abraham. Nor do all respond to the same treatments. Finding the best way to handle your PMS may require some trial and error. From the doctors who have worked most extensively with PMS come these recommendations.

**Don't worry, be happy.** A positive, confident attitude can help you cope and maybe even prevent future episodes of PMS, says Dr. Lark. If you feel PMS getting the best of you, she suggests reciting some positive affirmations. Sit in a comfortable position and repeat the following two or three times: "My body is strong and healthy. My estrogen and progesterone levels are perfectly regulated. I handle stress easily and competently."

## Do just 1 thing

Exercise. Experts agree that it may be your best PMS prescription. Moderate exercise increases your bloodflow, relaxes your muscles, and fights fluid retention, says Susan Lark, M.D.

What's more, says Edward Portman, M.D., exercise increases your brain's production of endorphins, natural opiates that make you feel better all over.

Walk at a fast pace in fresh air, swim, jog, take up ballet or karate–do something you enjoy on a daily basis, Dr. Portman suggests.

For best results, increase your level of activity for the week or two before PMS symptoms set in, says Dr. Lark.

**Destress your environment.** Women with PMS seem to be particularly sensitive to environmental stress, says Dr. Lark. Surrounding yourself with soothing colors and soft music can contribute to greater calm at this and other times of the month.

**Breathe deeply.** Shallow breathing, which many of us do unconsciously, decreases your energy level and leaves you feeling tense, making PMS feel even worse, says Dr. Lark. Practice inhaling and exhaling slowly and deeply.

**Sink into a tub.** Indulge yourself in a mineral bath to relax muscles from head to toe, Dr. Lark suggests. Add 1 cup of sea salt and 1 cup of baking soda to warm bathwater. Soak for 20 minutes.

**Be chaste.** Consider adding chasteberry to your arsenal of PMS treatments. Most experts recommend it as the top herbal remedy for PMS symptoms. Find it in a tea, tincture, or other preparation at a health food store. Drink a cup of chasteberry tea, or take 5 to 15 drops of tincture, mixed with a few ounces of water three times a day.

**Rely on rosemary.** According to herbal experts, certain compounds in rosemary may bring hormone levels into balance and reduce symptoms. To make

## Help from the Supplement Aisle

A number of vitamins, minerals, and even amino acids may help relieve PMS symptoms, some doctors say. Here's the lowdown on nutritional solutions.

**Vitamin B$_6$.** Research into vitamin B$_6$ and PMS has shown that increasing your intake of the nutrient can help alleviate symptoms such as mood swings, fluid retention, breast tenderness, bloating, sugar cravings, and fatigue, says Susan Lark, M.D. But, she cautions, don't experiment with the vitamin on your own. B$_6$ is toxic in high doses. Your doctor should supervise any vitamin therapy, including those mentioned below.

**Vitamins A and D.** These two vitamins work in tandem to improve the health of your skin. Because of their importance to the skin, they may play a part in suppressing premenstrual acne and oily skin, according to Dr. Lark.

**Vitamin C.** An antioxidant, vitamin C is believed to play a role in reducing stress. It may help relieve the stress felt during PMS, says Dr. Lark. And there's more. Vitamin C is also a natural antihistamine, says

Dr. Lark, and can help women whose allergies worsen before a period.

**Vitamin E.** Another antioxidant, vitamin E may have a powerful effect on the hormonal system, helping to relieve painful breast symptoms, anxiety, and depression, says Guy Abraham, M.D.

**Calcium and magnesium.** These two minerals work together to fight PMS, says Dr. Lark. Calcium helps prevent premenstrual cramps and pain, while magnesium helps the body absorb the calcium. She also believes that magnesium helps control premenstrual food cravings and stabilizes moods.

**L-tyrosine.** This amino acid is required for your brain's production of the chemical dopamine, your own natural antidepressant. Edward Portman, M.D., found that it helps some of his patients relieve the anxiety and depression associated with PMS.

**The PMS pill.** Your best bet for treating PMS with nutritional supplements is to take a balanced supplement every day, says Dr. Lark. Your drugstore may even sell products specially formulated for PMS symptoms.

rosemary tea, bring 1 cup of water to a boil and pour it over 1 teaspoon of dried rosemary leaves. Cover and steep for 10 to 15 minutes, then drink warm. During the week you expect your period, drink a cup before lunch and a cup before dinner for 3 days.

**Try a little romance.** The aching muscles and sluggish circulation that often accompany PMS can be relieved by having sex and reaching orgasm, says Dr. Lark. The stimulation helps move blood and other fluids away from congested organs.

**Get an advance from your sleep bank.** If insomnia is part of your PMS, prepare for it by going to bed a few hours earlier for a few days before PMS sets in, says Dr. Lark. It may help alleviate the tiredness and irritability that go hand in hand with insomnia.

**Stick to a schedule.** Set reasonable goals and schedules for each PMS day to avoid feeling overwhelmed, even if this means cutting back your routine, Dr. Lark suggests.

**Save social obligations for another time.** Postpone big plans, like holding a dinner party, until you feel you can handle it better. It'll only further frazzle an already-frazzled situation, says Dr. Lark.

**Don't hide the truth.** Talking about your PMS problems with your spouse, friends, or coworkers does help, says Dr. Lark. You may even find a PMS self-help group where you can share your experiences with others who have PMS. To find one in your area, ask your doctor or call a local women's medical center.

**Eat a little a lot.** Poor nutrition doesn't cause PMS, says Dr. Portman, but certain dietary factors can accentuate the problem. Several physicians recommend a hypoglycemic diet—small meals low in sugar several times a day—to help keep your body and psyche in better balance.

**Avoid empty calories.** Stay away from low-nutrient foods like soft drinks and sweets containing refined sugar, says Dr. Abraham. Giving in to a craving for sweets only makes you feel worse by contributing to anxiety and mood swings.

Try fresh fruit as a substitute, suggests Dr. Lark.

**Decrease dairy.** Eat no more than one or two portions per day of fat-free or low-fat milk, cottage cheese, or yogurt, Dr. Abraham says. Reason: The lactose in dairy products can block your body's absorption of the mineral magnesium, which helps regulate estrogen levels and increases its excretion.

**Restrict salt.** "Go on a low-sodium diet for 7 to 10 days before the onset of your period to offset water retention," suggests Penny Wise Budoff, M.D. "This means no restaurants, processed foods, Chinese food, commercial soup, or bottled salad dressing."

**Fill up with fiber.** Fiber helps your body clear out excess estrogens, says Dr. Abraham. Eat plenty of vegetables, beans, and whole grains.

Millet, buckwheat, and barley are high not only in fiber but also magnesium, adds Dr. Lark.

**Cut the caffeine habit.** Consume very limited quantities of coffee, tea, chocolate, and other caffeine-containing substances, says Dr. Abraham. Caffeine has been shown to contribute to painful breast tenderness, anxiety, and irritability.

---

## Those Crazy Cravings

Did you top off dinner tonight with a giant-size chocolate bar or a quart of ice cream? Don't put yourself down, especially if your menstrual period is around the corner. Chances are, your hormones made you do it.

"A woman doesn't overeat at this time of the month because of a weakness of character. Research shows that she's almost driven to it by the reaction of progesterone on her brain," says Peter Vash, M.D. What happens, researchers theorize, is that the high levels of progesterone released by the ovaries around the midpoint of a woman's menstrual cycle seem to affect those areas of the brain responsible for carbohydrate cravings.

As disturbing as the tendency is, it may actually be a primitive protective mechanism built into a woman's biology, Dr. Vash says. "When a woman is about to have her period,

she's going to lose a lot of fluid. Eating high-carbohydrate foods like potato chips and ice cream will cause her to retain fluid and also give her additional energy." Cravings for chocolate—a common pre-period occurrence—may result because of the brain's need for amino acids contained in that substance, he says.

Try to manage your cravings, says Dr. Vash, because giving in to them can make you feel worse. Here's how to steel yourself against the junk food.

**Be prepared.** "Know the cravings will occur for 7 to 10 days a month and mark your calendar," says Dr. Vash. "And know that they will stop, too. There's a limit. You can rise above them."

**Put up a fight.** Get adequate sleep, drink lots of fluids, and eat fruits and vegetables when your body asks for sweets and starches.

**Abstain from alcohol.** The depression that often accompanies PMS will be accentuated by alcohol, says Dr. Portman.

Alcohol can also worsen PMS headaches and fatigue and cause sugar cravings, says Dr. Lark.

**Say no to diuretics.** As a temporary antibloating measure, many women with PMS take diuretics, says Dr. Lark. But some over-the-counter diuretics draw valuable minerals out of your system along with water. A better approach is to stay away from substances like salt and alcohol that cause you to retain water in the first place.

## PANEL OF ADVISORS

**Guy Abraham, M.D.,** is a former professor of obstetrics and gynecologic endocrinology at the UCLA School of Medicine in Los Angeles and has conducted extensive research on PMS.

**Penny Wise Budoff, M.D.,** founded the Women's Medical Center in Bethpage, New York, and is author of *No More Hot Flashes and Even More Good News* and other related books.

**Susan Lark, M.D.,** is director of the PMS Self-Help Center in Los Altos, California, and author of *Dr. Susan Lark's Premenstrual Syndrome Self-Help Book.*

**Edward Portman, M.D.,** is a PMS consultant and researcher and was formerly the director of the Portman Clinic in Madison, Wisconsin.

**Peter Vash, M.D.,** is executive director of the Lindora Medical Clinic in Costa Mesa, California. He is also an endocrinologist and internist on the clinical faculty of the UCLA Medical Center in Los Angeles and a specialist in eating disorders.

# PROSTATE PROBLEMS
## 22 Gland Helpers

Call it nature's most irksome urge: frequent nighttime urination. It's a common complaint among men over 50, roughly half of whom have enlarged prostates to varying degrees, as do an estimated 80 percent of those age 80 and above.

Why are so many men plagued by prostate problems? The answer lies in the male anatomy. The prostate–the gland responsible for producing most of the fluids in semen–is situated directly beneath the bladder. Roughly the size of a pea at birth, it begins growing rapidly during puberty, when testosterone levels rise. In adults, it takes on the size and shape of a walnut. When a man hits his midforties, his prostate often begins to grow again, probably due to changes in hormone levels. The result? A condition called benign prostatic hyperplasia, or BPH, the technical term for enlarged prostate.

About one-half of men with BPH don't experience any overt symptoms. In others, the prostate presses up against the urethra, the tube through which urine passes out of the body. This creates a host of urinary difficulties, including frequency, urgency, reduction in flow, difficulty starting urination, discomfort when urinating, and a feeling that the bladder is not completely empty.

BPH isn't the only ailment that strikes the prostate. At one time or another, roughly 50 percent of all men develop prostatitis, a condition in which the prostate gland becomes inflamed. Prostatitis is a term given to three separate conditions. One, acute bacterial prostatitis, is a serious infection. (See "When to Call a Doctor" on page 480.) The second, chronic bacterial prostatitis, is a persistent low-grade infection with intermittent urinary symptoms, similar to those of BPH, along with pain after ejaculation, lower-back pain, and, possibly, semen tinged with blood. Antibiotics are usually needed to treat the infection. The third is a similar condition with identical symptoms, although no bacteria are present. Named chronic nonbacterial prostatitis, it is the most common form, although doctors aren't sure what causes it.

A proper diagnosis is critical for both BPH and prostatitis, since symptoms can mimic those of prostate cancer, and, in some cases, prescription drugs and even surgery may be warranted. Once you've been diagnosed, though, there's

## WHEN TO CALL A DOCTOR

Two prostate-related problems require immediate treatment: acute bacterial prostatitis and urinary retention. "If someone has acute prostatitis, he really needs medical attention because he can get very sick," cautions Martin K. Gelbard, M.D. "Fortunately, it's uncommon—but it's fairly dangerous." Acute prostatitis occurs when bacteria from the urethra travels to the prostate, creating an infection that must be treated with antibiotics. Unlike other forms of prostatitis, it comes on quickly, producing these severe symptoms:

● Fever, chills and flulike symptoms

● Pain in the prostate gland, scrotum, or lower back

● Urinary frequency and blood-tinged urine

● Painful ejaculation

Urinary retention is a complication associated with benign prostatic hyperplasia (BPH) and, rarely, prostatitis. It occurs when the gland enlarges to the point where it blocks the flow of urine, potentially damaging the kidneys. If you notice a diminished flow, are unable to completely empty your bladder, or have a continuous urge to urinate but can only produce a small trickle of urine, call your doctor immediately.

much you can do at home to treat both conditions. Here's what the experts recommend.

**Harvest the power of saw palmetto.** The berry extract of this southeastern United States palm tree is widely used to treat BPH. In 1998, scientists wondered if its reputation was warranted. They examined 18 clinical studies and concluded that saw palmetto yielded improvements similar to those produced by finisteride, a commonly prescribed testosterone-lowering drug, but with fewer side effects. Among the benefits are stronger urinary flow, fewer nighttime trips to the bathroom, less urine held in the bladder following urination, and less urinary frequency.

Why does it work? "The mechanism is not known yet," says Winston Craig, R.D., Ph.D. But it may be the phytosterols contained in saw palmetto—compounds similar to cholesterol, found in plants and thought to impart various health benefits, including aiding urinary difficulties. What's more, it appears to affect dihydrotestosterone, or DHT, a metabolite of the hormone testosterone. "High levels of DHT are associated with an enlarged prostate," explains Dr. Craig. Compounds in saw palmetto inhibit the production of DHT, and reducing DHT's growth-promoting effects eases urinary symptoms and increases urine flow, he notes.

Because saw palmetto is such an effective herbal remedy for this condition, you should consult your doctor for proper diagnosis and monitoring before using it to treat an enlarged prostate. Two to three 500-milligram capsules per day of saw palmetto extract should deliver improvement in 1 to 3 months.

**Try African pygeum.** Used extensively in Europe for the treatment of BPH, several studies find this fruit of an African evergreen tree effective, possibly because it diminishes inflammation. "The active extract seems to reduce symptoms of frequent nighttime urination and difficulty urinating," says Dr. Craig. Although African pygeum appears to be a safe herb, you should consult your doctor for proper diagnosis and monitoring before using it to treat a serious condition such as enlarged prostate. The standard dosage is usually 100 to 200 milligrams per day in capsule form.

**Rx with nettle root.** Nettle root extract appears to have steroidal and anti-inflammatory properties that benefit men with BPH, says Dr. Craig. Take up to six 300-milligram capsules per day, or take it in a combination supplement with saw palmetto.

**Think about zinc.** "Zinc is a high priority for natural therapy of the prostate gland," says Willard Dean, M.D. Since zinc is essential to the production of semen, a deficiency can lead to prostate problems. Take 30 milligrams per day. But beware—zinc and copper are linked in the body, so taking zinc for prolonged periods can throw off their balance. To avoid a potential imbalance, take a 2-milligram capsule or tablet of copper as well.

**Break open the Great Pumpkin.** Pumpkin seeds contain high levels of phytosterols and zinc—both critical for the prostate's well-being. Dr. Craig recommends taking 1 to 2 teaspoons of ground pumpkin seeds mixed with liquid twice a day. If you'd rather take a combination supplement with saw palmetto and African pygeum, follow the label recommendations for dosage amounts.

**Toss in some tomatoes.** Lycopene, the compound that tints tomatoes red, can do more than add color to your salad. In studies, higher tomato consumption is associated with a reduced risk of prostate cancer. Martin K. Gelbard, M.D., prescribes tomatoes for patients with BPH and prostatitis. "It helps relieve symptoms and may prevent the progression of prostate enlargement," he says. Dr. Gelbard suggests eating two or three tomatoes or tomato-based products a day.

**Watch what you eat.** Some foods and beverages can make matters worse for men with prostatitis. Avoid spicy foods, carbonated soft drinks, caffeinated beverages, and acidic foods such as citrus fruits and juices. "These items irritate the lining of the prostate," explains Dr. Gelbard. Hard liquor does the same, but beer and wine are okay.

**Keep on your toes.** Men with jobs that require long hours of sitting, especially occupations that constantly put pressure on the prostate area, such as truck driving, are more prone to both prostatitis and BPH. "Periodically throughout the day, take breaks from sitting," recommends Dr. Dean. Getting out of your seat helps prevent circulation from being diminished in that region of the body and helps relieve symptoms.

**Get some exercise.** "Men who exercise more are less likely to have symptoms of BPH," observes researcher Elizabeth Platz, Sc.D. Dr. Platz analyzed more than 30,000 participants of the Health Professionals Follow-Up Study, an ongoing prospective study of male dentists, veterinarians, optometrists, and other health professionals begun in 1986. In 1992 and 1994, the study asked participants about symptoms associated with BPH. Dr. Platz found that men who exercised regularly reported fewer symptoms. By contrast, their inactive counterparts—those who spent 41 or more hours per week watching TV—were 42 percent more likely to develop BPH and exhibited more severe symptoms.

Walking was the most common activity. According to Dr. Platz, walking for exercise for 2 or more hours per week yielded results.

**Cycle on a split seat.** If cycling is your preferred form of exercise, beware—it puts pressure on the prostate. This can lead to prostatitis or exacerbate an existing condition, says Dr. Gelbard. "Get a split bicycle seat," he recommends. A split seat is cushioned on either side, so your weight rests on the bones of your pelvis, keeping tension off the prostate.

**Quit smoking.** Men who smoke 35 or more cigarettes per day are more likely to report symptoms of BPH. That's what Dr. Platz concluded from the Health Professionals Follow-Up Study, which also examined the effects of smoking on BPH. Former smokers did not share the same risk.

**Consider alcohol.** Moderate alcohol consumption produces various health benefits—add to those possibly a reduced risk for symptomatic BPH. "Alcohol doesn't seem to contribute to a worsening of symptoms," Dr. Platz observes. She found that men who drank the equivalent amount of alcohol in two to three beers a day reported fewer symptoms of BPH. Researchers aren't sure why. Could be that muscle relaxation plays a role. "Alcohol tends to relax muscles. It might relax muscles important to bladder control," she suggests.

She cautions against drinking alcohol to reduce symptoms, but notes that early signs of BPH may not be reason to halt moderate drinking. Keep in mind, however, that alcohol can irritate the bladder and may aggravate some urinary symptoms, such as frequency. Talk to your doctor about whether moderate alcohol consumption is right for you, suggests Dr. Platz.

**Soothe it with a sitz.** A sitz bath, in which the lower half of your body rests in warm water, brings heat to the prostate gland and relaxes lower abdominal muscles. "It reduces inflammation and cuts down on pain and urgency," says Dr. Gelbard. Fill a tub with about a foot of warm water and soak for 15 minutes once a day.

**Buy loose cotton briefs.** Tight, restrictive underclothing also restricts bloodflow to the area surrounding the prostate. "Good bloodflow brings nutrients to the gland and carries out waste products," explains Dr. Dean. Similarly, while synthetic undergarments trap sweat, cotton wicks away moisture, allowing the skin to breathe. That means less accumulation of toxins in the skin directly over the prostate, which affects the underlying organs, he says.

**Make love more.** "Since the prostate is vitally involved in the production of semen, ejaculation can be therapeutic," counsels Dr. Dean. During ejaculation, muscles surrounding the prostate contract. "Think of it as exercise or gymnastics for the prostate," he says. "It's very good for bloodflow." Most likely to benefit are men who don't have regular sexual relations. Don't worry about passing the bacteria that caused the prostatitis on to your partner—the infection is not transmitted through sexual contact.

**Rub it out.** Reflexology is a natural healing therapy that can be effective in promoting health in certain disorders, including prostate ailments, says Dr. Dean. The principle behind reflexology is that the hands and feet contain sensors that connect to all other parts of the body. By massaging the reflex points related to the prostate, you send a signal to the gland that stimulates healing. The point for the prostate is located at the base of the heel on either side. (Charts showing actual points are available at most health food stores.)

Once you find the point, rub it with your thumb, a marble, or a pencil eraser. "Rub for 20 to 30 seconds a couple of times a day," says Dr. Dean. The spot may be sore at first, indicating the gland is in need of balance, he explains. With continued rubbing, it becomes less sensitive.

**Keep away from cold medicines.** Decongestants and antihistamines can cause the muscles that control urine flow to contract, making urination more difficult. In some cases, this can completely restrict the flow of urine, leading to a potentially life-threatening condition. If you experience allergies, ask your doctor to prescribe cold and allergy medications that don't contain antihistamines.

**Drink up.** If you're tempted to drink less because you're tired of so many trips to the bathroom, don't give in to the temptation, warns Dr. Gelbard. "Dehydration creates added stress," he explains. Drinking adequate amounts of water every day is important for proper functioning of the kidneys and can prevent urinary infections. Aim for six 8-ounce glasses a day.

**But not before bed.** Want to cut back on nightly bathroom visits? Don't drink any liquids after 6:00 P.M., advises Dr. Gelbard. Empty your bladder completely before hitting the sack.

**Heal with your mind.** The mind can be a very powerful tool for healing the body. Dr. Dean recommends trying these two techniques for improving prostate health.

*Visualization.* Put your imagination to good use—take time daily to create a mental picture of a robust prostate. "Visualize your prostate to be healthy and pink, and see the flow of blood carrying nutrients, with the white blood cells coming to heal, and the red blood cells bringing oxygen."

*Affirmations.* Tell yourself regularly that your condition is improving. When using this technique, how you frame your words is of vital importance. "Always keep things personal and positive," says Dr. Dean. For example, saying, "My prostate is getting better and better," is more powerful than saying, "My prostatitis is getting better and better," which places heavy focus on the illness.

## PANEL OF ADVISORS

**Winston Craig, R.D., Ph.D.,** is a professor of nutrition at Andrews University in Berrien Springs, Michigan.

**Willard Dean, M.D.,** is a holistic physician in Glorieta, New Mexico.

**Martin K. Gelbard, M.D.,** is an assistant clinical professor of urology at the University of California, Los Angeles, School of Medicine and the author of *Solving Prostate Problems.*

**Elizabeth Platz, Sc.D.,** is an assistant professor in the department of epidemiology at Johns Hopkins University Bloomberg School of Public Health in Baltimore.

# PSORIASIS
## 22 Skin-Soothing Remedies

Psoriasis is a disease in which the skin cells multiply like rabbits. Normally, skin renews itself in about 30 days—that's the time it takes for a new skin cell to work its way from the innermost layer of skin to the surface. In psoriasis, that cell reaches the top in just 3 days, as if the body has lost its brakes. The result is raised areas of skin called plaques, which are red and often itchy. After the cells reach the surface, they die like normal cells, but there are so many of them that the raised patches turn white with dead cells flaking off.

Psoriasis usually goes through cycles of flare-ups and remission, with flare-ups most often occurring in winter. Sometimes it disappears for months or years. The condition can improve or worsen with age.

Since the cause of psoriasis is unknown, the cure is also unknown. But many things can soothe the itching. Here are some strategies to try.

**Get a new attitude.** Philip Anderson, M.D., says that the most important thing is to accept that you have psoriasis and focus your attention on learning how to manage it and prevent it from getting serious. "Don't waste energy fussing over every bump," he says. "That's not a good idea."

Laurence Miller, M.D., agrees. "I see some of my psoriasis patients maybe twice a year," he says. "There is no law that says every person with psoriasis has to get rid of every flake on the body. I put my hands about a foot apart and tell them, 'It takes this much effort to get you 80 percent clear.' Then I stretch my arms out as far as I can and say, 'For the final 20 percent, this is what you

## WHEN TO CALL A DOCTOR

The impact of psoriasis on people's lives can range from mildly annoying to completely debilitating. If your condition causes you discomfort and pain, if performing routine tasks has become difficult, or if the appearance of your skin concerns you, go see a doctor.

have to do.' I never say, 'Learn to live with it.' When you think you've run out of treatments, you've gone from A to Z, you start over again at A. Mild psoriasis can be controlled totally by following some of these remedies."

**Feed your skin.** Emollients top every dermatologist's list of over-the-counter treatments. Psoriatic skin is dry, and that can mean a worsening of the psoriasis and increased flaking and itching. Emollients help your skin retain water. The emollient can be your favorite nonirritating body oil or something as mundane as vegetable shortening or petroleum jelly. It's most effective applied right after bathing, when you're still dripping wet. (For safety's sake, avoid bathing in bath oil, which can make the tub as slick as ice.) Dr. Miller recommends Sarna lotion, which contains menthol and camphor, to soothe itching. For a natural alternative, you may want to try a soothing herbal cream with calendula and beeswax to seal in moisture. An aloe vera–based cream may also be helpful.

**Turn on the lamp.** Get yourself a small ultraviolet A/ultraviolet B sunlamp to treat patches of psoriasis, suggests Dr. Miller. Each person's needs vary, so consult your doctor first. You may prefer the high UVA and low UVB light found in tanning parlors, but this light is weaker and needs much more time to work.

## Do just 1 thing

Get some sun. With regular doses of intense sun, 95 percent of people with psoriasis improve.

"The disease seems to be so much worse in wintertime or in a variable or humid climate that you should consider moving to a warm, dry area," says Philip Anderson, M.D. Ultraviolet waves seem to fight psoriasis, and the UVB rays work the fastest. But a catch-22 does exist. UVB's are also the rays that give you a sunburn and run up the risks for skin cancer. They can also cause people with psoriasis to break out in previously unaffected areas.

Sunscreen is your weapon of choice for blocking the sun's deadly rays. "The benefits of sunbathing can outweigh the risks of skin cancer and spreading psoriasis if you use sunscreens on the places where you don't have psoriasis and only expose the affected areas to the full force of the sun," says Laurence Miller, M.D.

**Use tar.** Over-the-counter (OTC) coal tar preparations are weaker than the prescription versions but can be effective in treating mild psoriasis, says Dr. Miller. You can apply the tar directly to the plaques or immerse yourself in tar bath oil and treat your scalp with tar shampoo. Since even the OTC tars can stain and smell, they're usually washed off after a certain amount of time, but some kinds can be left on the skin to enhance the effect of sunlight or UVB treatments. "Tar makes you more sensitive to the sun, so be careful," he warns.

Dr. Miller notes that some new tar products have been made a little more elegant and cosmetically acceptable in gel form. They don't smell like tar pits, and they can be used daily and wash off easily. He gives these precautions: "If any tar product causes burning or irritation, stop using it. Never use tar on raw, open skin."

**Get wet and warm.** "Baths and heated swimming pools are excellent for psoriasis," Dr. Miller says, by flattening plaques or cutting down scaling. "But hot water can actually make itching worse."

**Or get wet and cold.** A cold-water bath, maybe with a cup or so of apple cider vinegar added, is great for itching. "Another thing that really works is ice," Dr. Miller says. "Just dump some ice cubes into a small plastic bag and hold it against the afflicted skin."

**Try hydrocortisone for small areas.** "OTC topical hydrocortisone creams are weaker than their prescription cousins, but they're worth trying, and they're safer on the face and genital areas," Dr. Miller says. "But if you use it all the time in these areas, it will become less effective, and when you give up on it, the psoriasis can rebound. Just use it until you show some improvement, and then gradually wean yourself off."

**Seal off psoriasis.** Researchers have discovered that covering lesions with tape or plastic wrap for days or weeks can help clear up psoriasis, especially if cortisone cream is applied first.

"The cells on the surface get real soggy and damaged," Dr. Anderson explains. "It seems to slow down the proliferation." This treatment, however, is good only for small areas, no bigger than a half-dollar. You have to be careful because the skin can get gooey and infected, and then the psoriasis can get worse.

**Don't risk injury.** New lesions often appear on injured skin, Dr. Anderson

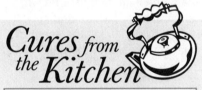

## Cures from the Kitchen

D'Anne Kleinsmith, M.D., offers the following kitchen cure if psoriasis is making a mess of your scalp.

First, heat olive oil until it is warm, but not hot. Massage the oil into your scalp. Leave the oil on for 20 to 30 minutes minimum or overnight, while wearing a shower cap. Wash out the oil with a dandruff shampoo. Do this nightly until your skin clears up, and then continue the treatment once or twice a week as needed.

## The Great Cover-Up

Hollywood to the rescue. Cosmetologist and Hollywood makeup artist Maurice Stein helps out clients referred to him by medical doctors across the country, as well as the standard must-be-perfect stars. Here are some of his recommendations.

- First of all, never try to cover up any open lesion, Stein says, echoing medical advice.

- "There's a very good over-the-counter cream, applied with a makeup sponge, that can be applied to the scalp to cover up the flaking," Stein says. "Get your doctor's approval first. It's called Couvré, and it comes in black; dark, medium, and light brown; auburn, blond, white, and gray. It works by darkening the scalp to match the color of the hair."

- For elbows and knees, Stein recommends Indian earth mixed with your favorite emollient and spread over the plaques with a makeup sponge. A rock, ground to face powder consistency, Indian earth can be bought in salons, department stores, health food stores, or online. "A dime-size portion is enough to do your whole body," he says. The emollient will keep the plaques moist, and the Indian earth will disguise their appearance. "If you have to wear clothes over it, pat it dry to remove the excess," Stein advises.

- If you can't find Indian earth, look for a cosmetic base with a lot of pigment, he says. "The best place to find and test them is at a local cosmetologist's."

says. Researchers believe the trauma to the skin may send the body into ungovernable overdrive. "People with psoriasis shouldn't go out picking blackberries, just like a man with a bad back shouldn't be a piano mover," he says. You can injure your skin with such things as tight shoes, watchbands, dull razors, and harsh chemicals.

**Lose weight if you're overweight.** While scientists can't swear that obesity worsens psoriasis, Dr. Anderson says, "it's one of the connectors. Weight loss helps many people with psoriasis. If you lose weight and maintain normal weight, the psoriasis is almost always better."

**Destress yourself.** "I saw a 13-year-old girl break out in psoriasis from head to toe after her father died," Dr. Miller reports.

Overwhelming evidence shows that stress can trigger psoriasis, agrees Eugene Farber, M.D. "If you lie on the beach in Hawaii for a week, you get better.

Even going into the hospital for surgery can make your psoriasis better. Although it's stressful, you're relaxing and being cared for. Any absence from your daily stresses, for any period of time, is helpful."

**Meditate mindfully.** If meditation is your thing, mindfulness meditation during light treatment helped people's skin clear up twice as fast in a current study. To try mindful meditation, look for a class at a meditation clinic.

**Avoid alcohol.** If you're a heavy drinker, the nutritional problems that accompany binge drinking will only make psoriasis worse.

**Try fish oil.** Adding fish oil capsules containing the fatty acid eicosapentaenoic acid (EPA) to your diet may help. Vincent Ziboh, Ph.D., is encouraged by what he's found. "About 60 percent of the people we studied responded well," he reports. The area and thickness of the plaques decreased, as did redness and itching.

But there are important cautions to consider. "A small number of people will not improve, and a small number will get worse," Dr. Ziboh says. "There's no guarantee." His original study was small and short-term, so the results are not conclusive. "We saw no adverse effects, but over a longer period of time, there could be some," he adds. For example, fish oil can cut down on blood clotting, so it can amplify the blood-thinning effects of other medications you may be taking. "If you take it, have your doctor monitor you," he warns.

Although the people in his study were taking 11 to 14 grams a day, he says, "I think you could do as well or better with half that dose." But make sure you check with your doctor first. While it's a good idea to eat fatty fish, such as salmon or mackerel, he adds, you'd have to eat at least 1 pound, perhaps even 2 pounds a day to get 5 grams of EPA.

**Grab some grape root.** Several herbalists recommend Oregon grape root as a treatment for psoriasis. The herb seems to have chemical constituents that fight bacteria and reduce skin eruptions. Look for extracts and capsules of Oregon grape root in your local health food store, and follow the dosage directions on the label.

**Treat infections.** A well-documented but unexplained link exists between infections and the initial onset of psoriasis. Existing psoriasis is also known to worsen when an infection strikes.

"We see children walk in with psoriasis covering their bodies 2 weeks after a strep throat," Dr. Miller says.

The key here, Dr. Anderson advises, is early and proper treatment of all infections, and extra attention to psoriasis when you have any type of infection.

# RASHES
## 15 Skin-Salving Solutions

Rashes sting and burn and come and go. And their causes can leave you scratching your head—not to mention the rest of your body.

Everyday materials that our skin comes in contact with are the most common cause of rashes—which is why dermatologists refer to the appearance of rashes as contact dermatitis. But if your rash is caused by a particular substance, then the phrase is "allergic contact dermatitis" and the triggers are called "allergens."

The five most common rash-producing allergens are the following, says Larry Millikan, M.D.

- Nickel, a metal often mixed with other metals to make costume jewelry
- Chromates, a chemical found in everyday home-improvement products such as cement, paints, and antirust products
- Preservatives or fragrance additives found in hand creams and lotions
- Rubber, found in products such as latex gloves, elastic waistbands, and shoes
- Urushiol, the oil in poison plants like ivy, oak, and sumac

These are just the most common allergens. Almost anything can cause a rash, though, including food and medications. Which is why figuring out what caused your rash may require that you and your doctor become detectives.

"The rash is sending a message that your body is not happy about something," says Dee Anna Glaser, M.D. The key is to go to your dermatologist appointment armed with a complete list of substances you've come in contact with that could have caused the rash. Once the doctor determines that cause, he can help you get rid of it.

In the meantime, here are some common causes and cures for what itches you.

## Nickel Rash

Nickel is a metal that is often mixed with other metals to make rings, necklaces, and bracelets. Costume jewelry is by far the most common cause of nickel reactions. The good news is that the nickel allergy is easy to diagnose because the rash springs up wherever nickel touches your skin, says C. Ralph Daniel III, M.D. For example, you may get a rash on your ears if you wear earrings with nickel in them. Here's what to do.

**Change your jewelry.** Many women have allergic reactions to costume jewelry with nickel, but this is an easy problem to solve. Stop wearing that particular jewelry, and the rashes should disappear, says Dr. Daniel.

## Rash Relief

Although millions of things can cause rashes, the treatments are pretty much the same. Here's what our experts suggest.

**Call on cortisone cream.** Start with 1 percent hydrocortisone cream, such as Cortaid, says C. Ralph Daniel III, M.D. Rub it on a mildly itchy or inflamed area two times per day for up to a week.

Use cortisone only if the rash is not infected, says Dr. Daniel. How do you know if it's infected? An infected rash may be more inflamed and swollen and possibly producing pus.

**Consider antihistamines.** They aren't just for hay fever anymore. Antihistamines will relieve some of your skin irritation, and if you take one of the older forms, it may even help you sleep.

**Soothe your skin.** Try a compress of cloth soaked in water or Domeboro, an over-the-counter astringent that you mix with water, to relieve the itch and inflammation. You may also want to try soaking in a bath with a special oatmeal bathing product designed to soothe inflamed skin.

**Just avoid it.** The best thing you can do is to minimize—or better yet, avoid—touching the allergens and irritants that will trigger an outbreak. If you do get an irritant on you or your clothing, wash it off as soon as possible with soap and warm water.

**Go for the gold.** Before the next gift-giving event, drop hints to your loved one to spring for a pure gold necklace or bracelet to replace the costume jewelry that's giving you problems. "I've never heard of anyone who's allergic to pure gold, that's for sure," says Dr. Millikan.

**Don't sweat in it.** Perspiration can aggravate the dermatitis in nickel-sensitive people. For instance, items containing nickel can cause an itchy, prickly sensation within 20 minutes after touching a sweaty palm. These same items can be worn for several hours without any problems, however, if you're not sweaty, says Dr. Daniel. So wear your nickel-containing jewelry to a movie but not to the gym.

## Chromate Rash

This is the most common cause of contact dermatitis in the workplace, says Dr. Millikan. This chemical is found in cement, paints, and antirust products. "People with certain blue-collar jobs are exposed to chromate all the time, as are people doing certain home-repair jobs on the weekends," he says.

**Wear gloves.** If you can't avoid the chemical, at least avoid getting it on your hands. Wear a sturdy pair of waterproof work gloves to keep the chromate from getting on, and then irritating, your skin.

**Wash up.** Make sure to wash your hands often when working with chromate to ensure that if any of the chemical does get on your skin, it's not on there very long. Since this much washing may dry out your skin, follow with a moisturizing cream or lotion.

**Use lighters.** Some matches also contain chromates, so touching unlit matches can contaminate your fingers. Even placing books of unlit matches in a pocket will contaminate that pocket lining of those pants. When you stick your hands in your pockets, bingo! A rash. Rely on a lighter instead.

## Additive Rash

Exposure to preservative and fragrance ingredients used in hand creams, lotions, and other skin-care products cause rashes in many people, says Dr. Millikan. "Make mental notes of what you were using at the time that the rashes started and report them to your dermatologist. It'll help your doctor get to the bottom of what's causing them more quickly."

Common culprits include:

- Neomycin, an ingredient found in many over-the-counter and prescription antibiotic creams, ointments, lotions, ear drops, and eyedrops
- Preservatives, such as ethylenediamine, added to creams to keep them from going rancid
- Chemicals in certain laundry detergents and fabric softeners such as sodium silicate, sodium phosphate, and sodium carbonate

Here's what to do.

**Read labels.** Once you realize that an additive causes you problems, scrutinize labels of other products and avoid that additive.

**Be consistent.** Find products that work for you and stick with them, says Dr. Daniel. "Use common sense. If you're using something in your laundry and an ingredient in it causes your skin to become irritated, switch to something else." "If you have something that works for you and doesn't cause you any problems, stick with it."

## Rubber Rash

Chemical additives in rubber products, especially latex gloves, can often cause allergic reactions and rashes, including itching, burning, and even welts. They're common among people who wear tight-fitting rubber gloves, such as medical workers. Here are some approaches to try.

**Try a different glove.** Powderless rubber gloves may be less allergenic, or vinyl (or other synthetic gloves) may be used as a substitute.

**Head to Victoria's Secret.** Undergarments with rubber stretch waistbands are common triggers of rubber rashes. Try lingerie made with spandex instead, and look for items without rubber-backed fasteners or edges.

**Check your shoes.** Many cases of allergic contact dermatitis are caused by ingredients used to make shoes, such as leather, certain dyes, adhesives, and, of course, rubber. But because so many parts of your shoe could be causing that foot rash, see your dermatologist for a patch test to determine what exactly you are allergic to before you purchase new shoes. And because hypoallergenic shoes are hard to find and tend to be rather costly, ask your dermatologist for a list of stores or Web sites that sell these shoes so that you can shop around easily.

## Poison Plant Rashes

If an incredibly itchy rash has popped up a few hours to a few days after gardening, a poison plant allergy could be the cause. See Poison Plant Rashes on page 468.

## PANEL OF ADVISORS

**C. Ralph Daniel III, M.D.,** is a clinical professor of dermatology at the University of Mississippi Medical Center in Jackson.

**Dee Anna Glaser, M.D.,** is an associate professor of dermatology at St. Louis University School of Medicine.

**Larry Millikan, M.D.,** is chairman of the department of dermatology at Tulane University Medical Center in New Orleans.

# RAYNAUD'S PHENOMENON
## 18 Toasty Tips

If you have Raynaud's phenomenon, then you know gloves and mittens are never enough. Not only are your fingers (and sometimes toes) often cold, but the reaction to sudden cold as your blood vessels constrict and bloodflow slows can be excruciatingly painful.

That's because when blood vessels to your extremities constrict, a spasm occurs. Beyond the pain are the color changes. As bloodflow slows to the affected area, the lack of oxygenated blood causes fingers and toes to pale, maybe even take on a bluish tinge.

Yet not everyone experiences Raynaud's in the same way. Some feel numbness from the lack of blood, then their fingers turn red again when the blood returns. In advanced stages of Raynaud's, poor blood supply can weaken the fingers and damage the sense of touch.

Cold isn't the only culprit. This odd but common affliction, which rough estimates show may affect 5 to 10 percent of the U.S. population, can result from injury to the blood vessels caused by vibrations from powerful equipment, like chain saws and pneumatic drills; hypersensitivity to drugs that affect the blood vessels; or disorders of the connective tissue or nerves.

Our experts provide some protective suggestions.

**Condition yourself to overcome chills.** Train your hands to heat up in the cold by adapting this technique devised by U.S. Army researchers in Alaska.

Choose a room that's a comfortable temperature and place your hands in a container of warm water for 3 to 5 minutes. Then go into a cold room and again dip your hands in warm water for 10 minutes. The cold environment would normally make your peripheral blood vessels constrict, but, instead, the sensation of the warm water makes them open. Repeatedly training the blood vessels to open despite the cold eventually enables you to counter the constriction reflex even without the warm water.

In the Army experiments, this procedure was repeated three to six times every other day on 150 test people. After 54 treatments, the results were impressive. Participants' hands were 7 degrees warmer in the cold than before.

"People are training on the rooftops in New York City, in freezer lockers, in grocery stores, and in hospitals and hotels," says Murray Hamlet, director of the army's cold research program.

**Twirl your arms to generate heat.** Force your hands to warm up through a simple exercise devised by Donald McIntyre, M.D. Pretend you're a softball pitcher. Swing your arm downward behind your body and then upward in front of you at about 80 twirls per minute. (This isn't as fast as it sounds; give it a try.)

The windmill effect, which Dr. McIntyre modeled after a skier's warmup exercise, forces blood to the fingers through both gravitational and centrifugal force. This warmup works well for chilled hands no matter what the cause.

**Eat iron-rich foods.** Lack of iron may alter your thyroid metabolism, which regulates body heat. That's what researchers at the USDA Human Nutrition Research Center in Grand Forks, North Dakota, suspect. They measured the effects of dietary iron on six healthy women when they entered a cold chamber. When the women took only one-third of the recommended amount of iron for 80 days, they lost 29 percent more body heat than when they were on an iron-rich diet for 114 days.

Iron-rich foods include poultry, fish, lean red meat, lentils, and leafy green vegetables. Orange juice is okay, too, since it increases your body's ability to absorb iron.

**Eat a hot, hearty meal.** The very act of eating causes a rise in core body temperature. This is called thermogenesis. So eat something before you go out to stoke your body's furnace. And eat something hot to give the stoking a boost. A bowl of hot oatmeal before your morning walk, a soup break, or a hot lunch helps keep your hands and feet toasty even in inclement weather.

**Drink up.** Dehydration can aggravate chills and frostbite by reducing your blood volume. Ward off the big chill by drinking plenty of warm fluids such as mulled cider, herbal teas, or broth.

**Pass on the coffee.** Coffee and other caffeinated products constrict blood vessels. The last thing you want when you have Raynaud's phenomenon is to interfere with your circulation.

**Avoid alcohol.** Don't be misled by the lure of a hot toddy either. Alcohol temporarily warms your hands and feet, but its detrimental effects outweigh its benefits as a hand and foot warmer.

Alcohol increases bloodflow to the skin, giving you the immediate perception of warmth. But that heat is soon lost to the air, reducing your core body temperature. In other words, alcohol actually makes you colder. The danger comes from drinking too much and then being subjected to unexpected cold for an extended period, which can lead to severe problems like frostbite or hypothermia.

**Dress smart.** To keep warm, you have to dress warmly. Common sense, yes, but many people will slap on gloves and footwear without taking equal precautions to maintain their core temperatures, which is really more important.

> ***Choose fabrics that wick away perspiration.*** Perspiration is an even bigger cause of cold hands and feet than temperature. Sweat is the body's air conditioner, and your body's air conditioner can operate in cold weather if you're not careful. Your hands and feet are especially susceptible because the palms and heels (along with the armpits) have the largest number of sweat glands in the body. That's why the heavy woolen socks and fleece-lined boots you bought to keep your feet warm may instead make them sweaty and chilly. Try a pair of polypropylene (a synthetic fabric) socks underneath your wool ones.

> ***Wear cotton-blend socks rather than pure cotton socks.*** All-cotton socks can soak up your perspiration and chill your feet. Those made of an Orlon-and-cotton blend, which wicks moisture away from your feet and insulates them, are a better choice.

> ***Make sure garments are loose.*** None of your garments should pinch. Tight-fitting clothes can cut off circulation and eliminate insulating air pockets.

> ***Dress in layers.*** If you're stepping out into the cold, the best warming measure you can take is to dress in layers. This helps trap heat and allows you to peel off clothes as the temperature changes. Your inner layer should consist of synthetic fabrics, like polypropylene, which wicks perspiration away from your skin. Silk or wool blends also are acceptable. The next layer should insulate you by trapping your body heat. A wool shirt is one of your best options.

> ***Waterproof your body.*** Choose a breathable, waterproof jacket or windbreaker. Gore-Tex shoes and boots are the best choice for keeping your feet warm and dry.

> ***Wear a hat.*** Your head is the greatest site of body heat loss. The blood vessels in your head are controlled by cardiac output and won't constrict like those in your hands and feet to keep in heat. So while your head may not feel as cold as those icy fingers and toes, it is important to keep it covered in order to keep in that precious body heat.

*Wear mittens.* Mittens keep you warmer than gloves because they trap your whole hand's heat, rather than one finger at a time.

**Try foot powder.** Clothes aren't the only way to keep dry. "Absorbent foot powders are excellent for helping keep feet dry," says Marc A. Brenner, D.P.M. He cautions people with severe cold-foot problems caused by diabetes and peripheral vascular disease to use a shaker can rather than a spray, since the mist from the spray can actually freeze your feet.

**Don't smoke.** Cigarette smoke cools you in two ways. It helps form plaque in your arteries and, more immediately, contains nicotine, which causes vasospasms that narrow the small blood vessels and restrict the amount of blood available to keep your hands and feet warm.

These effects can be especially hard on people with Raynaud's. "Raynaud's patients are sensitive even to other people's smoke," says Frederick A. Reichle, M.D.

**Chill out to warm up.** Staying cool and calm may help some people stay warm. Why? Stress creates the same reaction in the body as cold. It's the fight-or-flight phenomenon. Blood is pulled from the hands and feet to the brain and internal organs to enable you to think and react more quickly.

Calming techniques abound. Some, like progressive relaxation, in which you systematically tense and then relax the muscles from your forehead to your hands and toes, can be practiced at any time, in any place.

## PANEL OF ADVISORS

**John Abruzzo, M.D.,** is director of the division of rheumatology and a professor of medicine at Thomas Jefferson University in Philadelphia.

**Marc A. Brenner, D.P.M.,** is director of the Institute of Diabetic Foot Research in Glendale, New York; past president of the American Society of Podiatric Dermatology; and author and editor of various books.

**Murray Hamlet, D.V.M.,** is the former director of cold research at the U.S. Army Research Institute of Environmental Medicine in Natick, Massachusetts. He is now retired and is a consultant and lecturer on environmental medicine.

**Donald McIntyre, M.D.,** is a retired dermatologist in Rutland, Vermont.

**Frederick A. Reichle, M.D.,** has a practice affiliated with Mercy Suburban Hospital in Norristown, Pennsylvania. He was previously the chief of vascular surgery at Presbyterian–University of Pennsylvania Medical Center in Philadelphia.

# RESTLESS LEGS SYNDROME
## 20 Calming Techniques

Surveys in the United States and Canada have found that 15 to 25 percent of adults experience unpleasant feelings in their legs especially at night, at least some of the time. The problem appears to be more common in women than in men, and especially prevalent in the elderly.

According to the Restless Legs Syndrome Foundation, people describe the sensation as feeling like an electrical current flowing through the legs, a "creepy crawly" feeling, aching or itching bones, a sensation "like Coca-Cola bubbling through the veins," "crazy legs," and "the gotta moves." If this sounds all too familiar to you, chances are you have restless legs syndrome.

The condition, also known as Ekbom syndrome, is usually a chronic annoyance rather than a symptom of a larger disorder.

## WHEN TO CALL A DOCTOR

If you have restless legs syndrome, you probably don't have anything to worry about—except the sleep it sometimes causes you to miss.

But if you're experiencing symptoms for the first time—pronounced sensations in the legs, usually at night—see your doctor. The symptoms of restless legs syndrome can be warning signs for serious medical problems such as lung disease, kidney disease, diabetes, Parkinson's disease, and many neurological disorders.

So for safety—not to mention peace of mind—let your doctor make the diagnosis.

Also, if crawly legs are keeping you up at night and home remedies just aren't helping, your doctor may be able to prescribe something to help. Certain medications that act on brain chemistry have been shown to decrease the actual movements of the legs and patients' perceptions of unpleasant sensations, according to the Restless Legs Syndrome Foundation.

"Typically both lower legs are affected, although the thighs and even the arms can be involved," says Lawrence Z. Stern, M.D. It's not always symmetrical; sometimes it occurs in only one limb.

The origin of the sensations is unknown. Some researchers suspect that an imbalance in the brain's chemistry may be the root cause of the problem. A problem with iron metabolism may also be a contributor, and genetics are thought to play a role.

Whatever the cause, restless legs syndrome can be very frustrating to those who have it, and it can significantly interfere with sleep. Here are a few steps to quiet those jumpy legs.

**Take a multivitamin.** "Iron deficiency may be a cause of restless legs syndrome," says Ronald F. Pfeiffer, M.D. Several studies have found an association between iron deficiency and restless legs syndrome. Folate deficiency also has been implicated in restless legs syndrome.

Dr. Stern says that a daily multivitamin can protect you against deficiencies of both nutrients.

**Don't eat a big meal late.** Eating a lot late at night may get the legs really jumping. "It may be the activity of digesting a big meal that triggers something that causes symptoms," offers Dr. Stern.

**Avoid sleep-inducing medications.** They may provide short-term benefits, but many people build up a tolerance to them, and then they have two problems—restless legs syndrome *and* dependence on the drugs, says Dr. Stern.

**Don't use alcohol as a sedative.** Again, you set yourself up for double trouble, Dr. Stern says.

**Stop or dramatically reduce caffeine.** "Some studies have shown an association between relief of restless legs syndrome and stopping caffeine," Dr. Pfeiffer says.

**Avoid cold and sinus medications.** These have been reported to increase the symptoms, according to the Restless Legs Syndrome Foundation.

**Quit smoking.** Smokers were significantly more likely than nonsmokers to have restless legs syndrome in a University of Kentucky College of Medicine study of more than 1,800 men and women. That doesn't prove smoking causes restless legs syndrome, but it is worth noting that a Canadian doctor reported that for one of his patients, her symptoms were relieved a month after she stopped smoking, and she remained symptom-free months later.

**Come in from the cold.** Several studies have implicated prolonged exposure to cold as a possible cause of restless legs syndrome.

**Massage your legs.** "Right before bedtime, rubbing your legs may be beneficial," suggests Richard K. Olney, M.D. Mild stretching also may help.

**Wear cotton stockings or silk pajamas to bed.** These, and other rituals, seem to help some people feel better, says Dr. Olney.

**Take two aspirins before bedtime.** Doctors can't say why aspirin helps, but apparently it does reduce symptoms in some people.

**Lower your stress level.** Easier said than done, but certainly worth trying. "Stress just worsens the problem," says Dr. Stern. Being organized, giving yourself quiet time, taking deep breaths, and practicing various relaxation techniques are good ways to reduce stress.

**Walk before going to bed.** In some cases, this noticeably reduces bedtime bouts of restless legs syndrome, says Dr. Stern. "Exercise changes chemical balances in the brain—endorphins are released—and may promote more restful sleep," he adds.

**Get plenty of rest.** Symptoms may be more severe if you allow yourself to become overtired.

**Get up and walk.** Restless legs syndrome tends to strike at night, when you're at rest. When the urge to move hits, the quickest way to satisfy it is to comply with a stroll around the bedroom, says Dr. Pfeiffer.

**Wiggle your feet.** The idea is to move your feet back and forth when symptoms arise.

**Change positions.** "Some people seem to develop symptoms a lot more often sleeping in one position than another," says Dr. Stern. "Experiment with different sleeping positions. It's harmless and may prove to be worthwhile."

**Soak your feet in cool water.** "It works for some," Dr. Pfeiffer says. One caution: Do not follow a "more is better" theory and immerse your feet in a bucket of ice; you could cause nerve damage.

**Warm up.** While cold helps some people, others find using a heating pad more soothing and effective, Dr. Pfeiffer says.

**Rub your legs with an electric vibrator.** Some people say this reduces symptoms; in a few people, however, it could make symptoms worse.

## PANEL OF ADVISORS

**Richard K. Olney, M.D.,** is a professor of clinical neurology at the University of California, San Francisco.

**Ronald F. Pfeiffer, M.D.,** is professor, vice chairman, and director in the department of neurology at the University of Tennessee Health Science Center in Memphis.

**Lawrence Z. Stern, M.D.,** is a professor of neurology at the University of Arizona College of Medicine in Tucson.

# ROAD RAGE

## 14 Tips for a More Pleasant Drive

The terms *road rage* and *aggressive driving* are often used interchangeably.

But to those who study the ever-increasing vigilante performance of drivers on America's streets and highways, the terms are not synonymous.

Road rage is the deliberate, criminal attempt to hurt or kill a driver or pedestrian, by firing a gun, for example. And while aggressive driving isn't as overtly violent, it still results in about 28,000 deaths on U.S. roads each year, says Arnold P. Nerenberg, Ph.D.

While most people don't participate in road rage, says Leon James, Ph.D., we all are aggressive drivers.

"We are raised that way from childhood," Dr. James says. We acquire competitive and aggressive attitudes in the car, from parents and television, for example. By the time we start driving, our attitudes are pretty much set.

Few people, however, consider themselves aggressive behind the wheel, he says. In surveys, 80 percent of drivers say *others* are aggressive on the road, but only about 30 percent admit they're aggressive, too. "There's a 50 percent gap," says Dr. James. In other words, over half of all aggressive drivers don't realize they're aggressive drivers.

"We define aggressive driving as imposing your own preferred level of risk on others," says Dr. James's wife and co-researcher, Diane Nahl, Ph.D.

People who tailgate, for instance, may think that other drivers are slow. "If you get out of their way, they'll consider you to be a good driver," says Dr. Nahl. "If you don't, you're labeled a bad driver."

Some of the "symptoms" of aggressive driving include feeling stressed behind the wheel, cursing, acting hostile, speeding, yelling or honking, making insulting gestures, tailgating, cutting off others, wanting to let the other driver know how you feel, indulging in violent fantasies, or feeling enraged, competitive, or compelled to drive dangerously.

Anonymity is a major contributor to the problem, says Dr. Nerenberg. In cars, we tend to dehumanize each other, he says. "We don't think, 'This is a human being like myself, with fears, aspirations, love, and vulnerabilities. It's just some jerk that cut me off, and I'm going to teach him a lesson.'"

But there may be a price to pay, Dr. Nerenberg adds. An aggressive driver who contributes to a crash, injury, or death is likely to end up in court, or worse.

So here are some tips from the experts on how to relax behind the wheel, as well as some ways to steer clear of aggressive or angry drivers.

**Lend support.** Learn to accommodate other drivers, says Dr. James. Instead of competing with them, support them. "If they want to enter the lane ahead of you, make space. If they want to pass you, move over and let them. If they want to cut you off, slow down," he says.

"When you're a supportive driver, the stress not only vanishes, you begin to enjoy traffic," he says.

---

**What the Doctor Does ...**

Leon James, Ph.D., is a reformed aggressive driver. He often took risks on the road, such as weaving in and out of lanes.

"I acted like I was in a hurry all the time, even when I wasn't," he says. "It becomes a habit. People who have a habit of getting ahead of everybody else get panicky when they get stuck behind somebody."

Now, Dr. James is much more relaxed in the driver's seat.

It took several years of battling with his wife—who insisted that drivers should consider their passenger's feelings and safety—to realize that she was right.

"I carried a tape recorder in the car and spoke my thoughts out loud, then listened to it later," says Dr. James. From there, it was a matter of "one little skill at a time."

"The one thing that's most helpful is to learn to leave earlier," he says.

Dr. James regularly allows an extra 15 to 20 minutes to reach his destination.

"The same events do not stress me out as before," he says. "I am able to be patient."

**Do it right.** "Try life in the right lane," Dr. James suggests. People often avoid the right, or slower, lane because they fear losing time. But if you actually drive in the slow lane, you'll keep pace with less aggressive drivers and may realize it's not slow after all, he says.

Research shows that the average commute in the United States is 32 minutes. Driving in the fast lane generally saves about 10 percent of that time. So the average commuter who rushes gets to his destination only 3 to 4 minutes ahead of the slower driver. Don't believe it? Time yourself and see.

**Control yourself.** Don't let other drivers do it for you, says Dr. Nerenberg. He asks aggressive or angry drivers: "Do you want to turn control over to those people you're calling idiots, or do you want to keep control for yourself?" Losing your cool is turning control over to them. Once you become aware of what they're doing, it's easier to commit to keeping calm on the road.

**Empower your hours.** Dr. Nerenberg uses what he calls the "Power Thought System" to keep negative thoughts from arising and overpowering drivers. Remind yourself—hourly, if possible, and never fewer

## Do just 1 thing

Acknowledge your aggression. "It's a good first step, but it's a hard thing for people to do," says Diane Nahl, Ph.D.

People with road rage are often focused on other people—those on the outside of the windshield, she says. "We rarely focus on our own behavior."

One way to tune in: Talk behind the wheel.

"The act of speaking your thoughts out loud while you're driving creates awareness," she says.

Better yet, tape-record yourself while driving, and listen later. Research shows people often are surprised by what they've said.

Another option: Carry a notepad in the car. When you arrive at your destination, write down your thoughts and feelings about the drive. Over time, your observations will lend insight that may help you change aggressive patterns.

than six times a day—of how you want to be on the road. Think, for example: "I'm going to keep control over myself. I'm not turning control over to you." You'll learn to turn away destructive thoughts.

**Listen up.** "Backseat drivers have a bad reputation," says Dr. Nahl. But they may have a point. So listen to the "complaints" of your spouse, your children, and others who ride with you. They are witnesses to your driving.

**Be responsible.** To your passengers, that is. "A lot of drivers feel: 'I am the captain of my ship. You just put up with how I drive,'" says Dr. James. The driver controls the air conditioner, radio stations, speed, and just about everything else.

Instead, ask your passengers about their preferences. They'll likely appreciate the respect, and you'll feel better about yourself and calmer while driving.

**Get silly.** Feeling tense behind the wheel? Try making animal noises, machine sounds, or whatever you find amusing. "Laughter not only interrupts your negative thinking or anger but also unloads the stress," says Dr. Nahl.

**Forgive and forget.** If you are the "victim" of an aggressive driver, remind yourself that retaliation isn't worth it. Think about the people waiting for you to arrive at home. "You don't want to do anything that would endanger your life or anyone else's," says Dr. James. "Tell yourself, 'It's just not worth the hassle.'"

**Honk with care.** "Even honking has become a dangerous behavior," says Dr. Nahl. "People often take honking as a great insult, as a sign of disrespect." So be careful about when, where, and why you tap or lay on that horn.

**Don't get engaged.** Avoid confrontations. Never tailgate or make eye contact with an angry driver. Don't get out of the car or attempt to have a conversation. Similarly, don't go home or to work if someone is following you. "You don't want that person to know anything about you," Dr. Nerenberg says. If you feel frightened or threatened, go to a safe place, such as a police or fire station.

**Talk about it.** Meet with your family regularly, especially if you have teenagers, to talk about safe driving, says Dr. Nahl. Ask for feedback on your own driving, allow other family members to openly discuss driving habits or problems, and discuss potential scenarios and actions.

**Teach your children.** Babies and toddlers learn a lot in that car seat. "We call this the road-rage nursery," says Dr. Nahl. Before they even learn to speak, children absorb the attitudes of adults they ride with. They witness the yelling, the cursing, the gestures.

So learn to turn around those actions. Say something like: "Mommy just yelled at that other person. I really shouldn't do that." Also ask for your children's help. They might remind you to put on your seat belt, for example. Thank them, and encourage them. "You'll create a whole different culture in the car," Dr. Nahl says. That may pay off in the long run, and your children may be less aggressive when it's *their* turn to drive.

# ROSACEA
## 14 Face-Saving Steps

Quick . . . aside from spending lots of time in the public eye, what did former United States president Bill Clinton, the late Princess Diana, and the late comedian W. C. Fields all have in common?

They are three of the most famous people in the public eye to have had rosacea (pronounced "rose-AY-shah"), an inflammatory skin condition that often results in redness of the nose, cheeks, forehead, and chin. The skin condition affects an estimated 14 million Americans, but it is most common in people with fair complexions.

"I've seen it mostly in people of Scotch-Irish or British descent," says C. Ralph Daniel III, M.D. In some families of those nationalities, it's so common, it's considered a natural part of getting older.

"Rosacea is a common condition, but often the average person confuses it with adult acne or a skin allergy," says Dee Anna Glaser, M.D. It tends to be cyclical. It might be active for a while, then lessen in intensity, and then suddenly flare up again.

Left untreated, the redness becomes more permanent, and tiny blood vessels become visible. Bumps and pimples often develop, and in advanced cases, your nose may become bumpy, red, and swollen. In some cases, your eyes can appear watery or bloodshot, according to Dr. Glaser. That's why it's important to

**WHEN TO CALL A DOCTOR**

When a person starts to show early stages of rosacea, it's wise to see a dermatologist as soon as possible, suggests Dee Anna Glaser, M.D.

"A dermatologist can fully educate the person about rosacea—how to properly wash his or her face, how to deal with the things that trigger flare-ups, what should be avoided, and so forth," says Dr. Glaser. "The sooner the person gets that knowledge, the better."

get an early diagnosis and make the life changes necessary to keep the condition under control.

"The key is to know what triggers your flare-ups and to avoid those things as much as possible," says Dr. Glaser.

## Trigger Avoidance

As a rule, anything that causes a rosacea sufferer's face to get red or flush may trigger a flare-up. Among the most common trip wires are alcohol, heat, hot drinks, spicy foods, caffeine, stress, and sun exposure. To avoid a flare-up, make the following lifestyle changes.

**Be sun-savvy.** Sunscreens are helpful in decreasing rosacea. So you should use a quality sunscreen each and every time you go outdoors for an extended period of time, says Dr. Daniel.

Apply a broad-spectrum sunblock with a sun protection factor (SPF) of at least 15 to your face year-round, says Dr. Glaser. (Broad-spectrum sunblocks protect you from both the ultraviolet A and ultraviolet B waves of the sun.) Since perspiration and water can wash off your sunscreen, reapply it throughout the day.

**Cover your head.** If you're heading to the beach or spending extended time in the midday sun, wear a wide-brimmed hat, one with a 4-inch-wide brim, to keep the sun off your face and neck, says Dr. Glaser. Baseball caps, when worn with the bill in front, don't protect your ears, the back of your neck, or even most of your face from the sun.

**Follow the shade.** Minimize your midday sun exposure (10:00 A.M. to 3:00 P.M.), particularly during the summer months, or head to a shady spot on sunny days, says Dr. Daniel. At the beach or a backyard party, sit under a big umbrella. Also, if it's not too hot out, wear tightly woven clothing. It helps keep ultraviolet rays from penetrating your skin.

"Protecting yourself with sunblock and staying out of the sun are two ways to keep rosacea from cropping up again," says Dr. Daniel.

**Monitor your alcohol intake.** Alcoholic beverages can trigger flare-ups of rosacea. Use common sense: If alcohol aggravates your condition, reduce your intake or avoid alcohol entirely, says Dr. Daniel.

**Turn down the heat of your beverages.** A cup of piping hot coffee or hot chocolate may be a problem for some people with rosacea because hot beverages can make your face flush. Decreasing the temperature of your drink, even slightly, may be all that's required to keep enjoying coffee, tea, hot chocolate, or hot cider. "What triggers the rosacea to flare up can be different in different people, so it's up to you to figure out your triggers," says Dr. Glaser. "If it's hot coffee, try drinking it a little cooler. Or if you're a four-cup-a-day coffee drinker, then cut back to one or two cups instead or eliminate coffee entirely."

**Watch what you eat.** Hot, spicy food—seasoned with red and cayenne pepper, for instance—is a common rosacea trip wire. "If spicy foods make your rosacea worse, either eliminate or curtail your intake of them," says Dr. Daniel.

In some cases, other foods cause problems for people with rosacea, including avocados, broad-leafed beans and pods, cheese, chocolate, citrus fruit, eggplant, liver, sour cream, soy sauce, spinach, vanilla, vinegar, yeast extract, and yogurt.

"Keep a diary or make mental notes of what you eat and how it affects your rosacea," says Dr. Glaser. "Adjust your diet accordingly."

**Avoid high-intensity workouts.** Sure, exercise is an essential part of a healthy lifestyle, but too much exertion can cause rosacea to flare up, says Dr. Glaser. "You must still get exercise, but make adjustments. Exercise three times a day for 15 minutes rather than 45 minutes straight, to avoid overheating. Or in the summer months, exercise in an air-conditioned room or during the early evening hours when the sun isn't most intense," she says.

**Keep cool.** When exercising, drink cold fluids or chew on ice chips to keep from getting too overheated. Also, keep a bottle of cool water with you when you exercise either at home or at the gym. The water will keep you properly hydrated, and you can also spray it directly on your face for relief, says Dr. Daniel.

**Stay out of the sauna or hot tub.** The heat of hot tubs and saunas can bring on flushing and aggravate your condition, according to Larry Millikan, M.D.

**Be gentle when cleansing.** Begin each day with a thorough, but gentle cleansing of your face, says Dr. Millikan. Think "simple." People with rosacea get into trouble when they start using fancy soaps with fragrances, lots of preservatives, or harsh textures, he says.

So spread a gentle cleanser on your face softly with your fingertips. Then rinse your face with lukewarm, not hot, water to remove all dirt and soap, says Dr. Daniel.

Let your face air dry for a few minutes before applying any topical medication or skin-care products. Then allow the medication to completely dry for 5 to 10 minutes before applying a moisturizer or makeup.

Repeat the same cleansing process at night.

**Select skin-care products with care.** "Steer clear of products that include alcohol or other irritants, which may cause your face to burn, sting, or become red," says Dr. Glaser.

## Self-Esteem Boosters

The conspicuous redness, blemishes, and swelling caused by rosacea can take a psychological toll. It can make you camera-shy and even damage your self-esteem and self-confidence if you let it. Here are some tips to keep that from happening to you.

**Educate others.** If, during one of your flare-ups, you find yourself the object of stares or comments, turn this awkward situation into an educational situation by openly discussing your rosacea. Although the condition afflicts millions of people, many are unaware of it. So their actions may be simply caused by curiosity and a lack of knowledge on the subject.

**Wear the right clothes.** Avoid red or black-and-white garments, which accentuate your redness. Instead, opt for softer hues like blues, yellows, khakis, and other neutral colors.

**Keep makeup simple and natural.** Apply a contrasting concealer, usually a green tone, to offset rosacea's red appearance. Choose and apply a good foundation in the correct skin tone. Most people mistakenly match foundation to the back of their hand, but you'll get a truer color match by testing foundation colors under your chin. Follow with a loose powder to finish, making blemishes or redness less striking or noticeable.

## PANEL OF ADVISORS

**C. Ralph Daniel III, M.D.,** is a clinical professor of dermatology at the University of Mississippi Medical Center in Jackson.

**Dee Anna Glaser, M.D.,** is an associate professor of dermatology at St. Louis University School of Medicine.

**Larry Millikan, M.D.,** is chairman of the department of dermatology at Tulane University Medical Center in New Orleans.

# SCARRING

## 10 Ways to Decrease the Damage

Want to look mean and tough? Dress in black, smoke a fat cigar, carry a violin case, and—above all—have a big scar running down one cheek.

Of course, looking mean and tough may not be the look you're after. If that's the case, you've come to the right place. How you treat a cut can determine what kind of scar may develop. Then, how you care for that scar can determine how fast and to what extent it will fade over time. Here's what our experts suggest.

**Nip scars in the bud.** If you don't want dog hair on your sofa, don't own a dog. If you don't want cavities, don't eat sugar. And if you don't want scars, don't get cut. It's that simple. "Every time the skin gets cut, it scars,"

---

### WHEN TO CALL A DOCTOR

Generally, you'll be able to tell if a cut or scrape is severe enough to demand medical attention. Here are a few guidelines for those in-between situations, when you're not sure if a trip to the doc is appropriate or not. See a doctor if:

- Blood spurts or continues to flow after several minutes of pressure.
- Dirt or debris remains imbedded in the wound even after a thorough cleaning.
- You can't easily close the mouth of the wound.
- You notice any redness, drainage, warmth, or swelling—or the wound isn't healing properly.
- The wound is deep and dirty, and your last tetanus shot was more than 5 years ago.

---

says Gerald Imber, M.D. Some people, he says, tend to scar more than others. "It's a very personal thing."

However your body reacts, consider protecting your skin with gloves, long pants, and long sleeves whenever working around thorny, sharp, or jagged objects. If you cycle or skate, wear elbow and knee pads and wrist and shin guards to prevent accidental scrapes and abrasions.

**Don't pick at scabs.** Mom was right. Picking a scab off a healing wound could increase your chances of leaving behind a visible scar, says John F. Romano, M.D.

## Do just 1 thing

Thoroughly clean the wound. A wound that heals quickly and neatly is less likely to develop a scar than a wound that festers. Make sure that all your cuts and scrapes are properly cleaned, and try to keep the wound slightly moist with an antibiotic ointment while it is healing, says Jeffrey H. Binstock, M.D. If dirt and debris remain in the wound after washing, use tweezers cleaned with alcohol to remove particles.

**Close gaps with a butterfly bandage.** If you do get cut and the cut is large enough, you should go to a doctor for stitches, particularly if the cut is on the face where a scar would be most visible. But if a cut is small and you are concerned about scarring, consider using a butterfly bandage, says Dr. Romano. These bandages, available at most drugstores, can help keep the wound closed for better healing and minimal scarring. They should be used only after the wound has been thoroughly cleaned.

**Eat a well-balanced diet.** Wounds won't heal right unless your body has what it takes to *make* them heal right. What does it take? Protein and vitamins—obtained by eating a good, well-balanced diet—are essential. Of particular importance to wound healing is the mineral zinc. Good sources of zinc include roasted pumpkin and sunflower seeds, Brazil nuts, Swiss and Cheddar cheeses, peanuts, dark-meat turkey, and lean beef.

**Treat scars with tenderness.** Sweat glands, oil glands, and hair glands are all destroyed by a scar, leaving it much more at the mercy of the elements than the rest of your skin, says Paul Lazar, M.D. He advises keeping large scars, such as those from a third-degree burn, lubricated with a good skin cream to protect them from abrasions.

**Take it easy in the shower.** One common source of abrasions to tender scars is a washcloth in the hands of an overzealous washer. Dr. Lazar recommends cleaning scars very gently. If you shave in the shower, lather generously, and shave slowly. Replace your blade every three or four shaves to prevent cuts and skin irritation.

**Cover your scars with sunblock.** Scars have less pigment than the rest of your skin. They therefore lack the ability to develop a protective tan, and they are especially vulnerable to sunburn. Cover all scars with a strong sunscreen whenever you head outside on a sunny day, says Stephen Kurtin, M.D.

**Don't be overly alarmed.** Fresh scars are often quite noticeable, but don't be too concerned. Remember that the color of a scar typically fades over time all by itself, says Dr. Lazar.

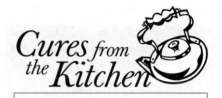

## Cures from the Kitchen

This kitchen cure actually comes from the sunny kitchen *windowsill.* Keep an aloe plant on your kitchen windowsill, and make the plant your ally for any minor cuts, scrapes, or wounds. Aloe is antibacterial, antifungal, antiviral, and an immune stimulant. Plus, the plant contains vitamins C and E and the mineral zinc, all nutrients shown to speed wound healing.

Studies suggest that commercial aloe preparations lose some of their wound-healing ability, so the plant is your best bet. Just snip off a leaf, slit it open, scoop out the gel, and apply it to your cut.

## PANEL OF ADVISORS

**Jeffrey H. Binstock, M.D.,** is an associate clinical professor of dermatologic surgery at the University of California, San Francisco, School of Medicine and a dermatologist in San Francisco and Mill Valley, California.

**Gerald Imber, M.D.,** is an attending plastic surgeon at New York–Presbyterian Hospital in New York City.

**Stephen Kurtin, M.D.,** is a practicing dermatologist and an assistant professor of dermatology at the Mount Sinai Hospital in New York City.

**Paul Lazar, M.D.,** is a professor emeritus of clinical dermatology at Northwestern University Medical School in Chicago. He is a former board member of the American Academy of Dermatology.

**John F. Romano, M.D.,** is a dermatologist and an assistant clinical professor of dermatology at New York Hospital–Cornell University Medical Center in New York City.

# SCIATICA
## 18 Strategies to Knock Out Nerve Pain

Nearly everyone experiences back pain on occasion, but only an unlucky few ever have to endure the agonizing pain of sciatica.

The sciatic nerve stretches down the lower back region, down the back of the legs to the ankles. Anything that puts pressure on the nerve, such as a herniated spinal disk, a bone spur, or spinal malalignment can result in sharp, shooting pains in the buttocks or legs.

A herniated disk is the most common cause of sciatica among young, active adults. This condition occurs when the outer wall of the disk, which normally functions as a shock absorber between the vertebrae, becomes torn, and the inner cushioning material moves into the spinal canal, where it compresses a nerve root.

Sciatica is often short-lived, but sometimes it persists for years. Even simple daily activities–bending over, sneezing, or having a bowel movement–can

---

### WHEN TO CALL A DOCTOR

About the only good thing concerning sciatica is that the pain is usually temporary. It often begins to feel better within 4 to 5 days, and most people will be well on the way to recovery within 6 weeks.

"There's no need to panic if you get sciatica, but it can be extraordinarily painful," says John G. Heller, M.D.

It's important to see a doctor right away, he adds. For one thing, you'll probably need medication to control the pain. You'll also want to be sure that you aren't risking permanent nerve damage.

One of the most serious warning signs is a loss of muscle function—your foot is dragging, for example, or you're stumbling when you walk. Even more serious is a loss of bowel or bladder control. If you have any one of these symptoms, don't wait to see your regular doctor, Dr. Heller advises. Go straight to an emergency room.

trigger attacks. Once the nerve has been irritated or damaged, the pain can persist even when you're lying still.

Because so many things can cause sciatica, and because the nerve can be permanently damaged without prompt treatment, it's essential to see a doctor at the first sign of symptoms. Surgery is sometimes required, but sciatica can usually be controlled with a combination of medications and home care. Here are a few ways to stop the pain and protect the nerve from additional harm.

**Ice it quickly.** At the first sign of pain, apply a cold compress (a small bag of ice cubes wrapped in a thin cloth) to the lower back for 15 to 20 minutes at a time, every 2 to 3 hours. Keep it cold for 24 to 48 hours. Cold reduces inflammation and helps prevent painful muscle spasms, says Andrew J. Cole, M.D.

The easiest approach is to use a gel pack, available at sporting goods and medical supply stores. The packs remain flexible even after they're chilled in the freezer. They mold themselves to the contours of your lower back, putting the cold right where you need it. In a pinch, you can even apply a bag of frozen peas or corn. Wrap it in a thin towel first to protect your skin.

**Use a heating pad.** After applying cold for a day or two, switch to heat, advises John J. Triano, D.C., Ph.D. Apply a hot-water bottle or a heating pad to your lower back for 15 minutes at a time. Repeat the treatment every hour, and keep doing it as long as it seems to help. Heat relaxes muscles and helps prevent painful spasms. It also increases circulation and helps flush pain-causing toxins from around the nerve.

# Do just 1 thing

Try stretching and flexibility exercises. They are among the best ways to reduce the inflammation and muscle spasms that often accompany sciatica, says John J. Triano, D.C., Ph.D.

Everyone responds differently to exercises. Some people do best with extension exercises, which include lying face-down, arching your back, and rising up on your elbows. Others require flexion movements—for example, lying on your back and bringing your knees to your chest. You'll have to experiment a bit to discover what works best for you.

"Stretching exercises encourage motion of the spine and associated joints, muscles, and ligaments, which can prevent adhesions or stiffness due to scar tissue formation after an injury," says John G. Heller, M.D. "If the exercises make you feel better, keep doing them. But they should never make pain worse or cause it to radiate down one or both legs. If they do, you'll know it's the wrong exercise for you and should seek professional advice."

No matter how much better heat makes you feel, don't use it for more than 15 minutes at a time. "Applying heat for longer can result in rebound swelling, which will make the pain worse later," says Dr. Triano.

**Take anti-inflammatory medications.** When you first feel the pain of sciatica, take aspirin, ibuprofen, or other nonsteroidal anti-inflammatory drugs (NSAIDs), Dr. Cole advises. They inhibit the body's production of prostaglandins, inflammatory chemicals that increase pain and swelling. Take the medications four times daily, following the dose listed on the label.

If aspirin or ibuprofen upset your stomach, it's fine to take acetaminophen—but keep in mind that it mainly works as a pain reliever. It has little effect on inflammation.

"I usually recommend naproxen (Aleve)," says Dr. Triano. "It's a good anti-inflammatory and is somewhat less likely than aspirin or ibuprofen to cause stomach upset."

**Go for a swim.** Or simply walk in water. The combination of warm water and gentle exercise will often loosen muscles and help relieve spasms and pain. Plus, water supports the body, which may relieve painful pressure on the back.

"Swimming and aquatic exercises are among the best rehabilitation tools available," says John G. Heller, M.D. It is especially effective for those who find exercise initially too painful by other means.

Most health clubs offer aquatics classes, he notes. Additionally, local arthritis associations often sponsor aquatics classes at community centers or YMCAs. The movements used in the classes are perfect for those with a history of back pain or sciatica, says Dr. Heller.

Swimming isn't recommended at the peak of an attack, but it's fine once the pain diminishes somewhat, Dr. Heller says. It's also a good preventive strategy for those who have had sciatica in the past.

**Walk if it's comfortable.** Walking is one of the best exercises for relieving and preventing sciatica. It keeps muscles limber and improves circulation throughout the body, including the area of the damaged nerve.

If you're in the acute stage of sciatica and walking causes sharp, stabbing pains, don't do it, Dr. Triano adds. "But if you've had the pain for more than a few days and it's mainly a dull, aching feeling, it's important to gently push through the discomfort with walking or other forms of gentle exercise."

**Strengthen your trunk muscles.** Also called the pelvic girdle, these are the muscles that surround and support the spine. "The basic curl-up is a good exercise for strengthening the muscles," says Dr. Cole.

Curl-ups are easy to do. Lie on your back with your pelvis tilted to flatten your back against the floor, your knees bent at about a 90-degree angle and your feet flat on the floor, and your arms at your side. Using your upper abdominal muscles, raise your head and shoulders off the floor. Your arms should be extended out in front. Then lower your shoulders to the floor in a slow, controlled motion. You don't want to raise your shoulders more than an inch or two, because that overtrains the muscle that links the lumbar spine to the legs and increases strain on the lower back, Dr. Cole explains.

**Get a massage.** It won't reverse underlying nerve or disk damage, but it can reduce muscle spasms and increase flexibility. "Massage makes people feel better, and that can allow their rehabilitation to advance," says Dr. Cole.

**Let your legs do the work.** Whether you currently have sciatica or have had it in the past, proper body mechanics—the ways you move every day—are essential. Bending from the waist, for example, is about the worst thing you can do. If you're doing anything more strenuous than picking up a sock, kneel or squat down and use your leg muscles to rise back up. Bending can trigger sciatica because it puts tremendous strain on the lower back, says Dr. Cole.

**Hold things close to your body.** Whether you're carrying a bag of groceries or a laundry basket, hold it as close to your body as possible, Dr. Cole advises. Holding weight close to your body takes some of the pressure off the lower spine.

**Support your lower back.** Sciatica can take weeks or even months to improve. In the meantime, giving your back extra support—by using a pillow or a rolled-up towel when you're sitting, for example—reduces pain and helps the injured area heal more quickly, says Dr. Triano.

Even better are pillows that inflate automatically with the turn of a valve. Available at camping stores and stores that specialize in back care, they allow you to easily change the firmness every 15 to 20 minutes. "They're a superb way of inexpensively minimizing back pain," says Dr. Triano.

Just don't think of back supports as a substitute for exercise and strong supporting muscles of the back, says Dr. Heller. Such muscles derived through disciplined exercise become your internal back support.

**Take frequent breaks.** Sitting is surprisingly hard on the lower back, especially when the sciatic nerve is inflamed and irritated. In fact, sitting without a back support can put about twice as much pressure on the spine as standing.

"If you have sciatica, your enemy is a prolonged, static posture," Dr. Triano says. "The elastic properties of your tissues are used up in about 20 minutes. After that, you're going to experience increased stress on the area."

If your job requires a lot of sitting, give your back a break by getting up at least every 15 to 20 minutes, or whenever your back starts feeling tense or tired. Walk around for a few minutes. Stretch. Give your muscles a chance to unwind before sitting back down again. "Keep this in mind during lengthy car or plane trips, too," notes Dr. Heller.

**Put a foot up.** The back naturally has a slight curve, but when you're standing flat-footed, the curve is accentuated, which can aggravate a sensitive sciatic nerve. A more "relaxed" posture affords slightly more room for the nerves.

"One of the best things you can do when you're standing is to alternately prop one foot up and then the other," says Dr. Triano. Elevating one foot slightly increases the "free" space around the sciatic nerve, and shifting from one foot to the other on a regular basis helps maintain elasticity in the spinal disks and surrounding tissues, he explains.

Whenever possible, rest your foot on a short stool or a step when standing. At the grocery store, rest one foot on the lower part of the shopping cart. On the street, use a curb or the base of a lamppost. Many people with sciatica find that elevating one foot even a few inches is often enough to temporarily eliminate the pain.

**Maintain a healthful weight.** The lower back supports a hefty amount of your body weight. The heavier you are, the more weight it has to carry—and the more likely you are to experience sciatica or other back problems.

"You can think of it as excessive loading of a structure. You might not pay a price for being overweight early on, but eventually it can be an aggravating factor for back problems and sciatica," says Dr. Heller.

**Stay out of the car.** Apart from the fact that most car seats are notoriously hard on the lower back, cars vibrate at four to five cycles per second—a frequency that can damage disks, increase muscle inflammation or spasms, and generally increase strain on the sciatic nerve.

Until your back is better, spend as little time in the car as possible. Even when you're out of pain, it's a good idea to limit driving time to 2 hours daily. Even then, get out of the car every 20 to 30 minutes to stretch and generally shake things up, says Dr. Triano.

**Find a position of comfort.** Everyone with sciatica has at least one posture or position that puts the least strain on the nerve. Some people experience less discomfort when their back is pitched slightly forward. Others do better when they stand military straight. Although good posture is important in the long run, don't obsess about it when you're in pain. Find whatever posture works best—and maintain it until the pain is gone.

Keep in mind, however, that a position of comfort has to be functional as well. If the only position that feels comfortable is flat on your back, or twisted around like a pretzel, work with a doctor or physical therapist to find a better alternative.

**Get plenty of sleep.** It's hard to do when you're hurting, but studies have shown that the body undergoes much of its healing during sleep. If pain is keeping you awake, try elevating your knees with a small pillow: It takes some of the pressure off the nerve, says Dr. Triano. If you usually sleep on your side, curl up and put a pillow between your knees.

**If you smoke, try to quit.** Cigarette smoke weakens the spinal disks and slows recovery if you're experiencing sciatica. If you need surgery for sciatica, smoking increases the risk that the operation won't be successful. "Some surgeons won't operate unless patients quit smoking," says Dr. Cole.

## PANEL OF ADVISORS

**Andrew J. Cole, M.D.,** is the medical director of the Spine Center at Overlake Hospital Medical Center and has a private practice with Northwest Spine and Sports Physicians in Bellevue, Washington. He was the director of Spine Rehabilitation Services at Baylor University Medical Center in Houston from 1993 to 1996, and coauthor of *Low Back Pain.*

**John G. Heller, M.D.,** is a professor of orthopedics surgery and director of the spine fellowship program at the Emory Spine Center at Emory University School of Medicine in Atlanta.

**John J. Triano, D.C., Ph.D.,** is director of the chiropractic division of the Texas Back Institute in Plano, Texas. His doctorate is in spine biomechanics. He specializes in prevention, treatment, and rehabilitation of neck and back disorders.

# SEASONAL AFFECTIVE DISORDER
## 15 Steps to a Brighter Outlook

Each autumn, as the days grow shorter, millions of people get the blues.

They may experience mild to severe depression, weight gain, lethargy, a desire to sleep more, and an increased appetite or cravings for carbohydrates such as cakes and cookies.

Almost magically in spring, their symptoms wane. They feel energized, sociable, and generally happy.

Their malady: seasonal affective disorder, or SAD, a form of depression most likely to occur in winter.

For about 5 percent of people, the condition is severe enough to interfere with daily activities, work, and relationships, says Norman E. Rosenthal, M.D. Another 15 percent experience milder symptoms known as subsyndromal SAD (S-SAD).

Scientists have studied SAD as a psychological disorder since the 1980s, when Dr. Rosenthal, formerly of the National Institute of Mental Health, named the illness.

Researchers don't fully understand what causes SAD, only that it is connected to light received by the brain through the eyes.

One theory is that light affects the hormone melatonin, which peaks in the brain at night and regulates your internal body clock. Another is that light tinkers with the neurotransmitter serotonin, a mood-regulating chemical in the brain.

There is no test for SAD. Diagnosis is based on the cluster of symptoms, which usually begin around October and fade around April and appear for two or more consecutive winters.

Because other conditions such as low thyroid functioning can mimic SAD, talk with your doctor before attempting to treat yourself, especially if you are severely depressed. Some of the suggestions below may complement treatment. If your symptoms are mild, try a few of these tips to dash the winter blues.

**Bring in the light.** Make your home shine, says Dr. Rosenthal. Add more lamps, brighten rooms with light-colored paint and carpets, raise window shades, and open draperies.

**Duplicate the sun.** Specially designed light fixtures, boxes, and visors offer full-spectrum lighting that replicate natural light without the harmful ultraviolet

## WHEN TO CALL A DOCTOR

Severe seasonal affective disorder can be helped by antidepressants such as selective serotonin reuptake inhibitors, or SSRIs. See a doctor if your symptoms are getting in the way of your work or relationships, says Norman E. Rosenthal, M.D.

Also get help if you feel despair about the future or are suicidal, or if you have major sleep or eating changes, such as a weight gain of 15 or 20 pounds.

"It's a matter of degree and a matter of dysfunction, versus unpleasantness or inconvenience," Dr. Rosenthal says. If self-help strategies aren't effective, seek guidance as well.

Don't use light therapy without consulting your physician and your eye doctor, says Brenda Byrne, Ph.D. Some medications may make your eyes sensitive to light.

rays. Light therapy is a proven treatment for SAD. Typically, people with SAD benefit from sitting in front of a light box for 30 minutes to 2 hours daily, Dr. Rosenthal says.

**Awaken to light.** If your symptoms are mild, put a bedroom light on a timer set to come on about an hour before you arise in the morning, says Dr. Rosenthal. "It helps people wake up in the morning, it helps them to feel better—even though it's just a regular bedside lamp—simply because the eyes are so very sensitive at that hour of the morning," he says. For more severe SAD, purchase a specially designed dawn simulator.

## Do just 1 thing

Walk outside. Go outdoors on a bright winter's day, and you'll naturally soak up some of that feel-good light, says Norman E. Rosenthal, M.D. Even on a cloudy day, you'll get more light than you would indoors. And it doesn't matter if you are bundled up—it's the light that is received through the eyes that helps to lift your mood. Aim for at least ½ hour daily for an emotional and physical boost.

**Take a window seat.** Sit by a window at work if you can. "Everybody wants a window seat," Dr. Rosenthal says. Even though the window's glass diminishes the sunlight's potency, you'll likely reap some mood-enhancing benefits.

**Get fit.** Whether you walk, jog, or cycle indoors or out, aerobic activity heightens mood-boosting brain chemicals that banish winter blues, says Dr. Rosenthal. For a one-two punch against SAD, combine exercise with light. For example, walk outside or set up a light box in front of your stationary cycle.

**Brave the weather.** "Winter weather can provide positive stimulation," says Andrew Weil, M.D. "Get out your cross-country skis or snowshoes on a brisk day," he says. "Find some outdoor chores to do when the sun turns the sky a brilliant blue." Enjoy the sensation of snowflakes on your cheeks. Be sure to dress warmly, and keep moving.

**Manage stress.** Don't set deadlines for winter if you have a choice. Similarly in winter, avoid long days of work that keep you out of the light. "Understand that winter is a time of year when you don't deal so well with stress," Dr. Rosenthal says.

**Prepare for winter.** Anticipate those months when your overall energy may flag, says Brenda Byrne, Ph.D. Instead of waiting until the holiday season to shop for gifts or address greeting cards, for example, complete those tasks in the warmer months, when you're likely to feel more energetic.

**Pencil in a vacation.** Then follow through. Even 3 to 4 days in a warm, sunny climate may pull you out of the doldrums, especially if your blues are mild. "Most people notice that within a few days, they really do feel better," says Dr. Byrne.

**Relocate.** If you're contemplating a move, think about heading south. The farther south you go, the lower the incidence of SAD and S-SAD. Researchers estimate, for example, that about 9.7 percent of people in New Hampshire experience seasonal blues, while in Florida only about 1.4 percent suffer similarly.

**Seek warmth.** Some experts believe that temperature affects seasonal changes in behavior, says Dr. Byrne. "Lots of people with SAD also hate cold weather and tell me they can't get warm in winter, no matter how many layers of socks they put on," she says. People who dislike cold may simply avoid the outdoors in winter and get less sunlight, worsening their blues. Some possible strategies for staying warmer: Nudge the thermostat upward, wrap yourself in an electric blanket, or sip hot beverages.

**Curb carbs.** "Many, many SAD patients claim to be carbohydrate addicts," says Dr. Rosenthal. But overdosing on carbohydrate-rich foods—comfort

## Lighten Up with These Resources

Norman E. Rosenthal, M.D., recommends these sources of full-spectrum lighting for the treatment of seasonal affective disorder (SAD) or winter blues.

- The SunBox Company, 19217 Orbit Drive, Gaithersburg, MD 20879. Call (800) 548-3962, or visit their Web site at www.sunboxco.com.
- Apollo Light Systems, 369 South Mountain Way Drive, Orem, UT 84058. Call (800) 545-9667, or go to www.apollolight.com.

- Bio-Brite, 4340 East-West Highway, Suite 401S, Bethesda, MD 20814. Call (800) 621-5483, or go to www.biobrite.com.

For more information on SAD, visit Dr. Rosenthal's Web site at www. normanrosenthal.com. Or contact the Society for Light Treatment and Biological Rhythms in San Francisco. Visit the society's Web site at www.sltbr.org.

# The Evolution of Seasonal Affective Disorder

The importance of light's influence on human behavior makes sense from an evolutionary point of view, says Norman E. Rosenthal, M.D.

"We evolved in a 24-hour day in which part is dark and part is light, and there's a whole different biology of what we do when it's dark and when it's light," he says. "When it's dark, we rest. We hunt and are active and explore the world when it's light. All that is based on our vision, on when it's safe to be out and about. And it's only safe when you can see."

Animals, too, are tuned in to seasonal changes. Some gain weight to prepare for winter's hibernation, for example. Others change color to camouflage themselves against the snow.

"The new development with seasonal affective disorder was the extension of this awareness of seasonality to humans," Dr. Rosenthal says. "In some extra-sensitive people, there is quite a complex set of behavioral changes that occur with the change in seasons."

foods like candy, cookies, cakes, potatoes, breads and pastas—can lead to lethargy and weight gain. Substitute protein-dense meals, especially in the morning and afternoon. Instead of cereal at breakfast, try an egg-white omelet. Rather than a sandwich at lunch, opt for a chicken Caesar salad without the croutons.

**Supplement your diet.** Reach for a daily multivitamin containing ample amounts of the B's, such as vitamin $B_6$, thiamin, and folic acid, says Dr. Rosenthal. Studies show that the B vitamins, in particular, can enhance mood.

**Try an herb.** St. John's wort benefits some people with winter depression. Try 300 milligrams of a standardized extract containing 0.3 percent hypericin (the active ingredient) three times daily, says Dr. Weil. "Since St. John's wort may take 6 to 8 weeks to work, start this well before the dark days of winter," he says.

*Note:* Do not combine St. John's wort with light therapy without consulting your physician and your eye doctor. The herb may make your eyes overly sensitive to the light.

## PANEL OF ADVISORS

**Brenda Byrne, Ph.D.,** is a psychologist and director of the seasonal affective disorder program of the light research program at Jefferson Medical College of Thomas Jefferson University in Philadelphia.

**Norman E. Rosenthal, M.D.,** is a clinical professor of psychiatry at Georgetown University in Washington, D.C., and a former senior researcher at the National Institute of Mental Health. He is author of *Winter Blues: Seasonal Affective Disorder* and *The Emotional Revolution.*

**Andrew Weil, M.D.,** is a clinical professor of medicine and director of the program in integrative medicine at the University of Arizona in Tucson. He is the author of several books, including *8 Weeks to Optimum Health.*

# SHINGLES
## 17 Tips to Combat the Pain

It's a medical mystery. Shingles arises when the long-dormant chickenpox virus, known as herpes zoster, suddenly reawakens in nerve cells, making its way to the skin in a swath of burning pain, tingling, and numbness. On the skin's surface, it may cause a painful rash and blisters, generally on the chest or back, but sometimes on the face, arms, legs, even inside the mouth.

Scientists just don't know why chickenpox leads, years later, to shingles in some individuals. Stress, illness, and a vulnerable immune system are thought to be contributing factors.

With the advent of the chickenpox vaccine in children, shingles will probably one day be just a footnote in medical history books. That offers little comfort to today's sufferers, many of whom are older adults. Among seniors over age 80, 50 percent may develop this frustrating and uncomfortable illness.

As if the rash, blisters, and pain of a shingles outbreak weren't enough, in some people shingles pain may persist long after the rash disappears. This complication, called post-herpetic neuralgia, results from damaged nerve fibers. It can be exceedingly painful and difficult to treat.

It's important to see your doctor for this complicated condition. Meanwhile, here's what you can do to make yourself as comfortable as possible.

### At the Outset

Here is what the experts recommend for the beginning stages of shingles.

**Reach for pain relief.** Jules Altman, M.D., favors Extra-Strength Tylenol, an aspirin substitute.

## WHEN TO CALL A DOCTOR

If you have symptoms of shingles and notice a rash beginning to develop, it's important that you see a doctor as soon as possible, preferably within 72 hours. That's because the three antiviral drugs approved to treat shingles need to be started early in the course of the illness. When they're taken right away, these drugs have been proven to shorten the time of viral activity, help the rash to heal more quickly, and reduce the intensity of shingles pain and the time it lasts.

What these drugs don't necessarily prevent is post-herpetic neuralgia, the nerve pain that lingers after the skin heals. Help is even available for those who have a chronic case of post-herpetic neuralgia. One of the relatively new medications is the Lidoderm patch. The medication in the patch penetrates the skin, reaching the damaged nerves just under the skin. If your shingles pain is more than you can stand, see your doctor as soon as possible. This is no time for stoicism. Ignore your discomfort, and you could end up with irreversible nerve damage and years of pain, says Leon Robb, M.D.

**Take St. John's wort.** This herbal remedy may help to reduce nerve pain and has antiviral properties as well explains Sota Omoigui, M.D. He recommends taking 200 to 300 milligrams of St. John's wort two or three times daily until the pain is gone.

**Give yourself a boost.** Both your immune system and your nerves will benefit from extra doses of vitamin C and B-complex vitamins, says John G. McConahy, M.D. He advises his shingles patients to take 200 milligrams of vitamin C five or six times a day to build immune power and a B-complex vitamin supplement to regenerate and rebuild nerve cells.

**Reach for olive leaf extract.** Similar to vitamins and minerals in its immune-boosting power, this herbal remedy is also an antiviral therapy notes Cynthia Mervis Watson, M.D. She recommends 500 milligrams three times a day from the time of diagnosis until the shingles outbreak is gone.

**Try lysine.** A number of studies show that the amino acid lysine can help inhibit the spread of the herpes virus. Not all studies on lysine point to that conclusion, however.

Taking lysine supplements at the onset of shingles can't hurt and might help, says Leon Robb, M.D.

# For Shingles Blisters

Once blisters appear, there are several ways you can get relief.

**Do nothing.** Leave the blisters alone unless your rash is really bad, says Dr. Robb. "You can retard healing if you irritate the skin by applying too many skin creams and ointments."

**Make a calamine liniment.** This recipe comes from James J. Nordlund, M.D. You may be able to get your local pharmacist to make it for you.

Add to calamine lotion, 20 percent isopropyl alcohol and 1 percent each of phenol and menthol. If the phenol is too strong or the menthol too cool, dilute the liniment with equal parts of water.

"Use this as often as you want in the course of a day until the blisters are dried and scabbed over," says Dr. Nordlund. "Then don't use it anymore."

**Try a chloroform/aspirin paste.** Mash two aspirin tablets into a powder. Add 2 tablespoons of chloroform and mix. Put the paste onto the affected area with a clean cotton ball. You can apply the paste several times a day. You can also ask your pharmacist to make this mixture for you, Dr. Robb says.

The chloroform is said to dissolve soap residue, oil, and dead cells in the skin. That leaves the aspirin to soak into the skin folds and desensitize the affected nerve endings. You should begin to feel better in 5 minutes. The relief can last for hours, even days. Skip this tip if allergic to aspirin.

**Apply a wet dressing to severe eruptions.** Take a washcloth or towel, dip it in cold water, squeeze it out, and apply it to the affected area, says Dr. Nordlund. "The cooler it is, the better it feels," he says.

**Stay cool.** Avoid anything that will make your blistered skin hotter. Heat will just macerate the skin, says Dr. Robb.

**Sink into a starch bath.** If you have shingles on your forehead, skip to the next tip. But if the problem is below your neck, this can help. Just throw a handful of cornstarch or colloidal oatmeal, such as Aveeno, into your bathwater and settle in for a good soak, says Dr. Nordlund.

"People find this helpful, although the relief may not last long," he adds. "I often have my patients do this 20 minutes before bed, then they take something for the pain to help them sleep."

**Zap the infection with hydrogen peroxide.** If the blisters become infected, try dabbing them with hydrogen peroxide. Don't dilute it. Straight out of the bottle is fine, says Dr. Robb.

**Use an antibiotic ointment.** But be careful about which one you choose. Neomycin and Neosporin are notorious as skin sensitizers, says Dr. Nordlund. Polysporin or erythromycin are better choices.

## Post-Blister Care

You may have some discomfort even when the blisters are gone. Here's what to do.

**Try Zostrix.** Zostrix is an over-the-counter remedy for shingles pain. Its active ingredient is capsaicin, a derivative of the red pepper used to make chili powder. Scientists believe it works by blocking the production of a chemical needed to transmit pain impulses between nerve cells.

Using this topical ointment on blistering skin, however, is "like putting red peppers on active shingles," says Dr. Altman. "The idea behind Zostrix is its counterirritant effect. It is for healed skin that has a pain sensation, not for an open, oozing infection."

**Get the benefits of capsaicin in your diet.** Using cayenne pepper on your food may speed pain relief, since it contains the same extract as the capsaicin in pain-relieving creams. Sprinkle cayenne pepper on eggs, soups, and casseroles, or use it in marinade sauces.

**Chill out with ice.** If you still have pain after the blisters have healed, put ice in a plastic bag and stroke the skin vigorously, says Dr. Robb. "What we're trying to do here is confuse the nerves."

**Seek emotional help.** Sometimes, for some people, long-lasting shingles pain may point to some underlying emotional need that's not being met, says Dr. Altman. Is the pain diverting your attention away from some other problem? Or is the pain diverting much-needed attention to you? It's an issue to consider, he says, and one which you may want to discuss with your doctor.

## PANEL OF ADVISORS

**Jules Altman, M.D.,** is a clinical professor of dermatology at Wayne State University in Detroit and a practitioner in Warren, Michigan.

**John G. McConahy, M.D.,** is a retired dermatologist in New Castle, Pennsylvania.

**James J. Nordlund, M.D.,** is a professor in the department of dermatology at the University of Cincinnati College of Medicine in Ohio.

**Sota Omoigui, M.D.,** is medical director of the L.A. Pain Clinic in Hawthorne, California.

**Leon Robb, M.D.,** is a pain-management specialist, anesthesiologist, and director of the Robb Pain Management Group in Los Angeles, where he treats patients with shingles and conducts research.

**Cynthia Mervis Watson, M.D.,** is a family practice physician in Santa Monica, California, who specializes in herbal therapy and homeopathy.

# SHINSPLINTS
## 13 Ways to Soothe Sore Legs

Shinsplints aren't hard to get.

Faulty posture, poor shoes, fallen arches, insufficient warmups, poor running mechanics, poor walking mechanics, and overtraining can lead to the telltale shin pain.

Shinsplints are one of the most common and disabling conditions in aerobics. Long-distance runners have probably suffered with them since the first road was paved.

Most people know when they have shinsplints, but very few—experts included—know what they are. Most doctors prefer the terms *tendinitis,* or *periostitis,* though they can't say for certain which of those terms, if either, actually describes the condition.

### WHEN TO CALL A DOCTOR

Because some experts believe shinsplints may actually be stress fractures in an early stage, telling the difference between the two is sometimes tricky. Even so, shinsplints can become full-blown stress fractures with continued abuse, so seeing your doctor for an early diagnosis is crucial.

"With a stress fracture, you're going to have pinpoint pain, about the size of a dime or quarter," says trainer Marjorie Albohm. "If somebody asks you where it hurts, you'll be able to go right to it, put one or two fingers on it, and tell them exactly where it is. It'll be right on or around a bony area, and it's point-specific. A shinsplint will be an aching discomfort up and down the whole lower leg."

Some say shinsplints are the start of a stress fracture. Others contend they are a muscle irritation. Still others think they are an irritation of the tendon that attaches muscle to the bone.

The symptoms of shinsplints are often confused with those of stress fracture. But shinsplints typically include pain in the shin of one or both legs, though there may or may not be a specific area of tenderness. Pain and aching will be felt in the front of the leg after activity, although it may occur during activity as the condition progresses.

The remedies here are designed to help keep that shinsplint condition from progressing to the point of stress fracture and to let you continue your active lifestyle without causing undue harm. Let pain be your guide. If anything recommended here causes increased discomfort, don't do it.

**Start with the ground.** Unyielding surfaces can produce shinsplints in an instant. "Start by looking at the surface," advises trainer Marjorie Albohm. "If you're walking, running, dancing, playing basketball, or whatever on a hard, unyielding surface, then you need to change that."

For those involved in aerobics, injuries are highest on concrete floors covered with carpet, while wood floors over airspace are the least damaging. If you must dance on a nonresilient floor, make sure that the instructor teaches only low-impact aerobics or that high-quality foam mats are provided. For runners, choose grass or dirt before asphalt, and asphalt before concrete. Concrete is very unyielding and should always be avoided.

**Then move to the shoes.** If you can't change your surface, or if you find that's not the problem, look at different footwear. Choose a shoe with good arch support, shock-absorption quality in the sole, and fit, says Albohm.

For those who participate in activities that cause a lot of forefoot impact such as aerobics, judge a shoe on its ability to absorb shock in that area. The best test is to try the shoes on in the store and jump up and down, both on the toes and flat-footed. The impact with the floor should be firm but not jarring.

For runners, the choice is a bit more difficult. Research has shown that about 58 percent of all runners with shinsplints also pronate excessively (meaning the foot rolls to the inside). Choosing a shoe for pronation control sometimes results in a loss of cushioning. If you're a pronator with shinsplints, motion-control shoes are probably what you need most. These shoes are rigid, durable, control-oriented running shoes that limit pronation.

**Choose shoes often.** One way to make sure your shoes retain as much cushioning ability as possible is to change them frequently. Runners who put in 25 miles a week or more need new shoes every 60 to 90 days, says Gary M. Gordon, D.P.M. Less mileage means new shoes every 4 to 6 months. Those who participate in aerobics, tennis, or basketball twice a week need new shoes two or three times a year, while those who participate up to four times a week need them every 60 days.

**Put it on RICE.** As soon as you notice shinsplint pain, follow the rules of RICE: rest, ice, compression, and elevation for 20 to 30 minutes a day. The experts swear by it.

Keep your icing routine simple, Albohm says. Just prop the leg up, wrap it with an elastic bandage, and place the ice pack on it for 20 to 30 minutes.

**Go for contrast.** A variation on the RICE treatment is the contrast bath, which seems especially effective for pain on the inner leg. With this method, alternate 1 minute of ice with 1 minute of heat. Do this before any activity that can cause shinsplint pain, and continue it for at least 12 minutes.

**Master massage.** "For shinsplints in the front of the leg, you want to massage the area right near the edge of the shin—not directly on it," says masseur Rich Phaigh. "If you work right on the bone, it just seems to make the inflammation worse."

To massage away shinsplint pain, sit on the floor with one knee bent and the foot flat on the ground. Start by lightly stroking both sides of the bone using the palms of your hands, gliding them back and forth from knee to ankle. Repeat this stroking motion several times. Then wrap your hands around the calf and, using the tips of your fingers, stroke deeply on each side of the bone from ankle to knee. Cover the area, using as much pressure as possible.

"What you want to do is restore length and relieve tightness in the tendons at the top and bottom of the shins," Phaigh says, noting that a good massage helps improve circulation in the area, too.

**Correct faulty feet.** Flat feet or very high arches can sometimes cause shinsplints, Dr. Gordon says. "If you have flat feet, the muscle on the inside of your calf has to work harder and gets fatigued quicker," he says, "making the bone take more of a pounding."

If you're flat-footed, you may need additional shock-absorbing material or arch support in your shoes. Inserts are available at sporting goods stores, but it might be best to see a podiatrist before adding inserts on your own.

Pain on the outside of the lower leg is sometimes associated with very high arches, Dr. Gordon says. "That requires a lot of stretching exercises, as well as strengthening the muscles and maybe adding orthotics."

**Stretch those calves.** Stretching the Achilles tendon and the calf muscles is an excellent preventive measure for shinsplints, Albohm says. "If you're a woman wearing 2-inch heels every day, you're not stretching either of those at all."

Stretching helps because shortened calf muscles tend to throw more weight and stress forward to the shins. Place your hands on a wall, extend one leg behind the other, and press the back heel slowly to the floor. Do this 20 times and repeat with the other leg.

**Now tend to the tendons.** Dr. Gordon offers this simple technique for stretching the Achilles tendon: Keep both feet flat on the ground about 6 inches apart. Then bend your ankles and knees forward while keeping your back straight. Go to the point of tightness and hold for 30 seconds. "You should feel it really stretching down in the lower part of the calf," he says. Repeat the exercise 10 times.

**Build muscle, reduce pain.** Shinsplint pain can sometimes be prevented by strengthening the muscles surrounding the shin. These muscles help decelerate the foot and reduce shock whenever you walk or run. Help strengthen them with the following.

- Try riding a bike with pedal clips. Concentrate on pulling up with the muscles in front of the shin every time you pedal. (Bicycling also gives you a good aerobic workout without aggravating shinsplints.)
- If you don't have access to a bike, walking around on your heels does much the same thing, forcing you to tighten and pull up with the muscles around the shin each time you take a step.
- If you're seeking a conditioning exercise that's a bit more strenuous, try this: Sit on the edge of a table that's high enough to keep your feet from touching the ground. Place a sock filled with coins over your foot, or make a 5-pound weight from an old paint can by filling it with gravel (place this over the foot with a shoe on so the wire doesn't hurt). Flex the foot upward at the ankle, then relax, then flex the foot upward again. Repeat this as many times as you can, tightening your shin muscles as you pull the foot up.

## PANEL OF ADVISORS

**Marjorie Albohm** is a certified athletic trainer at Orthopaedics Indianapolis. She served on the medical staffs for the 1980 Winter and 1996 Summer Olympics and the 1987 Pan American Games.

**Gary M. Gordon, D.P.M.,** has a sports medicine practice in Glenside, Pennsylvania, where he specializes in podiatric medicine and foot surgery.

**Rich Phaigh** is codirector of the American Institute of Sports Massage in New York City and the owner of a therapeutic massage clinic in Eugene, Oregon. He has taught more than 250 classes in advanced therapeutic technique in the United States and abroad. Phaigh has worked on the likes of running stars Alberto Salazar and Joan Samuelson.

# SIDE STITCHES
## 9 Ways to Avoid the Nuisance

A stitch or catch in the side—a sharp, temporary pain—is caused by a spasm of the diaphragm. It happens when the diaphragm, a muscle between the chest and abdomen, can't get the oxygen it needs.

This often happens to runners.

"Every time you raise your knee, you contract your belly muscles, which increases the pressure inside your belly," explains Gabe Mirkin, M.D. The end result: cramping of the diaphragm because the bloodflow is shut off.

You also can get side stitches from walking, or even laughing.

Here's how to handle them.

**Stop.** When the pain hits, stop whatever you are doing. You need to relax to calm your twitching muscle.

**Slow down and walk.** If you're running when you get a stitch, sometimes just slowing to a walk is enough to calm that jerking muscle, says Suki Munsell, Ph.D. When the twinge fades, speed up again.

**Press there.** Using three fingers, press on the area where the pain is the worst until the hurt stops. Or, use those three fingers to gently massage the painful area. Often this is enough to release the pain, says sports psychotherapist David Balboa.

**Exhale deeply.** As you begin to knead the cramp out of your diaphragm, take a breath, then purse your lips and blow it out as hard as you can. Take another breath and exhale again. The inhaling followed by a deep exhalation works like yoga, says Balboa, giving you an internal massage for your pinched muscle.

**Breathe in, breathe out.** Continue to massage your aching side and work to slow your breathing to a regular pace. Getting your breathing back to a steady rhythm will help stop the ache.

**Belly-breathe.** Before you go out to walk or run again, you need to know how to breathe to prevent stitches from taking sides.

Balboa suggests trying this test: Look down at your chest. Watch closely as you suck in a giant breath. What moved? If only your chest moved, you're breathing with your chest cavity and that's not enough. To fight side stitches, you want your diaphragm involved in the breathing exercise. One way to tell if you're using the right muscle is to get your chest *and* belly to move when you breathe. Keep an eye on your belly. Inhale. Exhale. It should move in and out. People need to get out of their military-style postures to exercise comfortably, says Balboa.

As you practice your belly breathing, take deep breaths. Exhale deeply. Be aware of your breathing while you exercise, and within a couple of weeks, diaphragmatic breathing will become habit.

**Massage your diaphragm.** Like any muscle, the diaphragm needs to be warmed up before it exercises. So before you stretch your legs, give your diaphragm a breath massage and get it in working order. Sit on the floor and place one hand on your chest, the other on your belly. As you breathe, both hands should move up and down, indicating you're using your full breathing capacity, including your diaphragm. A warmed diaphragm is less likely to stitch.

**Breathe all the time.** People naturally hold their breath when they are frightened or cold or when they want to avoid pain, says Balboa. If you allow yourself to feel your emotions and not try to avoid them by holding your breath, you're more likely to breathe naturally when exercise demands a constant flow of air, he suggests.

**Stop to go.** Even though side stitches are caused by a pinched diaphragm, some walkers and runners will get a similar feeling from trapped gas, says Dr. Munsell.

Any aerobic activity will slow or stop the digestive process while the blood rushes to help the muscles, says Balboa. That's why runners are told not to eat at least 2 hours before a race. It's also the reason runners sometimes get diarrhea if they drink a lot of water during a race.

Their advice? Be careful what and when you eat before you exercise. Eat plenty of fiber. Try to have a bowel movement before you begin any exercise if you are prone to side stitches.

## PANEL OF ADVISORS

**David Balboa, M.S.W.,** is a codirector of the Walking Project in New York City. He is an expert on walking and mind-body relationships.

**Gabe Mirkin, M.D.,** is an associate clinical professor of pediatrics at Georgetown University School of Medicine in Washington, D.C., and in practice at Mirkin Medical Consultants in Kensington, Maryland. He is the author of several sports medicine books, including *Women and Exercise*, and a syndicated newspaper columnist and radio broadcaster.

**Suki Munsell, Ph.D.,** a registered movement therapist, is president of the Dynamic Health and Fitness Institute in Corte Madera, California. A fitness consultant, her doctorate is in movement education and body transformations.

# SINUSITIS
## 16 Infection Fighters

Sinuses are air-filled pockets that serve as small air-quality-control centers under your cheekbones, above your eyes and nose, and behind your eye sockets. It's their job to help warm, moisten, purify, and generally condition the air you breathe before it hits your lungs. When they're functioning properly, entering bacteria get trapped and filtered out by mucus and minute nasal hairs called cilia that line your sinuses.

This little air-flow system may gum up, however, if something impedes the cilia, if a cold clogs the sinus openings, or if an allergen swells the sinus linings. Then air gets trapped, pressure builds, the mucus stagnates, and bacteria or other organisms can breed. Infection and inflammation of the sinuses can set in, a disorder called sinusitis.

When you try to sleep, it's as if you've sprung a slow leak. All night long, the drip, drip of nasal fluid trickles down your throat, sending you into coughing spasms.

Pressure and pain around the face, teeth, or eyes; headache; and a thick green or yellow nasal discharge are the hallmarks of acute sinusitis. You may run a fever as well. Acute sinusitis is usually caused by viruses or bacteria and can last a month or longer.

If you get clogged up too many times, you may wind up with a permanent thickening of the sinus membranes and a chronic stuffy nose. Less common than acute sinusitis, chronic sinusitis is caused by allergies—especially to dust, mold, pollen, and certain fungi—or other conditions and typically lasts longer than 8 weeks.

Doctors generally prescribe antibiotics to clear the infection if it's bacterial. But there are also a number of steps you can take to feel better. Here's what the doctors say you can do to unstuff your sinuses, reduce pain and pressure, and get the air flowing freely.

## WHEN TO CALL A DOCTOR

If you've tried self-treatment for 3 to 4 days and still have sinus pain, pressure, and stuffiness, you need to see a doctor to help clear up the infection and drain your sinuses, advises Terence M. Davidson, M.D. "Otherwise, your sinuses could abscess into your eye, or worse, into your brain."

You may also have chronic sinusitis, which can be a recurrent or prolonged disorder lasting for months or even years. Depending on the cause, you may need to take a longer course of antibiotics than for acute sinusitis or undergo a sinus drainage procedure or surgery to break up the blockage. A sinus specialist can perform x-rays or other tests to discover what's causing your congestion, be it bacteria, an obstruction like polyps, allergies, untreated acute sinusitis, or a sensitivity to medications such as birth control pills or aspirin.

**Get all steamed up.** "Humidity is the key to keeping the cilia working, the mucus flowing, and the sinuses drained," says Stanley N. Farb, M.D. Twice a day, stand in a shower hot enough to fog up the mirror. Or lean over a pan full of steaming water with a towel draped over your head, creating a steam tent. Inhale the vapors as they waft up toward your nostrils.

**Get steam on the run.** If stuffiness hits during the day when you're at work or on the run, get a cup of hot coffee, tea, or soup, cup your hands over the top of the mug, and sniff, suggests Howard M. Druce, M.D. It won't work as well as a steam bath, but it will provide some relief.

**Humidify your home.** Running a humidifier in your bedroom prevents your nasal and sinus passages from drying out, says Bruce Jafek, M.D. Just make sure you clean it once a week so that fungi don't invade your humidifier.

You can use either a cool-mist or warm-mist humidifier. Dr. Jafek suggests starting with a cool-mist machine. Though the room won't heat up like it would with a warm-mist unit, cool-mist machines may be safer since they won't burn if accidentally tipped over, he says.

**Bathe your nostrils daily.** To flush out stale nasal secretions, Dr. Jafek suggests using saline nasal sprays or drops, such as Breathe Right or Ayr, or mixing 1 teaspoon of table salt with 2 cups of warm water and a pinch of baking soda. Pour the liquid into a squirt bottle or medicine dropper, tilt your head back, close one nostril with your thumb, and squirt the solution into the open nostril while sniffing. Then blow that nostril gently. Repeat on the other side. You can also use a mister to spray the solution into your nos-

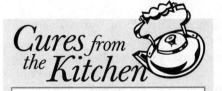

# Cures from the Kitchen

The way to find sinus relief may be through your stomach—eating foods that make your eyes water or nose run will help burst through your sinus blockage, says Howard M. Druce, M.D. Here's what he recommends.

**Garlic.** This pungent herb contains the same chemical found in a drug that makes mucus less sticky, says Dr. Druce.

**Horseradish.** This pungent root contains a chemical similar to one found in decongestants, he says. The bottled variety works just fine.

**Cajun spice seasoning.** You probably can't go wrong if you order Cajun food. These spicy dishes are made with cayenne chile peppers, which contain capsaicin, a substance that can stimulate the nerve fibers and may act as a natural nasal decongestant. Other hot peppers contain this potent compound as well. Look for the smaller varieties—they're usually hotter and have more capsaicin than the larger types—or use ground red pepper (cayenne) or other ground chiles in cooking.

trils, but keep your head in an upright position.

**Drink up.** Drinking extra water or other liquids—both hot and cold—throughout the day, thins out the mucus and keeps it flowing, says Dr. Farb. Sipping hot teas made with herbs such as fenugreek, fennel, anise, or sage may help move mucus even more.

**Blow one nostril at a time.** This helps prevent pressure buildup in the ears, which can send bacteria farther back into the sinus passages, Dr. Farb says.

**Go ahead and sniffle.** It turns out, says Dr. Farb, that sniffling is also a good way to drain the sinuses and escort stale secretions down the throat.

**Unstuff yourself with decongestant tablets.** The best over-the-counter medications to help drain sinuses are single-action tablets that contain only decongestants, such as Sudafed or Drixoral, says Dr. Farb. Decongestants constrict the blood vessels, which may reduce the swollen membranes. Air can then pass through the nose, and pressure is alleviated. You should avoid products containing antihistamines if you're stuffed up from an infection, he adds. "They work by drying nasal secretions and may plug you up more."

**Use medicated nasal sprays sparingly.** Medicated nose sprays or drops, such as Afrin or Neo-Synephrine, are fine to use in a pinch, but frequent use of these products could actually prolong the condition or even make it worse, warns Terence M. Davidson, M.D. It's what specialists call the "rebound effect."

Initially, the sprays shrink your nasal linings, explains Dr. Davidson. "But then the mucosa reacts by swelling even more than before, creating a vicious cycle of use. It can take weeks for the swelling to finally subside after you stop using the sprays."

**Take a walk.** Exercise, says Dr. Farb, may bring blessed relief because it releases adrenaline, which constricts the blood vessels, thereby possibly reducing swelling in the sinuses.

**Apply pressure.** Rubbing your sore sinuses brings a fresh blood supply to the area and soothing relief, suggests Dr. Jafek. Press your thumbs firmly on both sides of your nose and hold for 15 to 30 seconds. Repeat.

**Use heat.** Applying moist heat over tender sinuses, Dr. Druce says, is an easy way to wash away sinus pain. Apply a warm washcloth over your eyes and cheekbones and leave it there until you feel the pain subside. It may take only a few minutes.

**Stay where you are.** Some people decide to relocate if their allergies cause chronic sinusitis. It's not a wise move. "If you are allergy-prone," says Dr. Farb, "your sensitivities will follow you wherever you go, and sinusitis will reappear." In other words, you may eventually develop an allergy to desert dust if you move to the Southwest. Or, if you move to a humid climate like Miami, you may develop a sensitivity to mold. The solution? Control your exposure to allergens where you live now. (For some ideas on how to do it, see Allergies on page 15.)

## PANEL OF ADVISORS

**Terence M. Davidson, M.D.,** is a professor of head and neck surgery and director of the Nasal Dysfunction Clinic at the University of California, San Diego, Medical Center.

**Howard M. Druce, M.D.,** is an associate clinical professor of medicine in the division of allergy and immunology at the University of Medicine and Dentistry of New Jersey/New Jersey Medical School in Newark.

**Stanley N. Farb, M.D.,** is a retired chief of otolaryngology at Montgomery and Suburban Mercy Hospitals in Norristown, Pennsylvania.

**Bruce W. Jafek, M.D.,** is a professor in the department of otolaryngology at the University of Colorado School of Medicine in Denver. He served as chairman of the department for 22 years before returning to clinical practice and teaching. Dr. Jafek practices at University Hospital, Rose Medical Center, the Children's Hospital, and the Denver VA Medical Center.

# SNORING
## 10 Tips for a Silent Night

Snoring has long been the subject of jokes, cartoons, and sitcom episodes, but in a significant number of people, it is no laughing matter. Snoring can be a serious problem, disrupting normal sleeping patterns and disturbing partners as they try to sleep through the noise.

Snoring is extremely common, occasionally affecting 45 percent of normal adults. For 25 percent of Americans, snoring is a habitual problem, according to the American Academy of Otolaryngology/Head and Neck Surgery, whose members are physicians specializing in the ear, nose, and throat.

Clinically, moderate snorers are those who snore every night but perhaps only when on their backs or only part of the night, says Philip Westbrook, M.D.

A wind ensemble located in the back of the throat orchestrates the sound made by a snorer. "The tissue in the upper airway in the back of the throat relaxes during sleep," says Philip Smith, M.D. "When you breathe in, it causes this tissue to vibrate. The effect is very similar to a wind instrument."

A physician should evaluate heavy snorers to make sure they don't have a serious sleeping disorder called sleep apnea. For light or occasional snoring, here are a number of ways to have a silent night.

**Go on a diet.** Most snorers tend to be middle-aged, overweight men. Most women snorers are past menopause. Slimming stops snoring. "We've found that if a moderate snorer loses weight, the snoring becomes less loud, and in some people it actually disappears," says Earl V. Dunn, M.D.

"You don't have to be a 2-ton Tony to develop snoring. Just being a little overweight can bring on a problem," says Dr. Smith. But the more overweight you are, the more likely it is that your airway collapses while you sleep, causing snoring.

**Avoid having a nightcap.** "Alcohol before bed makes snoring worse," says Dr. Dunn. It relaxes all the muscles in the throat that vibrate. And it's dose-related—the more you drink, the louder you'll snore.

## WHEN TO CALL A DOCTOR

Modern science is now proving what Shakespeare wrote long ago in *The Tempest:* "Thou dost snore distinctly. There's meaning in thy snores." In general, says Philip Smith, M.D., the louder your snore, the more likely it's related to a medical problem.

One of the worst problems associated with snoring is a condition called sleep apnea, a potentially life-threatening disorder, in which breathing actually stops during sleep for at least 10 seconds and up to a minute, or even longer.

This can happen hundreds of times a night, contributing to high blood pressure, cardiovascular disease, memory problems, weight gain, impotency, and headaches. Sleep-deprived apnea patients have job-related problems and may be unsafe behind the wheel, according to the Washington D.C.–based American Sleep Apnea Association.

Sleep apnea afflicts more than 12 million Americans, especially overweight men over age 40. But women and children can have sleep apnea, too.

Symptoms of sleep apnea include loud snoring, that is, loud enough to be heard outside the room; snoring punctuated by periods of silence, gasping, or choking; and extreme tiredness during the day. If this sounds like you, see your doctor.

You also may find relief by going to a local sleep clinic. For the address of a sleep clinic near you, contact the American Academy of Sleep Medicine, One Westbrook Corporate Center, Suite 920, Westchester, IL 60154, or visit their Web site at www.aasmet.org.

**Stay away from sedatives.** Sleeping pills may make *you* sleep, but they will keep your partner awake. "Anything that relaxes the tissues around the head and neck will tend to make snoring worse. Even antihistamines will do it," says Dr. Dunn.

**Quit smoking.** Snuff snoring by snuffing cigarettes. "Smokers tend to be snorers," says Dr. Dunn. Smoking may cause swelling and inflammation of the throat tissues, rendering them more likely to vibrate and produce snoring.

**Change your sleep position.** Sleep on your side. "Heavy snorers snore in virtually any position," says Dr. Dunn. "But moderate snorers only snore when they are on their backs."

**Try the tennis ball trick.** In order to keep you from rolling over onto your back, sew a small pocket on the back of your pajamas. Then slip a tennis ball inside, suggests Dr. Dunn. "That way, when you roll over on your back, you hit this hard object and unconsciously you roll off your back."

**Toss your pillow.** Pillows only help elevate your snoring level. "Anything that puts a kink in your neck makes you snore more," Dr. Dunn says.

**Raise the head of your bed.** Elevating the bed can help minimize snoring. "Elevate the upper torso, not just the head," says Dr. Westbrook. "Put a couple of bricks under the legs at the head of your bed."

**Address your allergies.** Sneezing and snoring go together. "Snoring can develop because of allergies or colds," says Dr. Westbrook. "Use a nasal decongestant, especially if your snoring is intermittent and comes during hay fever season."

## The Search Goes On for a Sure Cure

Since 1874, the U.S. Patent and Trademark Office has issued more than 300 patents for so-called antisnoring devices.

Patent number 4644330, for instance, is a self-contained electronic device that's worn in the outer ear. It comprises a miniature microphone for detecting snoring sounds and the means for generating an aversive audio signal. What that means is that when you snore, an alarm blasts off in your ear, waking you up. (Its basis is the theory that people who are awake seldom snore.)

Then there's patent number 4669459. This device clamps onto one molar on each side of your mouth with a connecting button that "applies pressure to the soft palate to prevent vibration thereof."

Or number 4748702, which is a two-channel "antisnoring pillow." The inventor has placed "a relatively hard object" in the channel that holds the back of your head, and an object that is "not being relatively uncomfortable" in the area where the side of your face would go. Seems you get your choice. If you sleep on your back, you sleep on a rock; if you sleep on your side, it's something a bit softer. You choose.

While sleep experts say that some of the inventions may be based on sound snoring advice, they add that many of the inventions are untested and unproven. "There is very little scientific evidence supporting them," says Philip Westbrook, M.D.

## Consider Yourself Lucky!

Pity Mrs. Switzer. It seems her husband, Melvin, a 250-pound British dockworker, is the sovereign of snore.

Melvin trumpeted his way into the *Guinness Book of World Records* with a snore registered at 92 decibels, about the same intensity as a motorcycle engine being revved at full throttle.

And Mrs. Switzer? Unfortunately, the nightly snoring on the other side of the bed caused her to go deaf in one ear.

**Give your partner earplugs.** When all else fails, Dr. Westbrook says, the one on the receiving end of the nasal abuse can wear earplugs to bed. They're inexpensive and can be purchased at any drugstore.

## PANEL OF ADVISORS

**Earl V. Dunn, M.D.,** is a professor in the department of family medicine, faculty of medicine and health sciences, at the United Arab Emirates University in Al-Ain and a professor emeritus at the University of Toronto.

**Philip Smith, M.D.,** is a professor of medicine and a physician in the division of pulmonary and critical care, who specializes in sleep disorders, at the Johns Hopkins University School of Medicine in Baltimore.

**Philip Westbrook, M.D.,** is chairman of the board and medical director of Advanced Brain Monitoring, a company in Carlsbad, California, which develops software and technology that can be integrated into a portable device. He was founder and former director of the Sleep Disorders Centers at the Mayo Clinic in Rochester, Minnesota, and Cedars-Sinai Medical Center in Los Angeles, president of the American Academy of Sleep Medicine, and editor of the journal *Sleep*.

# SORE THROAT
## 26 Ways to Put Out the Fire

A burning, irritated throat can disrupt your sleep, interfere with your work, and make you feel generally miserable. Your raw throat may be an early warning sign of a cold, the flu, or some other viral or bacterial infection. Sometimes a sore throat is just a minor irritation caused by winter's low humidity or too much cheering at a football game.

Whatever the cause, here's how doctors say you can feel better fast.

**Suck on lozenges.** If your sore throat is caused by a viral infection, antibiotics won't help it. Most lozenges are only soothing, but medicated lozenges containing phenol, such as Cepastat, may do some good, says Hueston King, M.D. The phenol can kill surface germs, thereby keeping the invaders in check until your body has a chance to build up its resistance. Phenol's mild anesthetic action numbs raw nerve endings so that your throat doesn't feel as scratchy. These lozenges come in various strengths, so follow package directions to find out how often you should take them.

**Spray away pain.** By the same token, phenol-containing throat sprays, like Vicks Chloroseptic, can also give topical relief. But as Thomas Gossel, Ph.D., R.Ph., points out, the duration of contact between the spray and the irritated tissues is relatively brief. Lozenges simply last longer.

**Give zinc a chance.** Zinc lozenges can help the kind of sore throat that's associated with a cold, says Donald Davis, Ph.D. "We gave people one 23-milligram tablet of zinc gluconate every 2 hours—but we instructed them to let it dissolve slowly in their mouths rather than just swallowing it. The zinc relieved their sore throats as well as several other cold symptoms."

Another study, this one conducted at Wayne State University in Detroit, compared 25 cold sufferers receiving zinc with 23 who unknowingly received a lozenge containing no medication. Those who got the zinc had less severe sore throats. They also got over their colds in half the time. Use zinc lozenges, such as Cold-Eeze and Nature Made, according to label directions until your symp-

## WHEN TO CALL A DOCTOR

A strep throat is an extremely painful bacterial infection that may come on suddenly. Left untreated, it can lead to more serious problems like rheumatic fever and rheumatic heart disease. But there are many different viruses and bacteria that can cause severe sore throats. Fortunately, says Hueston King, M.D., the vast majority of bacterial infections, including strep, generally respond quite well to one course of an appropriate antibiotic. If this doesn't work, continued treatment with the same or another antibiotic has little chance of curing the infection, since it probably is viral in nature. At this point, your doctor may stop your antibiotic for 3 days and order a throat culture to identify the cause of the infection. Culturing before you try the antibiotic may allow time for a secondary bacterial infection to set in, explains Dr. King.

Other serious causes of sore throats include mononucleosis (a viral infection), tonsillitis, or epiglottitis, a dangerous bacterial infection in the voice box which causes swelling that closes the airway.

Because sore throats can have so many causes, some symptoms need to be evaluated by a doctor, says Jerome C. Goldstein, M.D. These include:

- Severe, prolonged, or recurrent sore throats
- Difficulty breathing, swallowing, or opening the mouth
- Joint pains, earache, or a lump in the neck
- Rash or a fever above 101°F
- Hoarseness lasting 2 weeks or longer
- Blood in saliva or phlegm

toms subside. Taking more than 40 milligrams a day can elevate your zinc levels, which impairs your body's ability to absorb copper.

**Gargle!** If it hurts when you swallow, the sore area may be high enough in your throat for gargling to bathe and soothe it, says Dr. King. So gargle frequently with one of the solutions below. But be aware that if you're hoarse or have a cough, the sore spot is further down, and gargling won't help.

*Salt water.* Mix 1 teaspoon of table salt in 2 cups of warm or room-temperature water, says Dr. Gossel. That's just enough salt to mimic the body's natural saline content, so you'll find it very soothing. Use every hour or so.

***Chamomile tea.*** Eleonore Blaurock-Busch, Ph.D., favors warm chamomile tea to relieve irritated membranes. Steep 1 teaspoon of dried chamomile in 1 cup of hot water. Strain. Let it cool to lukewarm and gargle as needed.

***Diluted lemon juice.*** Dr. Blaurock-Busch also suggests squeezing half of a lemon into an 8-ounce glass of lukewarm water. You can substitute bottled reconstituted lemon juice for fresh, using 1 tablespoon of juice and 4 to 8 ounces of water.

***Spirits.*** "Sometimes I add a spoonful of bourbon or whiskey to a large glass of warm water and use that to gargle," says Dr. Gossel. "It's just enough alcohol to help numb a sore throat."

**Humidify the room.** Sometimes a sore throat upon awakening is caused by sleeping with your mouth open. Ordinarily, your nose moistens air headed for your throat and lungs. But breathing through your mouth bypasses that step, leaving your throat parched and irritated.

Jason Surow, M.D., recommends a bedroom humidifier to keep the environment humid. "Use a bedside model even if your heating system has its own humidifier," he says. "Most built-in units don't do a good enough job, especially if you have a forced-air heating system, which is very drying in itself." You can use either a cool-mist or warm-mist machine, whichever is more soothing for you, he says. Humidifiers are available in drugstores and many other stores. Some brands are Vicks, Slant/Fin, and Robitussin.

**Get up a head of steam.** In the face of a worse-than-normal dry or sore throat, supplement your bedroom humidifier with steam inhalations, says Dr. Surow. Run very hot water in the bathroom basin to build up steam. With the water running, lean over the sink, drape a towel over your head to capture some of the steam, and inhale deeply through your mouth and nose for 5 to 10 minutes. Repeat several times a day if necessary. Personal facial steamers, such as HoMedics and Conair, are also available in department and discount stores and drugstores.

**Open your nose.** If part of the reason you're breathing through your mouth is that your nose is clogged, says Dr. Surow, open it with an over-the-counter medicated decongestant nasal spray or drops, such as Afrin and Neo-Synephrine. But limit its use to a day or two.

**Inhale sea breezes.** If you can't actually go someplace humid like the ocean, get the same sort of salty atmosphere from a saline nasal spray or drops, available at any drugstore. When you inhale the mist, says Dr. Surow, the salt-based spray moistens your nose and drips down the back of your throat to help increase humidity there. Among the brands available are Ocean, NaSal, and Ayr.

To make your own saltwater rinse, Robert Rountree, M.D., recommends stirring about ¼ teaspoon of sea salt and ⅛ teaspoon baking soda into 4 ounces of warm water. To apply, lean forward over a sink, start breathing through your mouth (to prevent the solution from coming out of your mouth and creating a very unpleasant choking sensation), and tilt your head to the left side. Pour the mixture into your right nostril. Tilt your head to the right to rinse the left nostril.

**Take a nonprescription pain reliever.** It doesn't occur to most people that a sore throat is a pain like any other physical discomfort, says Dr. Gossel. Aspirin, acetaminophen, or ibuprofen will help ease the pain.

**Increase your fluid intake.** Take in as much fluid as you can to hydrate your parched throat tissues, says Dr. Surow. Although it doesn't really matter *what* you drink, he says, here are a few things to avoid: Thick, milky drinks coat your throat and may produce mucus, making you cough and further irritating tissues; orange juice may burn an already inflamed throat; and caffeine-containing beverages have a counterproductive diuretic effect.

**Wrap your throat.** Dr. Blaurock-Busch finds that a warm chamomile poultice, applied directly to the throat, relieves discomfort. To make the poultice, add 1 tablespoon of dried chamomile flowers to 1 to 2 cups of boiling water. Allow it to steep for 5 minutes before straining. Soak a clean cloth or towel in this tea, wring out the excess, and apply to the affected area. Leave it on until the cloth is cold. Repeat if necessary with more warm liquid.

**Load up on garlic.** "Garlic is one of the best natural antibiotics and antiseptics," says Dr. Blaurock-Busch. She recommends taking 1,000 milligrams of garlic in capsule form a day.

**Use a Russian home remedy.** Irwin Ziment, M.D., mixes 1 tablespoon of pure horseradish, 1 teaspoon of honey, and 1 teaspoon of ground cloves in a glass of warm water and stirs. "Sip it slowly, keep stirring—as the horseradish tends to settle—and think happy thoughts," he says. Or use it as a gargle.

**Reach for vitamins.** Vitamin C may help build up your tissues to fight the germs that make your throat sore. "I usually tell people to take 500 milligrams in divided doses daily," says Dr. King. Another immunity booster is vitamin E. Dr. King recommends 400 milligrams natural vitamin E, labeled d-alpha-tocopherol, daily. Taking the combination of these vitamins while the infection is present is helpful with both viral and bacterial infections.

# Stage-Door Remedies

Actors can't afford to be upstaged by sore throats. So we asked some professionals how they perform comebacks when their throats are acting up.

- Several mentioned the time-honored salvo of lemon juice and honey in hot tea or water, sipped throughout the day.

- All had their favorite lozenges. Actor, director, and writer George Wolf Reily likes Ricola herbal mints from Switzerland. "They're great when you have to do two shows a day and your throat is hurting."

- Singer Geoffrey Moore prefers Halls Mentho-Lyptus drops. "They don't contain any anesthetics to dull the feeling in my throat."

- One of actor Norman Marshall's favorite remedies is a tablespoon of baking soda in a large glass of water. "I sip this throughout the day whenever my throat's irritated or I feel a cold coming on."

- Actress Elf Fairservis humidifies her sore throat with a facial sauna. "I just inhale the steam for about 10 minutes. If I can spare the time, I do it three times a day until I feel better."

- From a preventive standpoint, actor and singer William Perley protects his throat by "staying as healthy as I can and eating lots of carrots for their vitamin A. Also, I've been told by vocal teachers not to irritate my throat by clearing it too much."

**Toss your toothbrush.** Believe it or not, says Richard T. Glass, D.D.S., Ph.D., your toothbrush may be perpetuating—or even causing—your sore throat. Bacteria collect on the bristles, and any injury to the gums during brushing injects these germs into your system.

"As soon as you start feeling ill, throw away your toothbrush. Often that's enough to stop the illness in its tracks," he says. "If you do get sick, replace your brush *again* when you start to feel better. That keeps you from reinfecting yourself."

From a preventive standpoint, he recommends replacing your toothbrush every 2 weeks and storing it outside the moist, bacteria-prone bathroom. If you think it's expensive to buy so many brushes, he says, consider the cost of just one trip to the doctor's office. You'll do better in the long run to stay well.

**Tilt your bed.** Another cause of sore throat in the morning—besides sleeping with your mouth open—is a backup of stomach acids into your throat during the night. These acids are extremely irritating to sensitive throat tissues, says Jerome C. Goldstein, M.D. Avoid the problem by tilting your bed frame so that the head is 4 to 6 inches higher than the foot. (Try using bricks.)

Don't simply pile more pillows under your head; they can cause you to bend in the middle, increasing pressure on your esophagus and making the problem worse. As an extra precaution, don't eat or drink for an hour or two before retiring.

## PANEL OF ADVISORS

**Eleonore Blaurock-Busch, Ph.D.,** is associate laboratory director of King James Medical Laboratory and Trace Minerals International, both in Cleveland. She is also the director of Micro Trace Minerals in Hersbruck, Germany; cochairman of the International Association of Trace Elements and Cancer; and the author of several books.

**Donald Davis, Ph.D.,** is a research associate at the Biochemical Institute at the University of Texas at Austin.

**Elf Fairservis** is a New York City actress who's done Off-Broadway productions and commercials.

**Richard T. Glass, D.D.S., Ph.D.,** is director of the forensic graduate program and professor of oral pathology at Oklahoma State University, College of Osteopathic Medicine in Tulsa, Oklahoma. He is professor emeritus from the University of Oklahoma, Colleges of Dentistry, Graduate, and Medicine where he was professor and chairman of the department of oral and maxillofacial pathology and professor of pathology.

**Jerome C. Goldstein, M.D.,** is a visiting professor of otolaryngology/head and neck surgery at Georgetown University School of Medicine in Washington, D.C., and Albany Medical College in New York. He is also past executive vice president of the American Academy of Otolaryngology in Washington, D.C.

**Thomas Gossel, Ph.D., R.Ph.,** is a professor of pharmacology and toxicology at Ohio Northern University in Ada. He is an expert on over-the-counter products.

**Hueston King, M.D.,** is an associate clinical professor of otolaryngology at the University of Texas Southwest Medical Center in Dallas and the University of Florida in Gainesville. He is also an ear, nose, and throat specialist in Venice, Florida.

**Norman Marshall** is an actor who has worked in soap operas, movies, and children's theater. He formed the No Smoking Playhouse in New York City and directed it for 11 years.

**Geoffrey Moore** is a semiretired professional singer living in Ridgewood, New Jersey. He has a one-man program that he performs at nursing homes.

**William Perley** is an actor and singer. For the past several summers he has starred in the play *The Mark Twain Drama* in Elmira, New York, which has been aired on PBS.

**George Wolf Reily** is an actor, director, and writer who's done Off-Broadway and regional theater.

**Robert Rountree, M.D.,** is a holistic physician in Boulder, Colorado, and coauthor of *Immunotics*.

**Jason Surow, M.D.,** is an ear, nose, and throat specialist in both Teaneck and Midland Park, New Jersey. He's an attending otolaryngologist at both Valley Hospital in Ridgewood, New Jersey, and Holy Name Hospital in Teaneck.

**Irwin Ziment, M.D.,** is a professor of medicine in the department of pulmonary and critical care medicine at UCLA School of Medicine in Los Angeles.

# SPLINTERS
## 9 Ways to Get Them Out

In the well-known fable *Androcles and the Lion,* it was a tiny splinter that brought the mighty lion to his knees. And if you've ever had a spiky splinter puncture your tender skin, you can relate.

Getting a splinter in the hand or foot—or worse, someplace even more sensitive—pains even the strongest of us. Unfortunately, removing those little suckers can often be just as troublesome.

### WHEN TO CALL A DOCTOR

Call a health professional if the splinter is very large or deeply embedded and cannot be easily removed, says Dee Anna Glaser, M.D. Deep splinters may require the physician to make a small incision to remove it. "But, unless the splinter is removed, it will almost always become infected," she says.

Speaking of infection, those with diabetes or who are immune-compromised should see a physician if they have a deeply embedded splinter, suggests Dr. Glaser. "These people are at a greater risk for more serious infection."

If you see any signs of infection, including pain, redness, swelling, or red streaks, it may be a sign that the splinter has not been fully removed. Even with complete removal, infections may still occur in those whose immune system is compromised in some way, she cautions.

Yet another instance to make a doctor's visit is if the splinter is a piece of metal, not wood, and your last tetanus shot was more than 5 years ago, says Dr. Glaser.

"Splinters are small pieces of wood, glass, metal, or other matter that gets caught under your skin," says Dee Anna Glaser, M.D. "Even though they're often small, they tend to hurt. Whether they are buried deep or not, you need to remove them as soon as possible, so they don't cause infection."

Here's what some of the pros recommend for painless—or at least somewhat painless—removal to keep that splinter from becoming a real thorn in your side.

**Enlist some outside help.** First, get a loved one to sterilize a pair of tweezers by cleaning it in isopropyl rubbing alcohol or running it under a lighter or hot match. "It's hard to cause yourself pain, so ask a husband, wife, or someone else that cares about you to lend you a gentle, helping hand," says Dr. Glaser.

Once the tweezers are sterilized, grab the protruding end of the splinter with the tweezers and gently pull it out along the direction it entered, says Dr. Glaser. If the splinter is embedded in the skin, sterilize a needle with rubbing alcohol, a lighter, or a match, then make a small hole in the skin over the end of the splinter. Then, lift the skin up to expose the splinter, put the needle under the splinter until it can be grasped with the tweezers, and pull it out.

Last, have your helper check to make sure that the entire splinter has been removed. If not, repeat the steps above. "For really small splinters or if you don't get the entire splinter on the first try, use a magnifying glass to help get a closer look at the target," says Dr. Glaser.

**Let warm water do the work.** If probing for that splinter with a sterilized needle and tweezers won't do the trick, give the affected area a good soak in 2 quarts of warm water with 1 teaspoon of salt added. A 10- to 15-minute soak will cause the piece of wood to swell, which may help the splinter pop out on its own, says C. Ralph Daniel III, M.D.

**Try tape.** Dr. Daniel also suggests using adhesive tape first, if the thought of using tweezers or a needle makes you a little squeamish. Simply put the tape over the splinter, then pull it off. If the splinter hasn't penetrated too deeply into the skin, the adhesive tape will often stick to the splinter. Remove the piece of tape, and the splinter often comes out painlessly and easily. If that doesn't work, you'll have to turn to tweezers.

**Clean up your act.** After the splinter has been completely removed, clean the wound with hydrogen peroxide, allowing the bubbles to work on the area, says Joseph P. Bark, M.D.

Then apply a bandage, if needed, to keep the wound clean; otherwise, leave it open to the air, says Dr. Glaser. Either way, be on the lookout for signs of infection (redness, discharges of pus, increased pain, swelling, and even red streaking in that area). "Applying an antibiotic ointment once the area is cleaned will help the healing process," she says.

**Take preventive measures.** Dr. Glaser says that some splinters can be avoided with an ounce or two of prevention. She recommends the following:

- Wear shoes outdoors at all times and whenever you walk on unfinished wood floors, wooden decks, or boardwalks.
- Clean up all broken glass and metal shavings around the house immediately. Be careful when handling broken glass, and wear hard-soled shoes to protect your feet.
- Wear work gloves when handling plants with thorns, sharp tips, and spines.
- Be careful when applying friction to an object while performing tasks such as woodworking. "If you're not careful, a small portion of that wood can dislodge into your skin," says Dr. Glaser. "So again, wear gloves."

## PANEL OF ADVISORS

**Joseph Bark, M.D.,** is a dermatologist in Lexington, Kentucky, and the author of *Your Skin . . . An Owner's Guide.*
**C. Ralph Daniel III, M.D.,** is a clinical professor of dermatology at the University of Mississippi Medical Center in Jackson.
**Dee Anna Glaser, M.D.,** is an associate professor of dermatology at St. Louis University School of Medicine.

# SPRAINS
## 18 Self-Care Strategies

Ligaments are tough bands of tissue that wrap around your ankle and other joints, lending support and stability. They have a little bit of give, but only a little. If stretched beyond their usual limits, they can become damaged or inflamed—or, in other words, sprained.

"The usual time for a sprain to heal is about 6 weeks, but that's only if it's treated properly," says John M. McShane, M.D. "People tend to ignore sprains, which can result in chronic problems."

Many sprains can be treated at home without medical attention, Dr. McShane adds. Here's what you need to do.

## WHEN TO CALL A DOCTOR

All sprains are painful, and it's difficult even for doctors to tell right away if the injuries involve torn tissue, fractured bone, or other serious problems.

If there's a lot of swelling or bruising, or if the pain seems unusually severe, it's a good idea to get to an emergency room for x-rays, says Michael Osborne, M.D.

Sprains should start feeling better within a few weeks, Dr. Osborne adds. Even if the initial discomfort is mild, see your doctor if there isn't noticeable improvement within 2 to 4 weeks.

**Rest the joint.** Sprains don't necessarily hurt a lot at first, and people may assume it's okay to keep doing the activity that got them into trouble in the first place. But pushing an injured joint too hard makes the damage worse.

"Minor sprains need a couple of days of rest," says Dr. McShane. You don't have to limit your daily movements altogether, but you will want to avoid vigorous activities that stress the injured area.

**Ice it immediately.** Applying cold to a sprain deadens pain and reduces internal bleeding or the accumulation of fluids in the injured area. It's important to ice sprains immediately because swelling is hard to reverse once it's underway.

"Use ice cubes or crushed ice," Dr. McShane advises. "Put the ice in a resealable plastic bag, seal it, wrap it in a thin towel, and put it over the area. Keep icing the area as long as it's sore, especially if there's any swelling."

If you don't have ice, open the freezer and take out a bag of frozen vegetables. A vegetable bag with peas or corn is pliable enough to mold around the joint and apply cold right where it's needed, says Michael Osborne, M.D.

**Or use a gel pack.** Available at drugstores and sporting goods stores, gel packs stay flexible even when frozen and mold themselves to the contours of the joint. "Gel packs get colder than ice and can actually cause frostbite if they're put directly on the skin," Dr. McShane warns. So when using a gel pack, make sure to put a cloth between it and the skin, and don't leave it on for more than 15 minutes at a time.

**Wrap the joint.** Compressing the area with an elastic bandage helps prevent fluid from accumulating, which reduces swelling and pain. Wrapping a joint also restricts movement, which helps the injured ligaments heal.

Don't make the bandage so tight that it cuts off circulation, Dr. McShane adds. If the area beyond the sprain feels numb or cold, or if the bandage itself is uncomfortably tight, loosen it a bit.

"You should be able to slip a finger snugly under the bandage," Dr. McShane says.

### Use an air cast on the ankle.

Available at some drugstores and from mail-order catalogs, air casts can be pumped up with air to put even pressure on the ankle. "They help keep the swelling down and prevent the joint from moving too much," says Dr. McShane.

Another option is to use an elastic "tube" bandage. Available at some drugstores and most medical supply stores, the tubes come in different sizes for different joints. The problem with the elastic bandages mentioned above is that they can shift when you wear them, which may allow swelling in some areas. The tube bandages are preferred because they apply even compression all the way around the joint, says Dr. Osborne.

### Put gravity on your side.

For the first day or two after a sprain, elevate the area for as long as possible. If you've sprained your ankle, for example, put a few pillows underneath your calf. If you've sprained your wrist, keep your hand above chest level. Elevating the joint aids lymphatic drainage from the area and keeps swelling to a minimum, says Dr. Osborne.

## Do just 1 thing

Start with gentle exercises as soon as possible. It's normal for ligaments to be somewhat tight after a sprain. To prevent stiffness and restore joint mobility, it's helpful to do range-of-motion exercises once you're through the initial, painful phase.

Moving the joint may be painful at first, but that's okay. In fact, it's beneficial to gently push the joint slightly farther than it wants to go, says John M. McShane, M.D. "Ligaments actually heal better when they're slightly stressed," he explains.

If you're recovering from an ankle sprain, for example, use your foot to "sketch" the entire alphabet once or twice a day. Imagine that your big toe is the tip of a pen, he says. Using the ankle to move the foot, form each letter of the alphabet, from A to Z, in the air.

"That helps get the range of motion back, and it reduces swelling as well," says Dr. McShane.

### Take an over-the-counter anti-inflammatory.

Aspirin, ibuprofen, and other nonsteroidal anti-inflammatory drugs (NSAIDs) inhibit the body's production of prostaglandins, inflammatory chemicals that cause swelling and delay healing time. They are often used as the first treatment for overuse injuries.

"Acetaminophen is used for pain relief, but it doesn't have any effect on swelling," adds Dr. McShane. You'll get better results with aspirin, ibuprofen, or naproxen (Aleve). The drugs work equally well, but naproxen is more convenient because you only have to take it twice a day.

One caveat: If the injury is severe, wait until the bleeding has stopped or the swelling has stabilized before taking NSAIDs, because they also inhibit blood clotting and may complicate recovery time.

**Relieve stiffness with heat.** You don't want to treat a sprain with a heating pad or hot-water bottle in the first 48 to 72 hours after the injury, because heat increases circulation and may increase swelling. But after several days, when swelling has subsided, applying heat—or soaking the area in a whirlpool or hot bath—may help you feel more comfortable, says Dr. Osborne.

Heat also improves the flow of nutrients into the injured area while removing painful metabolic by-products.

**Wear a brace.** If you have a history of ankle sprains, consider wearing a brace. Available at drugstores, braces support and protect the joint, which can speed healing and reduce the risk of additional sprains. Some people with sprain-prone ankles wear braces whenever they do "risky" activities, such as play tennis or basketball.

**Get the right shoes.** If you've sprained your ankle once, you may have a higher risk of future sprains. One way to prevent problems is to buy shoes designed for the activities you do most. "Don't wear running shoes for playing basketball or racquetball," says Dr. McShane. "They don't provide ankle stability, and they may actually create a tendency for the ankle to roll in or out."

**Keep an eye on ground conditions.** Sprains would be a lot less common if the entire world were as flat as a running track. But hazards—everything from curbs in unexpected places to potholed playing fields—are everywhere. Whether you're walking, hiking, or playing sports, always check the ground to see what lies ahead. If you exercise outdoors at night, try to do it in well-lighted areas so that you can see where you're going.

**Strengthen the joint.** Once the sprain is better, it's worth taking the time to strengthen and condition the joint, which reduces stress on the ligaments. Because ankle sprains are so common, this is the area of the body that you may want to focus on—both for relieving stiffness and for preventing future problems.

"The ankle may be weak after a sprain, so you'll want to start with range-of-motion exercises, then progress to strengthening exercises," says Dr. Osborne. Try these exercises, for example.

- Put a few cans of soup or vegetables into a plastic grocery bag, slip your foot through the handles, and lift your toes toward the ceiling. Hold the weight for about 3 seconds, then lower it back down.

- Put your foot against a wall or another immovable object, and flex and relax the muscles. This type of isometric exercises improves bloodflow and exerts beneficial stress on the ligaments and other tissues.
- While sitting with your legs straight in front of you, flex the top of your foot back toward your body. Hold for a moment, then relax.
- While sitting, loop a towel or an elastic cord around your foot, then flex the muscles in different directions against the resistance.

**Stretch away tightness.** No one enjoys stretching very much, but it's worth getting in the habit, especially if you're recovering from a sprain and the muscles around the joint are tighter than they should be. At the very least, spend a few minutes a day stretching the muscles that cross the affected joint.

## PANEL OF ADVISORS

**John M. McShane, M.D.,** is an associate clinical professor of family medicine at Jefferson Medical College of Thomas Jefferson University and director of sports medicine at Thomas Jefferson University Hospital, both in Philadelphia.

**Michael Osborne, M.D.,** is senior associate consultant in the department of physical medicine and rehabilitation at Mayo Clinic Jacksonville, and an instructor at the Mayo Medical School in Jacksonville, Florida.

# STRESS
## 22 Tips to Ease Tension

Stress. It really should be a four-letter word. Here in the 21st century, it's as pervasive as the air that we breathe and as contagious as the common cold.

Since stress is so difficult to avoid, why not make it work *for* you instead of against you? Stress is a force you can turn to your advantage. You don't have to run from it, and you *don't* have to go to a stress-management seminar to find out how to manage it. The following doctor-tested tips show you how to combat stress—and win. For relief when the world has you in a headlock, read on.

**Get a new attitude.** "I think the single most important point you can make about stress is that in most cases it's not what's out there that's the problem, it's

## WHEN TO CALL A DOCTOR

Too much stress can directly threaten your health.

If your symptoms are new and have no obvious cause, especially if they interfere with your quality of life, see a doctor, says Paul J. Rosch, M.D.

Any of the following stress-related symptoms may indicate that you should seek medical help promptly.

- Frequent headaches, jaw clenching or pain
- Gritting or grinding teeth
- Stuttering or stammering
- Tremors, trembling of lips or hands
- Neck ache, back pain, or muscle spasms
- Light-headedness, faintness, or dizziness
- Ringing, buzzing, or "popping sounds"
- Frequent blushing or sweating
- Cold or sweaty hands and feet
- Dry mouth or problems swallowing

how you *react* to it," says Paul J. Rosch, M.D. How you react is determined by how you *perceive* a particular stress.

"Watch people on a roller-coaster ride," Dr. Rosch says. "Some sit in the back, eyes shut, jaws clenched. They can't wait for the ordeal in the torture chamber to end and to get back on solid ground. Up front are the wide-eyed thrill seekers who relish every steep plunge and can't wait to get on the very next ride. In between are those who are seemingly quite nonchalant or even bored.

"They're all having exactly the same experience—the roller-coaster ride—but they're reacting to it very differently: bad stress, good stress, and *no* stress."

Emmett Miller, M.D., draws on Chinese wisdom to make this point. "The Chinese word for crisis is *wuji*—two characters that separately mean 'danger' and 'opportunity.' Every problem we encounter in life can be viewed that way—as a chance to show that we can handle it."

The message from both doctors: Changing the way you think—viewing a difficult assignment at work as a chance to improve your skills, for example—can change a life of stress and discomfort into a life of challenge and excitement.

**Think about something else.** "Anything that will help you shift your perspective instantly is useful when you're under the gun," says Dr. Miller. "You want to distract yourself, to break whatever chain of thought is producing the stress. Thinking about almost anything else will do that."

**Think positive.** "Thinking about a success or a past achievement is excellent when you're feeling uncertain—before a presentation, for example, or a meeting with your boss," Dr. Miller says. "You're instantly reminded that you've achieved before, and there's no reason you shouldn't achieve this time."

**Take a mental vacation.** "Taking a mini-vacation in your mind is a very good way to relieve or manage stress," says Ronald Nathan, Ph.D.

"Imagine yourself lying in warm sand on a beach in the Bahamas, a gentle breeze coming off the ocean, the surf rolling in quietly in the background. It's *amazing* what this can do to relax you."

**Recite an antistress litany.** Stress can strike anytime, not just at work—in the bathroom before work, in the deli at lunchtime, in the car on the way home. To help yourself loosen up when unpleasant thoughts knot the muscles in your neck and tension mounts, recite the following litany, suggested by Dr. Miller.

- "There's no *place* I have to go at this moment in time."
- "There's no *problem* I have to solve at this moment in time."
- "There's nothing that I have to *do* at this moment in time."
- "The most important thing that I can experience at this moment in time is *relaxation.*"

It's necessary to think these thoughts consciously, Dr. Miller says, because doing so automatically changes the mindset that's producing the stress. If you're reciting the litany, you're *not* thinking about whatever was bothering you.

**Use affirmations.** Have a list of affirmations ready that you can start repeating when you feel stressed, Dr. Miller says. "They don't have to be complicated. Just chanting 'I can handle this' to yourself or 'I know more about this than anyone here' will work. It pulls you away from the animal reflex to stress—the quick breathing, the cold hands—and toward the reasoned response, the intellect, the part of you that really *can* handle it."

The result? You calm down.

**Count to 10.** Simply refusing to respond to a stress immediately can help defuse it, Dr. Nathan says. Making a *habit* of pausing and relaxing just for a few seconds before responding to the routine interruptions of your day can make a clear difference in the sense of stress you experience. When the phone rings, for example, breathe in deeply. Then as you breathe out, imagine you are as loose and limp as an old rag doll.

"One of the things pausing like this does is to give you a feeling of control," Dr. Nathan points out. "Feeling in control is generally less stressful than feeling out of control. Make a habit of using rapid relaxation during the pause before you answer the phone. Deliberately pausing can become an instant tranquilizer."

# The Way to Inner Peace

Transcendental meditation, yoga, Zen meditation—they *all* work by inducing something called the relaxation response, a body state first characterized and named by Herbert Benson, M.D.

"This phenomenon shuts off the distracting, stressful, anxiety-producing aspects of what is commonly called the fight-or-flight response," Dr. Benson writes in his book *Your Maximum Mind*.

In primitive situations, where dangers from wild animals might have been the order of the day, the fight-or-flight response was quite useful. In our own time, however, this response tends to make us more nervous, uncomfortable, and even unhealthy.

A person experiencing the relaxation response turns off all the hormones and behaviors that make him nervous. Basically any kind of meditation produces it, though most traditional forms require some degree of training and a good amount of self-discipline.

Dr. Benson suggests the following basic program for eliciting the response.

One, pick a focus word, phrase, or prayer ("peace," or "the Lord is my shepherd," for example) that is firmly rooted in your personal belief system. Two, sit quietly, close your eyes, and relax. And three, repeat your focus word each time you exhale. Continue for 10 to 20 minutes.

Tips: Practice at least once a day, and don't worry about how you're doing. If you realize that you've been distracted by thoughts, this is normal and should be expected. Simply say, "Oh, well," and return to your focus.

**Look away.** "If you look through a window at a far-distant view for a moment, away from the problem that's producing the stress, the eyes relax. And if the eyes relax, the tendency is for you to do the same," Dr. Nathan says.

**Get up and leave.** "Take a pot off the burner, and it quits boiling," says Dr. Nathan. "Leaving the scene can also give you a fresh perspective."

**Take several deep breaths.** Belly breathing is what some people call it. It's an old and useful trick for reducing anxiety and nervousness.

"The basic idea is act calm, be calm," says Bradley W. Frederick, D.C. "When you're experiencing stress, your pulse races, and you start breathing very quickly. Eastern medicine teaches us that we can control our autonomic nervous system and its responses. One example of this is respiration. By forcing yourself to breathe slowly and fully, you can change the body's automatic response to stress. This simple activity can slow the heart rate, bring needed oxygen to the brain and muscles, which eases tension and convinces the body that the stress is gone, whether it is or isn't."

The correct way to breathe? Abdominally–feeling your stomach expand as you inhale, collapse as you exhale. While there are many different breathing techniques to calm the mind, the simple "So Hum" meditation breathing is best for starters. Inhale deeply and say "soooooo," then slowly exhale with "hummmm." Pull your stomach in tight. Breathing slowly, fully, and calmly at the first signs of stress will change your attitude and life forever.

**Stretch.** "Essentially, every emotion we feel has a physical manifestation," says Dr. Frederick. "Tightening of the jaw and shoulder muscles is a common response to stress. Ideally, we'd prefer to eliminate the cause of the stress, rather than treat the symptoms. By stretching the muscles and keeping the spine mobile, however, you'll feel better, be healthier, and live longer. Given that we often can't do anything about the source of stress, that's important."

For many of us, that's all we need.

**Massage your target muscles.** "Most of us have particular muscles that knot up under stress," Dr. Miller says. "It's sort of a vicious circle: Stress produces adrenaline, which produces muscle tension, which produces more adrenaline, and so on. A good way to break the circle is to find out what your target muscles are–the ones that get tense under pressure, usually in the back of your neck and upper back–and massage them for a couple of minutes whenever you feel tense."

**Press on your temples.** This application of acupressure–the system that uses pressure points to relieve pain and treat a variety of ailments–works indirectly. Massaging nerves in your temples, says Dr. Miller, relaxes muscles elsewhere, chiefly in your neck.

**Drop your jaw and roll it left to right.** "People under pressure have a tendency to clench their teeth," says Dr. Miller. "Dropping the jaw and rolling it helps make those muscles relax, and if you relax the muscles, you reduce the sensation of tension."

**Stretch your chest for better breathing.** The tense musculature of a person under stress can make breathing difficult, according to Dr. Frederick, and impaired breathing can aggravate the anxiety you already feel. To relax your breathing, roll your shoulders up and back, then relax. The first time, inhale deeply as they go back and exhale as they relax. You may do this at the same time you are doing So Hum breathing. Repeat four or five more times, then inhale deeply again. Repeat the entire sequence four times.

**Relax all over.** Easier said than done? Not if you know how. A simple technique called progressive relaxation can produce immediate and dramatic reductions in your sense of stress by reducing physical tension.

Starting at top or bottom, tense one set of muscles in your body at a time, hold for a few seconds, then let them relax. Work your way through all major body parts—feet, legs, chest and arms, head and neck—and then enjoy the sense of release it provides. Dr. Frederick recommends learning at least one meditation technique. Fifteen minutes of meditation can give the body the rest of 1 hour of sleep.

**Take a hot soak.** Hot water works by defeating the stress response, says Dr. Frederick. When we're tense and anxious, bloodflow to our extremities is reduced. Hot water restores circulation, convincing the body it's safe and that it is okay to relax. Dr. Frederick recommends placing warm washcloths on your feet, hands, and forehead. "It feels great!" Cold water is a no-no for the opposite reason. It *mimics* the stress response, driving blood away from the extremities. The result: Tension increases.

An office alternative might be running hot water over your hands until you feel tension start to drain away.

**Move around.** Regular exercise, of course, builds stamina that can help anyone battle stress. But even something as casual as a walk around the block can help you throw off some of the tension that a rough business meeting or a family squabble leaves you carrying around.

"Exercise is what your body instinctively wants to do under stress: Run or fight," Dr. Miller says. "And it works. One, it burns off some of the stress chemicals tension produces. And two, a tired muscle is a relaxed muscle."

**Listen to a relaxation tape.** Relaxation, Dr. Miller says, is the opposite of tension—the antidote for stress. And the prerecorded relaxation tapes that he and others produce are very effective. (Dr. Miller's tapes have been used by such diverse organizations as the Mayo Clinic, Lockheed Martin, and Levi Strauss and Company.)

"Good relaxation tapes are very valuable," says Dr. Nathan. "They facilitate your relaxation response. And they're inexpensive."

Available tapes offer voice only, voice with music, or just natural sounds—wind in the trees, surf on the sand. All you need is a tape recorder and a headset to block out distractions and avoid disturbing others.

**Tune in the music.** Relaxation cassettes work, but they aren't your only option. The right music soothes as perhaps nothing else does.

"Music is an enormously powerful tool for fighting stress," Dr. Miller says. "You can use it in two basic ways—to relax or to inspire. New Age music is very relaxing."

**Beat stress with Siberian ginseng.** Herbalists refer to herbs that help combat stress as adaptogens because they help us adapt better to our stressors.

Try taking Siberian ginseng three times a day during periods of stress. Make sure you're using Siberian ginseng, and not its Asian or American cousins, which can wreak havoc on the menstrual cycle or worsen menopause symptoms in women, notes Douglas Schar, Dip.Phyt., M.C.P.P., M.N.I.M.H.

**Oust stress with oat straw.** Oat straw is a traditional remedy for nervous exhaustion and depression. You'll need to take it for at least a month before you notice its effects, but it's okay for long-term use, Schar says.

Take 1 teaspoon of 1:5 tincture three times a day.

## PANEL OF ADVISORS

**Herbert Benson, M.D.,** is an associate professor at the Mind-Body Medical Institute at Harvard Medical School and chief of the division of behavioral medicine at Beth Israel Deaconess Medical Center, both in Boston.

**Bradley W. Frederick, D.C.,** is a chiropractor and director of the International Institute of Sports Medicine in Los Angeles.

**Emmett Miller, M.D.,** is medical director for the Center for Healing and Wellness in Menlo Park, California. He is a nationally recognized expert on stress and mind-body medicine.

**Ronald Nathan, Ph.D.,** is a clinical professor at Albany Medical College in New York and coauthor of *The Doctors' Guide to Instant Stress Relief.*

**Paul J. Rosch, M.D.,** is a clinical professor of medicine and psychiatry at New York Medical College in Valhalla. He's also an adjunct clinical professor of medicine in psychiatry at the University of Maryland School of Medicine in Baltimore and president of the American Institute of Stress.

**Douglas Schar, Dip.Phyt., M.C.C.P., M.N.I.M.H.,** is a member of the National Institute of Medical Herbalists in the United Kingdom and an herbalist in Washington, D.C. He has a diploma in phytotherapy.

# SUNBURN
## 37 Cooling Treatments

Scarlett O'Hara was right. Wearing a wide-brimmed hat, carrying a parasol, and shunning the sun *are* good ideas. Anything to avoid the terrible pain, itching, and swelling of a sunburn.

If you found yourself outside without *your* trusty parasol and came away with a nasty sunburn, heed this advice from the experts.

**Apply soothing compresses.** Following a burn, the skin is inflamed. Cool it down with compresses dipped in any one of the following substances. If desired, you can direct a fan on the sunburned area to heighten cooling.

*Cold water.* Use either plain water from the faucet or add a few ice cubes, says Michael Schreiber, M.D. Dip a cloth into the liquid and lay it over the burn. Repeat every few minutes as the cloth warms. Apply several times a day for a total of 10 to 15 minutes each.

*Aluminum acetate.* If itching is intense, says Thomas Gossel, Ph.D., R.Ph., try mixing Domeboro's powder packets (available in drugstores) with water. The aluminum acetate in the powder keeps skin from getting too dry or itchy. Follow package directions.

### WHEN TO CALL A DOCTOR

A severe burn can take a lot out of you, says Rodney Basler, M.D. Consult a doctor if you experience nausea, chills, fever, faintness, extensive blistering, general weakness, patches of purple discoloration, or intense itching. Be aware that if the burn seems to be spreading, you could have an infection compounding the problem.

*Witch hazel.* Moisten a cloth with witch hazel, says Fredric Haberman, M.D. This incredible astringent has been shown to have long-lasting anti-inflammatory relief. Apply often for temporary relief. For smaller areas, dip cotton balls into the liquid and gently stroke on.

**Soak the pain away.** An alternative to compresses, especially for larger areas, is a cool bath. Add more liquid as needed to keep the water at the proper temperature. Afterward, gently pat your skin dry with a clean towel. Do not rub your skin, or you'll irritate it further. The following substances can reduce pain, itching, and inflammation.

*Vinegar.* Mix 1 cup of white or apple cider vinegar into a tub of cool water, says Carl Korn, M.D. A great astringent, it soothes sunburn pain.

## Do just 1 thing

Take some aspirin. This old standby can help relieve the pain, itching, and swelling of a mild to moderate burn. "Take two tablets every 4 hours," says Rodney Basler, M.D. The same dosage of Tylenol also would work. Or, if your stomach can tolerate it, you might try ibuprofen every 8 hours. Follow label instructions for dosages.

If you know you've gotten too much sun, try taking aspirin *before* the redness appears. "Some doctors recommend 650 milligrams of aspirin soon after sun exposure. Repeat every 4 hours for up to six doses," says Thomas Gossel, Ph.D., R.Ph.

*Aveeno powder.* If the sunburn involves a large area, use the premeasured packets or add ½ cup of Aveeno Bath Treatment, made from oatmeal, to a tub of cool water, says Dr. Schreiber. Soak for 15 to 20 minutes. Aveeno is a well-known remedy for itching.

*Baking soda.* Generously sprinkle baking soda into tepid bathwater, suggests Dr. Haberman. Instead of toweling off, let the solution dry on your skin. It is completely nontoxic, and it will soothe the pain.

**Go easy on soap.** Soap can dry and irritate burned skin. If you must use soap, says Dr. Gossel, use only a mild brand and rinse it off very well. Do not soak in soapy water. Likewise, stay away from bubble baths.

**Moisturize your skin.** Soaks and compresses feel good and give temporary relief, says Rodney Basler, M.D. But they can make your skin feel drier than before if you don't apply moisturizer immediately afterward. Pat yourself dry, then smooth on some bath oil.

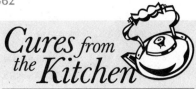

## Cures from the Kitchen

Common kitchen staples can be great sunburn soothers. Press the following into emergency action.

**Oatmeal.** Wrap dry oatmeal in cheesecloth or gauze. Run cool water through it. Discard the oatmeal and soak compresses in the liquid. Apply every 2 to 4 hours.

**Fat-free milk.** Mix 1 cup fat-free milk with 4 cups water, then add a few ice cubes. Apply compresses for 15 to 20 minutes; repeat every 2 to 4 hours.

**Cornstarch.** Add enough water to cornstarch to make a paste. Apply directly to the sunburn.

**Lettuce.** Boil lettuce leaves in water. Strain, then let the liquid cool several hours in the refrigerator. Dip cotton balls into the liquid and gently press or stroke onto irritated skin.

**Yogurt.** Apply yogurt to all sunburned areas. Rinse off in a cool shower, then gently pat skin dry.

**Tea bags.** If your eyelids are burned, apply tea bags soaked in cool water to decrease swelling and help relieve pain. Tea has tannic acid, which seems to ease sunburn pain.

Let it soak in for a minute, then apply a moisturizing cream or lotion, such as Eucerin. Some people like a topical cream called Wibi, which contains a little bit of cooling menthol.

**Chill out.** For added relief, try chilling your moisturizer before applying it.

**Seek hydrocortisone relief.** Soothe skin irritation and inflammation with a topical lotion, spray, or ointment containing 1 percent hydrocortisone, such as Cortaid or Cortizone-10, says Dr. Basler.

**Say goodbye with aloe.** "We're starting to see evidence in medical literature that aloe vera may really help wound healing," says Dr. Basler. Simply break off a leaf and apply the juice. But test a small area first, he cautions, to make sure you're not allergic to aloe.

**Guard against infection.** If you have an infection or are worried that one will develop, use an over-the-counter antibacterial ointment such as Polysporin or Neosporin, says Dr. Schreiber.

**Try a local anesthetic.** If your burn is mild, an over-the-counter anesthetic can relieve pain and itching, says Dr. Gossel. Look for brands that contain benzocaine, benzyl alcohol, lidocaine, or diphenhydramine hydrochloride. Aerosols are easier to apply than creams or ointments, but never spray them directly onto your face. Instead, put some on a piece of gauze or a cotton pad and pat it on your face to avoid contact with your eyes.

**Try an ice pack.** An ice pack can also provide relief if the burn is mild. Wrap it in a damp cloth and hold it over the sunburn. Improvise, if necessary, says Dr. Haberman. "You could even take a bag of frozen peas, for instance, and use that. But make sure to wrap it first so that you're not placing the icy package directly against your skin."

**Drink up.** It's a good idea to drink lots of water to help counteract the drying effects of a sunburn, says Dr. Gossel.

**Eat right.** Eat lightly but wisely, Dr. Gossel adds. A balanced diet helps provide the nutrients your skin needs to regenerate itself.

**Raise your legs.** If your legs are burned and your feet are swollen, elevate your legs above heart level to help stop the swelling, says Dr. Basler.

**Get a good night's rest.** Sleeping on a sunburn can be challenging, but you need rest for your body to recover from the burn. Try sprinkling talcum powder on your sheets to minimize chafing and friction, says Dr. Haberman. A waterbed or air mattress might also help you sleep more easily.

**Be careful with blisters.** If blisters develop, you have a pretty bad burn. If they bother you and they cover only a small area, you may carefully drain them, says Dr. Basler. But do not peel the top skin off—you'll have less discomfort and danger of infection if air does not come in contact with sensitive nerve endings.

To drain the fluid, first sterilize a needle by holding it over a flame. Then puncture the edge of the blister and press gently on the top to let the fluid come

---

**What the Doctor Does ...**

Rit Sun Guard is sun protection for your skin that you wash into your clothing. It is available at some supermarkets, drugstores, mass merchandisers, and online at www.DERMAdoctor.com. "This product increases the capability of fabric to prevent ultraviolet (UV) rays from reaching the skin and is the relative equivalent of a sun protection factor rating of 30 for sunscreen," says Audrey Kunin, M.D.

Simply add it to the wash cycle, rinse, and dry your clothes as usual. One treatment of Rit Sun Guard is good for more than 20 additional washings, says Dr. Kunin.

"Your typical T-shirt has an ultraviolet protection factor of 5, but by adding this Rit Sun Guard to the wash cycle, that same T-shirt will have a UV protection rating of 30," she says.

out. Do this three times in the first 24 hours, says Dr. Basler. Then leave the blisters alone.

**Beware ice and snow.** Don't let your guard down in winter, says Butch Farabee, former assistant superintendent of Montana's Glacier National Park. You can get a fierce burn from the sun's rays reflected off ice and snow. "I've even gotten the inside of my mouth sunburned when hiking up icy hills because I was breathing so hard that my mouth was open," he says. So cover up appropriately and wear sunscreen on all exposed areas.

**Don't make the same mistake twice.** After you've gotten burned, it takes 3 to 6 months for your skin to return to normal, says Dr. Schreiber. "When you get a sunburn and the top layer of skin peels off, the newly exposed skin is more sensitive than ever. That means you'll burn even faster than you did before if you're not careful."

**Follow the rules.** While the memory of your burn is still painfully fresh, brush up on your sun sense with these tips from Norman Levine, M.D.

- Apply a sunscreen about 30 minutes before going out, even if it's overcast. (Harmful rays can penetrate cloud cover.) Don't forget to protect your lips, hands, ears, and the back of your neck. Reapply as necessary after swimming or perspiring heavily.
- Pick a sunscreen with a sun protection factor (SPF) between 15 and 30. Sunscreens with SPF 15 protect against 94 percent of the sun's harmful rays, and those with SPF 30 protect against 97 percent. Also look for the ingredients zinc

## Are You Photosensitive?

We're not asking if you like to have your picture taken. The question is whether certain drugs increase your sensitivity to the sun and lead to a burnlike dermatitis.

Antibiotics, tranquilizers, and antifungal medications can cause reactions, says Rodney Basler, M.D. So can oral contraceptives, diuretics, drugs for diabetes, and even PABA-containing sunscreens. Always ask your doctor about potential side effects of any drugs you may be taking.

Even common foods can trigger a bad reaction. "Two young women I know tried to lighten their hair with lime juice," he says. "They didn't realize what a potent photosensitizer lime juice can be until they developed terrible dermatitis every place the juice had run down their faces and arms."

oxide, titanium dioxide, or avobenzone in your sunscreen. These block both ultraviolet A and B rays.

- Take extra care between the hours of 10:00 A.M. and 3:00 P.M. (11:00 A.M. and 4:00 P.M., daylight saving time), when the sun is at its strongest.
- Wear protective clothing when not swimming. Hats, tightly woven fabrics, and long sleeves help keep the sun off your skin.

## PANEL OF ADVISORS

**Rodney Basler, M.D.,** is a dermatologist and assistant professor of internal medicine at the University of Nebraska College of Medicine in Lincoln.

**Butch Farabee** is a former assistant superintendent of Montana's Glacier National Park in West Glacier. He had many years of field experience as a park ranger.

**Thomas Gossel, Ph.D., R.Ph.,** is a professor of pharmacology and toxicology at Ohio Northern University in Ada. He is an expert on over-the-counter products.

**Fredric Haberman, M.D.,** is an assistant clinical professor of medicine at the Albert Einstein College of Medicine of Yeshiva University in Bronx, New York, and director of the Haberman Dermatology Institute in Saddle Brook and Ridgewood, New Jersey, and New York City.

**Carl Korn, M.D.,** is an assistant clinical professor of dermatology at the University of Southern California in Los Angeles.

**Audrey Kunin, M.D.,** is a cosmetic dermatologist in Kansas City, Missouri, and the founder of the dermatology educational Web site DERMAdoctor.com.

**Norman Levine, M.D.,** is a professor of medicine in the department of dermatology at the University of Arizona College of Medicine in Tucson.

**Lia Schorr** is a skin-care specialist and director of Lia Schorr Institute of Cosmetics Skin-Care Training in New York City. She is the author of *Salonovations' Advanced Skin Care Handbook*.

**Michael Schreiber, M.D.,** is senior clinical lecturer in the department of internal medicine at the University of Arizona College of Medicine in Tucson and a dermatologist in Tucson.

# TACHYCARDIA
## 12 Ways to Calm a Rapid Heartbeat

It comes on suddenly. Seventy-two beats a minute become 120 . . . 180 . . . 200 beats in only seconds. The rapid heartbeat makes it hard to breathe and causes nausea and heavy perspiration.

This is tachycardia—more specifically, paroxysmal atrial tachycardia—which means that your heart is racing, beating faster than 100 beats per minute. This occurs when your atria—the chambers in your heart that receive blood from the veins and pump it into the ventricles—get a little out of control. The atria are still keeping a steady rhythm, but the rhythm can be three times faster than normal.

Here's how to put the brakes on tachycardia.

## WHEN TO CALL A DOCTOR

If your heart has lost its sense of timing, get to a doctor—as soon as possible. Only a doctor can distinguish between paroxysmal atrial tachycardia and more serious forms of heart arrhythmia, says Arthur Selzer, M.D.

Ventricular tachycardia is an example of a more serious, potentially life-threatening kind. That's what you have when one ventricle starts beating rapidly with a slightly irregular rhythm. (The ventricle is the heart chamber that pumps blood back into the arteries.) The amount of blood your heart returns to the arteries may drop markedly. You feel weak, sweaty; you may even faint.

Ventricular fibrillation, which sometimes occurs as a complication of ventricular tachycardia, is usually fatal. That's why we can't stress enough the importance of attending to any abnormal heart rhythms immediately. The right response to an attack depends on what the malfunction is.

A checkup may rule out ventricular tachycardia and all forms of heart disease, thyroid abnormalities, and pulmonary malfunctions.

**Slow down.** Think of that speeding heart as a flashing red light that says, "Stop what you're doing. Chill out. Rest." Rest, in fact, is your best mechanism for stopping an attack, says Dennis S. Miura, M.D., Ph.D.

**Try the vagal maneuver.** How fast your heart beats and how strongly it contracts are regulated by sympathetic nerves and parasympathetic nerves (or vagal nerves). When your heart pounds, the sympathetic network is dominant. (That's the system that basically tells your body to speed up.) What you want to do is switch control to the mellower parasympathetic network. If you stimulate a vagal nerve, you initiate a chemical process that affects your heart in the same way that slamming on the brakes affects your car.

One way to do this is to take a deep breath and bear down, as if you were having a bowel movement, says John O. Lawder, M.D.

**Reach for the right carotid artery.** Gently massaging the right carotid artery is another vagal maneuver. Be sure to have your doctor show you the right point and the right degree of pressure. You want to massage the artery where it connects in the neck, as far underneath the jaw as possible, says James Frackelton, M.D.

**Rely on the diving reflex.** When sea mammals dive into the coldest regions of the water, their heart rates automatically slow. That's nature's way of preserving their brains and hearts. You can call on your own diving reflex by filling a basin with icy water and plunging your face into it for a second or two.

"Sometimes, that will interrupt the tachycardia," says Dr. Miura.

**Break the coffee habit.** Ditto for cola, tea, chocolate, diet pills, or stimulants in any form. Overuse of stimulants can put you at risk for tachycardia, says Dr. Miura.

**Baby your hypothalamus.** What goes on in your head—your midbrain specifically—rules your heart, says Dr. Frackelton. That's why it's essential for you to give your hypothalamus the support it needs—through proper diet, exercise, a positive attitude—to maintain stability and control over your autonomic nervous system.

Stress, poor diet, and pollutants cause your hypothalamus to lose its grip on the autonomic nervous system, allowing the system to slip into high gear or what Dr. Frackelton terms *sympathetic overload.*

Here's how to help your hypothalamus retain control.

***Eat healthful, regular meals and go easy on the sweets.*** If you skip meals and then fill your stomach with a candy bar or soda, your pancreatic enzymes speed in to take care of the increased sugar intake, says Dr.

Frackelton. Then your insulin overshoots and you go into reactive hypoglycemia, or low blood sugar. Your adrenal glands bring adrenaline in to mobilize the stores of glycogen (sugar) in your liver to combat the low blood sugar levels. It's this adrenaline rush that stimulates a sudden increase in heart rate and the feeling of panic.

***Tailor your meal schedule to your metabolism.*** People who have a rapid metabolism should eat more protein foods, says Dr. Lawder. Proteins take longer to digest and help prevent your blood sugar from falling too low. When your blood sugar drops, it triggers the process discussed above.

***Let loose.*** Dr. Lawder says he's noticed a relationship between perfectionist, upwardly mobile, success-oriented individuals and tachycardia. "By and large, these are the same people who get migraine headaches," he says. "For people like this, the conduction mechanisms of the heart become highly exaggerated. There's chronic adrenaline overstimulation. When people are under a lot of stress, there is a breakthrough of autonomic conduction of the heart, a loss of rhythm."

How to compensate? Adopt a progressive relaxation program, practice biofeedback, or learn to visualize "serenity, tranquility, calmness, and peace," says Dr. Lawder.

### Get your fair share of magnesium.
In the muscle cells of the heart, magnesium helps balance the effects of calcium, which stimulates muscular contractions within the cell itself. Magnesium creates rhythmic contraction and relaxation, helping the enzymes in the cells pump calcium out, and making the heart less likely to get irritable, says Dr. Frackelton. Magnesium can be found in such foods as soybeans, nuts, beans, and bran.

### Keep potassium levels up.
Potassium is another mineral that helps slow heart action and reduce irritability of the muscle fibers, says Dr. Lawder. The mineral is found in fruits and vegetables, so getting enough shouldn't be difficult. But you can deplete it if your diet is high in sodium or if you use diuretics or overuse laxatives.

### Exercise.
"You can do a lot by getting into good tone," says Dr. Frackelton. "When you do the kinds of exercise that raise the heart rate, it tends to reset at a lower level. People who don't exercise usually have a heart rate around 80. When they begin to do a little bit of jogging, their heart rates go up to 160, 170. Then, with a little conditioning, they can bring the resting heart rate down to 60 to 65."

Exercise also makes you resistant to excess adrenaline release, he says. "It gets your aggressions out in a healthy way. You're using adrenaline release as part of a normal function."

## PANEL OF ADVISORS

# TEETHING
## 6 Ways to Soothe the Pain

Just one of the many miracles of life, an infant's teeth actually start developing months before birth. In fact, tooth buds begin appearing by the 7th week of pregnancy. By the time the baby is born, all 20 of the primary teeth that will sprout over the next $2\frac{1}{2}$ years are already present and accounted for in the jawbone.

Usually those first teeth start pushing for daylight 4 to 8 months after birth. Baby's gums become swollen and tender, and the little guy (or girl) becomes irritable and restless. Get ready—teething has begun.

### WHEN TO CALL A DOCTOR

"One of the most common myths is that babies will run a fever when teething," says pediatric nurse practitioner Linda Jonides. "If there's a fever, it means something else is going on in your baby's body. You should see your doctor."

An infant can react to this new sensation of teething in a variety of different ways.

"You could be in for nothing or for a little fussiness that goes along with the discomfort," says John A. Bogert, D.D.S. "Most infants are a little fussy and cranky with the first two to four teeth."

That doesn't sound so bad, but just in case your baby's teething gets a little more intense, here are a few helpful hints to see both of you through it.

**Cool those teeth.** "Chewing on teething rings, particularly those you can put in the refrigerator and keep cold, works very well and feels good on the baby's gums," says pediatric nurse practitioner Linda Jonides. "For a baby who's 6 months or older, even a clean, cold washcloth to chew on feels good," she adds. Avoid the teething rings with anything except water inside. They could break, and the liquid inside might not be safe. In addition, never tie a teething ring around a baby's neck. This could put your child at an unsafe risk of strangulation.

**Dab the drool.** Teething can cause a baby to drool, a lot. Use a warm washcloth often to wipe the drool off your baby's face to prevent a rash from developing.

**Gauze the gums.** Dentists and pediatricians advise cleaning your baby's mouth before the teeth appear. Use a lightly moistened, small gauze pad or even a soft baby washcloth wrapped around your forefinger to massage the gums.

Doing so removes bacteria buildup and gets the youngster used to having someone poking around inside her mouth. "That way, when that first tooth does come in, you can start brushing it right away without a lot of trauma," Dr. Bogert notes. Plus, daily massaging makes for much healthier gum tissue.

How soon should you start? "We actually recommend you start doing this the day you get the child home from the hospital," Dr. Bogert says. "But you're probably not too late if you begin today. A couple of times a day is good—especially at bedtime."

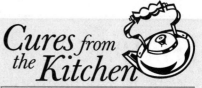

## Cures from the Kitchen

Instead of the typical teething ring, try giving your baby some frozen grapes or bananas in a product called Baby Safe Feeder. Designed to eliminate choking hazards for early eaters, the feeder looks similar to a pacifier with a small mesh bag (instead of a nipple) that can hold food for your baby to suck or chew. Most standard teething rings are flavorless, so just a little frozen fruit will give the baby an incentive to bite down and work those teeth through the gums.

When you do start brushing your infant's little teeth, make sure you use a child's soft toothbrush. And be gentle.

**Use over-the-counter products for pain and swelling.** "I recommend trying the types of things most parents already keep handy for pediatric pain," says Dr. Bogert. Usually, that's infants' Tylenol or Motrin. A number of topical anesthetics, such as Baby Orajel and Zilactin Baby, are also good for relieving teething pain and are available over the counter at any drugstore. Just wipe some on the gums for quick relief.

**Ban the bottle.** Well, not completely. But especially once she's teething, make sure your child doesn't fall asleep with a bottle in her mouth. The milk or juice can pool in the mouth and start the process of tooth decay and plaque.

## PANEL OF ADVISORS

**John A. Bogert, D.D.S.,** is a retired dentist in Chicago.

**Linda Jonides** is a pediatric nurse practitioner in Ann Arbor, Michigan.

**Helen Neville, R.N.,** is director of the Inborn Temperament Project at Kaiser Permanente Hospital in Oakland, California, and the author of *Temperament Tools*.

# TEMPOROMANDIBULAR DISORDERS
## 17 Ideas to Ease the Discomfort

Temporomandibular disorders, a group of diseases commonly known as TMD, are without a doubt among the most complex and controversial of all modern ailments.

While TMD is usually linked to problems with the muscles or joints (or a combination of the two), it sometimes involves related tissues, such as the ligaments or bone cartilage. Many experts believe that most cases have multiple causes. Trauma, stress, misaligned teeth, orthodontic treatment, and arthritis are just some of the factors associated with TMD. Other factors are yet to be discovered.

## WHEN TO CALL A DOCTOR

The most common signs of temporomandibular disorders (TMD)—among them, facial and jaw joint pain or swelling; headaches; toothaches; aching neck, shoulders, or back; and a clicking, grating, or popping noise or pain when opening or closing your jaw—are usually nothing more than minor to moderate annoyances that will go away when the condition is treated. Few people develop significant long-term effects.

Some symptoms, however, are considered more serious and should be investigated by your doctor, warns Harold T. Perry, D.D.S., Ph.D.

"If you can't open your mouth, can't brush your teeth, and are having sharp headaches, go see a doctor," he says. It's definitely a sign that your TMD is getting worse.

What is clearly known is that women appear to have TMD symptoms at about twice the rate of men. Fortunately, in the majority of cases, TMD pain is temporary and can be relieved with simple measures. Here are a few that our experts recommend.

**Apply heat or cold.** That is, do anything you can to increase bloodflow to the area. Heat is better for recurrent or prolonged conditions, but cold is more effective for relieving acute pain and reducing strain and swelling that go along with it, says Sheldon Gross, D.D.S. Don't interchange the two or use cold therapy for a prolonged period, since this could damage the tissues. For cold treatment, wrap an ice pack or a bag of frozen peas in a towel. Apply to the affected area for 5 to 10 minutes, or until it feels a little numb. Do not exceed 20 minutes. Repeat every 2 hours for up to 2 days, or until the pain is relieved. Apply heat therapy, using a warm compress, for the same length of time.

You can also try gently stretching and massaging the jaw as long as the muscles don't cramp up. If you get the blood flowing in the area, you are likely to alleviate some of your symptoms, says Dr. Gross. This will help gradually increase your range of motion and strengthen the joint.

**Take an anti-inflammatory and perform self-massage.** "Aspirin is a marvelous drug for any muscle or joint problem," says Harold Perry, D.D.S., Ph.D. He suggests one tablet followed up with a self-massage of the jaw several minutes later. You can also try other anti-inflammatories, such as ibuprofen or naproxen (Aleve), to relieve pain and reduce swelling.

**Check your body position.** If you work at a desk, check your body position throughout the day. Make sure that you, and especially your chin, are not leaning over the desk, says Owen J. Rogal, D.D.S. Your back should be supported. As a general guideline for sitting or standing, your cheekbone should be over your clavicle, and your ears should not be too far in front of your shoulders, he says.

If you have neck pain and headaches, Dr. Rogal suggests attaching an adjustable document holder to your computer monitor to minimize neck strain as you work.

**Throw away your head pillow.** Instead, tuck yourself in with a pillow under your knees. You can also use wedge-shaped pillows that are designed for reclining. Sleeping in this position—on your back throughout the entire night with your head, neck, shoulders, and upper back in alignment and less pressure on your lower back—can be very relaxing to your jaws and critical to overcoming TMD, says Dr. Rogal. But what if you generally sleep on your side? He suggests placing a beanbag on either side of your head to stop you from rolling over into that position.

**Limit your jaw movement.** If you feel a yawn coming, restrict it by holding a fist under your chin, says Andrew S. Kaplan, D.M.D. Yawning can stress the jaw.

**Don't chew gum.** Repetitive chewing can stress the jaw. Control other similar habits, such as biting your lips or fingernails, and use your pencil for writing, not chewing, advises Dr. Gross.

**Stop grinding your teeth.** Gnashing teeth, referred to by doctors as bruxism, is often associated with TMD and may be a factor that exacerbates existing symptoms, says Dr. Kaplan.

**Use a mouth guard.** Pick up the kind of mouth guard sold in sporting goods stores and drugstores that you soften in hot water and then bite down on to form a better fit in your mouth. It shouldn't feel loose or uncomfortable when you bite down. Wearing one during the day can help reduce grinding and clenching, says Dr. Gross.

If your symptoms seem worse in the morning, wear a mouth guard during the night, recommends Dr. Gross. You may be grinding your teeth while you sleep. In some cases, bruxism can lead to poor sleep habits and aggravate symptoms.

**Avoid hard, crunchy food.** If you have a lot of pain in and around your mouth, consider limiting yourself to soft and liquid food for a while, suggests Dr. Perry.

**Consider acupressure.** To find the point that will ease TMD cheek pain on the left side of your face, Albert Forgione, Ph.D., recommends the following:

## Seven Habits to Break

Overcoming temporomandibular disorders (TMD) is very much a matter of what you don't do, advises Andrew S. Kaplan, D.M.D. If any of these habits are yours—pay attention! These tips may be of help to you. Don't:

- Sleep on your stomach with your head twisted to one side
- Lie on your back with your head propped up at a sharp angle for reading or watching television
- Cradle the telephone between your shoulder and chin
- Prop your chin on one or both of your hands for too long
- Carry a heavy shoulder bag with the strap on the same shoulder for an extended period
- Avoid situations, such as painting a ceiling or sitting on the front row during movies, that require looking up for long periods of time
- Grind or clench your teeth

Lay your left forearm on a table with your palm flat down. Put the fingers of your right hand on your left forearm so that your index finger is in the fold of your elbow and the rest of your fingers lay next to each other. Wiggle your left middle finger and feel the corresponding ligament move at the edge of your right index fingertip. Press moderately hard on this point for 15 seconds (the point will feel quite sensitive and will hurt if you have found the right spot). You may have to do this three times in a row, pausing briefly in between. Switch sides to relieve pain on the right side of your face.

## PANEL OF ADVISORS

**Albert Forgione, Ph.D.,** is a pain specialist and director of research at the Gelb Craniomandibular Orofacial Pain Center at Tufts University School of Dental Medicine in Boston.

**Sheldon Gross, D.D.S.,** is a dentist in Bloomfield, Connecticut. He is a lecturer in Tufts University School of Dental Medicine's postgraduate orofacial pain program in Boston and the University of Medicine and Dentistry of New Jersey/New Jersey Dental School in Newark. He is also on the board of directors of the American Academy of Orofacial Pain, past president of the American Academy of Craniomandibular Disorders, and a member of both the American Pain Association and the American Headache Association.

**Andrew S. Kaplan, D.M.D.,** is an associate clinical professor of dentistry at the Mount Sinai School of Medicine of New York University and director of the TMJ and Facial Pain Clinic and attending dentist at Mount Sinai Hospital in New York City.

**Harold T. Perry, D.D.S., Ph.D.,** is a lecturer of orthodontics in the School of Dentistry at Marquette University in Milwaukee. He was a professor of orthodontics at the former Northwestern University Dental School in Chicago. He was also the editor of *The Journal of Craniomandibular Disorders* and a past president of the American Academy of Craniomandibular Disorders.

**Owen J. Rogal, D.D.S.,** is the director of the Pain Center in Philadelphia, which specializes in diagnosing and treating many types of pain, including TMD. He is a past executive director of the former American Academy of Head, Neck, and Facial Neck Pain, now called the American Academy of Craniofacial Pain.

# TENDINITIS
## 14 Soothing Remedies

Like simple muscle soreness from overuse, tendinitis—inflammation in or around a tendon—can be painful. But where simple muscle soreness is temporary, tendinitis is tenacious. It's soreness that doesn't go away with a few hours' rest and an ice pack.

## WHEN TO CALL A DOCTOR

If you only feel the pain of tendinitis during or after exercise, and if it isn't too bad, you may be thinking that you could run a race or swim laps with that same amount of pain—if you had to. Or maybe you already have.

In either case, you would be wise to realign your thinking. "You shouldn't play through pain unless your physician or physical therapist tells you otherwise," says the American Physical Therapy Association's Bob Mangine.

If pain is severe and you continue to abuse the tendon, it may rupture, says trainer Bob Reese. That could mean a long layoff, surgery, or even permanent disability.

In other words, exercising through tendon pain today could mean staying on the sidelines for the remainder of your tomorrows. To err on the safe side, back off if you're in pain, and see a physician if your pain is persistent.

The situation isn't hopeless, insists the American Physical Therapy Association's Bob Mangine. "But if you continue to use the tendon in the same repetitive motion that triggered the problem in the first place, it's going to be very difficult to get better." That applies to everyone from world-class marathoners to window washers and typists.

Still, it's possible to lessen the effects of tendinitis and prevent intense flare-ups, says Mangine. The key, he says, is unlocking your mind and freeing yourself to change some of your old ways.

**Give it a rest.** "That's a hard thing to get people to do," says Mangine. But a runner with Achilles tendinitis, for example, can't realistically expect any improvement if he doesn't take at least a couple of days away from the one-two pounding.

Of course, resting is easier said than done if the activity triggering your tendinitis is part of your job. If you have occupational tendinitis, it might not be a bad idea to save a day or two of vacation for those times when tendinitis is painfully persistent.

**But don't give it too long a rest.** "Muscles will start to atrophy," Mangine says. For athletes, "we never recommend absolute rest," adds Ted Percy, M.D. The key is to cross-train when possible. Choose an activity that doesn't reproduce the pain, so you can avoid the prolonged rest period and still maintain your cardiovascular endurance.

**Make a change.** If your tendinitis is exercise-induced, a new form of exercise may be just what your inflamed tendon needs. If you're a runner with tendon problems in the lower legs, for example, you can stay on the road if you're willing to hop on a bicycle, which will still give you a good upper-leg workout.

**Have a soak.** Taking a whirlpool bath or just soaking in warm bathwater is a good way to raise body temperature and increase bloodflow. Warming the tendon before stressful activity decreases the soreness associated with tendinitis, says Mangine.

**Use the ballerina treatment.** The New York Jets football team finds this method (inspired by a ballet dancer who had tendinitis) successful. Place a warm, moist towel over the tender tendon, then a plastic bag, then a heating pad, and last, a loose elastic wrap just to hold everything in place. Keep it on from 2 to 6 hours. To avoid burning yourself, keep the heating pad on low, advises former head trainer Bob Reese. For maximum success, your injured body part should be kept at a level higher than your heart.

**Warm with stretching.** The heat treatments above are only the first part of the warmup equation. You should always stretch before exercising at full speed, says Terry Malone, Ed.D. Stretching prevents the shortening of muscles and tendons that goes along with exercise.

In addition, says Mangine, some studies suggest that people who are less flexible are more prone to develop tendinitis. So stretching should be a regular part of your routine.

**Get braced for action.** Even a little extra support and warmth from a flexible brace or wrap can help during exercise and afterward, Mangine says. "There is no truth to the old wives' tale that wearing a brace will weaken the tendons and muscles, provided," he stresses, "you continue exercising."

**Use ice.** After exercising, ice is great for holding down both swelling and pain, Mangine says. People with heart disease, diabetes, or vascular problems, however, should be careful about using ice because ice constricts blood vessels and could cause serious difficulties in people with such problems. (For more information about using an ice pack, see page 550.)

**Wrap it up.** Another alternative for reducing swelling is to wrap your pain in an elastic bandage, says Dr. Percy. Just be careful not to wrap the inflamed area too tightly or to leave the area wrapped for so long that it becomes uncomfortable or interferes with circulation. (For more information about using an elastic bandage, see Sprains on page 550.)

**Raise the squeaky wheel.** Elevating the affected area above heart level is also good for controlling swelling.

**Wear a higher heel.** For Achilles tendinitis, wearing cowboy boots or high heels some of the time is a fine idea, according to Dr. Percy. "It lifts the heel off the ground," he says, "and the muscles and tendons don't have to work as hard."

**Go over the counter.** Aspirin, ibuprofen, and naproxen (Aleve)—nonprescription nonsteroidal anti-inflammatory drugs—are effective temporary pain relievers for tendinitis, Dr. Percy says. They also reduce inflammation and swelling.

**Strengthen your body.** "When we say strengthen, we're not asking people to be an Arnold Schwarzenegger," Mangine says, "just to get better defined muscles by working out at home with light weights. There's no difference between the training muscles or tendons and ligaments. All tissues develop simultaneously. You can even use pennies in a sock to work arm muscles." That's a lot cheaper than a set of weights.

**Take breaks.** This is a simple way to at least temporarily relieve physical stress at work, says Scott Donkin, D.C. "If you work in an awkward position," he says, "tendinitis can develop quite easily. Especially in the arms or wrists if you're working at a keyboard or typewriter all day."

## PANEL OF ADVISORS

**Scott Donkin, D.C.,** is a partner in the Chiropractic Associates in Lincoln, Nebraska. He is also an industrial consultant, providing tips on exercise to reduce stress for workstation users, and the author of *Sitting on the Job.*

**Terry Malone, Ed.D.,** is the director of physical therapy at the University of Kentucky in Lexington.

**Bob Mangine** is chairman of the American Physical Therapy Association's sports physical therapy section. He also is administrative director of rehabilitation at the Novacare Physical Rehabilitation in Florence, Kentucky, and author of *Physical Therapy of the Knee.*

**Ted Percy, M.D.,** is an associate professor emeritus of orthopedic surgery and sports medicine and head of the sports medicine section at the Arizona Health Sciences Center at the University of Arizona College of Medicine in Tucson.

**Bob Reese** is the former head trainer for the New York Jets and past president of the Professional Football Athletic Trainers Society. He is now an associate professor at the College of Health Sciences in Roanoke, Virginia.

# TINNITUS
## 17 Ways to Cope with the Din

The noise of the modern world is bad enough, but people with tinnitus have the added burden of hearing sounds in their own heads. This irritating condition causes people to hear clicking, roaring, ringing, or buzzing sounds when no external sounds actually exist.

Doctors and audiologists think tinnitus is caused by damage to the microscopic hairs on auditory cells in the inner ear, which in turn causes portions of the brain to generate its own sound.

Persistent exposure to ear-splitting music or other loud sounds is the main cause of tinnitus. It has also been linked to hearing loss, circulatory problems, and middle-ear problems. Tinnitus is often accompanied by an intense sensitivity to sounds called *hyperacusis*, explains Dhyan Cassie, Au.D., a doctor of audiology.

## WHEN TO CALL A DOCTOR

Because tinnitus can be caused by so many things, including a tumor, Lyme disease, and other medical problems that are potentially serious, it's essential to see a doctor at the first sign of symptoms, says Dhyan Cassie, Au.D.

If you've started experiencing tinnitus and you're also taking prescription or over-the-counter medications, talk to your doctor or pharmacist, Dr. Cassie adds. A number of drugs, including aspirin or antibiotics, can aggravate tinnitus in some people. Even drugs that help some people with tinnitus, such as antihistamines, may worsen it in others, she explains.

Of the 50 million Americans who experience tinnitus, 12 million have it seriously enough to seek medical help for their condition. It can sometimes be eliminated by treating underlying medical problems, or it sometimes goes away on its own, but the main approach is to help people cope with the persistent noise—and to prevent it from getting worse. Here's what doctors advise.

**Avoid loud noises.** Table saws, power motors, and the ear-pounding volume of rock 'n' roll are just a few of the things that can damage auditory cells and make tinnitus worse.

"If you're 8 feet from someone and have to raise your voice to make yourself heard, the environmental noise is probably too loud," says Douglas Mattox, M.D.

**Pick up some earplugs.** When you know you're going to be exposed to ear-splitting sounds—from a construction crew next door, for example—pick up some earplugs. Pharmacy earplugs work fine, but you'll do better with the type sold at music stores: They allow you to hear music or voices clearly, but at a greatly reduced volume, says auditory researcher Marshall Chasin.

"The earplugs you buy over the counter never fit very well," Chasin adds. "Custom-made earplugs, which are fitted to your ear, are a lot better. They fit like a good pair of shoes—you probably won't even be aware of them."

Customized earplugs are available at audiology clinics or businesses that specialize in hearing aids.

**Don a set of earmuffs.** If you don't like the sensation of earplugs, drop by the hardware store and pick up a set of foam-filled safety muffs, which form a tight seal over the ears. "They can make you feel hot and sweaty, but they're very effective," says Dr. Mattox. You probably won't wear these out in public, to a Billy Joel concert, for example, but they may come in handy while running your table saw in the privacy of your basement.

**Hum away noise.** One of the first lessons drummers learn is that humming for a few seconds during the loudest part of the song helps drown out the crashing sounds of cymbals. You can use the same technique whenever you're anticipating a loud noise—when you're walking past an idling bus, for example, or when you're using power tools at home.

Humming activates a muscle in the inner ear, which pulls tiny bones together and prevents some sound waves from getting through, Chasin says. "In evolutionary terms, the muscle may prevent our own voices from sounding too loud," he explains.

This protects you from tinnitus, because prolonged exposure to loud noises can cause tinnitus.

**Let your hair grow.** "If your hair is reasonably thick, wearing it over the ears will provide three or four decibels of protection," Chasin says. "That may not sound like much, but reducing sound by three decibels essentially means that you can be exposed to the sound for twice as long before damage occurs." This could help keep your tinnitus from getting worse.

## Do just 1 thing

Distract yourself. It can be hard to ignore the sounds of tinnitus, but it's worth making the effort. The more you focus on the sounds, the more likely it is your brain will build additional neural pathways to make your listening more efficient. In other words, you may wind up hearing the annoying sounds even more, says Douglas Mattox, M.D.

"The most important thing is to keep the auditory system busy doing other things," Dr. Mattox advises. "When you're working or doing other quiet activities, create a little ambient noise, like the sound of a small water fountain or an inexpensive noise generator."

An even easier solution is to turn on the radio. Just be sure to keep the volume low, Dr. Mattox advises. "You don't necessarily want sounds that you'll pay attention to or that you'll find distracting."

**Give your ears a rest.** A single loud noise could potentially result in tinnitus, but persistent loud noises are more likely to be a problem. It's important to let the ears "rest" for about 16 hours after exposure to loud sounds. If you spent the morning vacuuming, for example, don't fire up the weed trimmer the same afternoon, Chasin says.

**Obtain a hearing aid if necessary.** About 90 percent of those with severe tinnitus also have hearing loss. Using a hearing aid often helps both problems at the same time.

"As long as the auditory pathway is occupied by outside sounds, you'll be less likely to hear the tinnitus," Dr. Cassie explains.

**Sleep with static.** The sounds of tinnitus aren't really louder at night, but they often seem as though they are because of the relative silence of the surroundings. Creating a little background sound—the static of a radio set between stations, for example, or the whir of a small fan, for example—helps mask the sounds of tinnitus and makes it easier to rest, Dr. Cassie says.

**Get a wearable sound generator.** Available from audiologists, sound generators are hearing-aid-like devices that fill the ears with a soft white noise. "As long as the auditory pathways are occupied, the brain can't concentrate on the sounds of tinnitus, and it will eventually learn to ignore it," Dr. Cassie explains.

**Watch what you eat.** Red wine, chocolate, pickles, and other processed foods that contain chemicals called sulfides may increase tinnitus in some people, Chasin says.

**Eat less salt.** Tinnitus is sometimes caused by Ménière's disease, a condition which results in excessive amounts of fluid in the ear. People with this condition should restrict their daily sodium intake to 2,000 milligrams by limiting the use of table salt, for example, and buying low-sodium soups, condiments, and other packaged foods.

**Cut back on caffeine.** If you drink a lot of coffee, tea, or cola, you might experience higher levels of tinnitus. That's because caffeine constricts blood vessels and temporarily raises blood pressure, which can make the sounds of tinnitus louder. Giving up caffeine isn't likely to eliminate the problem, but it might make a small difference in some people, says Dr. Mattox.

**Don't smoke.** The nicotine in cigarettes and cigars has the same effect as caffeine: It constricts blood vessels and may make tinnitus sounds more noticeable.

**Reduce the noise with baby oil.** Buildups of earwax can impair hearing and potentially make the sounds of tinnitus louder. One solution is to apply a few drops of baby oil with an eyedropper once or twice a day for several days. Once the wax softens, gently flush the ear canal with warm water, using a bulb syringe. Repeating this several times removes excessive wax from the ear canal.

Get your doctor's okay before using baby oil and water to flush the ear canal, Dr. Cassie adds. "There could be a ruptured eardrum behind the wax, and the treatment could cause additional problems," she explains.

**Try "tinnitus retraining."** Studies have shown that when people subject themselves to a quiet sound—static or white noise from a sound generator that's just loud enough to mask the tinnitus sounds—the internal noise may diminish or even disappear.

"Over a period of months, you'll find that the volume of sound needed to mask the tinnitus keeps getting lower," Chasin says.

**Practice stress control.** "When people are under stress, they feel it in the weakest part of the body," says Dr. Cassie. "If you already have tinnitus, high levels of stress are likely to make the sounds seem even louder."

Everyone controls stress in different ways. Some people exercise. Others meditate, practice yoga, or retreat to the movies for the afternoon. "I'm a big fan of self-hypnosis," Dr. Cassie says. You can buy audiotapes or CDs that explain how to do it. Or you can see a professional hypnotist or other therapists who will help you find ways to unwind on your own.

## PANEL OF ADVISORS

**Dhyan Cassie, Au.D.,** is a doctor of audiology and coordinator of the Tinnitus/Hyperacusis Management Clinic for Speech and Hearing Associates at the College of New Jersey in Ewing.

**Marshall Chasin** is an audiologist and director of auditory research at the Musicians' Clinics of Canada in Toronto and the author of *Musicians and the Prevention of Hearing Loss*.

**Douglas Mattox, M.D.,** is chairman of the department of otolaryngology–head and neck surgery at Emory University School of Medicine in Atlanta.

# TOOTHACHE
## 12 Tips for Pain Relief

It's no wonder dentistry may have been one of the earliest medical specializations in ancient Egypt. Toothaches can be excruciatingly painful. The Egyptians used some bizarre methods to ward off tooth pain—for example placing a live mouse on the gums of a person with tooth pain. Mice have such good teeth, they reasoned, there should be some effect. By Roman times, things were only marginally better. One ancient scholar noted that a frog tied to the jaws would make teeth firmer, and that toothaches responded to ear drops made from boiling earthworms in olive oil.

The good news is, no rodents, amphibians, or worms need to be harmed to follow the advice we've gathered from *modern* dentists. Here's what they suggest for tooth pain.

**Rinse.** Take a mouthful of tepid water and rinse vigorously, says Jerry F. Taintor, D.D.S. If your toothache is caused by trapped food, a thorough rinse may dislodge the problem.

---

### WHEN TO CALL A DOCTOR

A toothache can be a symptom of a wide range of problems, says Philip D. Corn, D.D.S. The pulp of your tooth or the gums around your throbbing cuspid could be infected. There could be decay in a molar. You may have a cracked bicuspid.

An injury, a piece of food caught between two teeth, or even a sinus problem may be at the root of your pain, adds Jerry F. Taintor, D.D.S. The bottom line? If you have tooth pain, it's important to find out why. See a dentist whenever you have tooth pain, even if the pain subsides.

---

**Floss gently.** If swishing doesn't work, try to pry a small bit of food like a pop-corn hull from between your teeth by flossing, says Dr. Taintor. Be gentle! Your gums are likely to be sore.

**Swish with alcohol.** Hold a swig of whiskey over the painful tooth, says Philip D. Corn, D.D.S. Your gums will absorb some of the alcohol, and that will numb the pain.

**Rinse with salty water.** After each meal and at bedtime, stir 1 teaspoon of salt into an 8-ounce glass of tepid water, says Dr. Corn. Hold each mouthful; roll it around your mouth. Spit.

**Try a hand massage.** Wrap a thin cloth around an ice cube and rub into the V-shaped area where the bones of the thumb and forefinger meet. Gently hold the ice on the area for 5 to 7 minutes. Amazingly, this technique can ease toothache pain. In a study, Ronald Melzack, Ph.D., found that ice massage eased toothaches in 60 to 90 percent of the people who tried it. His research shows this procedure works by sending rubbing impulses along the nerve pathways that the toothache pain would normally travel on. Since the pathways can carry only one signal at a time, rubbing outweighs the pain.

**Use oil of cloves.** People have been using this remedy for many years, says Richard Shepard, D.D.S. Drop a little directly onto the tooth, or dab a little on a cotton ball and pack it next to the problem tooth.

---

## Be Gentle to Tooth Sensitivity

"If you can't even touch the tooth, that's an ache," says Roger P. Levin, D.D.S. "But if the tooth is merely reacting to heat or cold, then it's a problem with sensitivity."

More than 40 million Americans have "dentinal hypersensitivity," and it begins when the dentin underneath the tooth enamel becomes exposed—usually at the gumline.

Age, receding gums, surgery, and overzealous brushing with harsh toothpastes and hard brushes can expose dentin. Sometimes plaque attacks the tooth enamel and exposes the dentin.

Philip D. Corn, D.D.S., recommends an over-the-counter toothpaste made especially for people with sensitive teeth, applied with a soft nylon-bristle brush. Such toothpastes include Sensodyne, Aquafresh, Colgate, and Biotene.

Of course, if you're noticing sensitivity for the first time, it makes good sense to see your dentist to make sure you have no other problem.

**Don't bite.** If the toothache is caused by an injury to the tooth, try not to use that area when you eat, says Dr. Corn. If nothing is damaged, resting the tooth may ease the ache.

**Ice it.** Treat the problem as you would treat a bruise with ice, says Dr. Corn. Place ice in a small resealable plastic bag, seal it, wrap a thin cloth around it, and put it on the aching tooth or the adjacent cheek for 15-minute intervals at least three or four times a day.

**Keep your mouth shut.** If cold air moving past the tooth is a problem, just shut off the flow, says Roger P. Levin, D.D.S.

But don't clench your teeth. Some toothaches happen when a person's bite isn't quite right. In that case, says Dr. Levin, avoid shutting your mouth as much as possible until the dentist can take a look.

**Swallow aspirin.** Don't believe that old-time remedy calling for placing an aspirin directly on the aching gum. This can cause an aspirin burn, says Dr. Taintor. For pain relief, take an aspirin every 4 to 6 hours as required, unless you're allergic.

**Avoid heat.** Keep heat away from your aching cheek even if it makes the toothache feel better, warns Dr. Corn. "If it's an infection, the heat will draw the infection to the outside of the jaw and make the infection worse."

## PANEL OF ADVISORS

**Philip D. Corn, D.D.S.,** has a practice in Philadelphia. He is a former director of the Pennsylvania Academy of General Dentistry.

**Roger P. Levin, D.D.S.,** is the chief executive officer of the Levin Group, a dental practice in Baltimore.

**Richard Shepard, D.D.S.,** is a retired dentist in Durango, Colorado. He is also the executive director of the Holistic Dental Association.

**Jerry F. Taintor, D.D.S.,** is chairman of endodontics at the University of Tennessee College of Dentistry in Memphis. He is the author of *The Complete Guide to Better Dental Care.*

# TOOTH STAINS
## 11 Brightening Ideas

Coffee, tea, colas, smoke, acidic juices, certain medications, and highly pigmented foods can take a dingy toll on pearly whites.

Not that teeth were ever meant to be totally white. The natural color of teeth is actually light yellow to light yellow-red, says Roger P. Levin, D.D.S. But as you age, your teeth tend to darken even more.

Over time, surface enamel cracks and erodes, exposing dentin, the less dense interior of the tooth, which absorbs food color. Stains also latch onto the plaque and tartar buildup on and between teeth, finding anchorage in crevices.

Many things can stain teeth, says Ronald I. Maitland, D.M.D., including antibiotics, quirks in individual metabolism, even a high fever.

The yellower your tooth stains, the easier it will be to remove them. Deep brown stains, such as those brought on by long-term use of the antibiotic tetracycline, can be very difficult to erase.

The good news is that many common stains—the coffee and cigarette variety—can often be washed away between professional cleanings. Here's how.

**Brush after every meal.** If you clean your teeth regularly and conscientiously, you have less chance of keeping stains on your teeth, says Dr. Levin.

**Polish with baking soda.** Mix baking soda with just enough hydrogen peroxide to make a mixture the consistency of toothpaste, says Dr. Levin, then brush stains away. Be sure not to use too much peroxide, as it can burn.

**Check your plaque quotient.** Rinse with a disclosing solution from your dentist to show where plaque remains on your teeth after brushing. Those spots are where your teeth will stain if you don't improve your brushing technique, says John D. B. Featherstone, Ph.D.

**Rinse often.** After every meal, rinse the food from your teeth, says Dr. Maitland. If you can't get to a restroom, pick up your water glass, take a swig, then rinse and swallow at the table.

**Switch to an electric toothbrush.** They're better at motivating reluctant brushers to clean their teeth more often than manual toothbrushes, says the Academy of General Dentistry. But when it comes to plaque removal, it depends more on the quality of your brushing than the type of toothbrush you're using.

**Be choosy about your mouthwash.** All mouthwashes are fine for rinsing, but mouthwashes that have an antibacterial action will reduce stain-catching plaque, says Dr. Featherstone.

**Use a whitening toothpaste or tooth polish.** Dentists used to warn patients away from over-the-counter whitening products because they contained gritty abrasives that could erode the tooth enamel. But manufacturers have gotten better at using peroxide instead of abrasives to give you a slightly brighter after-brushing effect, says Dean Lodding, D.D.S.

But don't expect miracles. Because peroxides in toothpastes or polishes only stay on the tooth surface for a brief period of time, you'll only get a bit of lightening, Dr. Lodding notes.

**Scrub gently.** Just as abrasive products could scrub away enamel, overly aggressive brushing can expose the deeper-hued dentin, which, ironically, could make your teeth look even dingier.

**Try tooth strips.** These products look like package sealing tape, but fit across your teeth. They keep peroxide on the teeth a little bit longer than a tooth polish, so they'll get them a bit whiter, says Dr. Lodding. "They're simple, inexpensive, and safe. You have nothing to lose," he says. Regular use can lighten your teeth 2 to 3 shades, compared to the 8 to 10 shades of lightening you can get from a dentist-directed home-bleaching program or in-office treatment.

**Sleep with a bleach tray.** One of the most effective means of bleaching teeth is a home-bleaching program. Your dentist custom fits you with a mouthguard-like tray that fits over your teeth. You fill it each night with a concentrated bleach solution and wear it while sleeping for 2 to 3 weeks. This option costs between $300 and $500. While more expensive, the results are dramatically more effective than you can obtain with over-the-counter products.

Some companies make over-the-counter products that use bleach in trays that fit onto your teeth. The problem is that these one-size-fits-all trays don't actually conform to the surfaces of your teeth and gums. Not only will they distribute the peroxide unevenly over your tooth surfaces, they may also irritate your gums. The reason professional bleaching methods work better is that they use a higher concentration of peroxide that penetrates the thousands of tiny tubules that run from the outside of your tooth into the dentin, where they oxidize the discoloration harbored there, says Dr. Lodding.

**Do it all in one visit.** If you're impatient, a dentist can bleach your teeth in a 1- to 2-hour appointment by using a concentrated carbamide peroxide solution and a special light that "powers the material into the dentin," says Dr. Lodding. The only downside is the cost, which can be $400 to $800.

## PANEL OF ADVISORS

**John D. B. Featherstone, Ph.D.,** is a professor and chairman of the department of preventive and restorative dental sciences in the School of Dentistry at the University of California, San Francisco.

**Roger P. Levin, D.D.S.,** is the chief executive officer of the Levin Group, a dental practice in Baltimore.

**Dean Lodding, D.D.S.,** is a dentist in Elgin, Illinois, and past president of the American Academy of Cosmetic Dentistry.

**Ronald I. Maitland, D.M.D.,** is a New York City dentist who specializes in cosmetic dentistry. He is chairman of the Greater New York Dental Meeting and an expert on dental stains.

# ULCERS
## 16 Tips for Quick Relief

The surprising thing about ulcers isn't how common they are—about 4 million American adults have an ulcer, and approximately 350,000 new cases are diagnosed each year. What's surprising is that we don't get them more often.

Every time you eat, your stomach bathes foods in acids to continue digestion that was begun in the mouth. The same acids that break down protein and fat are actually strong enough to damage the stomach and the duodenum, the portion of the small intestine nearest the stomach. The only reason they don't is that the tissues are coated with a protective, spongelike mucous lining that resists the acidic onslaught.

Sometimes, however, the tissues break down. Most ulcers—small, painful sores that are generally about the size of a pencil eraser—occur when a corkscrew-shaped bacterium called *Helicobacter pylori* bores through the lining of the duodenum or stomach and allows acids to damage the delicate tissue underneath. Over-the-counter medications such as aspirin and ibuprofen can strip away the stomach's protective lining and cause similar problems.

Gastric and duodenal ulcers often may go away on their own within 1 to 3 weeks once aspirin or other tissue-damaging medications are stopped. Ulcers can recur sporadically unless the bacteria are treated, which lowers the recurrence rate to less than 3 percent. The pain in the meantime, however, can be intense. To stop the pain of ulcers or prevent recurrences, here's what doctors advise.

**Take an antacid.** During ulcer flare-ups, taking an antacid is the quickest way to relieve the pain, says Samuel Meyers, M.D.

Antacids contain calcium, aluminum, magnesium, or a combination. Aluminum causes constipation in some people, while magnesium can lead to diarrhea. "I advise people to evaluate their overall bowel habits, and choose an antacid based on that, as well as their overall calcium requirement," says Dr. Meyers.

**Reduce acid production.** Over-the-counter medicines called H$_2$ blockers are among the best ways to treat ulcers, says Dr. Meyers. Drugs in this class include—Pepcid AC, Tagamet HB 200, Axid AR, and Zantac 75. They reduce the output of acid-secreting cells in the stomach, which reduces discomfort and helps ulcers heal more quickly.

"I usually recommend Pepcid because it doesn't interact with other medications that people may be taking," he adds.

One of the best ways to get relief from ulcer pain is to *combine* antacids with

$H_2$ blockers. Antacids will ease discomfort within 10 to 15 minutes, and $H_2$ blockers provide longer-term protection, says Dr. Meyers.

"If you're using $H_2$ blockers, don't take antacids at the same time, because they'll interfere with absorption," Dr. Meyers adds. Take the $H_2$ blocker at the recommended times, then wait an hour or two before using antacids, he advises.

**Swig the pink stuff.** The active ingredient in Pepto-Bismol is bismuth sub-salicylate: It protects the lining of the stomach and intestine and decreases *H. pylori* populations in the digestive tract.

"I advise people with ulcers to take two tablets or 1 ounce of liquid four times daily," says Philip Miner, M.D. Pepto-Bismol is unlikely to cause side effects, but it may cause stools to turn black while you're using it, he adds.

**Give up orange juice for a while.** Doctors aren't sure why, but oranges—along with tomatoes and possibly grapefruit—may trigger the release of pain-causing chemical messengers, or neurotransmitters, in those with ulcers, says Dr. Miner.

**Don't fall for the milk myth.** For a long time, doctors encouraged people with ulcers to drink milk. They thought milk's smooth texture would coat and soothe painful ulcers. Research has shown, however, that the protein and calcium in milk stimulate acid production and can make ulcers worse, says Dr. Meyers.

**Soothe with yogurt.** Although milk can aggravate an ulcer, yogurt can actually soothe one. Researchers from Sweden analyzed the diets of 764 people with ulcers and 229 people without. They found that the men and women who ate the most yogurt reduced their risk of ulcers by 18 percent, compared with those who ate the least. The *friendly* bacteria in yogurt, such as *Lactobacillus bulgaricus* and *L. acidophilus*, may be the therapeutic substance.

**Guard with garlic.** Long known as a natural antibiotic, some alternative experts suspect that garlic may also in-

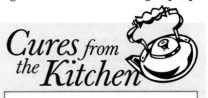

*Cures from the Kitchen*

Folk healers have traditionally advised people to drink cabbage juice during ulcer flare-ups. It might be worth a try because cabbage contains an amino acid called glutamine, which is thought to speed intestinal healing.

Some alternative experts recommend juicing half a head of cabbage and drinking it once daily. Eating the same amount of raw cabbage will have similar effects—but don't bother with cooked cabbage, because heat cancels the beneficial effects.

hibit the growth of *H. pylori.* In one laboratory study, the extract from the equivalent of two cloves of garlic was able to stop the growth of this ulcer-causing bacterium.

**Ask your doctor about licorice.** It's a traditional folk remedy for ulcers, and there's some evidence that it's effective. Licorice contains glycyrrhizic acid, a compound that is thought to strengthen the intestinal lining and help ulcers heal more quickly, says Dr. Miner.

The problem with licorice is that long-term daily use can cause high blood pressure. Also, read the label on the package: Most "licorice" in the United States is actually made with licorice flavoring, which won't have the same effects as the real thing. The average daily dose is 1.5 to 3 grams, says Dr. Meyers, but talk to your doctor before taking this amount, because the risk of high blood pressure is high. Licorice should not be used on a regular basis for a prolonged time—no more than for 4 to 6 weeks.

**Eat more frequently.** Even though the stomach's acid production increases during and after meals, the presence of food in the stomach helps buffer the corrosive effects. Eating also increases bloodflow to the stomach, which helps protect it from digestive acids. Rather than having two or three large meals a day, eat five or six small meals daily, Dr. Miner advises.

**Reduce the stress in your life.** For a long time, emotional stress was thought to be a leading cause of ulcers. Doctors now know that stress doesn't cause ulcers—but anxiety, tension, and a high-strung approach to life can increase the brain's perception of pain, says Dr. Meyers. If you already have an ulcer—or have had one in the past—it makes sense to include stress reduction in your overall treatment plan.

Everyone controls stress in different ways. Vigorous exercise—walking, running, or biking, for example—is a great way to dispel tension at the end of hectic days. Others turn to more formal stress reduction strategies, such as deep breathing, meditation, or prayer. The idea isn't to eliminate stress entirely, but simply to find ways to prevent it from taking over your life—or disrupting your insides.

**Try a different pain reliever.** Aspirin and ibuprofen are among the most effective over-the-counter painkillers ever discovered, but the long-term use of these medications is a common cause of stomach ulcers, says Dr. Miner. Along with other nonsteroidal anti-inflammatory drugs (NSAIDs), aspirin and ibuprofen inhibit the body's production of prostaglandins, chemicals that help maintain the stomach's protective lining. About 20 percent of people who use these drugs regularly go on to develop ulcers.

If you need long-term pain relief—because of arthritis, for example—your doctor may advise you to switch to acetaminophen. It's just as effective as the

NSAIDs, such as aspirin or ibuprofen, for easing many types of pain but is less likely to damage the stomach lining.

**Quit smoking.** People who smoke are much more likely to get ulcers than those who don't, Dr. Meyers warns. Smoking slows the healing time of ulcers, increases the risk of relapses, and also may make the body more susceptible to infection-causing bacteria.

**Drink alcohol in moderation.** Alcohol can erode the stomach's protective lining, resulting in inflammation and bleeding. It is even more likely to cause problems if you also smoke or take aspirin regularly, says Dr. Meyers. For men, the daily alcohol limit should be two drinks; for women, the upper limit is one drink daily. If ulcers continue to cause problems, you may want to give up alcohol altogether.

**Cut back on coffee.** Both regular and decaffeinated coffee increase levels of stomach acids. Coffee is unlikely to *cause* ulcers, but it can increase discomfort while an ulcer is healing, Dr. Meyers says.

**Drink a lot of water.** Drink at least 2 quarts of water daily when ulcers are "active"—and have a full glass whenever you experience discomfort. "Drinking water helps dilute acid in the stomach," Dr. Meyers explains. "Unlike milk, it doesn't stimulate the production of more acid."

## PANEL OF ADVISORS

**Samuel Meyers, M.D.,** is a gastroenterologist and clinical professor of medicine at the Mount Sinai School of Medicine of New York University in New York City.
**Philip Miner, M.D.,** is a gastroenterologist and the president and medical director of Oklahoma Foundation for Digestive Research in Oklahoma City.

# URINARY TRACT INFECTIONS
## 17 Germ-Fighting Strategies

Urinary tract infections are easy to treat, but that's hardly reassuring when you're rushing to the bathroom every 15 minutes to urinate—and experiencing burning, excruciating pain.

Most urinary tract infections (UTIs) occur when bacteria from outside the body enter the urethra, the tube that carries urine from the bladder out of the body. Sex is a common cause of UTIs because intercourse can "massage" external bacteria into the urethra. UTIs are also common after menopause, when declines in estrogen make tissues in the vagina and urethra drier and, thus, more vulnerable to bacteria.

One in five women will get a UTI—in the urethra, bladder, or kidneys—at some point in her life. Some women get them over and over again. Men are much less likely to get UTIs because their extra inches of anatomy make it harder for bacteria to get inside.

Antibiotics are necessary to knock out urinary tract infections, says Larrian Gillespie, M.D. Once you start taking the drugs, the discomfort will usually disappear within a day or two. In the meantime, here are a few steps that will reduce discomfort and help prevent the infection from coming back.

**Drink a lot of water.** The more you drink, the more you urinate—and frequent urination helps flush harmful bacteria from the bladder. "If you keep

## WHEN TO CALL A DOCTOR

Urinary tract infections respond very quickly to antibiotics, so call your doctor at the first sign of symptoms. It's especially important to make the call if you're having fever, chills, or nausea, along with the usual sensations of burning or urgency. These are signs of a kidney infection, which can be serious without prompt treatment, says Larrian Gillespie, M.D.

filling your bladder and flushing it out, you can reduce the number of bacteria," says Diana Koster, M.D.

Water also dilutes the concentrated salts in urine, which can reduce discomfort when you have an infection, Dr. Koster adds. Try to drink at least 64 ounces of water each day.

**Fight bacteria with baking soda.** At the first sign of symptoms, drink a solution made with ¼ teaspoon of baking soda mixed in 8 ounces of water. Continue this once a day until you can get a culture done at a doctor's office or clinic and can get on antibiotics. Baking soda makes the bladder environment more alkaline, which reduces the ability of bacteria to multiply, says Dr. Gillespie.

**Drink Evian water.** It contains the same bicarbonate as baking soda but without the extra sodium. It neutralizes acid in the bladder and helps reduce painful nerve irritation, Dr. Gillespie explains.

**Dilute the burn.** The concentrated salts in urine can cause stinging pain when you have a UTI. You can reduce discomfort by pouring body-temperature water over yourself while you urinate, says Dr. Koster.

**Relax with a heating pad.** Applying heat to the abdomen is a great way to reduce cramps or painful pressure that sometimes accompanies UTIs, says Dr. Gillespie. If you don't have a heating pad, a hot-water bottle or washcloth soaked in hot water works just as well.

**Avoid orange juice for a few days.** Along with strawberries, grapefruit, and pineapple, orange juice has a high acid content. When you have a UTI, it will increase the burn when you urinate, says Dr. Gillespie.

**Don't drink coffee or alcohol.** When you have an infection, coffee and alcohol can make it painful to urinate, says Dr. Gillespie. Caffeine and alcohol also stimulate the muscular walls of the bladder, which may increase urinary "urges" and cause additional discomfort.

**Take vitamin C for prevention.** "If you already have a urinary tract infection, taking vitamin C to acidify the urine is like putting out a fire with gasoline," says Dr. Gillespie. "But if you want to prevent bacteria from adhering to the bladder wall in order to prevent infections, you want the urine to be more acidic."

For preventing UTIs, she advises 1,000 to 2,000 milligrams of vitamin C daily. "Once you have a urinary tract infection, stop taking vitamin C," Dr. Gillespie adds.

**Drink cranberry juice.** Once you've had a UTI, you won't want to ever have another one. Acquire a taste for cranberry juice. It's a traditional remedy for preventing UTIs, and scientific research suggests it works. Cranberry juice is rich in proanthocyanidins, chemical compounds that appear to help prevent bacteria from sticking to cells in the urinary tract. It also changes the acidity, or pH, of the urine and makes it a less friendly environment for bacteria to grow, says Beverly Kloeppel, M.D. You should avoid cranberry juice, however, if you have an overactive bladder, because it can irritate the bladder and make it more sensitive.

If you get frequent UTIs, drink one glass of cranberry juice daily for a few months to see if it makes a difference. While you're at it, add some blueberries to your breakfast cereal or morning smoothie—they're related to cranberries and contain the same active compounds.

**Eat more yogurt.** The research isn't conclusive, but there's some evidence that the organisms in live-culture yogurt, *Lactobacillus acidophilus*, may help prevent unwanted bacteria from multiplying in the urinary tract and prevent UTIs, says Mary Jane Minkin, M.D.

Yogurt is especially helpful if you're taking antibiotics. While these drugs are very effective at killing harmful bacteria, they also kill "good" germs, which can lead to UTIs. Eating a cup of live-culture yogurt daily helps replenish beneficial bacteria while keeping the "bad" bugs away.

**Wash before sex.** It's impossible to eliminate infection-causing bacteria from around the anus, but you can prevent them from gaining entry into the urinary tract by washing the genital area before having sex, suggests Dr. Minkin. This helps prevent the bacteria from being pushed up into the vaginal area and urethra.

**Urinate after sex.** It washes out bacteria that may have made it inside the urethra during intercourse, says Dr. Kloeppel.

**Use a lubricant.** If you're experiencing vaginal dryness, it's important to use a water-based lubricant during sex. By decreasing friction, the extra lubrication lessens the possibility of inflammation in the external urethral area, which in turn makes it more difficult for bacteria to cause infection.

**Change birth control methods.** Studies have shown that women who use diaphragms and spermicides for birth control have a higher risk of UTIs, probably because use of these products irritates the urethral lining. If you get infections frequently, you may want to talk to your doctor about other forms of birth control.

**Use regular tampons.** Women tend to get more infections around the time of their periods. This is partly because the warmth and moisture of the blood provides a favorable environment for germs. In addition, super-size tampons can obstruct the bladder and prevent it from emptying completely. It's easier for bacteria to multiply when urine stays in the bladder for a long time, Dr. Gillespie explains.

It's a good idea to use pads or regular-size tampons, says Dr. Gillespie. Change tampons every time you urinate, she adds.

**Always wipe backward.** After using the bathroom, wiping from front to back helps ensure that anal bacteria doesn't get pushed forward toward the urethra, says Dr. Kloeppel.

**Don't use "feminine" products.** The chemicals in douches and deodorant sprays may irritate tender tissues in the urethra and vagina, making it easier for bacteria to thrive, says Dr. Koster.

## PANEL OF ADVISORS

**Larrian Gillespie, M.D.,** is a retired assistant clinical professor of urology and urogynecology and president of Healthy Life Publications. She is the author of *You Don't Have to Live with Cystitis.*

**Beverly Kloeppel, M.D.,** is associate director of the Student Health Center at the University of New Mexico in Albuquerque.

**Diana Koster, M.D.,** is vice president of medical affairs and medical director of Planned Parenthood of New Mexico.

**Mary Jane Minkin, M.D.,** is a clinical professor at Yale University School of Medicine and an obstetrician-gynecologist in New Haven, Connecticut.

# VAGINAL AND YEAST INFECTIONS
## 12 Comforting Steps

Think "yeast" and what do you think of? The magical multiplying qualities it brings to flour and water that turn it into bread? Ironically, those same qualities can wreak such havoc in women, when a vaginal fungus called *Candida albicans*, also known as yeast, gets out of control. Typically, *Candida* is kept in check by other organisms that also inhabit the vagina, much like salt prevents the yeast in bread dough from going overboard. But when conditions are right, *Candida* multiplies, causing the painful itching, irritation, or white cottage-cheese-like discharge of a yeast infection. About 75 percent of women will get at least one yeast infection, and more than 45 percent will have two or more at some time in their lives.

Luckily, there are numerous ways to reduce the discomfort and prevent the infections from returning.

## WHEN TO CALL A DOCTOR

Women often assume that every vaginal infection is caused by yeast—and then proceed to use over-the-counter medications inappropriately. Experience has shown, however, that women often misdiagnose their own infections, says Diana Koster, M.D.

If you haven't had vaginal infections in the past, see your doctor at the first sign of symptoms, Dr. Koster advises. The infection might turn out to be yeast—or it could be caused by trichomoniasis, a sexually transmitted parasite, or by bacteria that will require treatment with antibiotics.

You'll also want to talk to your doctor if you get four or more yeast infections a year. You could have a resistant strain of yeast that won't get better without the use of prescription medications.

**Visit the drugstore.** Often, women who have had several yeast infections in the past are pretty savvy about the symptoms, says Diana Koster, M.D., but you may want to see your doctor first to be sure it's truly a yeast infection. While some strains of yeast require treatment with prescription drugs, others can be controlled with the active ingredients in over-the-counter creams or suppositories.

Over-the-counter products for controlling yeast usually contain clotrimazole (such as Gyne-Lotrimin). The drugs are equally effective, but read the labels before using them, because they may have to be used for different lengths of time.

"The research on 3-day products indicates they work as well as those that are used for 7 days," says Dr. Koster.

Don't skimp on the medication, especially if the outer vaginal tissues are irritated. Dr. Koster advises women to put a dab of the medication on their finger and apply a little to the external areas as well as inside the vagina.

**Ease irritation with an oatmeal bath.** Available in drugstores, colloidal oatmeal (such as Aveeno) is ground to a fine powder, which enables it to stay suspended in water. Added to a warm bath, it's very soothing for itchy, irritated tissues.

## Do just 1 thing

Wear loose clothes. The yeast fungus thrives in a warm, moist environment. Women who get frequent infections should do everything possible to make the vagina just a little less hospitable by keeping it cool and dry, advises Diana Koster, M.D.

Start by wearing loose clothes instead of skin-tight jeans. If you swim or work out, change into dry clothing as soon as you're done. "If you make the vaginal area a little less warm and moist, it might shift the balance of organisms just enough that you'll get fewer infections," she says.

It's also helpful to sleep in the nude, or to wear a skirt without panties when you're home. Anything that increases air circulation keeps the vaginal area drier. This can help reduce discomfort if you have a vaginal infection, and it will also help prevent future problems, says Dr. Koster.

"It's not a cure, but it might relieve some of the discomfort," says Dr. Koster.

**Apply a cool compress.** When you're feeling unusually itchy or sore, apply a cool, damp washcloth to the outer part of the vagina. Both the moisture and the cool temperature will temporarily ease the discomfort.

**Pat yourself dry.** After showers or baths, rubbing yourself dry with a towel can be irritating. Gently pat yourself dry, or simply lounge around in the nude and allow the area to air-dry.

**Wear cotton next to your skin.** Unlike nylon and other synthetic fabrics, cotton panties–or nylons with cotton crotches–"breathe." In other words, they allow air to get in and moisture to get out, which will reduce your risk of infection, says Larrian Gillespie, M.D.

**Avoid scented bath products.** Scented soaps, bath oils, and other fragrant products contain chemicals that can irritate vulvar tissues and make you even more uncomfortable. You'll be less vulnerable to yeast or other infections if you wash with water and a mild soap, like Ivory or Dove.

"We're not meant to have harsh chemical scents near tender parts of our bodies," says Dr. Koster. "They can cause irritation."

**Don't douche.** The vagina is essentially self-cleaning, so douching is unnecessary, at best. It can also be harmful because it disrupts the natural balance of organisms in the vagina and increases the risk of infections, says Dr. Gillespie.

**Wipe with care.** Vaginal infections often occur when bacteria that normally inhabit the anal area move–or are pushed–into the vagina. This can also result in uncomfortable and potentially dangerous infections of the bladder, kidneys, or urethra (the tube that carries urine out of the body).

One way to keep anal bacteria where they belong is to wipe from front to back after urinating or having a bowel movement. It's also a good idea to wash around the vagina with soap and water prior to sex to keep bacteria from being pushed into the vagina.

**Identify changes in your life.** It's not uncommon for women who have never had vaginal infections in the past to suddenly start getting them. Try to figure out if you're doing something different, Dr. Koster advises. "If you get irritated by using a new type of condom or even a different lubricant, switch to another product," she explains.

**Eat live-culture yogurt.** It won't help if you already have a yeast infection, but researchers believe that the live-culture bacteria in yogurt may reduce the risk of future infections.

Yogurt appears to help in several ways. It contains *Lactobacillus acidophilus*, which helps the vagina maintain a healthy acid/alkaline balance. In addition, the beneficial bacteria in yogurt find their way into the vaginal canal, where they "crowd out" yeast.

One 6-month study found that women who ate 8 ounces of live-culture yogurt daily were much less likely to develop yeast infections than those who didn't eat yogurt.

If you already have an infection and are taking antibiotics, it's helpful to eat a cup or two of live-culture yogurt daily. It replenishes helpful bacteria in the intestine that are killed by antibiotics, helping prevent diarrhea or bloating.

**Practice good glucose control.** Some women with diabetes get more vaginal infections than those without the disease because they may have abnormally high levels of glucose (blood sugar) in the blood. Higher-than-normal glucose levels can reduce the vagina's natural protective abilities.

If you have diabetes, it's essential to keep glucose levels under strict control by eating more fruits, whole grains, and other healthful foods, and by exercising, maintaining a healthful weight, and taking medication, if necessary.

Even if you haven't been diagnosed with diabetes, you may want to get yourself checked if you've been getting frequent vaginal infections. Diabetes can reduce the ability of the immune system to combat yeast and other infections, says Beverly Kloeppel, M.D.

## PANEL OF ADVISORS

**Larrian Gillespie, M.D.,** is a retired assistant clinical professor of urology and urogynecology and president of Healthy Life Publications. She is the author of *You Don't Have to Live with Cystitis.*

**Beverly Kloeppel, M.D.,** is associate director of the Student Health Center at the University of New Mexico in Albuquerque.

**Diana Koster, M.D.,** is vice president of medical affairs and medical director of Planned Parenthood of New Mexico.

**Mary Jane Minkin, M.D.,** is a clinical professor at Yale University School of Medicine and an obstetrician-gynecologist in New Haven, Connecticut.

# VARICOSE VEINS
## 17 Helpers and Healers

Most people don't even see varicose veins as a disease—they think of them only as something cosmetic.

Actually, this is far from the case. "People with varicose veins have a disease, a disease with a cosmetic aspect," says Brian McDonagh, M.D.

Blue, swollen, lumpy-looking veins—and their cousins, the crimson "spider veins"—are only the most evident signs of varicose vein disease. Veterans of this condition know all too well that these visible veins often come with achy, tired, listless legs.

The condition is usually not life-threatening, so there's no reason to panic or rush to a doctor. If you have varicose veins, however, you—and your poor legs—will be better off knowing how to manage them.

Here's what our experts suggest.

## WHEN TO CALL A DOCTOR

One hundred years ago, doctors yanked out varicose veins with hooks. Luckily, the treatment today is much more humane—and helpful. Today, injection therapy is used with resounding success against even the wiliest varicose veins.

But when do varicose veins warrant a trip to the doctor? Brian McDonagh, M.D., says that varicose veins present two major complications: vein clotting and rupture.

How do you recognize a clot? "It will become very painful, sore, and tender—it just hurts," says Dr. McDonagh. Clots are usually visible as red lumps in the veins that don't decrease in size even when you put your legs up.

Varicose veins around the ankle areas are more inclined to rupture and bleed. This is much more dangerous than clotting because you can lose blood very rapidly. If this happens, put pressure on it to slow the bleeding and get to your doctor.

**Don't feel guilty.** By far the greatest risk factor for varicose veins is having a parent with the problem, says Dr. McDonagh. Myths abound to explain the existence of this largely hereditary disease—the largest myth being that varicose veins are caused by crossing your legs.

"That's nonsense," says Dr. McDonagh. Most people with varicose veins are simply one of the 17 percent of all Americans who possess the culprit genes. And most just happen to be women.

**Get gravity on your side.** Varicose veins are weakened veins that lack the strength they once had to return blood to the heart. Veins in the legs are the most susceptible, for they are farthest—and straight downhill—from the heart. You can make their job much easier by putting gravity on your side. It's easy. Using a couch, pillows, or an easy chair, raise your legs above hip level whenever they ache, and the discomfort should start to go away, says Dudley Phillips, M.D.

**Wear support hose.** They help provide relief. These stockings, available in

## Do just 1 thing

Try yoga. The ancient system of yoga has much to offer people with varicose veins, says John Clarke, M.D.

This yogic breathing practice can be done without instruction, without danger, and with a good chance that it will relieve your discomfort from varicose veins, he claims. Try this exercise right now. Lie flat on your back and prop your feet up on a chair. Breathe slowly and evenly from your diaphragm, through your nose. That's it!

While gravity is pulling excess blood out of your raised legs, your full, steady inhalations create negative pressure in your chest that helps pull in air to the chest cavity, as well as blood from all over the body, including your blood-gorged legs, Dr. Clarke says.

drugstores and department stores, resist the blood's tendency to pool in the small blood vessels closest to the skin, explains Dr. Phillips. (Instead, the blood is pushed into the larger, deeper veins, where it is more easily pumped back up to the heart.)

**Throw those veins a one-two punch.** Dr. Phillips suggests that people with varicose veins combine the powers of gravity and support hose in the following exercise: Slip on your support hose. Then lie flat on your back and raise your legs straight up in the air, resting them against a wall. Hold this position for 2 minutes. This allows the blood to flow out of the swollen leg veins and back toward your heart. Repeat throughout the day, if possible, as often as needed.

**Tilt your bed.** Make gravity work for you through the night by raising the foot of your bed several inches, says Paul Lazar, M.D. He cautions, however, that if you have a history of heart trouble or if you have any difficulty breathing during the night, consult a doctor before adjusting your bed.

**Wear sensible shoes.** Varicose veins are discomforting enough to the legs. Don't give your dogs any extra trouble by wearing high heels or cowboy boots, says Dr. Phillips.

**Buy a pair of elastic stockings.** These special stockings, generally sold in medical supply stores rather than in drugstores, are to support hose what a .45 Magnum is to a BB gun. Specially fitted elastic stockings, worn up to knee level, can give you considerable relief, depending on the severity of the varicose veins, says Dr. McDonagh. Get measured for a good-quality stocking.

**Watch your weight.** Added body weight means more pressure on your legs, one reason pregnant women often get varicose veins. Keep your weight down, and chances are you'll have fewer problems with bulging veins, says Lenise Banse, M.D.

**Stay away from tight-fitting clothes.** Tight garments, particularly a too-tight girdle or panty hose that are too constricting in the groin area, can act like tourniquets and keep blood pooled in your legs, says Dr. Banse.

**Be suspicious of the Pill.** Hormonal imbalances, which sometimes occur with birth control pills, can be the cause of spider veins. If your problem appeared after you started the Pill, there may be a connection, says Dr. McDonagh.

**Don't smoke.** A report from the Framingham Heart Study noted a correlation between smoking and the incidence of varicose veins. The researchers conclude that smoking may be a risk factor for varicose veins.

**Go for a walk.** Prolonged sitting or standing can cause problems in your legs because the blood tends to pool.

## Cures from the Kitchen

Strangely enough, a high-fiber diet may be the kitchen's key to preventing varicose veins. Straining to have a bowel movement puts pressure on the veins in your lower legs. Over time, this pressure promotes the development of varicose veins.

A high-fiber diet can stop this gradual decline before it's too late. Fiber keeps waste moving freely through the system, so to speak, preventing straining and thus preventing varicose veins in the long run. Try to get around 25 grams a day from sources like bran cereals, beans, and whole grains.

A little bit of exercise throughout the day, particularly walking, can often prevent this, says Eugene Strandness Jr., M.D. In fact, the Framingham study found that sedentary adults were more likely to have varicose veins than those who were active.

**Try some herbs.** Horse chestnut and butcher's broom are the two top-shelf herbs when it comes to varicose vein relief. Take 600 milligrams of a commercially prepared horse chestnut extract whenever you put your legs in a stressful situation, such as by walking all day or sitting through a long flight, says Mindy Green, director of education at the Herbal Research Foundation. She also suggests taking 16 to 33 milligrams of a standardized butcher's broom extract or tincture three times a day to help strengthen and constrict the walls of varicose veins.

**Find relief with water.** Relief for varicose veins may be as close as your shower. While showering, alternate between applications of hot and cold water on your legs, advises Green. Change temperatures at 1- to 3-minute intervals, and repeat the switch three times. The changing temperature gets blood moving by expanding and contracting the blood vessels.

**Don't hide from your problem.** Much of the discomfort and pain of varicose veins can be masked with pain pills. Don't do it, says Dr. McDonagh. "Varicose veins are a problem that should not be dealt with by hiding the pain," he says. If you've gone down the list of tips and nothing helps, seek medical attention.

## PANEL OF ADVISORS

**Lenise Banse, M.D.,** is a dermatologist in Clinton Township, Michigan, where she is director of the Northeast Family Dermatology Center. She has special expertise in cutaneous oncology as well as cosmetic dermatology.

**John Clarke, M.D.,** is presently a consultant in Milton, Massachusetts, and was formerly a cardiologist with the Himalayan International Institute in Honesdale, Pennsylvania.

**Mindy Green** is director of education at the Herbal Research Foundation in Boulder, Colorado.

**Paul Lazar, M.D.,** is a professor emeritus of clinical dermatology at Northwestern University Medical School in Chicago. He is a former board member of the American Academy of Dermatology.

**Brian McDonagh, M.D.,** is a phlebologist (vein specialist) based in Chicago. He is the founder and medical director of Vein Clinics of America, the largest medical group in the country dedicated solely to the treatment of vein disorders.

**Dudley Phillips, M.D.,** of Darlington, Maryland, has practiced family medicine for more than 40 years. He is now retired.

**Eugene Strandness Jr., M.D.,** was a professor of surgery at the University of Washington School of Medicine in Seattle.

# WARTS
## 20 Healing Secrets

After acne, warts are the most common dermatological complaint.

At any one time, about 10 percent of people have a wart, says Robert Garry, Ph.D. About 25 percent will get one sometime in their lives.

Warts are benign skin tumors that can occur singly or in large packs on just about any part of the body. They come in several different varieties, each bearing its own special name, each caused by various strains of the papillomavirus. The virus masterfully tricks the body into providing it with free room and board in a sheltered "house"–the wart.

Unfortunately, standard medical treatments are often violent–burning, scraping, cutting, freezing, injecting, or zapping the wart with a laser. Many are also painful. Some even leave scars. The irony is, these techniques are not always effective. To add insult to injury, warts often reappear, no matter what treatment is used.

Knowing all this, you may want to try some home remedies before heading to the doctor's office. But, by all means, heed the advice of Thomas Goodman Jr., M.D. "Don't injure yourself with wart treatments. Start with simple measures and persist for several weeks before proceeding to stronger ones."

Unless otherwise noted, the following are effective for both common warts and plantar warts (those found on the foot).

## WHEN TO CALL A DOCTOR

If you have the slightest doubt about what you're dealing with, see a doctor. It could be a corn, callus, mole, or cancerous lesion.

In general, warts are pale, skin-colored growths with a rough surface, even borders, and blackened surface capillaries. Normal skin lines do not cross a wart's surface. And contrary to popular opinion, warts are very shallow growths—they don't have "roots" or "runners" that go down to the bone.

**Leave 'em alone.** According to one estimate, 40 to 50 percent of all warts eventually disappear on their own–typically within 2 years. Children, in particular, often lose warts spontaneously.

Warts constantly shed infectious virus, though, cautions Marc A. Brenner, D.P.M. If left untreated, they may get larger or spread to other areas. So if your warts start multiplying, take action.

**Call in the A-team.** Dr. Garry has had great success applying vitamin A directly to warts. Simply break open a capsule containing 25,000 IU of natural vitamin A from fish oil or fish-liver oil, squeeze some of the liquid onto the wart,

---

# How to Avoid a Wart

Warts are caused by a virus. It's in the air, and you pick it up the same way you do any viral infection. If you're susceptible to the virus and you have an appropriate cut or crack in the skin for it to take hold, you'll get a wart. It's that simple. Even so, there are a few things that you can do to lessen your chances of sprouting a wart.

**Keep your shoes on.** The wart virus thrives in a very moist environment, says Suzanne M. Levine, D.P.M., so always wear plastic thong sandals around swimming pools, health clubs, and locker rooms to avoid foot contact with it. By not going barefoot, you also sidestep minute cracks or cuts in your feet through which the virus could easily enter.

**Change shoes frequently.** Since the wart virus breeds in moist places, you should change your shoes frequently and allow shoes to dry out between wearings, says Dr. Levine.

**Clean up.** "At a health club or gym, you might even want to clean the shower out first with a product like Lysol," says Dr. Levine. "Even just household bleach works to kill viruses and bacteria."

**Look but don't touch.** "Warts spread easily," says Marc A. Brenner, D.P.M. "So if you have one on the bottom of your foot, for instance, try not to touch it with your hand. If you have even a small cut on your finger, you risk getting a wart there."

**Pamper your cuticles.** If the wart virus enters a cut or opening around your cuticle, it can cause a particularly nasty type of wart. Called periungual warts, they're very difficult to treat, says Dr. Levine. "If you do get a cut in the cuticle, put on a topical antibiotic cream (such as Bacitracin) and then cover it with a bandage until it heals."

**Play it cool.** "My own feeling is that people seem to be more susceptible to warts when they're under stress and eating poorly," says Dr. Levine. "And the warts seem to spread more then." So try to take it easy.

and rub it in. Apply once a day. He emphasizes that the vitamin should be applied to the skin only. Taken orally in large doses, vitamin A can be toxic.

Different warts respond differently to this treatment. Juvenile warts can disappear in a month, others in 2 to 4 months, but plantar warts might take 2 to 5 months longer, he says.

Dr. Garry recalls one woman who had more than 200 warts on her hand. By persisting with the vitamin A therapy for 7 to 8 months, she was able to get rid of all but one stubborn wart under her fingernail.

### "C" what another vitamin can do.

Apply a paste of crushed vitamin C tablets and water to the wart and then cover with a bandage so that the paste doesn't rub off. Although no formal research has been done in this area, there is some evidence that the high acidity of vitamin C can kill the wart-producing virus, according to Jeffrey Bland, Ph.D., who spent many years studying vitamin C at the Linus Pauling Institute in Corvallis, Oregon. Keep in mind, however, that vitamin C may irritate your skin, so apply the paste only to the wart.

### Stay dry.

Warts thrive on moisture, so keeping your feet very dry may help eliminate plantar warts. To try banishing a plantar wart without chemicals, change your socks at least three times a day, says Dr. Brenner. At the same time, apply a medicated foot powder such as Zeasorb-AF frequently—10 times a day if necessary.

### Opt for a nonprescription product.

Probably the most popular commercial wart remedies are the over-the-counter (OTC) salicylic acid preparations. Salicylic acid is believed to work against warts by softening and dissolving them. These products come

## Cures from the Kitchen

When all is said and done, you never know just what will cure any particular wart. The remedy that so neatly dispatched one little growth might leave another completely unscathed. So perhaps your most powerful weapon in the war of the warts is an open mind. That's why you shouldn't overlook the healing potential of so-called folk cures, treatments that have never undergone formal scientific scrutiny but have worked just fine for many people. Here are a few that some folks swear by.

- Apply clove oil or the milky juice of unripe figs directly to the wart.

- Soak lemon slices in apple cider with a little salt. Let stand 2 weeks. Then rub the lemon slices on the wart.

- Rub with a piece of chalk or a raw potato.

- Tape the inner side of a banana skin to a plantar wart.

# Mind Games: Who's in Control Here?

**Go into a trance.** "You are getting very sleepy—soon you will be in a deep trance—soon your warts will disappear." Hogwash? No, hypnosis. And it may be a formidable weapon against warts.

According to psychiatrist Owen Surman, M.D., "Hypnosis does seem to be a scientifically validated tool for treating warts. Why it would be is subject to guesswork. Currently, people are very interested in this area called psychoneuroimmunology. It's attractive to think that mental phenomena could affect immune function."

In one study, Dr. Surman hypnotized 17 people who had warts on both sides of their bodies for a series of five sessions and told them that their warts would disappear from one side only. Another 7 people were not hypnotized and were instructed to abstain from using any wart remedies on their own. Three months later, more than half of the hypnotized group had lost at least 75 percent of their warts. The people who hadn't been hypnotized still had their warts.

Although the warts that did go away disappeared from *both* sides of the hypnosis group's bodies, "we felt the experiment was a success," says Dr. Surman.

**Imagine your warts away.** The power of suggestion alone—without hypnosis—may be equally effective at wasting warts. Perhaps the most research in this area has been done by Nicholas Spanos, Ph.D. "We tell patients to imagine that their warts are shrinking, that they can feel the tingling as their warts dissolve and their skin becomes clear. Initially, we give them about 2 minutes of this type of imagery, then we have them practice on their own at home for 5 minutes a day.

"Believe it or not, we can actually predict who will achieve results based on the very first session. People who report really vivid imagery that first day are more likely to lose warts than those who say their imagery was relatively weak."

**Be a believer.** Other doctors have had plenty of informal success with the power of suggestion. Says Christopher McEwen, M.D., "I've treated a couple of kids who could not tolerate freezing, which is how we usually remove warts. So I gave them a harmless substance to use and impressed upon them that it was a very strong medicine that would knock out the warts. And it worked." Strong belief in a cure may also explain the continued popularity of such offbeat, old-fashioned folk remedies as rubbing the wart with a penny and then burying the penny under the porch.

in liquid, gel, pad, and ointment form. Don't use them if you have diabetes or impaired circulation.

Follow these three rules for dealing with an acidic OTC, says Glenn Gastwirth, D.P.M. "First, be certain that it *is* a wart you're treating (see "When to Call a Doctor" on page 605). Second, follow package instructions to the letter. And third, if the wart does not respond within a reasonable amount of time—say, a week or two—see a doctor."

Liquid products like Compound W are effective on small warts, says Christopher McEwen, M.D. One good thing about Compound W is that it contains a little oil, which makes it less irritating to the skin than some other salicylic acid products, adds Suzanne M. Levine, D.P.M.

Dr. Brenner advises, however, that the liquid and gel products, which typically contain only about 17 percent salicylic acid, may not be strong enough to work on plantar warts, which have thick calluses covering them.

**Pad the wart.** "If I had to pick one over-the-counter product," says Dr. McEwen, "I'd go with a 40 percent salicylic acid in a plaster vehicle such as Compound W Pads. It works fairly well for plantar warts and can also be effective on hand warts, although it's harder to keep the patch in place on the hand."

"The main drawback to pads," says Dr. Levine, "is that people often use too large a piece, which exposes the surrounding skin to serious irritation. And they put on a new pad every day. Pretty soon they have an ulcer around the wart that's far worse than the wart they started with. The best course of action is to follow the directions on the label."

To ensure a good fit, cut out a little cardboard template in exactly the shape and dimensions of your wart. Then use that template to precut a supply of patches from the adhesive plaster. Lightly coat the perimeter of the wart with petroleum jelly to prevent any medication from touching your skin.

**Go with an ointment.** Rounding out the salicylic acid arsenal is 60 percent ointment. For best results, advises Dr. Levine, soak the wart area in lukewarm water for about 10 minutes to allow for greater penetration. Dry well, then apply a drop of the ointment to the wart. Cover with a bandage. If you're dealing with a plantar wart, do this at bedtime so that you won't have to walk around on the wart and rub off the ointment. In the morning, soak the area again and lightly pumice off any softened skin.

## PANEL OF ADVISORS

**Jeffrey S. Bland, Ph.D.,** is president and chief science officer of Metagenics, a leading health sciences company in Gig Harbor, Washington.

**Marc A. Brenner, D.P.M.,** is director of the Institute of Diabetic Foot Research in Glendale, New York; past president of the American Society of Podiatric Dermatology; and author and editor of various books.

**Robert Garry, Ph.D.,** is a professor of microbiology and immunology at Tulane University School of Medicine in New Orleans.

**Glenn Gastwirth, D.P.M.,** is executive director of the American Podiatric Medical Association.

**Thomas Goodman Jr., M.D.,** is a dermatologist and former assistant professor of dermatology at the University of Tennessee Health Science Center in Memphis. He is the author of *Smart Face*.

**Suzanne M. Levine, D.P.M., P.C.,** is a podiatrist and a podiatric attending physician at New York–Presbyterian Hospital. She is the author of *Your Feet Don't Have to Hurt*.

**Christopher McEwen, M.D.,** is a dermatologist in Baton Rouge, Louisiana.

**Nicholas Spanos, Ph.D.,** is a former professor of psychology at Carleton University in Ottawa, Canada.

**Owen Surman, M.D.,** is an assistant professor of psychiatry at Harvard Medical School and a psychiatrist at Massachusetts General Hospital in Boston.

# WEIGHT PROBLEMS
## 29 Ways to Win the Battle of the Bulge

On any given day, about half the women and a third of the men in America are trying to shed pounds. That's 106 million dieters!

We spend more than $30 *billion* every year on diet products, programs, and paraphernalia. Yet from the looks of our growing obesity epidemic, we don't seem to be getting our money's worth.

In the early 1990s, when *The Doctors Book of Home Remedies* was first published, about 12 percent of the population was obese—meaning, in most cases at least 30 pounds over their ideal weight. Now that figure has more than doubled, and more than *half* of the general population is overweight. If you're unsure how you fit into the equation, see page 611 for instructions on how to calculate your ideal weight.

As the population has grown heavier, diseases related to excess weight have also risen. An estimated 300,000 adults die each year from diabetes, heart disease, stroke, high blood pressure, and other obesity-related complications, second only to tobacco-related deaths.

On one hand, it's not as if we're not trying to lose the weight. We're caught up in diet crazes, "boot camp" workout programs, and low-fat cookies, but still we let out our belts, notch after notch, year after year.

Where's the disconnect? Experts point to several insidious causes.

First, we live in a society where it's just very easy to get large. Consider the fast-food phrase that's become standard English: supersize. It refers to the way restaurants appeal to our sense of frugality by tempting us with more food for our dollar.

"I think the environment's tougher than it was 10 to 15 years ago," says Gary Foster, Ph.D. All-you-can-eat buffets and the accessibility of cheap, high-fat, big-portion foods make it much more difficult to stay at a healthy weight.

Big servings also rub Mary Friesz, R.D., Ph.D., the wrong way.

"Restaurants never supersize salads or vegetables!" she says. "Who needs a bucket of fries at one time?"

Larger helpings often continue at home when we dish out the same portion

## How Much Is Too Much?

Most health professionals use a tool called the body mass index (BMI) to determine if someone falls into either the "overweight" or "obesity" categories. The BMI measures body weight relative to height, which usually correlates to the amount of body fat you have. People who have a BMI of 30 or higher are classified as obese—meaning, in most cases, at least 30 pounds overweight. This category includes a person who is 5 feet 4 inches and weighs 174, or a 5-foot 10-inch person who tips the scales at 209 pounds.

People with a BMI of 25 to 30 are considered overweight, because they weigh more than the standard for their height. The excess weight can come from muscle, bone, or body water as well as fat. This means that certain individuals, such as a bodybuilder or person with a large frame, can be overweight but not overfat. BMI values below 25 and down to 18.5 are considered normal or healthy weight.

You can calculate your own BMI by dividing your weight in pounds by your height in inches squared, then multiplying by 703. Or go to the Web site of the National Heart, Lung, and Blood Institute and use the automatic BMI calculator available there. You will also find tables that have the BMIs already calculated at that site.

Another key tool to determine overweight is waist circumference, which is an obvious indicator of abdominal fat. You can determine your waist circumference by standing and placing a measuring tape snugly around your waist. Health risks rise as waist measurement increases, especially if it's greater than 35 for women or 40 for men.

**WHEN TO CALL A DOCTOR**

It's a good idea to talk with your doctor if you think you may need to lose weight. Doing so is especially important if you have reached or are near menopause or if you have risk factors for developing a chronic disease associated with overweight and obesity, such as a smoking habit, a sedentary lifestyle, high blood sugar, or abnormal blood fats. Weight loss during menopause may increase the rate at which bone density is lost. So your doctor should be aware of your efforts to lose weight—you may need supplemental calcium.

sizes we remember from eating out, she says. Your body can only use so much fuel at one time. Eat more than that, and you store it away as fat.

Second, today's society has grown very sedentary. While our ancestors plowed fields and churned butter as part of their workday, nowadays many of us tap keyboards for a living, then go home at the end of the day to watch television, Dr. Foster says.

Countless "labor-saving devices" spare us effort and exercise, he points out. Escalators zip us to the next floor at the mall. Remote controls allow us to change channels from our recliner. *Getting* too many calories is no problem, but we have to *look* for ways to burn them off.

Even with the challenges society presents, the "secret" to weight loss is so basic: Burn more calories than you consume. The following pages show how to use your mind, mouth, and muscles to control your weight.

## Use Your Mind

Many weight-loss efforts fail from our improper mindset, says Dr. Foster, who views the weight-loss process from a psychologist's perspective. Here's how to use your mind to lose your girth.

**Resist the hard sell.** Regardless of all the get-thin-quick pitches you see stapled to telephone poles and hear on the radio, the best way to lose weight and keep it off is to make permanent changes to your eating and exercise habits, says Marsha Marcus, Ph.D.

Easy answers to a difficult task like losing weight and keeping it off are certainly appealing. But if a weight-loss pitch sounds too good to be true—no matter how convincing—then it is.

**Choose goals wisely.** Despite the inspiring advertisements of skinny people holding up the huge clothes they used to wear, the best goal for weight loss is to lose *10 percent of your body weight*, Dr. Foster says.

It's hard to think small in our more-is-better culture. In one of Dr. Foster's studies, a group of obese women reported how successful they would consider different amounts of weight loss. They called a 25 percent weight loss one they wouldn't be happy with, and a 17 percent weight loss one they could not view as successful in any way. Such unreliable expectations can seriously undermine motivation and the ability to maintain long-term weight loss, Dr. Foster explains.

People who set themselves up by shooting for too high a goal, like losing 100 pounds, do one of two things. Many engage in superhuman behaviors, eating even less, exercising even more, which leads to eventual perceived failure because nobody can continue living that way long term. Others just give up from the get-go and say, "To heck with it if this is the best I can do."

Instead, Dr. Foster recommends figuring out how much 10 percent of your body weight is and shooting for that. For example if you weigh 150 pounds, you'd strive to lose 15 pounds. For most people, it will take about 6 months to achieve this initial goal, adds Dr. Foster.

**Remember that a little goes a long way.** Once you've figured out how much weight to lose at first, plan on losing ½ to 1 pound a week, advises Joanne Larsen, R.D. "When we go on a very low calorie diet or get way too much exercise and lose more than 2 pounds per week, our body goes into starvation mode. When our body's in starvation mode, it burns fewer calories," she says, and it resists your efforts to lose more weight.

**Enjoy your success.** Once they've shed 20 pounds or so, many clients tell Dr. Foster that they sleep better, can climb stairs more easily, and have more energy to play with their grandkids.

Take time to notice and celebrate these successes. Treat yourself to a new dress or a manicure.

**Plan to get by on less.** An aggravating fact of weight loss is that the smaller you get, the fewer calories you can consume and still maintain that new weight, Dr. Foster says. After you've lost 10 percent of your weight, you'll have to eat roughly 10 percent fewer calories each day than you do now to stay at that weight, he says.

But most people don't think of how they're going to maintain their weight loss. They diet awhile, lose the weight, and return to their old eating habits. The weight comes right back, Dr. Foster says. The idea is not to get to your goal and go back to the way you used to eat.

**Go awhile and rest.** Once you've reached your goal of losing 10 percent of your body weight, your next goal should be to simply maintain that loss for a while.

"Try to stay at that weight for at least another 6 to 8 months or a longer period of time than it took to lose that initial amount. Really get a sense of what it is to live in your skin at that weight," Dr. Foster says. If the time is right and you're ready and willing for even more weight-loss effort, *then* start peeling off another reasonable amount. Before attempting additional weight loss, think about your motives for losing weight, how difficult it was, and what else is going on in your life, he explains. The day after moving across the country, for example, would not be a good time to start.

"You'll be in a much better position to know what's required to lose weight after you've maintained it. If I'm not banging my head against the wall just to maintain my weight, then the prospects of losing more weight is a little more appealing," he says.

No one knows for sure how much someone should lose after they have been successful on the first attempt. Dr. Foster suggests trying for 5 percent of your body weight. Everyone will lose at a different rate, so there's no way to predict how long it will take.

**Make changes you can live with.** Even if you can totally cut out fast food, greasy movie-theater popcorn, and other tempting foods while you're losing weight, you'll need to learn that you can enjoy all foods, including those, in moderation for the rest of your life.

"I think that for people with weight problems, it's a question of a lifetime of self-management. That's not to say that one has to *diet* over one's lifetime. We have to say yes to ourselves and enjoy our food, but we also have to learn to say no," Dr. Marcus says.

**Become more aware of your eating behavior.** In order to *change* your eating behavior, you first have to *learn* what that behavior is. It's a two-step process, explains Dr. Marcus. First, start paying attention to what, when, where, and with whom you're eating, how you feel, and what kind of activities you're doing throughout the day. Next, think about what triggers the eating. Dr. Marcus recalls seeing the comics character Cathy clinging on to a parking meter because "she could smell the bread and hear the bakery calling her in." Other triggers could be the sight of a certain food, boredom, or aggravation.

It's very easy to go through our days without paying attention to such details, Dr. Marcus says. A lot of us eat all the time without thinking about it. Keep a food diary to record the information, so you can read it over later, she suggests.

**Make a good reflection.** Hang a full-length mirror in your home, Larsen suggests. Overweight people often use mirrors that only reflect their face, and they don't see the full image that everyone else sees.

You can find full-length mirrors in department stores for less than $20. Take a good look into it regularly.

## Use Your Mouth

Sure, it's easy to say that the secret to weight loss is to eat fewer calories than you burn. Sadly, because of our fast-paced, sedentary lifestyle, eating well isn't that simple in daily life.

Larsen knows firsthand how precious little that people know about healthy living. A dietitian and computer guru, she's operated a nutrition information Web site since 1995.

"My inbox right now has 30,092 e-mail messages," she says. The vast majority of them deal with weight issues. "I'd say most people are just beginning to learn about nutrition. People ask even basic questions like 'What are carbohydrates?'"

**Figure out what you need.** An estimate of how many calories you should consume each day to lose weight safely is 10 calories per pound of body weight per day. If you weigh 180 pounds, try to get 1,800 calories per day.

Your individual needs may differ from this, however, depending in part on your body composition and activity. Gender and genetics have a strong impact on how your body uses and stores food. For example, women's hormones tend to encourage fat deposition. A dietitian can help you figure out a more precise number, Larsen suggests. Ask at your local hospital for a referral or check out the "Find a Dietitian" link on the Web site of the American Dietetic Association. You can also use the "Healthy Body Calculator" at www.dietitian.com.

**Eat a balanced diet.** High-protein/low-carbohydrate diets, which cut out the bread, pasta, and fruit and bump up the meat, have enjoyed a wave of popularity.

Though people might lose weight while enjoying steak, eggs, and beef jerky, it's partly due to fluid loss from the unusual way their body must turn food into energy, and partly because they're eating fewer calories. Using so much protein as fuel can leave you fatigued and constipated and puts more demands on your kidneys as they filter excess protein, posing special risks to those with diabetes, Dr. Friesz says.

A diet that's ultra-low in fat isn't good either. In reasonable amounts, the fat in your food makes you feel full, so you want to stop eating. For example, when you choose fat-free ice cream, you may wind up eating more because it's less satisfying—and get more calories than if you'd eaten a bit of regular ice cream. In the end, it's the calories that count, Dr. Friesz says.

The balanced diet that experts recommend for weight loss or weight maintenance is simple. Each day, try to get about *half* of your calories from carbohydrates. Good sources of carbohydrates include fruits, vegetables, whole grain breads, pasta, rice, and milk.

About a *quarter* of your calories should come from protein. Good sources include lean cuts of beef, chicken breast, fish, and beans. If you're a vegetarian, have rice in the same day as beans to ensure that you receive complete proteins.

The last *quarter* of your calories should come from fats and oils. The best are olive and canola oils. These are the healthiest for your heart, but they're still high in calories, so don't go overboard with them.

**Keep track of your calories.** Larsen suggests using a food diary, whenever possible, to record what you've eaten each day, how many calories the foods contain, along with the other details of your eating behavior.

"Keeping food records is the only way to know whether you're on track or not. Here's a comparison," she says. Imagine that you write checks and put money in your checking account, but you don't write down the amount of the check, and you never balance your checking account. You'd have no idea where you're at financially. It's the same thing with losing weight.

**Eat frequently.** Instead of eating all your food for the day in two or three sittings, eat four to six smaller meals throughout the day, Dr. Friesz suggests. When you eat smaller, more frequent meals each day as opposed to a couple of belly busters, your body is more likely to use the calories instead of packing them away as fat, she says. You'll also ensure that you aren't starving when you pull up to the table, which increases your chances of wolfing down more than you need.

Just make sure that the total calories in your small meals, when added up, don't exceed the amount of calories you should be consuming each day.

**Be creative at the restaurant.** You know when you eat out that the waiter is likely to drop a calorie bomb onto your table that can devastate your hips for months to come. "If you're full when you leave the table, you ate too much. That's your body's way of saying, 'There's too much here for me to digest at one time,'" Dr. Friesz says. You need to stop before that, when you still have room for food but don't have that hunger feeling. Instead of eating until you hurt:

• Split an entrée with your spouse or friend.

• Order a child-size entrée.

• Ask the waitress to immediately box up half the meal so that you can take it home and enjoy later.

• If you order a meal served atop a bed of pasta, ask for the pasta separately. Side servings of pasta are usually about $1\frac{1}{2}$ cups, but bottom servings can be twice that amount, explains Dr. Friesz.

• If you get a stuffed baked potato, ask for the butter, sour cream, and other toppings separately, and add just enough for flavoring. If you can still taste the potato, you're doing well.

# To the Extreme

Plenty of us have some weight that we'd like to lose, but we don't always take the healthiest approach in getting there. When eating patterns control a person's life, it's possible that an eating disorder is at play.

The two main eating disorders are bulimia nervosa and anorexia nervosa. By current estimates, fewer than 5 percent of women will suffer from bulimia in their lifetime. Most people with bulimia endure a pattern of binge eating followed by behavior to make up for the binge, such as vomiting; using diuretics, enemas, or other medications; fasting; or excessive exercise; and then finally relief. Although they are typically in the normal weight range, since their behavior after a binge prevents weight gain, people with bulimia don't want to overeat. But they have a sense of being out of control and feel disgusted and ashamed during their binging, says Marsha Marcus, Ph.D. Purging or other behaviors are often performed secretly.

Binge-eating disorder is another type of bulimia, marked by similar out-of-control feelings. The most important difference, however, between these two illnesses is that people with binge-eating disorder do not perform compensatory behavior after a binge, such as overexercising or purging, so many of them are overweight. This leads to shame and self-disgust, starting the cycle over again.

Anorexia nervosa is an eating disorder that rarely occurs in men and older women. But about 1 percent of American teenage girls develop this disorder, and up to 10 percent of those may die from the disease. Typically, people with anorexia are extremely worried about being overweight, even though they're already too thin (usually at least 15 percent under their ideal weight). Because they still see themselves as overweight and intensely fear gaining weight or becoming fat, they starve themselves and may purge, engage in excessive exercise, or use other methods to control their weight.

People with anorexia won't admit they have a problem to anyone, most of all themselves, or they deny the seriousness of problem, says Dr. Marcus. In fact, that's one of the ways doctors diagnose it.

If you suspect that you or someone you care about may have an eating disorder, seek professional help immediately. For more information on eating disorders, contact:

National Association of Anorexia
　Nervosa and Associated Disorders
PO Box 7
Highland Park, IL 60035
(847) 831-3438
www.anad.org

National Eating Disorders Association
603 Stewart Street, Suite 803
Seattle, WA 98101
(800) 931-2237
www.nationaleatingdisorders.org

**Strive for 25.** Eating at least 25 grams of fiber each day is especially important if you're trying to lose weight. Foods rich in fiber tend to be nutritious, filling, lower-calorie choices, Larsen says.

You can accumulate a total of 25 grams of fiber in a day by having a cup of bran flakes for breakfast, toasting a whole wheat English muffin for your morning break, tossing ½ cup of chickpeas onto your lunch salad, snacking on a large apple, and stir-frying ½ cup of broccoli for dinner.

**Guzzle—don't gobble.** Drink eight 8-ounce glasses of water each day. Keeping some water in your stomach most of the time can help fool it into thinking it's full, Larsen says.

## Use Your Muscles

The last key component of any weight-loss program is exercise. Activity burns calories, allowing you to eat more and weigh the same, or eat the same and weigh less. Exercise combined with diet is the most effective approach for weight loss and is an integral part of long-term weight maintenance. Here's how to wield the power of exercise to your advantage.

**Go for a blend.** The best exercise program combines aerobic exercise, strength training, and stretching, says Joseph Chromiak, Ph.D. Aerobic exercise that is continuous, such as biking, walking, and swimming, strengthens your heart and is best for reducing your risk of many chronic diseases. "Stop-start" activities, such as racquetball, are not as beneficial.

Strength training, such as calisthenics or weight lifting, makes your muscles stronger and helps maintain muscle mass. This becomes more important as we get older, because our muscle mass starts diminishing in our early twenties. If you don't use your muscles, they decline in size. Since muscle tissue significantly contributes to a person's daily calorie expenditure, the more muscle mass you have, the more calories you expend. The daily difference isn't large, but it's huge over time, explains Dr. Chromiak.

Stretching helps prepare your muscles for a workout and increases flexibility. But the best time to stretch for long-term results is after exercise, when your muscles are warmed up, advises Dr. Chromiak. Try to stretch for 10 to 15 minutes at least three times a week.

**Don't go for all-or-nothing.** Initially, plan to exercise for 20 minutes for a minimum of 3 days a week, Dr. Chromiak says. Build up to 30 to 40 minutes at a time. The more days you exercise, the better, but 3 days is a good starting point if you haven't been exercising.

If your size or fitness level prevents you from working out for 20 minutes a day, start with just 15 minutes and gradually work your way up, he suggests. Don't put off exercising if time is an issue. Even exercising for 10 to 15 minutes intermittently through the day helps strengthen your heart. And just a few minutes of exercise done regularly will eventually make it easier to go for longer periods.

**Find exercises you enjoy.** Think of all the activities you might enjoy, then alternate among them whenever you wish, Dr. Chromiak suggests. Adding variety may make it easier to stick with your program.

**Be able to speak.** While you're doing aerobic exercise, exert yourself at a moderate intensity level. You should be able to carry on a conversation punctuated by moderately heavy but not comfortable breathing, Dr. Chromiak says.

**Play these numbers in the weight room.** Adults get the greatest gains in muscle strength and muscle endurance by using weights that they can comfortably lift for a set of 8 to 12 repetitions, Dr. Chromiak suggests. If you can't lift a weight 8 times, decrease the weight. If you can easily lift it 12 times, bump up the weight a few pounds.

Ideally, you should lift weights three times a week. If you can hit the gym or exercise at home that often, you only need to do each set of repetitions once. If you can only lift weights 2 days a week, do two to three sets of each exercise, he suggests.

**Seek help.** It's a good idea to talk to a qualified trainer to ensure that you're choosing the right exercises to safely work all the major muscles in your body. If you don't belong to a gym, hire a personal trainer for a few sessions to get you started. Look for someone who is certified by the National Strength and Conditioning Association (NSCA) as a certified strength and conditioning specialist or certified personal trainer.

**Make a priority.** If you're not accustomed to exercising regularly, schedule it in advance as an appointment on your calendar or electronic planner, Dr. Friesz suggests. Otherwise, you'll forget or find an excuse not to do it. After 3 months, it should become a habit, she says.

## PANEL OF ADVISORS

**Joseph Chromiak, Ph.D.,** is an assistant professor in the department of health, physical education, recreation, and sport at Mississippi State University in Starkville and a certified strength and conditioning specialist.

**Gary Foster, Ph.D.,** is clinical director of the weight and eating disorders program at the University of Pennsylvania in Philadelphia.

**Mary Friesz, R.D., Ph.D.,** is a nutrition and wellness consultant and a certified diabetes educator in Boca Raton, Florida.

**Joanne Larsen, R.D.,** designs nutrition software and food and ingredient data-bases for software companies. She also has a nutrition information Web site at www.dietitian.com.

**Marsha D. Marcus, Ph.D.,** is an associate professor of psychiatry and psychology and chief of the behavioral medicine and eating disorders program in the department of psychiatry at the University of Pittsburgh School of Medicine.

# WRINKLES
## 15 Age-Defying Secrets

The quality of many fine wines and single-malt scotches improves dramatically with age, as do the value of *most* 401(k) plans. Unfortunately, our skin doesn't. Rather, it loses moisture, elasticity, and resiliency as we age, causing it to wrinkle.

Skin undergoes two types of aging, says Coyle S. Connolly, D.O. The first, intrinsic aging, is genetically programmed. You can't do much about that without the help of a dermatologist. The second—extrinsic aging, or photoaging—is the result of damage primarily due to the sun.

You can fight photoaging every step of the way by making smart choices. Here's what the experts advise to keep wrinkles—those reminders of how much mileage you have on your odometer—from taking too much of a toll on your skin.

**Sleep on your back.** Sleeping on your side or belly with your face mashed into the pillow causes wrinkles, says D'Anne Kleinsmith, M.D. Some stomach sleepers develop a diagonal crease on their foreheads, running above their eyebrows. Sleeping on your back may eliminate this problem.

**Gotta wear shades.** One real problem area for wrinkles is around the eyes, says Dr. Kleinsmith. These wrinkles, called crow's-feet, often result from squinting. One way to avoid them or lessen their severity is to wear sunglasses whenever you go outside.

**Keep a stone face.** Excessive frowning or smiling, or any other much-repeated facial expression, aggravates wrinkles, says Dr. Kleinsmith. "I'm not saying that you should not smile or frown, but try to be aware of how often you're doing it—especially frowning."

For the same reason, Dr. Kleinsmith and other experts advise *against* facial exercises.

Facial exercises build facial muscles just like biceps curls build biceps, says Audrey Kunin, M.D. Normal, everyday repeated movements cause enough wrinkles. Smiling causes crow's-feet, frowns result in deep crevices between your brows, and lifting your brows in surprise leaves you with lines across your forehead.

**Lay off the cigarettes.** "Smokers have more wrinkles than people who don't smoke, especially around their lips," says Dr. Kleinsmith. That's because smoking robs the complexion of oxygen, decreasing blood circulation to facial skin and thus resulting in premature lines and wrinkles. Plus, anyone puffing on a cigarette essentially does a lot of repetitive facial movements that add even more wrinkles.

**Be sun smart.** Whether it's achieved indoors or outside, today's tan leads to tomorrow's wrinkles. "Obviously, excessive exposure to sunlight is going to increase your chances of developing wrinkles," says Dr. Kunin. Wear your sunscreen, preferably with a sun protection factor (SPF) of 30 and with both ultraviolet (UV) A and B protection (also known as broad-spectrum). Also sport a pair of UV-coated glasses (melanoma can form at the back of the eye), and you may even want to wash your clothing in Rit Sun Guard.

Rit Sun Guard is sun protection for your skin that you wash into your clothing. "This product increases the capability of fabric to prevent UV rays from reaching the skin and is the relative equivalent of an SPF 30 rating for sunscreen," she adds.

Simply add it to the wash cycle, rinse, and dry your clothes as usual. One treatment of Rit Sun Guard is good for more than 20 washings, says Dr. Kunin. "Normal cloth only has an SPF of 4, making it worthless when it comes to screening out the longer UVA rays. While these rays may not cause a sunburn like UVB, they are more likely to cause skin damage that leads to wrinkles and skin cancer down the road," she says.

**Ban tanning beds.** Twenty minutes of tanning-bed use is equivalent to an entire day at the beach without sunscreen. Avoid them like the plague to keep from damaging your skin, suggests Dr. Kunin. "If you want to look tan, use a self-tanner lotion and perhaps a bronzer with your foundation," she says.

**Wear a hat.** Whether you're heading to the beach or spending extended time in the midday sun, put on a hat with a 4-inch-wide brim to keep the sun off your face and neck, says Dr. Kunin.

But steer clear of straw hats that are unlined and loosely woven. They allow the sun's rays to penetrate directly through the hat. Also keep in mind that baseball caps don't protect your ears, the back of your neck, or even most of your face from full-bore sun.

Choose a hat with an extra-long bill and sun-protective cloth inside, says Dr. Kunin. "It gives you the extra protection you need to limit your chances of developing wrinkles."

**Stay out of the midday sun.** That's 10:00 A.M. to 4:00 P.M. during spring, summer, and fall, or 10:00 A.M. to 2:00 P.M. during winter. These peak hours are when the ultraviolet radiation is the strongest, says skin-care expert Joni Keim Loughran. She cautions that sunblock is needed even during winter and on cloudy days and recommends titanium oxide or zinc oxide with an SPF of 8 to 15.

**Be a shady person.** Since wrinkles are caused by excessive sun exposure, periodically retreat to a shady spot on sunny days, says Loughran.

At the beach or in your backyard, sit under a large umbrella. While on hikes or on the water, if it's not too hot out, wear tightly woven clothing. It helps keep UV rays from penetrating your skin.

**Use a moisturizer.** If you have dry skin, daily use of a moisturizing lotion can plump up your skin and temporarily hide smaller wrinkles that form on the skin surface, says Dr. Connolly. "It's not a long-term solution for wrinkles, but it will give your skin a healthier look."

**Give me a "C."** Apply a topical vitamin C cream or ointment on a daily basis. You'll notice a marked improvement in your skin's overall quality, says Dr. Connolly. "Vitamin C creams help build collagen and gobble up free radicals, which if left unchecked will cause your skin to age or wrinkle," he says. Vitamin C creams and ointments are available over the counter in many drugstores.

**Try an active treatment.** Active skin-care creams contain one or more of six ingredients that do more than just moisturize the skin. They also help reduce wrinkles, make skin look brighter and more youthful, and stimulate fibroblasts (connective tissue cells that make collagen), which helps reduce fine lines, blotchy skin discoloration, and so forth—all those signs of skin aging. The ingredients to look for and some product samples are vitamin C (found in many topical creams); GHK copper peptides (Neutrogena Visibly Firm); glycolic acid (Total Skin Care Glycolic Gel); tretinoin, a vitamin A derivative (RoC Retinol Actif Pur Anti-Wrinkle Treatment); N6 furfuryladenine (Kinerase cream or lotion); and alpha lipoic acid (Z. Bigatti Re-Storation Deep Repair Facial Serum).

Using an "active agent" helps hydrate the skin, says Dr. Kunin. If your skin still feels dry even after using the active cream with a sunscreen, add a moisturizer, she says.

**Slough off the cells.** Alpha hydroxy acids (AHAs), found in plants and fruits, are available in creams, lotions, and gels. They act by defoliating dead skin cells on the surface to uncover the younger cells underneath. And, in plumping up the skin, they fill in the areas that cause wrinkles. Glycolic acid is the most common AHA, and there are fragrance-free versions of AHAs for sensitive skin around the eyes.

If your skin is too sensitive for AHAs, you might try beta hydroxy acids (BHAs), such as salicylic acid. It's available in moisturizers and cleaners, and it exfoliates the skin like an AHA but with less irritation.

**Dine on fish and flaxseed.** Two dietary adjustments can help to maintain proper skin moisture. Eat fish such as salmon, trout, whitefish, and tuna, which are rich in omega-3 fatty acids, at least twice a week to help replenish moisture to dry skin. Flaxseed oil, which also is loaded with omega-3s, can be mixed into fruit juice or drizzled on salad and vegetables. It is perishable, so it must be refrigerated.

**Put on some papaya.** Try using a papaya peel twice a month. The same protein-eating enzymes that make this tropical fruit a good digestive agent can also break down your outer layer of skin. Grind 2 tablespoons of washed and peeled papaya in a food processor, and add 1 tablespoon of dry oatmeal (the oatmeal helps to remove debris from the skin). Pat this mixture onto clean skin and let it set for 10 minutes. Then remove it with a wet washcloth, using an outward, circular motion.

## PANEL OF ADVISORS

**Coyle S. Connolly, D.O.,** is an assistant clinical professor at the Philadelphia College of Osteopathic Medicine and a dermatologist in Linwood, New Jersey.

**D'Anne Kleinsmith, M.D.,** is a cosmetic dermatologist at William Beaumont Hospital in Royal Oak, Michigan, and is an expert on wrinkles.

**Audrey Kunin, M.D.,** is a cosmetic dermatologist in Kansas City, Missouri, and the founder of the dermatology educational Web site DERMAdoctor.com.

**Joni Keim Loughran** is a skin-care expert in Petaluma, California.

# GUIDELINES FOR SAFE USE OF HERBS, VITAMINS, AND SUPPLEMENTS

Although most herbs, vitamins, and supplements are generally safe and cause few, if any, side effects, doctors caution that you should use them responsibly. After all, every product has the potential to cause adverse reactions.

If you are under a doctor's care for any health condition or are taking any medication, talk with your doctor before using herbs and supplements. Certain natural substances can change the way your body absorbs and processes medications.

Also, if you are pregnant, do not treat yourself with any natural remedy without the consent of your obstetrician or midwife. The same goes for nursing mothers and women trying to conceive.

## Herbs

Following are cautions for the herbs mentioned in this book that may be more likely than others to cause adverse reactions in some people. Though such occurrences are rare, you should be aware of what they are and discontinue use of the herb if you experience an unusual reaction. Also, do not exceed the recommended dosages—more is not better.

| Common Name | Botanical Name(s) | Safety Guidelines and Possible Side Effects |
| --- | --- | --- |
| **Aloe** | *Aloe barbadensis* | May delay wound healing; do not use gel externally on any surgical incision. Do not ingest the dried leaf gel, as it is a habit-forming laxative. |
| **American ginseng** | *Panax quinquefolius* | May cause irritability if taken with caffeine or other stimulants. Do not take if you have high blood pressure. |

*(continued)*

| Common Name | Botanical Name(s) | Safety Guidelines and Possible Side Effects |
| --- | --- | --- |
| **Arnica** | *Arnica montana,*<br>*Arnica* spp. | Do not use on broken skin. |
| **Black cohosh** | *Actea racemosa* | Do not use for more than 6 months. |
| **Cascara sagrada** | *Rhamnus purshianus* | Do not use if you have any inflam-matory condition of the intestines, in-testinal obstruction, or abdominal pain. Can cause laxative dependency and diar-rhea. Don't use for more than 14 days. |
| **Chamomile** | *Matricaria recutita* | Very rarely, can cause an allergic reaction when ingested. People allergic to closely re-lated plants such as ragweed, asters, and chrysanthemums should drink the tea with caution. |
| **Chasteberry (vitex)** | *Vitex agnus-castus* | May counteract the effectiveness of birth control pills. |
| **Dandelion** | *Taraxacum officinale* | If you have gallbladder disease, do not use dandelion root preparations without med-ical approval. |
| **Echinacea** | *Echinacea angustifolia,*<br>*E. purpurea,*<br>*E. pallida* | Do not use if allergic to closely related plants such ragweed, asters, and chrysanthemums. Do not use products with echinacea flowers. Do not use if you have tuberculosis, or an autoimmune condi-tion such as lupus or multiple sclerosis be-cause echinacea stimulates the immune system. |
| **False unicorn root** | *Chamaelirium luteum* | May cause nausea and vomiting in doses higher than 5 to 15 drops of tincture or ½ cup of infusion. |
| **Fennel** | *Foeniculum vulgare* | Do not use medicinally for more than 6 weeks without supervision by a qualified practitioner. |
| **Feverfew** | *Tanacetum parthenium* | If chewed, fresh leaves can cause mouth sores in some people. |
| **Flax** | *Linum usitatissimum* | Do not take if you have a bowel obstruc-tion. Take with at least 8 ounces of water. (Note: This caution pertains to flaxseed only. Flaxseed oil is considered safe.) |

| Common Name | Botanical Name(s) | Safety Guidelines and Possible Side Effects |
|---|---|---|
| **Garlic** | *Allium sativum* | Do not use supplements if you're on anticoagulants or before undergoing surgery, because garlic thins the blood and may increase bleeding. Do not use if you're taking hypoglycemic drugs. |
| **Gentian** | *Gentiana lutea* | May cause nausea and vomiting in large doses. Do not use if you have high blood pressure, gastric or duodenal ulcers, or gastric irritation and inflammation. |
| **Ginger** | *Zingiber officinale* | May increase bile secretion, so if you have gallstones, do not use therapeutic amounts of the dried root or powder without guidance from a health care practitioner. |
| **Ginkgo** | *Ginkgo biloba* | Do not use with antidepressant MAO inhibitor drugs such as phenelzine sulfate (Nardil) or tranylcypromine (Parnate), aspirin or other nonsteroidal anti-inflammatory medications, or blood-thinning medications such as warfarin (Coumadin). Can cause dermatitis, diarrhea, and vomiting in doses higher than 240 mg of concentrated extract. |
| **Goldenseal** | *Hydrastis canadensis* | Do not use if you have high blood pressure. |
| **Guggul** | *Commiphora mukul* | Rarely, may trigger diarrhea, restlessness, apprehension, or hiccups. |
| **Hawthorn** | *Crataegus oxycantha,* *C. laevigata,* *C. monogyna* | If you have a cardiovascular condition, do not take hawthorn regularly for more than a few weeks without medical supervision. You may require lower doses of other medications, such as high blood pressure drugs. If you have low blood pressure caused by heart valve problems, do not use without medical supervision. |
| **Horse chestnut** | *Aesculus hippocastanum* | May interfere with the action of other drugs, especially blood thinners such as warfarin (Coumadin). May irritate the gastrointestinal tract. |

*(continued)*

| Common Name | Botanical Name(s) | Safety Guidelines and Possible Side Effects |
| --- | --- | --- |
| **Kava kava** | *Piper methysticum* | Do not take with alcoholic beverages. Do not use if taking prescription or over-the-counter drugs or if you have a history of liver disease. Do not exceed 300 mg kavalactones per day or take more than the recommended dose on package. Use caution when driving or operating equipment, as this herb is a muscle relaxant. Discontinue use of kava and seek medical attention if you experience symptoms associated with jaundice, such as nausea, fever, or dark urine. |
| **Licorice** | *Glycyrrhiza glabra* | Do not use if you have diabetes, high blood pressure, liver or kidney disorders, or low potassium levels. Do not use daily for more than 4 to 6 weeks, because overuse can lead to water retention, high blood pressure caused by potassium loss, or impaired heart and kidney function. |
| **Meadowsweet** | *Filipendula* spp. | Do not take if you need to avoid aspirin, because its active ingredient, salicin, is related to aspirin. |
| **Myrrh** | *Commiphora myrrha* | Can cause diarrhea and irritation of the kidneys. Do not use if you have uterine bleeding for any reason. |
| **Nettle** | *Urtica dioica* | If you have allergies, your symptoms may worsen, so take only one dose a day for the first few days. |
| **Oats** | *Avena sativa* | Do not use if you have celiac disease (gluten intolerance), as it contains gluten, a grain protein. |
| **Parsley** | *Petroselinum crispum* | Do not use if you have kidney disease, because it increases urine flow when used in therapeutic amounts. Safe as a garnish or ingredient in food. |
| **Psyllium** | *Plantago ovata* | Do not use if you have a bowel obstruction. Take 1 hour after other drugs. Take with at least 8 ounces of water. |

| Common Name | Botanical Name(s) | Safety Guidelines and Possible Side Effects |
|---|---|---|
| **Rosemary** | *Rosmarinus officinalis* | May cause excessive menstrual bleeding in therapeutic amounts. Considered safe when used as a spice. |
| **Sage** | *Salvia officinalis* | Used in therapeutic amounts, can increase sedative side effects of drugs. Do not use if you are hypoglycemic or undergoing anti-convulsant therapy. |
| **Sarsaparilla** | *Smilax orata* | May speed elimination of prescription medications thereby requiring an increase in the effective dose. |
| **St. John's wort** | *Hypericum perforatum* | Do not use with antidepressants or other prescription medicine without medical approval. May cause photosensitivity; avoid overexposure to direct sunlight. |
| **Turmeric** | *Curcuma domestica* | Do not use if you have high stomach acid or ulcers, gallstones, or bile duct obstruction. |
| **Valerian** | *Valeriana officinalis* | Do not use with sleep-enhancing or mood-regulating medications, because it may intensify their effects. May cause heart palpitations and nervousness in sensitive individuals. If such stimulant action occurs, discontinue use. |
| **White willow** | *Salix alba* | Can cause stomach irritation, especially when consumed with alcohol. |
| **Yarrow** | *Achillea millefolium* | Rarely, handling flowers can cause skin rash. |

# Vitamin and Mineral Supplements

Although serious side effects from vitamin and mineral supplements are not common, they can happen. The guidelines presented here are designed to help you use the supplements mentioned in this book safely and wisely.

The vitamin and mineral doses listed below are the Daily Values or the suggested daily intakes (noted in *italics*). Also given below are the safe upper limits for adults, above which harmful side effects can occur. These amounts are the total from both food and supplements. Do not take more than the safe upper limit of any vitamin or mineral without first consulting your physician. (Note: mg = milligrams; mcg = micrograms; IU = international units)

| Vitamin or Mineral Supplement | Daily Value (DV) or *Suggested Daily Intake* | Safe Upper Limit | Cautions and Other Information |
|---|---|---|---|
| **Biotin** | 300 mcg | 2,500 mcg | A healthy, balanced diet provides enough of this nutrient to meet your body's needs. |
| **Calcium** | 1,000 mg (the DV) *1,200 mg for people over age 50* | 2,500 mg | Taking more than 2,500 mg a day can cause serious side effects such as kidney damage. For best absorption, avoid taking more than 500 mg at one time. If you are over age 50, look for a formula that contains vitamin D as well as calcium, since you may need more vitamin D than is supplied by a multivitamin alone. Some natural sources of calcium, such as bonemeal and dolomite, may be contaminated with lead and other dangerous or undesirable metals. |
| **Copper** | 2 mg | 10 mg (10,000 mcg) | For best absorption, use supplements containing copper sulfate or cupric sulfate rather than copper oxide or cupric oxide. |
| **Magnesium** | 400 mg | 350 mg from supplements only | Check with your doctor before beginning supplementation in any amount if you have heart or kidney problems. Doses exceeding 350 mg a day can cause diarrhea in some people. |
| **Niacin** | 20 mg | 35 mg | Taking more than the safe upper limit of 35 mg a day can cause flushing and itching. Because serious side effects, including liver damage, can occur from doses above 500 mg, high doses of niacin should be taken only under your doctor's supervision. When selecting a B-complex supplement, |

| Vitamin or Mineral Supplement | Daily Value (DV) or *Suggested Daily Intake* | Safe Upper Limit | Cautions and Other Information |
|---|---|---|---|
| | | | check the label for the amount of each ingredient to help you determine its safe use. |
| **Vitamin A** | 5,000 IU | 10,000 IU (3,000 mcg) | Taking more than 10,000 IU a day can cause headache, double vision, drowsiness or fatigue, nausea, or vomiting. |
| **Vitamin B₆** | 2 mg | 100 mg | Taking more than 100 mg a day can cause reversible nerve damage. When selecting a B-complex supplement, check the label for the amount of each ingredient to help you determine its safe use. |
| **Vitamin B₁₂** | 6 mcg | 3,000 mcg | None |
| **Vitamin C** | *100 to 500 mg* (DV is 60 mg) | 2,000 mg | Taking more than 2,000 mg a day can cause diarrhea in some people. To help maintain levels of vitamin C throughout the day, take half of the recommended dose in the morning and half at night. |
| **Vitamin E** | *100 to 400 IU* (DV is 30 IU) | 1,500 IU (natural form, d-alpha-tocopherol) or 1,100 IU (synthetic form, dl-alpha-tocopherol) from supplements only | Because it acts like a blood thinner, consult your doctor before taking vitamin E if you are already taking aspirin or a blood-thinning medication, such as warfarin (Coumadin). |
| **Zinc** | 15 mg | 40 mg | Taking more than 40 mg a day can cause nausea, dizziness, or vomiting. When levels of zinc are elevated, the absorption of copper can become impaired. |

# Supplements

Reports of adverse effects from supplements are rare, especially when compared to prescription drugs, and supplement manufacturers are required by law to provide information on labels about reasonably safe recommended dosages for healthy individuals. Be aware that the potency and dosing strategy can vary significantly among products.

You should note, however, that little scientific research exists to assess the safety or long-term effects of many emerging supplements, and some supplements can complicate existing conditions or cause allergic reactions in some people. Take supplements with food for best absorption and to avoid stomach irritation, unless otherwise directed. Never take them as a substitute for a healthy diet, since they do not provide all the nutritional benefits of whole foods.

| Common Name | Safety Guidelines and Possible Side Effects |
| --- | --- |
| **Activated charcoal** | If taken for more than 2 days, may interfere with absorption of nutrients or pose risk of gastrointestinal obstruction. May interfere with the absorption of oral medications or other supplements if not taken at least 2 hours apart. Do not take more than the recommended label dosage, since it may cause stomach upset, diarrhea, constipation, or vomiting. |
| **Bromelain** | May cause nausea, vomiting, diarrhea, skin rash, and heavy menstrual bleeding. Can also increase the risk of bleeding in people taking aspirin or anticoagulants (blood thinners). Do not take if you are allergic to pineapple. |
| **Coenzyme Q$_{10}$** | Discuss supplementation with your doctor if you are taking the blood thinner warfarin (Coumadin). On rare occasions, it may reduce warfarin's effectiveness. Supplementation should be observed by a knowledgeable naturopathic or medical doctor if taken for more than 20 days at levels of 120 mg per day or higher. Side effects are rare, but tend to be heartburn, nausea, or stomachache, which can be prevented by consuming the supplement with a meal. |
| **Curcumin** | May cause heartburn in some people. |
| **Fish oil** | Do not take if any of the following apply: You have a bleeding disorder, uncontrolled high blood pressure, or an allergy to any kind of fish, or you take anticoagulants (blood thinners) or aspirin regularly. People with diabetes should not take fish oil because of its high fat content. Increases bleeding time, possibly resulting in nosebleeds and easy bruising, and may cause upset stomach. |
| **Glucosamine** | May cause upset stomach, heartburn, or diarrhea. |

| Common Name | Safety Guidelines and Possible Side Effects |
|---|---|
| **Lysine** | Don't take arginine and lysine at the same time, as they compete for absorption in the body. |
| **Quercetin** | Doses above 100 mg may dilate blood vessels and cause blood thinning in some people. Should be avoided by individuals at risk for low blood pressure or problems with blood clotting. |
| **SAM-e** | May increase blood levels of homocysteine, a significant risk factor for cardiovascular disease. |

# COMBINATIONS TO AVOID

The following guide can help you avoid mixing common drugs with herbs, supplements, and foods that can cause problems. Please note that this list is not comprehensive. If you're taking a different drug for any of these conditions, consult your doctor or pharmacist about possible interactions. To be safe, be sure to tell your doctor about all the medicines you're taking and any medicinal herbs or foods you use therapeutically (such as garlic or ginger).

| If You Have . . . | And Are Taking . . . | Then Steer Clear Of . . . | Because . . . |
|---|---|---|---|
| **Allergies** | Antihistamines such as diphenhydramine (Benadryl), hydroxyzine (Atarax), or astemizole (Hismanal) | Sedative herbs such as passionflower, skullcap, and valerian | They may increase the drug's sedative effects. |
| **Angina** | Beta-blockers such as propranolol (Inderal) | The herbs broom and fumitory | They increase the drug's effects. |
| **Anxiety** | Hypnotic and mild sedative drugs such as flurazepam (Dalmane), diazepam (Valium), or alprazolam (Xanax) | Cowslip, mistletoe, and yohimbe Sedative herbs such as passionflower, skullcap, and valerian | They increase the drug's effects. They may increase the drug's sedative effects. |
| | Triazolam (Halcion) | Grapefruit juice | It boosts the absorption of the drug. |

*(continued)*

| If You Have . . . | And Are Taking . . . | Then Steer Clear Of . . . | Because . . . |
|---|---|---|---|
| **Asthma** | Theophylline (Theo-Dur) | Charcoal | It decreases the drug's effects. |
| | | Guarana | It increases the drug's effects. |
| | | St. John's wort | It may lower blood levels of the drug. |
| | | Ephedra | It intensifies the drug's effects. |
| | Ephedrine or pseudoephedrine | Tannin-containing herbs such as black tea, green tea, and uva-ursi | They may interfere with the drug's absorption. |
| **An auto-immune disorder, an inflammatory disease such as tendinitis, or allergies or asthma** | Drugs that suppress the immune response such as corticos-teroids, including prednisone (Deltasone) | Immune-enhancing herbs such as astra-galus, echinacea, maitake, and reishi | They may counteract the drug's effects. |
| | Aspirin or other nonsteroidal anti-inflammatory drugs | Ginkgo | It may increase the blood-thinning effects of these medications. |
| **Congestive heart failure or atrial fibrillation** | Cardiac glycosides such as digitalis medi-cations, including xdigitoxin (Crys-todigin) or digoxin (Lanoxin) | Coltsfoot, golden-seal, hawthorn, and motherwort | They can affect the cardiovascular system. |
| | | Aloe, fumitory, goldenseal, haw-thorn, licorice, lungwort, night-blooming cereus, Queen Anne's lace, and Siberian ginseng | They increase the drug's effects. |
| | Digoxin (Lanoxin) | St. John's wort | It lowers blood levels of the drug. |
| | | Licorice | It causes potassium loss, which can in-crease the risk of the drug's toxicity. |
| **Constipation** | Laxative drugs such as docusate (Colace) or polycarbophil (FiberCon) | Aloe, cascara sagrada, plantain, rhubarb, senna, and yellow dock | They also have a laxative effect. |

| If You Have . . . | And Are Taking . . . | Then Steer Clear Of . . . | Because . . . |
|---|---|---|---|
| **Cough or pain** | Codeine | Tannin-containing herbs such as black tea, green tea, red raspberry tea, and uva-ursi | They may interfere with the drug's absorption. |
| **Depression** | SSRI (selective serotonin reuptake inhibitor) antidepressants such as fluoxetine (Prozac), sertraline (Zoloft), or paroxetine (Paxil) | Broom and yohimbe Sedative herbs such as passionflower, skullcap, and valerian | They increase the drug's effects. They may increase the drug's sedative effects. |
| | | St. John's wort | It can cause "serotonin syndrome," lethargy, and confusion. |
| | MAO (monoamine oxidase) inhibitor antidepressants such as phenelzine (Nardil) or tranylcypromine (Parnate) | Butcher's broom, capsicum, galanthamine, ginkgo, ginseng, and tonka bean | They may increase the drug's effects or cause toxic reactions. |
| **Headache or fatigue** | Drugs containing caffeine, such as Excedrin, No Doz, or Vivarin | Creatine | It decreases the drug's effects. |
| | | Asian ginseng, ephedra, guarana, yerba maté, and yohimbe | They exacerbate anxiety, insomnia, high blood pressure, and rapid heart rate. |
| **Heart attack, atrial fibrillation, venous thrombosis, pulmonary embolism, or stroke** | Anticoagulants such as warfarin (Coumadin) | Angelica, black haw, bogbean, bromelain, buchu, cat's claw, chamomile, chondroitin, dan shen, devil's claw, dong quai, fenugreek, feverfew, garlic, ginger, ginkgo, ginseng, horse chestnut, Irish moss, kelp, khella, lungwort, papaya, pau d'arco, poplar, prickly ash, | They increase the drug's effects. |

*(continued)*

| If You Have . . . | And Are Taking . . . | Then Steer Clear Of . . . | Because . . . |
|---|---|---|---|
| | | red clover, tonka bean, wintergreen, and yarrow | |
| | | St. John's wort | It may lower blood levels of the drug. |
| **Heartburn caused by gastro-esophageal reflux disease (GERD)** | The gastrointestinal stimulant cisapride (Propulsid) | Grapefruit juice | It can inhibit intestinal enzymes that help your body absorb the drug. |
| | | Menthol-containing herbs such as peppermint | They may make the reflux worse. |
| **High blood pressure** | Diuretics such as furosemide (Lasix) or indapamide (Lozol) | Buchu, cornsilk, dandelion, uva-ursi, and yarrow | They also act as diuretics, and they increase the drug's effects. |
| | | Cowslip, cucumber, dandelion, and horsetail | They increase the drug's effects. |
| | | Stimulant laxative herbs such as aloe, cascara sagrada, and senna | They promote potassium depletion. |
| **High blood pressure or congestive heart failure** | Calcium channel blockers such as amlodipine (Norvasc), diltiazem (Cardizem), or nifedipine (Procardia) | Grapefruit juice | It boosts the absorption of the drug. |
| | | Betony, black cohosh, cat's claw, dandelion, fumitory, goldenseal, Irish moss, kelp, khella, Queen Anne's lace, and yarrow | They increase the drug's effects. |
| | | Arnica, blue cohosh, and capsicum | They decrease the drug's effects. |
| | | Ephedra and licorice | They may raise blood pressure. |
| | | Garlic and hawthorn | They may lower blood pressure. |

| If You Have ... | And Are Taking ... | Then Steer Clear Of ... | Because ... |
|---|---|---|---|
| | Felodipine (Plendil) | Grapefruit juice | It boosts the absorption of the drug. |
| | ACE (angiotensin converting enzyme) inhibitors such as captopril (Capoten) or enalapril (Vasotec) | The herb pill-bearing spurge Ephedra and licorice Garlic and hawthorn | It increases the drug's effects. They may raise blood pressure. They may lower blood pressure. |
| **High cholesterol** | HMG-CoA reductase inhibitors, or statins, such as atorvastatin (Lipitor), simvastatin (Zocor), or pravastatin (Pravachol) | Grapefruit juice | It can inhibit intestinal enzymes that help your body absorb the drug. |
| **Menopausal symptoms** | Ethinyl estrodiol (Estinyl), conjugated estrogens (Premarin), or estradiol (Estrace) | Grapefruit juice | It boosts the absorption of the drug. |
| | Conjugated estrogens (Premarin) | Isoflavone-containing herbs such as red clover | They may interfere with the drug's absorption or increase its effects. |
| **Nicotine addiction** | Drugs containing nicotine | Blue cohosh | It increases the drug's effects. |
| **Pain** | Aspirin | Angelica, black haw, bogbean, bromelain, buchu, cat's claw, chamomile, chondroitin, dong quai, fenugreek, feverfew, garlic, ginger, ginkgo, horse chestnut, Irish moss, kelp, khella, lungwort, pau d'arco, poplar, prickly ash, red clover, tonka bean, wintergreen, and yarrow | They reduce the clotting tendency of the blood and can thin it too much. |

# INDEX

# H

M

O

# S

# W